ESSENTIALS OF CLINICAL GERIATRICS

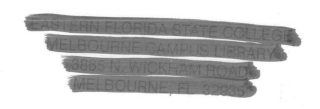

NOTICE

Medicine is an ever-changing science. As new research and clinical experience broaden our knowledge, changes in treatment and drug therapy are required. The authors and the publisher of this work have checked with sources believed to be reliable in their efforts to provide information that is complete and generally in accord with the standards accepted at the time of publication. However, in view of the possibility of human error or changes in medical sciences, neither the authors nor the publisher nor any other party who has been involved in the preparation or publication of this work warrants that the information contained herein is in every respect accurate or complete, and they disclaim all responsibility for any errors or omissions or for the results obtained from use of the information contained in this work. Readers are encouraged to confirm the information contained herein with other sources. For example and in particular, readers are advised to check the product information sheet included in the package of each drug they plan to administer to be certain that the information contained in this work is accurate and that changes have not been made in the recommended dose or in the contraindications for administration. This recommendation is of particular importance in connection with new or infrequently used drugs.

ESSENTIALS OF CLINICAL GERIATRICS

EIGHTH EDITION

Robert L. Kane, MD
Professor and Minnesota Endowed Chair in Long-Term Care and Aging
School of Public Health
University of Minnesota
Minneapolis, Minnesota

Joseph G. Ouslander, MD
Professor and Senior Associate Dean for Geriatric Programs
Chair, Department of Integrated Medical Sciences
Charles E. Schmidt College of Medicine
Florida Atlantic University

Barbara Resnick, PhD, CRNP, FAAN, FAANP
Professor
University of Maryland School of Nursing
Sonya Gershowitz Chair in Gerontology
Baltimore, Maryland

Michael L. Malone, MD
Medical Director, Aurora Senior Services & Aurora at Home
Director of Geriatric Medicine Fellowship, Aurora Health Care
Clinical Adjunct Professor, University of Wisconsin School of Medicine & Public Health
Milwaukee, Wisconsin

New York   Chicago   San Francisco   Athens   London   Madrid   Mexico City
Milan   New Delhi   Singapore   Sydney   Toronto

Essentials of Clinical Geriatrics, Eighth Edition

1 2 3 4 5 6 7 8 9   DSS   22 21 20 19 18 17

ISBN 978-1-259-86051-5
MHID 1-259-86051-5

This book was set in Adobe Garamond Pro by Cenveo® Publisher Services.
The editors were Karen G. Edmonson and Cindy Yoo.
The production supervisor was Richard Ruzycka
Project management was provided by Raghavi Khullar, Cenveo Publisher Services
RR Donnelley was printer and binder.

This book is printed on acid-free paper.

Library of Congress Cataloging-in-Publication Data

Names: Kane, Robert L., 1940- author. | Ouslander, Joseph G., author. |
    Resnick, Barbara., author. | Malone, Michael L., author.
Title: Essentials of clinical geriatrics / Robert L. Kane, Joseph G.
    Ouslander, Barbara Resnick, Michael L. Malone.
Description: Eighth edition. | New York : McGraw-Hill Education, [2018] |
    Preceded by Essentials of clinical geriatrics / Robert L. Kane ... [et al.]. 2013. |
    Includes bibliographical references and index.
Identifiers: LCCN 2017006766 | ISBN 9781259860515 (pbk. : alk. paper) |
    ISBN 1259860515 (pbk. : alk. paper)
Subjects: | MESH: Geriatrics | Aged | Geriatric Assessment |
    Aging—physiology | Aging—psychology
Classification: LCC RC952 | NLM WT 100 | DDC 618.97—dc23 LC record available at
https://lccn.loc.gov/2017006766

IN MEMORIAM

On March 6, 2017, we in the field of geriatrics lost a brilliant, witty, and irreverent leader, mentor, and passionate advocate for the most vulnerable of our patients. As colleagues and coauthors, we will feel the sadness of Bob Kane's sudden death for many years. Each of us had the honor to work with him on this book and many other projects, and we respectfully dedicate this edition, which he coauthored and edited, to his memory.

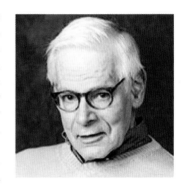

Essentials of Clinical Geriatrics was Bob's idea. In 1980, after he and other leaders at UCLA made the nation aware of the growing need for the field of geriatrics, he recognized the need for a text that succinctly summarized the key aspects of clinical care for older adults as a critical step in defining the field and in improving the care of this population. Although geriatrics in the United States was in its infancy, Bob wanted to disseminate a resource that could make a difference while the field grew and matured. Admittedly not an experienced practicing clinician, Bob engaged Itamar Abrass, then Director of the Geriatric Research Education and Clinical Centers (GRECCs) at the Sepulveda VA, and one of us (JGO) to coauthor the book. Its success over the past three decades, in terms of book awards, reviewer accolades, and sales around the world, speaks for itself.

Each of us would like to share a few of many memories of working with Bob.

JGO: Bob was a relentless mentor, whose "feedback" could be brutally honest. I vividly remember the day I met with him to review my first draft of the first chapter I authored for the first edition of this text. He shoved it across the table and said: "I can't read this. Go get a book called *The Elements of Style* and learn to write a sentence properly, and then rewrite the chapter and give it back to me." He was right. Like many young physicians just out of fellowship, I had no idea how to write proper, efficient English for the medical literature. He helped me get better at it for the next 30 years. Then there was the time about 10 years later when I was on a panel with him speaking at a meeting of geriatric nurse practitioners. As I was speaking, Bob was listening attentively and taking notes. I thought to myself, "Wow, my mentor is taking notes on my presentation." When I finished, he handed me a list of all the typos and grammatical errors on my slides. He always pushed me hard, and I am forever indebted to him for doing so.

BR: When Bob first invited me to join in authoring this book, I was both honored and a bit hesitant, fearing that I would never be able to meet his expectations. I worked harder on those book chapters than any other I ever wrote and was thrilled to have Bob's approval of each. Moreover, his editorial recommendations were always written in a productive manner, were appropriate, focused on including all members of the interdisciplinary team, and had the older patient in mind. His focus was always on how to ensure that new clinicians would understand the current system and management approaches, and that they would think about ways to improve on those approaches. On a personal note, when Bob heard about my own recent experience with cancer he called me to discuss it further. He wanted to learn more about my experience and how it might help others. We commiserated about the system and the way in which health-care providers approach patients in the acute care setting and the impact it has on the patient. We also discussed thoughts about death and dying when faced with potentially life-threatening illnesses, and the challenges to being able to enact personal preferences and choices. It is a great consolation to me personally, as it should be to us all, that Bob didn't have to endure the indignities of a long stay in the acute or long-term care setting.

MLM: We recently offered Bob the chance to teach as the national geriatrics expert at a monthly case conference for geriatrics fellows on the East Coast. He agreed without hesitation. The case discussion focused on the very complex clinical care of an older man with dementia, who had refused care. Bob expressed clear teaching points that none of the participants had considered. Bob simply outlined his recommendations: (1) make a time-graph of the important events of the patient; (2) define what you know, what you do not know, and the overarching problem that requires attention first; (3) define the patient's capacity to take care of himself; and (4) define what his family is willing to do to help him. All the fellows and faculty noted the clarity of his teaching. We appreciated his direct, commonsense approach. Bob was a straight-talking communicator. His teaching was clear and his points made you reflect on many of the things that you would not have otherwise considered. At the last AGS meeting, while I was in a cab with him, he said: "It sure sucks when the problems of aging start happening to you." Physically disabled from longstanding musculoskeletal problems and too stubborn to use a wheelchair, Bob had fallen earlier in the day and suffered a painful hematoma around his knee. I joined Joe and Lynn Ouslander in attending to his injury. Despite the discomfort, Bob was persistent in his wish to attend the JAGS Editorial Board dinner, yet many of us were worried about him. He was so appreciative of his friends and colleagues making sure that he was as comfortable as possible under the circumstances. The next day he gave a remarkable presentation on how to successfully publish a manuscript. He enjoyed teaching, even when he physically was not at his best. Bob sent a very kind note after he had returned home, thanking us for the assistance we provided.

Bob died physically frail, but as intellectually active as ever. One of us (JGO) was on a call about papers in review and in development just 4 days before he died, and he could not have been sharper. He remained involved in so many important projects with so many colleagues despite his physical challenges right up until the day he died. He left a tremendous legacy of writings and intellectual challenges to the field of geriatrics and to our society advocating for the need for humane, compassionate, and high-quality, yet not overly medicalized, care for people in the last stages of life. We hope that all he touched will help finish the work left behind by his untimely death. This book is one contribution to that goal.

Joseph G. Ouslander
Barbara Resnick
Michael L. Malone

CONTENTS

List of Tables and Figures xi

Preface xxiii

PART I

THE AGING PATIENT AND GERIATRIC ASSESSMENT

1. Clinical Implications of the Aging Process 3
2. The Geriatric Patient: Demography, Epidemiology, and Health Services Utilization 23
3. Evaluating the Geriatric Patient 43
4. Chronic Disease Management 79

PART II

DIFFERENTIAL DIAGNOSIS AND MANAGEMENT

5. Prevention 107
6. Delirium and Dementia 139
7. Diagnosis and Management of Depression 169
8. Incontinence 201
9. Falls 243
10. Immobility 263

PART III

GENERAL MANAGEMENT STRATEGIES

11. Cardiovascular Disorders 301
12. Decreased Vitality 333
13. Sensory Impairment 381

14. Drug Therapy 405

15. High-Value Health Services 427

16. Nursing Home Care 471

17. Ethical Issues in the Care of Older Persons 499

18. Palliative Care 523

Appendix   Selected Internet Resources on Geriatrics 541

Index 547

TABLES AND FIGURES

CHAPTER ONE

Table 1-1.   Pertinent Changes That Commonly Occur With Aging....................7
Table 1-2.   Nine Hallmarks of Aging...10
Table 1-3.   Web-Based Resources for Health Promotion and Aging.................19

CHAPTER TWO

Figure 2-1.   Change in the relationship of older persons and workers................24
Figure 2-2.   Age-adjusted death rates for selected leading causes of death:
              United States, 1958–2013 25
Figure 2-3.   Medicare spending by function and chronic disease.....................27
Table 2-1.   Changes in Most Common Causes of Death, All Ages and Those
              65 Years and Older 28
Figure 2-4.   Life expectancy at age 65 by sex and race/ethnicity 29
Table 2-2.   Percentage of Medicare Beneficiaries Reporting Difficulty With
              Common Activities, by Age Group: 2012...............................31
Figure 2-5.   Living arrangements by age and sex, 2015 32
Figure 2-6.   Percentage of Medicare FFS beneficiaries by number of chronic
              conditions and age: 2010..33
Figure 2-7.   30-day readmission rates for five diseases 34
Table 2-3.   Hospital Discharge Diagnoses and Procedures for Persons
              Aged 65 Years and Older, 2010 35
Table 2-4.   Postacute Care Used Within 30 Days in 2008, for the Top Five
              Diagnostic-Related Groups 36
Table 2-5.   Percentage of Office Visits by Selected Medical Conditions, 2012 37
Table 2-6.   Factors Affecting the Need for Nursing Home Admission 39

CHAPTER THREE

Figure 3-1.   The Kaiser Pyramid...44
Figure 3-2.   Components of assessment of older patients............................45
Table 3-1.   Examples of Randomized Controlled Trials of Geriatric Assessment 46
Table 3-2.   Potential Difficulties in Taking Geriatric Histories 48
Table 3-3.   Important Aspects of the Geriatric History..............................49
Table 3-4.   Geriatric Screening Questions and Recommendations for Further
              Assessment 52
Table 3-5.   Essential Elements of Person-Centered Care 54

Table 3-6.   Common Physical Findings and Their Potential Significance
in Geriatrics 55

Table 3-7.   Laboratory Assessment of Geriatric Patients 58

Table 3-8.   Important Concepts for Geriatric Functional Assessment 61

Table 3-9.   Purposes and Objectives of Functional Status Measures 61

Table 3-10.   Examples of Measures of Physical Functioning. 62

Table 3-11.   Important Aspects of the History in Assessment of Pain 65

Table 3-12.   Important Aspects of the Physical Examination in Assessment of Pain . . . 65

Figure 3-3.   Samples of two pain intensity scales that have been studied
in older persons. Directions: Patients should view the figure without
numbers. After the patient indicates the best representation of his or
her pain, the appropriate numerical value can be assigned to facilitate
clinical documentation and follow-up 66

Table 3-13.   Assessment of Body Composition 66

Table 3-14.   Critical Questions in Assessing a Patient for Malnutrition. 67

Table 3-15.   Factors That Place Older Adults at Risk for Malnutrition 67

Table 3-16.   Medicare Initial Preventive Physical Examination. 68

Table 3-17.   Medicare Annual Wellness Visit 69

Table 3-18.   Example of a Screening Tool to Identify Potentially Remediable
Geriatric Problems. 71

Table 3-19.   Questions on the Probability of Repeated Admissions Instrument for
Identifying Geriatric Patients at Risk for Health Service Use. 72

Table 3-20.   Suggested Format for Summarizing the Results of a Comprehensive
Geriatric Consultation 73

Table 3-21.   Preoperative Assessment Checklist 73

Table 3-22.   Potential Manifestations of Caregiver Stress. 75

CHAPTER FOUR

Figure 4-1.   Paths to chronic disease catastrophe. 80

Table 4-1.   Chronic Care Tenets 80

Figure 4-2.   Narrowing of the therapeutic window. This diagram portrays in a
conceptual manner how the space between a therapeutic dose
and a toxic dose narrows with age. 81

Figure 4-3.   A conceptual model of the difference between expected and
actual care. The heavier line represents what is usually observed in
clinical chronic care. Despite good care, the patient's course
deteriorates. The true benefit, represented by the area between
the dark line and the dotted line, is invisible unless some means is
found to display the expected course in the absence of good care.
Such data could be developed based on clinical prognosis,
or they could be derived from accumulated data once such a system
is in place. 82

Figure 4-4.   Clinical glidepath models. (**A**) In this model, the expected course (solid line) calls for gradual decline. The confidence intervals are shown as dotted lines. Actual measures that are within or better than the glidepath are shown as *o*'s. When the patient's course is worse than expected, the *o* changes to an *x*. The design shown uses confidence intervals with upper and lower bounds, but actually only the lower bound is pertinent. Any performance above the upper confidence interval boundary is very acceptable. (**B**) The design of the glidepath can also take another form. It may be preferable to think in terms of reaching a threshold level within a given time window (eg, in recuperating from an illness) and then maintaining that level. 86

Table 4-2.   Team Models. 91

Table 4-3.   Team Composition 92

Table 4-4.   The Two-Step Discharge Decision-Making Process. 93

Table 4-5.   Rationale for Using Outcomes. 96

Table 4-6.   Outcomes Measurement Issues 97

Table 4-7.   Geriatric Outcome Categories 98

Table 4-8.   *Choosing Wisely* Recommendations. 100

Table 4-9.   ACOVE Recommendations 102

CHAPTER FIVE

Table 5-1.   Considerations in Assessing Prevention in Older Patients 108

Table 5-2.   Preventive Strategies for Older Persons 109

Table 5-3.   Healthy People 2020 Report Card Items Most Relevant for Older Adults 110

Table 5-4.   U.S. Preventive Services Task Force (USPSTF) Recommendations for Screening Older Adults. 111

Table 5-5.   Additional Preventive Services From U.S. Preventive Services Task Force (USPSTF) (May Be Suitable for Older Adults) 114

Table 5-6.   Requirements for the Welcome to Medicare Visit and Annual Wellness Visit. 119

Table 5-7.   Measurement of Psychosocial Factors Among Older Adults. 122

Table 5-8.   Types of Exercises 124

Figure 5-1.   MyPlate for older adults. 126

Table 5-9.   Efficacy of Common Biphosphonates for the Prevention of Fractures . . . 129

Table 5-10.   Common Iatrogenic Problems of Older Persons 132

Figure 5-2.   Narrowing of the therapeutic window. This diagram portrays in a conceptual manner how the space between a therapeutic dose and a toxic dose narrows with age. 132

Table 5-11.   Potential Complications of Bed Rest in Older Adults 134

CHAPTER SIX

Table 6-1.	Key Aspects of Mental Status Examination.	140
Table 6-2.	NIA–AA Core Clinical Diagnostic Criteria for Mild Cognitive Impairment	142
Table 6-3.	Diagnostic Criteria for Delirium	143
Table 6-4.	Predisposing and Precipitating Factors for Delirium From Validated Predictive Models	144
Table 6-5.	The Confusion Assessment Method Diagnostic Algorithm	145
Table 6-6.	Differentiating Delirium, Dementia, Depression, and Acute Psychosis	146
Table 6-7.	Common Causes of Delirium in Geriatric Patients	147
Table 6-8.	Drugs That Can Cause or Contribute to Delirium and Dementia	148
Table 6-9.	Interventions for Risk Factors for Delirium	149
Table 6-10.	NIA-AA Core Clinical Diagnostic Criteria for All-Cause Dementia and Dementia Due to Alzheimer Disease	150
Table 6-11.	Potentially Reversible Conditions That Can Contribute to Cognitive Impairment and Dementia	152
Table 6-12.	Causes of Dementia	153
Table 6-13.	Clinical Features of Common Dementias	154
Figure 6-1.	Primary degenerative dementia versus multi-infarct dementia: comparison of time courses. (1) Recognized by patient, but detectable only on detailed testing. (2) Deficits recognized by family and friends. (3) See text for explanation. (4) Exact time courses are variable; see text.	156
Table 6-14.	Symptoms That May Indicate Dementia	156
Table 6-15.	Evaluating Dementia: The History	157
Table 6-16.	Evaluating Dementia: Recommended Diagnostic Studies	159
Table 6-17.	Key Principles in the Management of Dementia	160

CHAPTER SEVEN

Table 7-1.	Factors Associated With Suicide in the Geriatric Population	171
Table 7-2.	Factors Predisposing Older People to Depression	172
Table 7-3.	Examples of Physical Symptoms That Can Represent Depression	175
Table 7-4.	Key Factors in Evaluating the Complaint of Insomnia	176
Table 7-5.	Medical Illnesses Associated With Depression	179
Table 7-6.	Drugs That Can Cause Symptoms of Depression	180
Table 7-7.	Some Differences in the Presentation of Depression in the Older Population, as Compared With the Younger Population	181
Table 7-8.	Summary Criteria for Major Depressive Episode	182
Table 7-9.	Major Depression Versus Other Forms of Depression	183
Table 7-10.	Examples of Screening Tools for Depression	184

Table 7-11.   Diagnostic Studies Helpful in Evaluating Depressed Geriatric
                Patients With Somatic Symptoms. 186

Table 7-12.   Evidence-Based Treatment Modalities for Depression. 187

Table 7-13.   Antidepressants for Geriatric Patients. 191

Table 7-14.   General Treatment Approaches for Use of Antidepressants 193

Table 7-15.   Characteristics of Selected Antidepressants for Geriatric Patients. 196

CHAPTER EIGHT

Figure 8-1.   Prevalence of urinary incontinence (UI) in the geriatric population.
                "Regular UI" is more often than weekly and/or the use of a pad.
                (Percentages range in various studies; those shown reflect
                approximate averages from multiple sources.). 202

Table 8-1.   Potential Adverse Effects of Urinary Incontinence. 202

Table 8-2.   Requirements for Continence 203

Figure 8-2.   Structural components of normal micturition. 204

Figure 8-3.   Peripheral nerves involved in micturition.. 205

Figure 8-4.   Simplified schematic of the dynamic function of the lower urinary
                tract during bladder filling (*left*) and emptying (*right*). As the bladder
                fills, true detrusor pressure (*thick line at bottom*) remains low (<15 cm
                H$_2$O) and does not exceed urethral resistance pressure (*thin line
                at bottom*). As the bladder fills to capacity (generally 300–600 mL),
                pelvic floor and sphincter activity increase as measured by
                electromyography (EMG). Involuntary detrusor contractions (illustrated
                by *dashed lines*) occur commonly among incontinent geriatric patients
                (see text). They may be accompanied by increased EMG activity in
                attempts to prevent leakage (*dashed lines at top*). If detrusor pressure
                exceeds urethral pressure during an involuntary contraction, as shown,
                urine will flow. During bladder emptying, detrusor pressure rises,
                urethral pressure falls, and EMG activity ceases in order for normal
                urine flow to occur (*right side of figure*). 206

Figure 8-5.   Simplified schematic depicting age-associated changes in pelvic floor
                muscle, bladder, and urethra–vesicle position, predisposing to stress
                incontinence. Normally (*left*), the bladder and outlet remain anatomically
                inside the intra-abdominal cavity, and rises in pressure contribute to
                bladder outlet closure. Age-associated changes (eg, estrogen deficiency,
                surgeries, childbirth) can weaken the structures maintaining bladder
                position (*right*); in this situation, increases in intra-abdominal
                pressure can cause urine loss (stress incontinence). .206

Table 8-3.   Reversible Conditions That Cause or Contribute to Geriatric Urinary
                Incontinence. 208

Table 8-4.   Medications That Can Cause or Contribute to Urinary Incontinence 209

Table 8-5.   Mnemonic for Potentially Reversible Conditions 209

Table 8-6.   Basic Types and Causes of Persistent Urinary Incontinence............211

Table 8-7.   Components of the Diagnostic Evaluation of Persistent Urinary
               Incontinence..213

Table 8-8.   Key Aspects of an Incontinent Patient's History.....................214

Figure 8-6.   Example of a bladder record for ambulatory care settings..............215

Figure 8-7.   Example of a record to monitor bladder and bowel functions in
               institutional settings. This type of record is especially useful for
               implementing and following the results of various training
               procedures and other treatment protocols............................216

Table 8-9.   Key Aspects of an Incontinent Patient's Physical Examination..........217

Figure 8-8.   Example of a simplified grading system for cystoceles..................218

Table 8-10.   Criteria for Considering Referral of Incontinent Patients for Urological,
               Gynecological, or Urodynamic Evaluation 220

Figure 8-9.   Algorithm protocol for evaluating incontinence.......................222

Table 8-11.   Treatment Options for Geriatric Urinary Incontinence..................223

Table 8-12.   Primary Treatments for Different Types of
               Geriatric Urinary Incontinence......................................224

Table 8-13.   Examples of Behavioral Interventions for Urinary Incontinence 225

Table 8-14.   Example of a Bladder Retraining Protocol.............................227

Table 8-15.   Example of a Prompted Voiding Protocol for a Nursing Home 229

Table 8-16.   Drug Treatment for Urinary Incontinence and Overactive Bladder 230

Table 8-17.   Indications for Chronic Indwelling Catheter Use 235

Table 8-18.   Key Principles of Chronic Indwelling Catheter Care 235

Table 8-19.   Causes of Fecal Incontinence..236

Table 8-20.   Causes of Constipation..237

Table 8-21.   Drugs Used to Treat Constipation.....................................238

CHAPTER NINE

Table 9-1.   Complications of Falls in Older Patients...............................244

Figure 9-1.   Multifactorial causes and potential contributors to falls in
               older persons..244

Table 9-2.   Age-Related Factors Contributing to Instability and Falls...............245

Table 9-3.   Causes of Falls..247

Table 9-4.   Common Environmental Hazards......................................248

Table 9-5.   Factors Associated With Falls Among Older Nursing Home Residents ...248

Table 9-6.   Evaluating the Older Patient Who Falls: Key Points in the History........252

Table 9-7.   Evaluating the Older Patient Who Falls: Key Aspects of the Physical
               Examination...253

Table 9-8.   Example of a Performance-Based Assessment of Gait and Balance
               (Get Up and Go)...255

Table 9-9.   Principles of Management for Older Patients With Complaints
              of Instability and/or Falls 257

Table 9-10.   Examples of Treatment for Underlying Causes of Falls...................258

CHAPTER TEN

Table 10-1.   Factors That Influence Immobility 264

Table 10-2.   Complications of Immobility 266

Table 10-3.   Assessment of Immobile Older Patients 268

Table 10-4.   Example of How to Grade Muscle Strength in Immobile
              Older Patients...269

Table 10-5.   Clinical Features of Osteoarthritis Versus Inflammatory Arthritis.........271

Figure 10-1. Characteristics of different types of hip fractures. 273

Table 10-6.   Recommended Treatment Options for Venous Thromboembolism
              Prophylaxis in Immobility..274

Table 10-7.   Drugs Used to Treat Parkinson Disease 276

Table 10-8.   Clinical Characteristics of Pressure Sores..............................279

Table 10-9.   Principles of Skin Care in Immobile Older Patients 280

Table 10-10. Pain Categories and Management Options............................283

Table 10-11. Examples of Drug Groups and Associated Drugs Commonly
              Used to Treat Pain...286

Table 10-12. CDC Recommendations for Determining When to Initiate or
              Continue Opioids for Chronic Pain..291

Table 10-13. Basic Principles of Rehabilitation in Older Patients 293

Table 10-14. Physical Therapy in the Management of Immobile Older Patients.......294

Table 10-15. Occupational Therapy in the Management of Immobile
              Older Patients...295

CHAPTER ELEVEN

Table 11-1.   Resting Cardiac Function in Persons Aged 30 to 80 Years Old
              Compared With That in Persons Aged 30 Years Old 302

Table 11-2.   Performance at Maximum Exercise in Sample Screened for
              Coronary Artery Disease Aged 30 to 80 Years 302

Table 11-3.   Initial Evaluation of Hypertension in Older Adults......................303

Table 11-4.   Secondary Hypertension in Older Persons.............................304

Table 11-5.   Thiazide Diuretics for Antihypertensive Therapy 307

Table 11-6.   Antihypertensive Medications..309

Table 11-7.   Stroke...312

Table 11-8.   Outcome for Survivors of Stroke......................................312

Table 11-9.   Modifiable Risk Factors for Ischemic Stroke 313

Table 11-10.   Transient Ischemic Attack: Presenting Symptoms 314

Table 11-11.   Factors in Prognosis for Rehabilitation 316

Table 11-12.   Stroke Rehabilitation 317

Table 11-13.   Presenting Symptoms of Myocardial Infarction 318

Table 11-14.   Differentiation of Systolic Murmurs 320

Table 11-15.   Manifestations of Sick Sinus Syndrome 324

Table 11-16.   Calculation of the Ankle–Brachial Index 326

CHAPTER TWELVE

Table 12-1.   Common Noninsulin Medications for Diabetes Mellitus
               in Older Adults 339

Table 12-2.   Common Clinical Conditions to Consider in the Care of Older
               Individuals With Diabetes Mellitus 344

Figure 12-1.   Flow diagram for treatment of hospitalized (nonintensive care unit)
               patients with type 2 diabetes mellitus. CHF, congestive heart failure;
               NPH, neutral protamine Hagedorn (insulin); NPO, nothing by mouth;
               PO, by mouth; TPN, total parenteral nutrition 348

Table 12-3.   Thyroid Function in Normal Older Adults 350

Table 12-4.   Laboratory Evaluation of Thyroid Disease in Older Persons 350

Table 12-5.   Thyroid Function Tests in Nonthyroidal Illness 351

Figure 12-2.   An algorithm for the management of subclinical hypothyroidism.
               LDL, low-density lipoprotein. 353

Table 12-6.   Myxedema Coma 353

Table 12-7.   Laboratory Findings in Metabolic Bone Disease. 356

Table 12-8.   Signs and Symptoms of Anemia. 358

Table 12-9.   Differential Tests in Hypochromic Anemia 360

Table 12-10.   Nutritional Requirements in Older Persons. 362

Table 12-11.   Factors Predisposing to Infection in Older Adults 366

Table 12-12.   Pathogens of Common Infections in Older Adults 368

Table 12-13.   Clinical Presentation of Hypothermia 371

Table 12-14.   Clinical Presentation of Hyperthermia 372

Table 12-15.   Complications of Heat Stroke. 373

CHAPTER THIRTEEN

Table 13-1.   Physiological and Functional Changes of the Eye With
               Advancing Age. 382

Table 13-2.   Ophthalmological Screening Covered by Medicare Fee-for-Service 383

Table 13-3.   Restoring Vision After Cataract Surgery—Intraocular Lenses 384

Table 13-4.   Signs and Symptoms Associated With Common Visual Problems
in Older Adults 386

Table 13-5.   Potential Adverse Effects of Ophthalmic Solutions 387

Table 13-6.   Aids to Maximize Visual Function 389

Table 13-7.   Functional Components of the Auditory System. 391

Table 13-8.   Assessment of Hearing 391

Table 13.9.   Initial Evaluation of an Older Patient With Acute or Subacute
Hearing Loss 392

Table 13-10.   Effects of Aging on the Hearing Mechanism and Hearing
Performance in Older Adults 393

Table 13-11.   Health Implications of Hearing Loss in Older Adults 393

Table 13-12.   Medical Conditions That Present With Hearing Loss in Older Adults 396

Table 13-13.   Factors to Consider in Evaluation of an Older Adult for a Hearing Aid . . . 397

Table 13-14.   Some Advantages and Disadvantages of Various
Styles of Hearing Aids 398

Table 13-15.   Essential Points That a Health Professional Should Know About
Over-the-Counter Wearable Hearing Devices 399

Table 13-16.   Strategies to Improve a Health Professional's Communication
With an Older Patient Who Has a Hearing Impairment 400

Table 13-17.   Essential Points That a Health Professional Should Know
About Cochlear Implants 400

CHAPTER FOURTEEN

Figure 14-1.   Factors that can interfere with successful drug therapy. 406

Figure 14-2.   Example of a basic medication record recommended by the U.S.
Food and Drug Administration. 408

Table 14-1.   Strategies to Improve Adherence With Drug Therapy in the
Geriatric Population 410

Table 14-2.   Examples of Common and Potentially Serious Adverse Drug
Reactions in the Geriatric Population 412

Table 14-3.   Examples of Potentially Clinically Important Drug–Drug Interactions. . . . 414

Table 14-4.   Examples of Potentially Clinically Important
Drug–Patient Interactions 415

Table 14-5.   Age-Related Changes Relevant to Drug Pharmacology 416

Table 14-6.   Renal Function in Relation to Age 418

Table 14-7.   General Recommendations for Geriatric Prescribing 419

Table 14-8.   Examples of Antipsychotic Drugs. 420

Table 14-9.   Examples of Sedative–Hypnotics Approved for Insomnia by
the U.S. Food and Drug Administration 421

CHAPTER FIFTEEN

Figure 15-1.   Measuring the effects of good chronic care. Both trajectories show decline, but the slope of expected care is steeper. The yellow area between the lines represents the effects of good care............428

Figure 15-2.   Medicare fee-for-service expenditures and percentage distribution, by Medicare program and type of service: calendar years 1995–2014. . .432

Table 15-1.   Summary of Major Federal Programs for Older Patients.................442

Figure 15-3.   Living arrangements of older people with disabilities by age group, 2012...........................445

Table 15-2.   Essential Elements of Person-Centered Care 446

Figure 15-4.   Disability prevalence and the need for assistance by age: 2010 448

Figure 15-5.   Change in ADLs and IADLs from 1992 to 2013..........................449

Figure 15-6.   Long-term care spending by payer, 2013 450

Table 15-3.   Potential Symptoms of Caregiver Stress.................................450

Figure 15-7.   Change in the rate of nursing home use by age group, 1973–2004.....452

Figure 15-8.   Use of different types of institutional long-term care by age group, 1985 and 2004 453

Figure 15-9.   ADLs limitations by living situation. Estimates based on CMS National Health Expenditure Accounts data for 2013 453

Figure 15-10   Institutional use by disability................................454

Table 15-4.   Remaining Lifetime Use of Long-Term Supportive Services (LTSS) by People Turning 65 in 2005..454

Table 15-5.   RUG-IV Classification System...457

Table 15-6.   Home Care Provided Under Various Federal Programs 460

Figure 15-11   Core components of long-term care....................................463

Figure 15-12A   Personal care pyramid...464

Figure 15-12B   Medical needs pyramid..464

Table 15-7.   Examples of Community Long-Term Care Programs 465

Table 15-8.   Variations in Case Management 467

CHAPTER SIXTEEN

Table 16-1.   Goals of Nursing Home Care 472

Figure 16-1.   Categories of individuals in nursing homes. In this chapter, short-stayers are generally referred to as "patients" and long-stayers as "residents" due to the different nature of their conditions and goals for care...473

Table 16-2.   Factors That Distinguish Assessment and Treatment in the Nursing Home From Assessment and Treatment in Other Settings 474

Table 16-3.   Common Clinical Disorders in the Nursing Home Population...........476

Table 16-4.   Important Aspects of Various Types of Assessment in the
Nursing Home 478

Figure 16-2.   Example of a face sheet for a nursing home record.. 484

Table 16-5.   SOAP Format for Medical Progress Notes on Nursing
Home Residents. 486

Table 16-6.   Screening, Health Maintenance, and Preventive Practices in the
Nursing Home 488

Figure 16-3.   Example of an INTERACT VERSION 4.0 care path for managing acute
change in condition in a nursing home 492

Table 16-7.   Common Ethical Issues in the Nursing Home. 496

CHAPTER SEVENTEEN

Table 17-1.   Major Ethical Principles. 500

Table 17-2.   Components of a Durable Power of Attorney for Health Care. 504

Table 17-3.   Step Approach to Discussions With Patients Around EOL Care 510

Table 17-4.   Details and Goals of Care and Symptom Management at the
End of Life. 511

Table 17-5.   The Older Americans Reauthorization Act of 2016 (S. 192) 516

Table 17-6.   Evidence of Abuse or Neglect 517

CHAPTER EIGHTEEN

Table 18-1.   Hospice Services 524

Table 18-2.   A Five-Step Framework for Discussing Care Choices at the End
of Life. 525

Table 18-3.   Signs and Symptoms of Frailty. 528

Table 18-4.   Principles for End-of-Life Decision Making in Frail Older Adults 529

Table 18-5.   Assess ABCDE to Determine Level of Cultural Influence in EOL
Decisions. 530

Table 18-6.   Management of Symptoms Noted at End of Life 532

Table 18-7.   Adjuvant Pharmacologic Treatments for Pain Management. 534

PREFACE

As we prepare the eighth edition of this book, the trajectories of demography and geriatrics seem to be moving in opposite directions. Just as the baby boom is producing a bumper crop of older persons, geriatrics has encountered serious problems in recruiting participants from either medicine or nursing. If ever there was a time when health-care providers with expertise in the care of older adults were needed, it is now.

One thing seems clear, especially in light of the demographic forecasts: we cannot simply try harder to do what we have always done. Ingenuity will be essential. We need to take greater advantage of a variety of technologies to support care by persons less steeped in geriatrics. This book is one small step in that direction.

Since the first edition of this book in 1984, modern American geriatrics has struggled to define its role. The establishment of the National Institute on Aging was designed to make aging an academic discipline. From the outset several paths were proposed. Was geriatrics a specialty, a primary care discipline, or a largely academic enterprise that would "gerontologize" other practice disciplines? The promoted clinical realm of geriatrics publicly wavered between primary care and specialty care. There were other calls for recasting geriatrics as chronic disease care expertise. In 2005, the American Geriatrics Society (AGS) Task Force on the Future of Geriatric Medicine identified five goals for the field: ensuring high-quality care for older adults, expanding the geriatrics knowledge base, increasing the number of health-care professionals employing geriatrics principles, increasing the number of geriatricians and other geriatrics providers, and advocating for better public policy to serve older adults. In 2012 the editor in chief of the *Journal of the American Geriatrics Society (JAGS)* urged geriatrics to focus on care of the oldest old. Geriatrics, however, covers the entire aging continuum, caring for those who are healthy older adults as well as those who have multiple comorbidities as well as facilitating end-of-life care.

Geriatrics is a meta-discipline that transcends and informs all other disciplines. It is essentially the merger of gerontological principles and methods for effective chronic care. Geriatricians are the experts in complex chronic care, especially multimorbidity, offering key prototypes for the kind of care needed today. The field of geriatrics has developed useful tools and approaches for managing complex problems, beginning with geriatric assessment and management. More recently it has created a number of approaches to coordinating care for the most challenging patients—for example, those with multimorbidty, who use a disproportionate amount of resources.

While the context of health care for older adults is evolving, basic bedside care remains focused on patients and their caregivers. As its name describes, this book is intended to provide health professionals with essential clinical information to provide excellent care for older adults. The book was written with the health professional in mind. References, suggested readings, and selected websites should support the reader.

One thing has not changed. This is an authored, not edited, book. Our goal was to make it clinically useful and to speak with a single voice. We use figures and tables to summarize material whenever possible.

The eighth edition of this book reflects some changes in authorship. With the last edition we added a distinguished nurse practitioner to the authors. This edition marks the retirement of one of our founders, Itamar Abrass. His role has been ably filled by an accomplished geriatrician, Michael Malone, who serves as the Medical Director of Senior Services and Aurora at Home at Aurora Health Care in Wisconsin. He is a Clinical Adjunct Professor of Medicine at the University of Wisconsin School of Medicine and Public Health.

We are confident that this book will help all health-care professionals work across disciplines to provide the innovative, cost-effective and person-centered care that older people and their caregivers deserve.

THE AGING PATIENT AND GERIATRIC ASSESSMENT

CHAPTER 1

Clinical Implications of the Aging Process

Geriatrics stands at the intersection of three forces:

1. Gerontology (both basic and applied)
2. Chronic disease management, especially multimorbidities
3. End-of-life care

Principles of gerontology can help explain insights of geriatric care. For example, the presentation of disease is often different in older persons because the response to stress is different. A hallmark of aging is a decreased ability to respond to stress. The body's stress response is what typically generates the symptoms of an illness. Older people fail to respond as actively. Hence, they may not have spiking fevers or elevated white blood cell counts in the face of an infection. Heart disease may be silent.

Chronic disease management is difficult on its own. Age itself is the strongest risk factor for several chronic diseases such as heart disease, cancer, stroke, diabetes mellitus, and pneumonia (Miller, 2002). Management is much more difficult when an older patient suffers from multiple simultaneous diseases. Basic care guidelines may not work. Indeed, they may pose a threat (Boyd et al, 2005).

Much of the emphasis in care planning is directed at containing disease and maintaining function and identifying how to make the end of life meaningful (Gawande, 2014). Death is a part of old age. Geriatrics must address that reality and help patients and families deal with end of life, helping them make informed decisions that reflect their goals and preferences. But geriatrics cannot focus exclusively on end-of-life care. One compromise has been the evolution of palliative care (discussed in Chapter 18). To this triad, some might also add a role for advocating reasonable preventive actions (see Chapter 5).

This chapter describes the aging process, changes associated with normal aging, as well as hallmarks of aging at the cellular level. We then introduce the topic of frailty, and the concepts of resilience and homeostenosis. We posit the link between aging and multimorbidity. Next we describe geriatric syndromes and the atypical presentation of common clinical problems. Finally, we put it all together by describing clinical implications of the aging process.

THE AGING PROCESS

Whereas most people think of age as a chronological phenomenon, gerontologists assess age based on the force of mortality—how much longer can an individual be expected to live. *Aging* is defined as the time-dependent sequential deterioration that occurs in most living beings, including weakness, increased susceptibility to disease and adverse environmental conditions, loss of mobility and agility, and age-related physiological changes (Goldsmith, 2006). At least in vitro, it is clear that the "aging clock" can be reset (Rando and Chang, 2012). Somatic cell nuclear transfer of the nucleus of a mature somatic cell into an enucleated oocyte can give rise to mature, fertile animals.

It is important to distinguish life expectancy from life span. The former refers to what proportion of the possible maximum age a person may live. The latter suggests a biological limit to how many years a species can expect to survive. In general, geriatrics may contribute to improving life expectancy, but new genetic breakthroughs may ultimately affect life span as well. Another helpful distinction is between chronological aging and gerontological aging. The latter is calculated based on the risk of dying, the so-called force of mortality. Thus, two people of the same chronological age may have very different biological ages, depending on their health state. Some of that propensity for death is malleable; some is simply predictable.

The term *health span* is also an important concept for the geriatrics health professional to understand. This term refers to the number of years that are spent free of functional limitations, morbidity, and chronic pain. The extension of health span is the goal of most "best practice" approaches (also called geriatrics models of care). These interventions try to slow or prevent adverse events over time. Models of care are based on efforts to improve function and hence increase health span, as compared to life span or life expectancy. The idea that the amount of disability can decrease as morbidity is compressed into the shorter span between the increasing age of onset of disability and the fixed occurrence of death is called "compression of morbidity" (Fries, 1980).

Unraveling the process of aging poses intriguing challenges. From a medical perspective, we cannot determine whether aging is a feature of an organism's design that has evolved over time and is beneficial to the survival of species, or aging is a disease or defect that confers no survival benefit. Even more important to medical management of aging is the question of whether there are medically treatable factors that are common to the various manifestations of aging we see. Could aging treatments delay the signs and symptoms of aging? The "geroscience hypothesis" posits that targeting fundamental mechanisms may be able to decrease the likelihood of multiple aging processes. Some medications (eg, metformin, acarbose, ARBs, and rapamycin) are being studied as key strategies to target fundamental aging processes across multiple organ systems simultaneously.

The distinction between so-called normal aging and pathologic changes is critical to the care of older people. We wish to avoid both dismissing treatable pathology as simply a concomitant of old age (eg, the onset of urinary incontinence) and treating natural aging processes as though they were diseases (eg, difficulty recalling the name of a new neighbor after a brief introduction). The latter is particularly dangerous because older adults are vulnerable to iatrogenic effects of well-intentioned interventions.

There is growing appreciation that everyone does not age in the same way or at the same rate. The changing composition of today's older adults compared with that of a generation ago may actually reflect a bimodal shift wherein there are both more people with disabilities and more healthy older people. We continue to learn more and more about healthy or successful aging through hearing the stories of the growing number of centenarians. The consensus is that moderation in all areas (eg, food intake, alcohol intake), regular physical activity, and an engaging social life are critical to successful aging. A large actuarial study (Gavrilova and Gavrilov, 2005) further suggested that environmental factors may also be relevant. Social factors can also play a strong role (Banks et al, 2006). The challenge is to recognize and appreciate aging changes while using resources to prevent or halt further changes and to overcome aging challenges.

CHANGES ASSOCIATED WITH "NORMAL" AGING

Clinicians often face a major challenge in attributing a finding to either the expected course of aging or the result of pathologic changes. This distinction perplexes the researcher as well. There is no universal marker of aging per se. We currently lack precise knowledge of what constitutes normal aging. Much of our information comes from cross-sectional studies, which compare findings from a group of younger persons with those from a group of older individuals. Such data may reflect differences other than simply the effects of age, such as those associated with lifestyle behaviors (physical activity, alcohol intake, smoking, and diet), as well as prophylactic medication management. For example, older adults in the coming century may present with less evidence of osteoporosis because of prophylactic lifelong intake of high-calcium and vitamin D diets, regular physical activity, and early interventions with bisphosphonates and potentially future treatments for osteoporosis. Statins can drastically affect the course of cardiovascular disease.

Many of the changes associated with aging result from a gradual loss of homeostatic mechanisms ("homeostenosis"). These losses may often begin in early adulthood, but—thanks to the redundancy of most organ systems—the decrement does not become functionally significant until the loss is fairly extensive.

The concept of aging, or at least what constitutes old age, has changed as life expectancy has increased, although the biology has not. Based on cross-sectional comparisons of groups at different ages, most organ systems seem to lose function at about 1% a year beginning around age 30 years. Other data suggest that the changes in people followed longitudinally are much less dramatic and certainly begin well after age 70 years. In some organ systems, such as the kidney, a subgroup of persons appears to experience gradually declining function over time, whereas others' function remains constant. These findings suggest that the earlier theory of gradual loss must be reassessed as reflecting disease rather than aging. Given a pattern of gradual deterioration—whether from aging or disease or both—we are best advised to think in terms of thresholds.

The loss of function does not become significant until it crosses a given level. Thus, the functional performance of an organ in an older person depends on two principal factors: (1) the rate of deterioration and (2) the level of performance needed. It is not surprising then to learn that most older persons will have normal laboratory values. The critical difference—in fact, the hallmark of aging—lies not in the resting level of performance but in how the organ (or organism) adapts to external stress. For example, an older person may have a normal fasting blood sugar but be unable to handle a glucose load within the normal parameters for younger subjects.

This failure to respond to stress explains the atypical presentation of many diseases in older patients. Many of the signs and symptoms of disease are actually the body's response to those assaults. For example, a depressed response may mean not having a high white blood cell count with an infection or even pain with a heart attack. Instead, older patients may present with ill-defined symptoms like confusion. Clinicians need to apply a different set of a priori expectations and interpretations when providing care for older patients.

The same pattern of decreased response to stress can be seen in the performance of other endocrine systems or the cardiovascular system. An older individual may have a normal resting pulse and cardiac output but be unable to achieve an adequate increase in either with exercise.

Sometimes the changes of aging work together to produce apparently normal resting values in other ways. For example, although both glomerular filtration and renal blood flow decrease with age, many older persons have normal serum creatinine levels because of the concomitant decreases in lean muscle mass and creatinine production. Thus, serum creatinine is not as good an indicator of renal function in older adults as in younger persons. Knowledge of kidney function is critical in drug therapy. Therefore, it is important to get an accurate measure of kidney function. A useful formula for estimating creatinine clearance based on serum creatinine values in older individuals was developed (Cockcroft and Gault, 1976). (The actual formula is provided in Chapter 14.) Table 1-1 summarizes some of the pertinent changes that occur with aging. For many items, the changes begin in adulthood and proceed gradually; others may not manifest themselves until well into advanced age.

HALLMARKS OF AGING

Nine hallmarks of aging are important for a practicing geriatrics health professional (Lopez- Otin et al, 2013). Table 1-2 summarizes these concepts and simplifies many of the principles as they relate to a clinician. First, aging is associated with an accumulation of DNA damage and delayed repair of DNA throughout life. Stress from environmental or endogenous stressors could result in a lesion to the DNA. This process of "irreversible growth and proliferation arrest induced by stress" was described by Hayflick in 1965. This lesion on the DNA is typically repaired with no detrimental outcome. If unrepaired, the DNA lesion could lead to an error in transcription or to an error in replication. Such errors could lead to cellular dysfunction, genetic instability, and cell death. Hence, defects in the repair of DNA or excessive damage that overcomes the repair capacity are more likely to occur with aging and may cause aging phenotypes and age-related disease.

In the second hallmark, aging is described as telomere attrition. With each cell division, a portion of the terminal end of chromosomes (called the telomere) is not replicated and therefore shortens. It is proposed that telomere shortening is the

TABLE 1-1. Pertinent Changes That Commonly Occur With Aging

System	Common age changes	Implications of changes
Cardiovascular	Atrophy of muscle fibers that line the endocardium Atherosclerosis of vessels Increased systolic blood pressure Decreased compliance of the left ventricle Decreased number of pacemaker cells Decreased sensitivity of baroreceptors	Increased blood pressure Increased emphasis on atrial contraction with an S_4 heard Increased arrhythmias Increased risk of hypotension with position change Valsalva maneuver may cause a drop in blood pressure Decreased exercise tolerance
Neurological	Decreased number of neurons and increase in size and number of neuroglial cells Decline in nerves and nerve fibers Atrophy of the brain and increase in cranial dead space Thickened leptomeninges in spinal cord	Increased risk for neurological problems: cerebrovascular accident Parkinsonism Slower conduction of fibers across the synapses Modest decline in short-term memory Alterations in gait pattern: wide based, shorter stepped, and flexed forward Increased risk of hemorrhage before symptoms are apparent
Respiratory	Decreased lung tissue elasticity Thoracic wall calcification Cilia atrophy Decreased respiratory muscle strength Decreased partial pressure of arterial oxygen (Pao_2)	Decreased efficiency of ventilatory exchange Increased susceptibility to infection and atelectasis Increased risk of aspiration Decreased ventilatory response to hypoxia and hypercapnia Increased sensitivity to narcotics
Integumentary	Loss of dermal and epidermal thickness Flattening of papillae Atrophy of sweat glands Decreased vascularity Collagen cross-linking Elastin regression Loss of subcutaneous fat Decreased melanocytes Decline in fibroblast proliferation	Thinning of skin and increased susceptibility to tearing Dryness and pruritus Decreased sweating and ability to regulate body heat Increased wrinkling and laxity of the skin Loss of fatty pads protecting bone and resulting in pain Increased need for protection from the sun Increased time for healing of wounds

(continued)

PART I

TABLE 1-1. Pertinent Changes That Commonly Occur With Aging (*continued*)

System	Common age changes	Implications of changes
Gastrointestinal	Decreased liver size Less efficient cholesterol stabilization and absorption Fibrosis and atrophy of salivary glands Decreased muscle tone in bowel Atrophy of and decrease in number of taste buds Slowing in esophageal emptying Decreased hydrochloric acid secretion Decreased gastric acid secretion Atrophy of the mucosal lining Decreased absorption of calcium	Change in intake caused by decreased appetite Discomfort after eating related to slowed passage of food Decreased absorption of calcium and iron Alteration of drug effectiveness Increased risk of constipation, esophageal spasm, and diverticular disease
Urinary	Reduced renal mass Loss of glomeruli Decline in number of functioning nephrons Changes in small vessel walls Decreased bladder muscle tone	Decreased GFR Decreased sodium-conserving ability Decreased creatinine clearance Increased BUN Decreased renal blood flow Altered drug clearance Decreased ability to dilute urine Decreased bladder capacity and increased residual urine Increased urgency
Reproductive	Atrophy and fibrosis of cervical and uterine walls Decreased vaginal elasticity and lubrication Decreased hormones and reduced oocytes Decreased seminiferous tubules Proliferation of stromal and glandular tissue Involution of mammary gland tissue	Vaginal dryness and burning and pain with intercourse Decreased seminal fluid volume and force of ejaculation Reduced elevation of the testes Prostatic hypertrophy Connective breast tissue is replaced by adipose tissue, making breast examinations easier
Musculoskeletal	Decreased muscle mass Decreased myosin adenosine triphosphatase activity Deterioration and drying of joint cartilage Decreased bone mass and osteoblastic activity	Decreased muscle strength Decreased bone density Loss of height Joint pain and stiffness Increased risk of fracture Alterations in gait and posture

(*continued*)

TABLE 1-1. Pertinent Changes That Commonly Occur With Aging (*continued*)

System	Common age changes	Implications of changes
Sensory: Vision	Decreased rod and cone function Pigment accumulation Decreased speed of eye movements Increased intraocular pressure Ciliary muscle atrophy Increased lens size and yellowing of the lens Decreased tear secretion	Decreased visual acuity, visual fields, and light/dark adaptation Increased sensitivity to glare Increased incidence of glaucoma Distorted depth perception with increased falls Less able to differentiate blues, greens, and violets Increased eye dryness and irritation
Sensory: Hearing	Loss of auditory neurons Loss of hearing from high to low frequency Increased cerumen Angiosclerosis of ear	Decreased hearing acuity and isolation (specifically, decreased ability to hear consonants) Difficulty hearing, especially when there is background noise, or when speech is rapid Cerumen impaction may cause hearing loss
Sensory: Smell, taste, and touch	Decreased number of olfactory nerve fibers Altered ability to taste sweet and salty foods; bitter and sour tastes remain Decreased sensation	Inability to smell noxious odors Decreased food intake Safety risk with regard to recognizing dangers in the environment: hot water, fire alarms, or small objects that result in tripping
Endocrine	Decreased testosterone, GH, insulin, adrenal androgens, aldosterone, and thyroid hormone Decreased thermoregulation Decreased febrile response Increased nodularity and fibrosis of thyroid Decreased basal metabolic rate	Decreased ability to tolerate stressors such as surgery Decreased sweating and shivering and temperature regulation Lower baseline temperature; infection may not cause an elevation in temperature Decreased insulin response, glucose tolerance Decreased sensitivity of renal tubules to antidiuretic hormone Weight gain Increased incidence of thyroid disease

BUN, blood urea nitrogen; GFR, glomerular filtration rate; GH, growth hormone.
For more information see Schmidt, 1999.

TABLE 1-2. Nine Hallmarks of Aging

Hallmark	Mechanisms	Manifestations
Genomic instability	Spontaneous mutagenesis Failure in DNA repair systems	Copying errors
Telomere attrition	With each cell division the terminal end of the chromosome called the telomere is shortened.	Telomerase is an enzyme that adds DNA bases back to telomeres. Telomere length may be associated with function and health in oldest old.
Epigenetic alteration	Changes in gene expression, instead of changes in the underlying sequence.	Changes to how cells read genes.
Loss of proteostasis	Impaired building, stability, and function of proteins.	Failure to refold or degrade the unfolded proteins leads to their piling up and results in damage.
Deregulated nutrient-sensing	Dietary restriction affects the somatotrophic axis involving growth hormone and insulin/IGF-1 signaling pathway.	Decreased nutrients in rodents prolonged aging, but mixed benefits noted in primates.
Mitochondrial dysfunction	Mitochondria are key to energy production via electron transport system and ATP generation.	As cells age, the efficiency of the respiratory chain tends to decrease.
Cellular senescence	Over time, cells, exhaust their ability to regenerate.	DNA damage accelerates aging.
Stem cell exhaustion	Over time, cells exhaust their ability to replicate.	In the hematopoietic system there is increased incidence of anemia and myelodysplasia.
Altered intracellular communication	Signaling becomes dysregulated by inflammation.	Inflammaging—altered intracellular communication with resultant impact on multiple organ systems.

For more information see Lopez-Otin et al, 2013.

clock that results in the shift to a senescent pattern of gene expression and ulti-mately cell senescence (Fossel, 1998). Pathological telomere dysfunction accelerates aging in mice and in humans. Stimulation of telomeres can delay aging in laboratory mice, which shows that the telomere fulfills the key features of an important aspect of aging. Telomerase is an enzyme that acts by adding DNA bases to telomeres.

Transfection of the catalytic component of this enzyme into senescent cells extends their telomeres as well as the replicative life span of the cells and induces a pattern of gene expression typical of young cells. The extent to which telomere shortening is relevant to cellular senescence and aging in vivo, however, remains unknown. In contrast, telomerase inhibitors may be potent anti-cancer therapies. The role of replicative senescence in aging and associated chronic disease processes is now being explored. Studies of the oldest old have not demonstrated any relationship between telomere length and mortality. However, telomere length may be associated with function and health rather than exceptional longevity, as healthy centenarians had significantly longer telomeres than did unhealthy centenarians (Terry et al, 2008). The findings were similar in a population-based cohort study of individuals aged 70 to 79 years (Njajou et al, 2009).

The third hallmark describes aging as associated with changes in gene expression that do not involve a change to the underlying DNA sequence. These changes, called epigenetic changes, in turn affect how cells read genes. Epigenetic alterations that contribute to aging include DNA methylation, histone modifications, and chromatin remodeling.

Fourth, there is evidence that aging is linked to impaired stability and functioning of proteins. These proteins, which are made within the cells, must be correctly folded, stable in their location, and working. This process of normal building, stabilizing, and functioning of proteins is referred to as proteostasis. Endogenous or exogenous stress causes the unfolding of proteins. Likewise, stress can impair proper folding during protein synthesis. Disrupted intracellular proteins are usually refolded or removed and degraded. Failure to refold or degrade unfolded proteins can lead to their piling up and this process causes damage to the cell and is associated with aging.

The fifth hallmark involves deregulated nutrient-sensing. Metabolic alterations such as dietary restriction can affect aging in yeast, worms, flies, and rodents. While one group has reported health and mortality benefits from caloric restriction in primates (Colman et al, 2009), a more recent study did not find similar benefits (Maxmen, 2012). The somatrophic axis involving growth hormone and the insulin/ insulin growth factor 1 (IGF-1) signaling pathway are remarkably stable in aging. Decreased nutrients can impact this pathway and extend longevity. Pharmacological manipulation of this mechanism that imitates a state of nutrient availability (such as rapamycin) can extend longevity in mice.

Sixth, mitochondrial dysfunction can accelerate the aging process in mammals. Mitochondrial function and the clinical implications on muscle strength are key areas of interest to frailty researchers.

The seventh hallmark of aging highlights that cells exhaust their ability to regenerate over a period of time. This arrest of the cell cycle is called cellular senescence and is in part caused by telomere shortening. DNA damage that becomes deleterious accelerates aging when tissues exhaust their regenerative capacity.

Eighth, stem cell exhaustion is a feature of aging. An example of this is the hematopoietic stem cells which decline with aging and the resultant increased incidence of anemia and increased risk of myelodysplasia.

Finally, intercellular communication is a normal part of physiology through the endocrine system and via neurohormonal signaling. This signaling becomes dysregulated in aging as inflammation increases. Several inflammatory markers increase with advancing age and these inflammatory markers may affect multiple organ systems simultaneously (eg, muscle, bone, arteries, and brain). Age-associated alteration in intracellular communication is called "inflammaging." The inflammation noted may be caused by the accumulation of pro-inflammatory tissue damage, or the failure of a dysfunctional immune system to clear pathogens, or the activation of the NF-κB transcription factor, or the occurrence of a defective autophagy response. These inflammatory agents have multiple triggers, seem to be correlated with altered intracellular communication, and result in the dysregulation of multiple physiological systems.

FRAILTY AS THE CLINICAL FEATURE OF THE AGING PROCESS

Frailty is an important concept to discuss in detail in the discussion of aging. Frailty may represent the clinical manifestation of the hallmarks of aging (Fedarko, 2011), which were outlined above.

The frailty phenotype is characterized by dysregulation of multiple organ systems (Fried, 2007). In this concept, frail individuals have decreased physiological reserves and increased vulnerability to stressors and distinct changes (in functional performance and in biomarkers) when compared to nonfrail individuals. Frailty phenotype is defined by the presence of three or more of these characteristics: (1) unintentional weight loss of 10 pounds or more in the last year; (2) sense of exhaustion (felt last week that "everything I did was an effort" or "I could not get going"; (3) poor grip strength, as measured by a hand dynamometer; (4) slow walking speed for 15 feet (with cutoff depending on sex and height); and (5) poor physical activity (Fried, 2016). Having one or two of these features would be consistent with prefrailty.

The Canadian Study of Health and Aging (CSHA) Clinical Frailty Scale is another tool that has been used to define older individuals who are vulnerable to institutionalization and death. The scale frames the assessment of an older person into one of the following seven categories: (1) very fit/robust—active, energetic folks who commonly exercise and are the most fit for their age; (2) well—without active disease, but less fit than people in the first category; (3) well—with treated comorbid disease symptoms that are well controlled; (4) apparently vulnerable—individuals who are not frankly dependent, yet may complain of being "slowed up" or have disease symptoms; (5) mildly frail—individuals with limited dependence on others for instrumental activities of daily living; (6) moderately frail—need help for both instrumental activities of daily living and basic activities of daily living; and (7) severely frail—completely dependent on others for basic activities of daily living, or terminally ill. The CSHA scale provides the clinician a reference to compare a patient's clinical performance, while the frailty phenotype has the clinician assess for five clinical characteristics to meet a threshold above which the condition of frailty exists. Each increase from one category to the next of the CSHA scale increases the risk of death within about 6 years and entry into an institution (Rockwell et al, 2005). This measure of frailty is feasible to implement in clinical practice. While the CSHA Clinical Frailty Scale seems to lump the concepts of frailty with functional dependency, the frailty phenotype alternatively may connote a gradation of vulnerability prior to the loss of function.

The prevalence of frailty based on the phenotype at baseline among a large cohort of community-dwelling older individuals in the Cardiovascular Health Study increased with advancing age, from 3% among individuals aged 65 to 70 to 16% for individuals aged 80 to 84. Generally, older women were more likely to be frail than older men. The cohort of older black women had roughly twice the rate of frailty when compared to the original cohort of women. Individuals were assessed at 3 and 7 years to define the incidence of adverse outcomes associated with frailty. Frail individuals at baseline, when compared to intermediate, and not frail older persons: (1) were more likely to die, (2) were more likely to have been hospitalized, (3) were more likely to have fallen, (4) were more likely to require assistance in self-care, and (5) were more likely to have a worsened mobility disability. Frail patients, those having four or five of the previously noted characteristics, undergoing elective surgery had an increased risk of postoperative complications (Makary et al, 2010). The frail group stayed in the hospital longer (after their surgery) and were more likely to be discharged to a skilled nursing facility. In short, frailty is a marker of an older adult who is vulnerable to stressors (Fried et al, 2004). In practice, oncologists and cardio-thoracic surgeons often use frailty tools, in conjunction with functional assessment, to develop a plan of care for older patients receiving care in each setting. Care plans in these settings generally use interdisciplinary teams to define and work toward patients' goals and preferences. An additional discussion of the clinical approach to frailty is found in Chapter 12.

RESILIENCE AND HOMEOSTENOSIS

Resilience is defined by the rapidity and completeness with which an individual recovers from stressors and the return to meeting the criteria for success (Rowe and Kahn, 1997). A resilient older individual in the context of her or his life demonstrates a stable response to social or behavioral stressors. Kuchel has described the concept of resilience by using the analogy of the San Francisco Golden Gate Bridge (Kuchel, 2016). The weight of the roadway is hung from two cables that pass through the two main towers and are fixed in concrete at each end. Resilience of the bridge comes from the multiple components of the design which work together to recover from stress (eg, caused by wind and weight). Multiple components of the bridge would need to be compromised for the structure to fail. If there were numerous areas of damage to such a structure, the smallest weight, or even the weight of the road itself, would cause the bridge to fail. Likewise, the resilient older individual has multiple systems in place to withstand stress. Further, the loss of multiple key systems simultaneously may cause an irreversible cascade of decline.

Homeostenosis is characterized by a diminished capacity to respond to varied homeostatic stressors. Further, there may be an additive effect of the failures in multiple organ systems, which eventually results in an overall cascade of decline, which becomes irreversible. Homeostatic dysregulation is generally featured by a loss of physiological reserve, enhanced basal activity, poor end-organ responsiveness, higher basal activity, and a loss of negative feedback inhibition. Clinical examples of homeostenosis include elevated temperature in response to high ambient temperature, and a drop in blood pressure in response to volume depletion and arising from sitting to standing position. Researchers believe that sarcopenic obesity may likewise describe a group with a diminished capacity to respond to stressors. In this clinical syndrome individuals have features of obesity, poor physical performance, low muscle mass, and poor muscle quality. Further, sarcopenic obesity is independently associated with and precedes a decline in the ability to perform instrumental activities of daily living (IADLs) (Baumgartner et al, 2004). These patients are at a high risk for developing functional decline over time. The hypothesis of the diminished response to stressors is that of high levels of IL-6 and other inflammatory markers associated with the obesity. The chronic inflammation results in poor response to stress and muscle wasting. The muscle wasting may then lead to physical disability which in turn leads to decreased activity levels. As the muscles have decreased stimulus there is further wasting and decline.

THE LINK BETWEEN AGING AND MULTIMORBIDITY

While younger adults may develop important chronic illnesses, the single best predictor of many chronic diseases is advancing age. Many older individuals develop multiple comorbid illnesses. Thirty-five percent of the population in the United States aged 65 to 79 years reports two or more diseases and this rate increases to 70% at age 80 years and older. Two-thirds of all older Medicare beneficiaries have two or more chronic conditions and one-third have four or more. Comorbidity is associated with high health-care utilization and expenditures (Fried et al, 2004). Further, comorbidity increases the risk of disability and mortality. Comorbidity and frailty are each independent predictors of disability. Comorbidity may represent the aggregation of the physiological damage that leads to diseases, while frailty may represent the aggregate of subclinical losses of reserve across multiple physiological systems. There are shared risk factors for illness across organ systems that are important to take into account (eg, risk factors like smoking, hypertension, and diabetes for coronary artery disease and for stroke, and chronic kidney disease). The treatments for several diseases likewise can improve outcomes for other organ systems.

GERIATRIC SYNDROMES

Because comorbid illnesses often do not tell the whole story in geriatrics, it is more helpful to think in terms of presenting problems. One aid to recalling some of the common problems of geriatrics uses a series of I's:

- Immobility
- Instability

- Incontinence
- Intellectual impairment
- Infection
- Impairment of vision and hearing
- Irritable colon
- Isolation (depression)
- Inanition (malnutrition)
- Iatrogenesis
- Insomnia
- Immune deficiency
- Impotence

The list is important for several reasons. Especially with older patients, the expression of the problem may not be a good clue to the etiology. Conversely, a problem may occur for a variety of reasons.

For example, immobility may be caused by a variety of underlying physical and emotional problems. The older individual may have sustained a fractured hip or congestive heart failure, a recent fall and fear of falling, or significant pain caused by degenerative joint disease, any or all of which may cause immobility. It is important to explore with the individual the underlying cause(s) so that appropriate interventions can be implemented. It may be necessary, for example, to alleviate patients' pain and address their fear of falling before initiating therapy or engaging the individual in a regular exercise program.

Several themes of geriatric syndromes should be highlighted. While they are common in older adults, and age itself may predispose to the condition, they are not a part of normal aging. Also, geriatric syndromes often have multiple etiologies and may have shared risk factors. Geriatric syndromes and functional dependence may result when decline in multiple domains compromises the person's compensatory capacity (Tinetti et al, 1995). Geriatric syndromes predispose older persons to worse health outcomes. They are usually treatable with nonpharmacological and medical treatments that can improve the patient's function and quality of life. Part II of this book provides details on multiple geriatric syndromes.

ATYPICAL PRESENTATION OF COMMON CLINICAL PROBLEMS

One of the greatest challenges in the care of older adults is the atypical presentation of many diseases. Because older people may lose resilience and response to strength, they may not demonstrate typical manifestations of diseases. Most signs and symptoms are actually the result of the body's response to a physiological insult. Decreased responsiveness leads to atypical presentations.

It is not unusual for the first sign of an acute problem such as an infection (urine, respiration, or wound being the most common) to present with an atypical finding such as confusion, functional change, worsened appetite, or a fall, rather than more typical symptoms such as urinary burning, cough, or fever. When the older individual has an underlying cognitive impairment, these changes may be very subtle, and caregivers may report that "he just isn't himself today" without providing more specific clinical signs. It is not unusual for independent and cognitively intact older individuals to come into the office with complaints that they just didn't feel right or didn't feel like making their bed and, on examination, are in new onset of atrial fibrillation. Any report of this type of new or sudden change in the individual's behavior or function should be approached as an acute medical problem, and a comprehensive evaluation should be initiated. Further, health professionals should take into account that they may be assessing a patient with an atypical presentation early in the course of their illness. Reassessing the patient after a short interval may provide a better picture of the trajectory of the patient's illness. In uncertain clinical presentations, the clinician should alert the patient and family to "red flag" signs and symptoms that would signal a worsening in condition.

The presentation of a new problem is further complicated by the presence of extant comorbidity. It may be hard to detect the new event in the context of manifestations of other problems.

The first and principal task of the health professional is to identify a correctable problem and address it. No amount of rehabilitation, compassionate care, or environmental manipulation will compensate for missing a remediable diagnosis. However, diagnoses alone are usually insufficient. Older adults often have multiple comorbid chronic conditions that must be managed in the context of their lives. The individual and his or her family make decisions about chronic illness most often when they are not in the setting of a health professional. The clinician and clinical team are charged with teaching patients about their illness and guiding their plan of care. The process of geriatrics is thus threefold: (1) careful clinical assessment and management to identify acute and remediable problems, (2) ongoing management of underlying chronic illnesses, and (3) careful evaluation for evidence of geriatric syndromes (as per the I's discussed previously). It is only through addressing the biopsychosocial needs that the individual will be able to optimize the use of resources (eg, environmental interventions, social interactions) and achieve his or her highest level of health and function.

CLINICAL IMPLICATIONS—PUTTING IT ALL TOGETHER

As we apply the biology of aging to the clinical care of older patients there are several points to consider. The first point to note is the variability within a group of older persons. This means that within a cohort of older individuals there can be a wide range of health and of function. To demonstrate this point, if a clinician were to join a clinical practice setting in a retirement community, his or her responsibilities would vary from efforts to maintain the health and vitality of independent residents in their own apartments to caring for older individuals with multiple comorbid illnesses and a need for assistance with their daily self-cares. This book outlines topics that span the wide range of health needs of older adults.

The second clinical implication of biological aging is the need to approach the whole person. This person-centered care may be in contrast to the specialty care for older adults (eg, in surgery or in cardiovascular disease). In both of these examples, the specialist needs to remain keenly focused on the clinical aspects of the discipline that pose great risk to the patient. At times, however, such effort may not be sufficient. A clinical example would be an 88-year-old woman with rib fractures from a fall who becomes anxious and short of breath. Assessing and addressing the whole patient's needs will help improve the patient's care in the periprocedure course. A paradigm that can take into account the entire biopsychosocial needs of an individual is the Wisconsin Star method (taught by Dr Timothy Howell at University of Wisconsin–Madison School of Medicine and Public Health). The approach helps the clinician address the complex needs of the patient by specifically assessing (1) the medical needs of the patient; (2) the medications; (3) the social needs of the individual—including his or her function; (4) the behavioral health needs; and finally (5) the meaning of the illness/situation to the individual. The most challenging aspect of the case is defined and often written in the middle of the star. This approach helps a clinician (1) assess the essential aspects of the entire patient, (2) understand the interaction between different points of the star (eg, assessing the medical aspects of the above case scenario led to determining that the patient had a low oxygen level from a mucous plug, whereas simply treating the anxiety with benzodiazepine medications would not have been sufficient); and (3) better understand the gaps in the clinician's assessment of how the patient's health problem affects their lives. This approach works exceedingly well in the care of older persons with complex needs. Further, this approach allows the patient to define goals and preferences and the clinician to work toward them.

Function is the cornerstone of the third key clinical aspect of biological aging. Function was mentioned in the prior two points and serves as a compass in decision making. Knowing the patient's baseline and current functional status can help define if a patient can return home from the emergency department visit for an acute problem or likewise be transitioned home after a hospital admission. Geriatric best-practice models are directed to sustain or improve function. Multiple chapters of this book outline key areas of the functional status of older adults in an effort to help maintain or regain functional independence. Functional assessment tests are particularly useful for a variety of assessments in older adults. Many of these have been collected in a book produced annually by the American Geriatrics Society (Reuben et al, 2016). This resource is available for purchase at the app store for your tablet or smartphone.

In treating an older adult, it is useful to keep in mind that an individual's ability to function depends on a combination of his or her characteristics (eg, innate capacity, motivation, pain tolerance, or fear) and the setting in which that person is expected to function. The same individual may be functional in one setting and dependent in another. Think of how well you would do if you were suddenly transported to a country where you could not speak the language or understand the customs. It is critical to allow the older adult to independently perform all activities during clinical encounters to facilitate a true assessment of capability and function. For example, observing the patient's ability to get up and down from an examination chair or table, walk into the examination room, and don and doff a shirt are critical components of the examination. Physicians and other primary health-care providers should serve as role models to encourage optimal function among older individuals. Unfortunately, caregivers, both formal and informal, may tend to provide unnecessary care for the older individual in an effort to decrease his or her risk of trauma or fatigue. This propagates a dependent status and can cause functional impairment and disability.

Fourth, clinicians must use the notion of variability in aging to help individuals make lifestyle and treatment choices to optimize their aging. An example of this might be an older person who wishes to remain in her own home in the community, in spite of family efforts to prepare for a move to an independent apartment. Her quality of life at her current setting is valued greater than the trade-off of living in a retirement community. Honoring her choices respects her autonomy as she ages.

Fifth, special consideration should be given to the older adult's physical and social environment. Multiple environmental assessment tools can be used to consider the fit between the individual and his or her environment (Gallo et al, 2006). The Housing Enabler (www.enabler.nu/) is a tool that helps the clinician conduct such a comprehensive evaluation considering not only the environment and the environment risks, but the match of the person's functional abilities with that environment. Again, once evaluated, the team can be used to identify interventions to decrease risks of falls and optimize function.

Sixth, evidence supports the benefit of lifestyle interventions (specifically diet and physical activity) to help overcome some of the physical changes that can occur with age and may improve overall health and quality of life. With regard to diet, there are protective effects to diets low in saturated fats and high in fruits and vegetables. Likewise, engaging in regular physical activity, at least 30 minutes daily, has been noted to have both physical and mental health benefits. Numerous resources help clinicians prescribe and motivate older adults to change prior behaviors and/or continue to engage in health-promoting activities (Table 1-3).

Seventh, it is impossible to address aging without considering the psychosocial aspects that occur in addition to the more visible biological and physical changes (Rowe and Kahn, 1987). Transitions associated with aging are commonly noted around retirement. Aging is a time of loss: loss of social position, a spouse or significant other, pet, home, car and ability to drive, as well as the loss of sensory function (hearing and vision), or ambulatory ability or capacity. Many fear the loss of independence with age and cognitive decline, and worry about having an acute catastrophic problem such as a hip fracture or stroke. Conversely, many older adults are quite resilient in the face of these losses and have much to teach the younger generation on how to respond to loss, optimize remaining function and ability, and adjust.

Eighth, it is critical when working with older adults to be well aware of one's own beliefs with regard to theories of aging, attitudes about the aging process, and philosophies about how to age successfully. Recognizing these beliefs, clinicians must be open to evaluating their patient's beliefs and attitudes about aging and match interventions and recommendations with those beliefs. Gawande's book (2014)

TABLE 1-3. Web-Based Resources for Health Promotion and Aging

Agency for Healthcare Research and Quality Guidelines from the U.S. Preventative Services Task Force	www.ahrq.gov/clinic/uspstfix.htm
American Academy of Family Physicians: Summary of Policy Recommendations for Periodic Health Examinations	www.aafp.org/exam.xml
Canadian Task Force on Preventive Health Care	www.phac-aspc.gc.ca/cd-mc/ctfphc-gecssp-eng.php
Centers for Disease Control and Prevention: Healthy Living	www.cdc.gov/HealthyLiving/
MedPAC Data Book on Health Care Spending and the Medicare Program, June 2016	www.medpac.gov/docs/default-sourc/data-book/june-2016
National Center for Health Statistics	www.cdc.gov/nchs
National Cholesterol Education Program	www.nhlbi.nih.gov/health-pro/guidelines/current/cholesterol-guidelines/final-report
National Guideline Clearinghouse	www.guideline.gov
The Eighth Report of the Joint National Committee on Prevention, Detection, Evaluation, and Treatment of High Blood Pressure (JNC-8)	www.aafp.org/afp/2014/1001/p503.html
Web-based resources related to exercise facilitation in older adults (accessed 11/14/16)	
AgePage: Exercise: Feeling Fit for Life	www.iamfitforlife.com/
American Heart Association	www.heart.org
Fitness Past 50 Materials	www.fitnesspastfifty.com/articles.html
International Council on Active Aging (ICAA)	www.icaa.com/
International Counsel on Active Aging	www.icaa.cc/
National Blueprint: Increasing Physical Activity Among Adults Age 50 and Older	www.agingblueprint.org/tips.cfm
National Institute of Aging: Exercise: A Guide From the National Institute of Aging	www.nia.nih.gov/HealthInformation/Publications/ExerciseGuide/
President's Council on Physical Fitness and Sports	www.fitness.gov/
The Exercise Assessment and Screening for You Tool	www.easyforyou.info
YMCA Programs Such as Active Older Adults (AOA)	www.ymca-austin.org/aoa.htm

provides a clear paradigm of successful aging. From a diagnostic perspective, this is particularly important because older adults, who assume that with age it is normal to be short of breath, forgetful, and fatigued, may not report these symptoms as significant and thereby won't provide the health-care provider with the necessary information to facilitate a diagnosis. This requires the provider working with older adults to develop keen assessment skills and to use objective measures appropriately developed for older individuals.

Common examples of missed diagnoses occur related to cognitive impairment and depression. Older individuals, particularly those who have strong social skills and were well educated and engaged in social and professional activities throughout their life, may appear to be cognitively intact in the course of a social interaction and even a brief medical visit. However, on closer evaluation and with the use of standardized screening measures of memory, it may become evident that the individual has significantly impaired short-term memory.

Finally, the clinician's primary responsibility is to diagnose any acute clinical problems and alleviate all treatable symptoms. Once the patient's physical and psychological health has been optimized, the health-care provider has the opportunity to engage all members of the health-care team (nursing, physical and occupational therapy, social work, etc.) to help the patient achieve his or her highest level of function and quality of life.

REFERENCES

Banks J, Marmot M, Oldfield Z, et al. Disease and disadvantage in the United States and in England. *JAMA*. 2006;295:2037-2045.

Baumgartner RN, Wayne SJ, Waters DL, et al. Sarcopenic obesity predicts instrumental activities in daily living disability in the elderly. *Obesity Research*. 2004;12(12):1995-2004.

Boyd CM, Darer J, Boult C, Fried LP, Boult L, Wu AW. Clinical practice guidelines and quality of care for older patients with multiple comorbid diseases: implications for pay for performance. *JAMA*. 2005;294:716-724.

Cockcroft DW, Gault MH. Prediction of creatinine clearance from serum creatinine. *Nephron*. 1976;16:31-41.

Colman RJ, Anderson RM, Johnson SC, et al. Caloric restriction delays disease onset and mortality in rhesus monkeys. *Science*. 2009;325:201-204.

Fedarko NS. The biology of aging and frailty. *Clin Geriatr Med*. 2011;27(1):27-37.

Fossel M. Telomerase and the aging cell: implications for human health. *JAMA*. 1998;279:1732-1735.

Fried LP. Interventions for human frailty: physical activity as a model. *Cold Spring Harb Perspect Med*. 2016;6:a025916.

Fried LP, Ferrucci L, Darer J, Williamson JD, Anderson G. Untangling the concepts of disability, frailty, and comorbidity: implications for improved targeting and care. *J Gerontol Med Sci*. 2004;59(3):255-263.

Fried LP, Tangen CM, Walston L. Cardiovascular Health Study Collaborative Research Group. Frailty in older adults: evidence for a phenotype. *J Gerontol Med Sci*. 2007;61:262-266.

Fries JF. Aging, natural death, and the compression of morbidity. *N Engl J Med*. 1980;303:130-135.

Gallo JJ, Bogner HR, Fulmer T, et al. *Handbook of Geriatric Assessment.* 4th ed. Rockville, MD: Aspen; 2006.

Gavrilova NS, Gavrilov LA. Search for predictors of exceptional human longevity. In: *Living to 100 and Beyond Monograph.* Schaumburg, IL: The Society of Actuaries; 2005:1-49.

Gawande A. *Being Mortal—Medicine and What Matters in the End.* New York, NY: Metropolitan Books Henry Holt and Co; 2014.

Goldsmith TC. *The Evolution of Aging.* 2nd ed. Annapolis, MD: Azinet Press; 2006.

Hayflick L. Biological aging is no longer an unsolved problem. *Ann N Y Acad Sci.* 2007;1100:1-13.

Kuchel G. Adaption to stress—resilience. Lecture at the 2016 GEMSTAR U13 Conference on Models and Studies of Aging, September 24, 2016, and personal conversation September 25, 2016.

Lopez-Otin C, Blasco MA, Partridge L, Serrano M, Kroemer G. The hallmarks of aging. *Cell* 2013;153(6):1194-1217.

Makary MA, Segev DL, Pronovost PJ, et al. Frailty as a predictor of surgical outcomes in older patients. *J Am Coll Surg.* 2010;210(6):901-908.

Maxmen A. Calorie restriction falters in the long run. *Nature.* 2012;488:569.

Miller RA. Extending life: scientific prospects and political obstacles. *Milbank Q.* 2002;80(1):155-174.

Njajou OT, Hsueh W-C, Blackburn EH, et al. Association between telomere length, specific causes of death, and years of healthy life in health, aging, and body composition, a population-based study. *J Gerontol A Biol Sci Med Sci.* 2009;64:860-864.

Rando TA, Chang HY. Aging, rejuvenation, and epigenetic reprogramming: resetting the aging clock. *Cell.* 2012;418:46-57.

Reuben DB, Herr KA, Pacala JT, et al. *Geriatrics at Your Fingertips.* New York, NY: American Geriatrics Society; 2016.

Rockwood K, Song X, MacKnight C, et al. A global clinical measure of fitness and frailty in elderly people. *CMAJ.* 2005;173(5):489-495.

Rowe JW, Kahn RL. Human aging: usual and successful. *Science.* 1987;237:143-149.

Rowe JW, Kahn RL. Successful aging. *Gerontologist.* 1997;37(4):433-440.

Schmidt K. Physiology and pathophysiology of senescence. *Int J Vitam Nutr Res.* 1999;69:150-153.

Terry DF, Nolan VG, Andersen SL, et al. Association of longer telomeres with better health in centenarians. *J Gerontol Biol Sci Med Sci.* 2008;63:809-812.

Tinetti ME, Inouye SK, Gill T, Doucette JT. Shared risk factors for falls, incontinence, and functional dependence: unifying the approach to geriatric syndromes. *JAMA.* 1995;273(17):1348-1353.

SUGGESTED READINGS

Caldo RT, Young NS. Telomere diseases. *N Engl J Med.* 2009;361:2353-2365.

Campisi J, Vijg J. Does damage to DNA and other macromolecules play a role in aging? If so, how? *J Gerontol A Biol Sci Med Sci.* 2009;64A:175-178.

Goldsmith TC. *The Evolution of Aging.* 2nd ed. Annapolis, MD: Azinet Press; 2006.

Hoeijmakers JHJ. DNA damage, aging, and cancer. *N Engl J Med.* 2009;361:1475-1485.

CHAPTER 2

The Geriatric Patient: Demography, Epidemiology, and Health Services Utilization

By all demographic accounts, geriatric business will be good for some time. Medical practice will serve a growing number of older adults. Today persons aged 65 years and older currently represent a little more than one-third of the patients seen by a primary care physician; in 40 years, we can safely predict that at least every other adult patient will be aged 65 or older. The relative rate of growth varies with age. The older the old, the faster their relative numbers grow. Those over 85 are the most rapidly growing group of older individuals, with a growth rate twice that of those aged 65 years and older and four times that of the total population. This group now represents approximately 10% of the older population and is anticipated to grow from 5.7 million in 2010 to over 19 million by 2050 (Census Data, 2010). Among this old-old group, those aged 90 and above will show an even steeper rise. People in this old-old group tend to have poorer physical activity, be more dependent in activities of daily living, and have more cognitive impairment (Zhao et al, 2010).

The growth in aging spawns several concerns around numbers and dollars. As shown in Figure 2-1, the growing numbers of older people are not matched by growth in those following them. Hence, there will be fewer people to support programs like Social Security and Medicare, and fewer people to provide needed care. We hear a great deal of talk about the incipient demise of Social Security, the bankrupt status of Medicare, the death of the family as a social institution, and dire predictions of demographic cataclysms. There is, indeed, cause for concern but not necessarily for alarm. The message of the numbers is straightforward: we cannot go on as we have; new approaches are needed. The shape of those approaches to meeting the needs of growing numbers of older persons in this society will reflect societal values.

Americans who view aging as a problem can take some solace in knowing that we are not aging as fast as many other countries. Indeed, we rank 48th of 228 countries and areas in the world. The costs associated with an aging society have already stimulated major changes in the way we provide care. If we face a dearth of caregivers (paid and unpaid), we will need more creative approaches to giving care.

There is actually some basis for optimism. The rate of dementia has been falling for decades. Compared to the incidence in the late 1970s and early 1980s, the incidence declined 44% during the late 2000s and early 2010s (Satizabal et al, 2016) The incidence of hip fractures has been falling steadily. Rates of heart disease and stroke have been declining for several decades. Some of this decline can be attributed to better medical care (and the use of medications such as beta blockers and

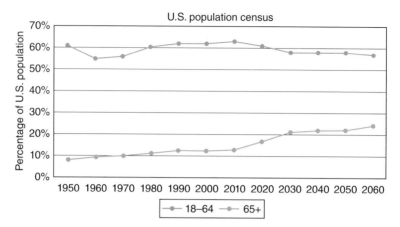

FIGURE 2-1 Change in the relationship of older persons and workers. (*Data from Colby SL, Ortman JM: Projections of the Size and Composition of the U.S. Population: 2014 to 2060. US Census Bureau; March, 2015.*)

bisphosphonates), but much of the reason for the decline remains a mystery. Data from the National Long-Term Care Survey show a decline in the rate of disability among older people. Overall, this rate has decreased by 1% or more annually for the last several decades. However, the growth in the aging population more than offsets this gain. The number of persons with disabilities aged 65 years and older in 1982 was 6.4 million. It increased to 7 million in 1994, and in 1999, the projected level of disability applied to population projections called for was about 9.3 million. It remains to be seen whether this trend toward lower disability rates can be sustained, but if so, it will greatly offset the effects of an aging population. Death rates from major killers have been falling in some areas. As seen in Figure 2-2, death in older persons from cardiovascular and cerebrovascular diseases has dropped remarkably, but death from cancer overall has not changed much. The rapid rise in Alzheimer disease deaths is likely due to more aggressive detection and reporting. As noted, the incidence of this disease is now falling.

The current obesity epidemic may alter longevity among current adults. Obesity appears to reduce life expectancy at age 50 years by 1.5 years for women and by 1.9 years for men (Preston and Stokes, 2011). Likely related, the number of patients with type 2 diabetes is increasing rapidly, and is associated with premature death (van Dieren et al, 2010). Consequently, life expectancy in the United States is anticipated to drop lower than that experienced in other countries.

Aging is associated with increased disability, which in turn leads to more health care. However, aging is not the only contributor to the rapidly escalating costs of care. Although older people use a disproportionately large amount of medical care, most of the growth in costs is traceable to tremendous expansion in medical technology, both diagnostic and therapeutic. We have potent, but often expensive tools at our disposal. Much of this technology imposes risks as well as benefits. In some ways,

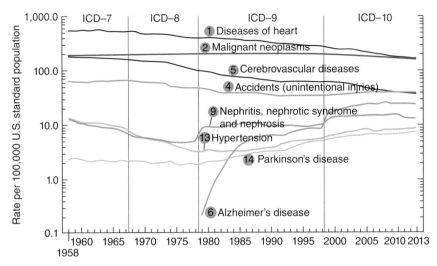

FIGURE 2-2 Age-adjusted death rates for selected leading causes of death: United States, 1958–2013. Note: ICD is the *International Classification of Diseases.* Circled numbers indicate ranking of conditions as leading causes of death in 2013. (*Reproduced with permission from Xu J, Murphy SL, Kochanek KD, et al: Deaths: Final Data for 2013, Natl Vital Stat Rep. 2016 Feb 16;64(2):1-119.*)

we can be said to be reaping the fruits of our success. While a substantial number of older people live to enjoy many active years, some persons who might not have survived in earlier times are now living into old age and bringing with them the chronic disease burden that would have been avoided by death. A noted British geriatrician, Bernard Isaacs, described this phenomenon as "survival of the unfit test."

Public policy has been directed at countering financial effects of this trend. While increasing insurance coverage for those under age 65, the Patient Protection and Affordable Care Act (PPACA) and the Reconciliation Act contain provisions designed to reduce Medicare program costs. Health care is evolving. Value-based purchasing is an overt goal. Various approaches to bundling payment and defining accountability more broadly are being tested. There is even talk about better integrating social and medical care. It is thus an exciting time for geriatricians and other members of the health-care profession to rethink how care is provided to best meet the needs of an aging America. Increasingly, there will be an emphasis on quality of life that at least parallels quantity of care. One subtle approach to rationing is the press to increase the use of advance directives (ADs) to avoid futile care, in the name of enhancing autonomy. (ADs are discussed more thoroughly in Chapter 18.)

Patient-centered care is *de rigeur*, but not everyone wants to steer his or her own ship. Overwhelmed by choices, older adults and their caregivers will be looking to clinicians to help them with decisions about screening practices, such as when to stop going for mammography, as well as treatment decisions, such as whether or not to undergo cancer treatment or invasive surgical interventions.

GROWTH IN NUMBERS

A look at a few trends helps focus the problem. The numbers of older people in this country (and in the world) have been growing in both absolute and relative terms. The absolute growth in numbers can be traced to the advances in medical science that have improved survival rates from specific diseases, whereas the relative growth reflects the birth rate. The relative numbers of older persons are primarily the result of two birth rates: (1) the one that occurred 65 or more years ago and (2) the current one. The first one provides the people, most of whom will survive, to become old. The second means that the proportion of those who are old depends on how many were born subsequently. This ratio is critical in estimating the size of the workforce available to support an elderly population. The looming demographic crisis is based on the forecast of a large number of older persons increasing through the first half of the next century as a result of the post–World War II baby boom. That group of people, born in the late 1940s and early 1950s, reached seniority beginning in 2010. The relative rate of growth increases with each decade over age 75 years. Indeed, many older persons are now surviving longer; it is not rare to encounter a centenarian. In fact, the United States currently has the greatest number of centenarians of any nation, estimated at 72,000 in 2014, but China will soon eclipse that distinction. This corresponds to a national prevalence of 1 centenarian per 4400 people.

Although these forecasts can vary with the future birth and death rates, they are likely to be reasonably accurate. Thus, since the turn of the twentieth century, we have gone from a situation in which 4% of the population was aged 65 or older to a time when more than 12% has reached 65 years. By the year 2030, that older population will have almost doubled. Put another way, in 2030 there will be as many people older than 75 years as there are today who are older than 65 years. When that observation is combined with the reduction in births in the cohort behind the baby boomers, the social implications become more obvious. There will be fewer workers to support the larger older population. This demographic observation has led to several urgent recommendations: (1) redefine retirement age to recognize the increase in life expectancy and thereby reduce the ratio of retirees to workers (retaining workers may not only postpone retirement costs, it may also alleviate the shortages in critical areas like personal care); (2) encourage younger persons to personally save more for their retirement to avoid excessive dependency on public funds (the current rate of savings for most people suggests that they will have a hard time affording retirement, let alone long-term care [LTC] costs); (3) encourage volunteerism among older adults to augment services in libraries, health-care facilities, and schools as well as provide professional services (von Bonsdorff and Rantanen, 2011) (although for the reasons just cited, older people may need to keep working for pay to afford retirement); and (4) change public programs to address the needs of an aging society (however, with fewer taxpayers and growing demands for public support of a variety of programs, this political argument may be hard to make).

Because older people use more health-care services than do younger people, there will be an even greater demand on the health-care system and a concomitant rise in total health-care costs. Because Medicare beneficiaries use more institutional services (ie, hospital and nursing home care), their health-care costs are higher than those for younger groups. The 12% of the population aged 65 years and older accounts for over one-third of health expenditures.

As seen in Figure 2-3, health expenditures increase substantially with disability and with numbers of chronic diseases.

The growth in the number of aged persons reflects improvements in both social living conditions and medical care. Estimates suggest that well less than half of the gain has resulted from better medical care. Much of health reflects behaviors such as eating, drinking, and exercising. Over the course of the last century, we have moved from a preponderance of acute diseases (especially infections) to an era of chronic illnesses. Today at least two-thirds of all the money spent on health care goes toward chronic disease. (For older people that proportion is closer to 95%.) Changes in the health-care system proposed within the PPACA are facilitating an increased focus on chronic care and management of not only single but multiple chronic illnesses (Boult and Wieland, 2010). Indeed, multimorbidity is the medical challenge of our time. Table 2-1 reflects the changes in the most common causes of death from 1900 to 2014. Many of those common at the turn of the twentieth century are no longer even listed. Today, the pattern of death in old age is congruent to that of the population as a whole. The leading causes are basically the same, but there are some differences in the rankings. The leading causes of death are heart disease, cancer, stroke, chronic obstructive pulmonary disease, and influenza/pneumonia. Alzheimer disease features prominently.

Although the most dramatic reduction of mortality has occurred in infants and mothers, there has been a perceptible increase in survival even after age 65. Our stereotypes of what to expect from older people may therefore need reexamination.

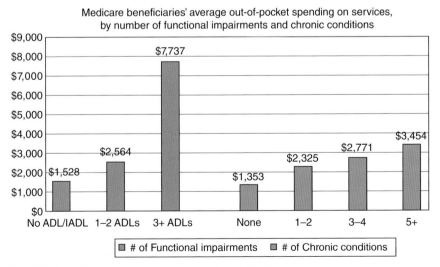

FIGURE 2-3 Medicare spending by function and chronic disease.

TABLE 2-1. Changes in Most Common Causes of Death, All Ages and Those 65 Years and Older

	Rate per 100,000					
	All ages				Age 65+	
	1900	Rank	2014	Rank	2014	Rank
Diseases of heart	13.8	4	193	1	1060	1
Malignant neoplasms	6.4	8	185	2	896	2
Cerebrovascular diseases	10.7	5	41	5	245	4
Chronic lower respiratory diseases	4.5	9	47	3	270	3
Influenza and pneumonia	22.9	1	18	8	97	8
Diabetes mellitus	1.1		24	7	117	6
Alzheimer disease			267	6	200	5
Nephritis, nephritic syndrome, and nephrosis	8.9	6	15	9	86	9
Accidents	7.2	7	41	4	105	7

Reproduced with permission from 1900 data: Anderson and Smith, 2005; 2014 data: National Vital Statistics System, National Center for Health Statistics, CDC.

The average 65-year-old woman can expect to live another 19.2 years and a 65-year-old man another 16.3 years. Even at age 85, there is an expectation of more than 5 years. Life expectancy at age 65 continues to increase for both men and women, and the gender gap is narrowing (Fig. 2-4). Women continue to do better than men. Whites do better than blacks, but Hispanics do best.

However, this gain in survival includes both active and dependent years. Indeed, one of the great controversies of modern gerontological epidemiology is whether the gain in life expectancy brings with it equivalent gains in years free of dependency. The answer lies somewhere between. Although increased survival may be associated with more disability, the overall effect has been a pattern of decreasing disability (Cutler, 2001). Moreover, not all disability is permanent. Some older people experience transient episodes.

A debate continues about the relationship of mortality and morbidity. Fries' concept of compression of morbidity argues that active prevention can delay the onset of disability without extending life expectancy (Fries, 1980). Hence, people would enjoy good health until shortly before they die. But others maintain that the actions that promote health also postpone death, and hence the timing gap persists.

DISABILITY

Some analysts have used disability as the basis for defining quality of life. They have then seized on the concept of active life expectancy to create a concept of quality-adjusted life-years (QALYs). Under this formulation, which is especially popular

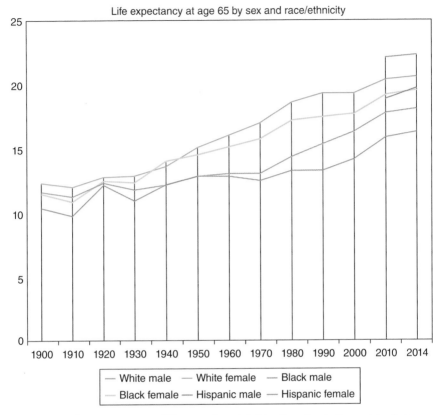

FIGURE 2-4 Life expectancy at age 65 by sex and race/ethnicity. (*Reproduced with permission from Centers for Disease Control (CDC)*)

with economists who are seeking a common denominator against which to weigh all interventions, the goal of health care is to maximize individuals' periods of disability-free time. However, such a formulation immediately raises concerns about the care of all those who are already frail; both younger persons with disabilities and frail older people start from a lower baseline, and thus even longevity gains are discounted. They would derive no benefit from any actions on their behalf unless they could convert them to a disability-free state. Frail older people face a double whammy: they will likely benefit less and have fewer years remaining.

The World Health Organization used to distinguish among impairments, disabilities, and handicaps, but the latter term raised such an outcry from the disability community that it was abandoned. A disease may create impairment in organ function. That failure can eventually lead to a reduced ability to perform certain tasks. This inability to perform may become a handicap when those tasks are necessary to carry out social activities; this is now rolled into the concept of disability.

Hence, a disability is the result of external demands and may be mitigated by environmental alterations. The distinction can provide a useful framework within which to consider the care of older persons.

Sensory impairment and orthopedic problems increase with age. Because they tend to accumulate over time, the prevalence of chronic conditions increases with age. However, the nature of survivorship produces the occasional twist that undermines the association between prevalence and age. Those living with diabetes and those with chronic lung disease, for example, do not survive as readily to age 85 and above. The majority of older adults have one or more chronic conditions, including common problems such as hypertension (53%), degenerative joint disease (50%), heart disease (31%), cancer (21%), and diabetes (18%). Despite having more chronic conditions and impairments, older people tend to report their health as generally good, although 3 out of 10 Medicare beneficiaries rate their health as fair or poor. In the 75- to 84-year age group, 24% of individuals rate their health as fair or poor, with the remainder rating their health as good, very good, or excellent. This increases such that among those aged 85 years and older, 30% rate their health as fair or poor, and the remainder indicate that they have good, very good, or excellent health. This contrast highlights the coping abilities of older persons discussed in Chapter 1.

The more recent pattern is mixed. Compared to the current senior population when they were middle-aged, the next wave of seniors smokes about half as much but has a 55% higher prevalence of diabetes and a (not unrelated) 25% higher prevalence of obesity. Over the past 3 years, obesity among seniors has increased 9%. Perhaps as a result, the emerging elders have a 9% lower prevalence of very good or excellent health status (United Health Foundation, 2016).

Because physicians provide health care for those who are sick, they may tend to form a distorted picture of senior citizens. Most older persons are indeed self-sufficient and able to function on their own or with minimal assistance.

Those who need the most help are likely to be the very old; many suffer from multiple diseases. Functioning can be measured in a variety of ways. Commonly, we use the ability to perform specific tasks as a reflection of independence. These are grouped into two classes of measures. The term *instrumental activities of daily living (IADLs)* refers to tasks required to maintain an independent household. IADLs include such tasks as using the telephone, managing money, shopping, preparing meals, doing light housework, and getting around the community. They generally demand a combination of both physical and cognitive performance. The ability to carry out basic self-care activities is reflected in the so-called activities of daily living (ADLs). Dependencies in terms of ADLs—which include such tasks as eating, using the toilet, dressing, transferring, walking, and bathing—are less common than IADL losses. As shown in Table 2-2, even among the oldest groups, the prevalence of ADL dependency is generally low. As with the decline in health ratings, there is a decline in ability to perform ADLs and IADLs among those in the 85+ age group. Approximately 23% of those aged 65 to 84 years and 48% of those aged 85 years and older indicate that they need help with ADLs. Similarly, with regard to IADLs, 23% of those aged 65 to 84 years and 43% of those aged 85 years and older need

TABLE 2-2. Percentage of Medicare Beneficiaries Reporting Difficulty With Common Activities, by Age Group: 2012

	Percent		
	Under 65	65–84	85+
	Percent n = 7,285,372	Percent n = 32,398,008	Percent n = 4,814,713
ADLs			
Walking	52.3	24.5	50.5
Getting in/out of bed/chair	33.2	11.8	25.0
Bathing	23.9	8.6	25.8
Dressing	21.2	6.5	17.0
Toileting	14.2	4.4	12.8
Eating	10.4	2.9	6.9
IADLs			
Doing heavy housework	65.5	28.8	54.1
Shopping	34.7	10.7	32.2
Doing light housework	34.5	9.6	54.1
Preparing meals	25.1	7.3	22.5
Paying bills	23.4	5.3	20.3
Using the telephone	11.0	5.2	20.0

Note: Excludes beneficiaries with end-stage renal disease or residing in a facility.
Reproduced with permission from Medicare Current Beneficiary Survey, Data Brief #002, July 2014

help with IADLs. Overall, men tend to be less likely to independently perform ADLs and IADLs across all age groups (Cubanksi et al, 2010).

SOCIAL SUPPORT

An important feature in determining an older person's ability to live in the community is the extent of support available. The family is the heart of LTC. Family and friends provide the bulk of services in each category with, or more often without, the help of formal caregivers. Informal care is largely provided by women, be they daughters or spouses, but men provide about 40% of all care for older persons.

Because women are both the major givers and receivers of LTC, a natural coalition has formed between those advocating for improved LTC and women's organizations. Even as women are entering the workforce in large numbers, they continue to bear the majority of the caregiving load. Largely because they outlive men, over twice as many older women, as compared with men, live alone (Fig. 2-5), but the gap narrows by age 85. Wives and daughters are the most important source of family support for older persons. Those who are unmarried are more likely to live in LTC facilities, as are those who are female and older than age 85.

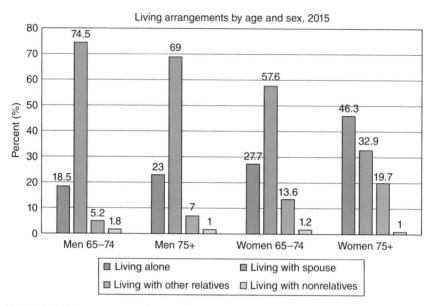

FIGURE 2-5 Living arrangements by age and sex, 2015. (*Data from Current Population Survey*)

Survey data suggest that more than 70% of persons aged 65 and older have surviving children. (Remember that the children of persons aged 85 and older may themselves be aged 65 or older.) These "children" provide more than a third of the informal care.

The difference between needing and not needing a nursing home can depend on the availability of such support. Extrapolating from available data, we estimate that for every person older than age 65 in a nursing home, from one to three people are equally disabled living in the community. The importance of social support must be kept constantly in mind. Formal community supports will continue to rely heavily on family and friends to see that adequate amounts of care are provided to maintain an elderly individual in the community. Efforts to reduce the burden of caregiving include encouraging respite care and providing direct assistance to the caregivers, both formal care to share the burden and pragmatic instruction about how to cope with the behavioral problems of older persons with dementia.

Clinicians must work together to help caregivers provide the type and level of care needed to maintain older individuals in their least restrictive living situation and to avoid high-cost LTC. They need to include caregivers (and care recipients) in all decision making. They need to respond to caregivers' questions. They need to convey respect and appreciation for all the caregivers do to maintain the older person's functioning lifestyle. They need to pay attention to caregivers' (often vague but insightful) observations that the older person just isn't herself.

USE OF SERVICES

Aging is associated with chronic disease. Figure 2-6 shows the distribution of older persons with varying numbers of concomitant diseases. Thus, the use of health-care services increases with age. One exception is dental care; it is not clear whether this reflects the lack of coverage under Medicare or a loss of teeth, but probably is at least greatly influenced by the former. Older people are more likely to see physicians because of chronic problems.

Hospitalizations account for nearly one-third of the $2 trillion spent on health care in the United States annually. Nearly 20% of these hospitalizations are rehospitalizations occurring within 30 days of discharge. Reducing readmissions has now become a major focus of the Medicare program. Hospitals are penalized for high rates of readmission, and are now holding other parts of the system (eg, nursing homes) accountable as well. Seven conditions are responsible for almost 30% of spending on readmissions:

- Heart failure
- Chronic obstructive pulmonary disease
- Pneumonia
- Acute myocardial infarction (heart attack)
- Coronary artery bypass graft
- Percutaneous transluminal coronary angioplasty
- Other vascular diseases

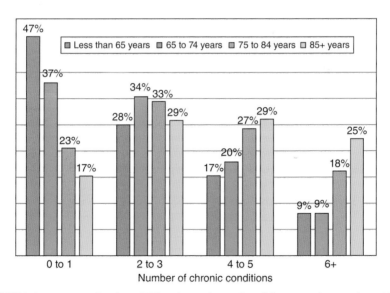

FIGURE 2-6 Percentage of Medicare FFS beneficiaries by number of chronic conditions and age: 2010.

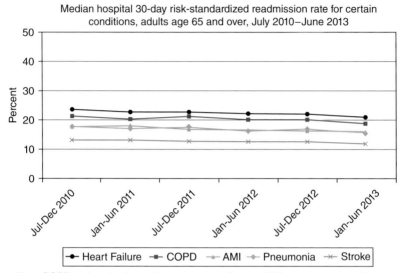

Key: COPD = chronic obstructive pulmonary disease; AMI = acute myocardial infarction.
Denominator: Expected number of readmissions for Medicare fee-for-service patients age 65 years and over for each disease type given the hospital's case mix.

FIGURE 2-7 30-day readmission rates for five diseases. Note: For this measure, lower rates are better. Readmission refers to an unplanned admission to a hospital for any condition or procedure 30 days after discharge. (*Reproduced with permission from Centers for Medicare & Medicaid Services, 2014 Medicare Hospital Quality Chartbook*)

Figure 2-7 traces the change in readmission rates for five of these high-risk diseases. Between 2010 and 2013 there was a modest decline in all. Just around that time a new incentive/penalty system was introduced to discourage readmissions.

The introduction of a prospective payment system (PPS) for hospitals under Medicare in 1984 was associated with shorter lengths of stay and decreased admission rates, but the pressure for rapid discharges may exacerbate the readmission issue. Table 2-3 shows the most common discharge diagnoses and surgical procedures in 2010. Heart disease, cancer, stroke, and pneumonia continue to dominate the scene. The growth of technology can be seen in the frequent use of procedures, especially catheterization and endoscopy.

The introduction of PPS greatly spurred the use of postacute care (PAC). Patients discharged earlier from hospitals often needed someplace to recuperate. As a result, Medicare began paying twice for hospital care. It paid a fixed amount for shorter stays and then often again for the posthospital care. PAC has been the fastest-growing segment of Medicare. It can be delivered in a variety of settings, including home health care, skilled nursing facilities, and inpatient rehabilitation facilities—IRFs. Each has its own method of providing this care; some rules have been established for certain sectors. For example, patients in IRFs must be able to tolerate at least 3 hours of therapy a day. Concerns over the variation in care provided by different venues has

TABLE 2-3. Hospital Discharge Diagnoses and Procedures for Persons Aged 65 Years and Older, 2010

Diagnoses	Rate per 10,000 population
Fracture, neck of femur	634
Diabetes mellitus	489
Congestive heart failure	178
Cerebrovascular disease	164
Pneumonia	153
Malignant neoplasms	146
Osteoarthritis	141
Cardiac dysrhythmias	124
Chronic bronchitis	98
Coronary atherosclerosis	92
Acute myocardial infarction	87
Psychoses	52
Volume depletion	37
Procedures	
Arteriography and angiography using contrast material	297
Endoscopy of small intestine	139
Cardiac catheterization	124
Total knee replacement	95
Insertion, replacement, removal of cardiac pacemaker	75
Reduction of fracture	71
Endoscopy of large intestine	69
Balloon angioplasty of coronary artery	63
Insertion of coronary stent	57
Coronary artery bypass graft	57
Total hip replacement	41
Cholecystectomy	35
Prostatectomy	18
Treatments/Tests	
Respiratory therapy	169
Diagnostic ultrasound	133
Hemodialysis	86
Insertion of endotracheal tube	80

Reproduced with permission from National Center for Health Statistics – National Hospital Discharge Survey.

led to work on the development of a single assessment instrument. At least 60% of IRF admissions must come from one of the following 13 conditions:

• Stroke
• Brain injury
• Spinal cord injury
• Femur fracture (hip)
• Congenital deformity
• Major multiple trauma
• Neurologic disorders
• Burns
• Amputations
• Active polyarticular rheumatoid arthritis, psoriatic arthritis, and seronegative arthropathies
• Systemic vasculitis with joint inflammation
• Severe advanced osteoarthritis
• Knee or hip replacement immediately preceding the IRF admission (and also must meet additional criteria)

As shown in Table 2-4, the most common reasons for postacute care were hip procedures (fractures), joint replacements, stroke, kidney disease, and pneumonia. The latter two are not among the mandatory 16.

Ambulatory care visits for those 65 years of age and older are higher than for all other age groups with the exception of infants (CDC, 2008). Table 2-5 describes the patterns for ambulatory visits at various ages. Despite the general principle that bad things are more common with increasing age after age 75, not all diagnoses increase with age. Close to half (41%) of all visits for older adults are due to chronic versus acute medical problems.

There is some evidence of improvements in care between 2014 and 2015, including a 9% decrease in preventable hospitalizations and an 8% decrease in the prevalence of full-mouth teeth extractions. Hip fractures decreased 5% from 6.2 to 5.9 hospitalizations

---

TABLE 2-4. Postacute Care Used Within 30 Days in 2008, for the Top Five Diagnostic-Related Groups

	Any PAC	SNF	LTCH	HHA	Therapy
Hip procedure	95	68	0.4	8	2
Joint replacement	94	37	2.0	37	10
Stroke	75	37	0.1	17	8
Kidney, urinary tract infection	44	58	0.4	29	11
Pneumonia	36	51	0.9	38	9

HHA, home health care; LTCH, long-term care hospital; PAC, postacute care; SNF, skilled nursing facility; Therapy, rehabilitation.

TABLE 2-5. Percentage of Office Visits by Selected Medical Conditions, 2012

	Age 45–64 years	Age 65–74 years	Age 75+ years
Hypertension	32.5	46.8	52.7
Arthritis	17.3	21.7	23.8
Diabetes	13.9	21.3	19.7
Depression	12.2	9.4	7.7
Obesity	8.8	8.0	3.6
Chronic obstructive pulmonary disease	3.7	7.4	8.0
Ischemic heart disease	3.4	7.3	9.4
Congestive heart failure	1.1	3.2	5.8

Reproduced with permission from Centers for Disease Control and Prevention, 2012

per 1000 Medicare beneficiaries. Between 2012 and 2015, there was an 18% increase in the availability of home health care workers, a 40% increase in hospice care use, and a 29% decrease in hospital deaths (United Health Foundation, 2016). Between 2000 and 2009 the proportion of deaths among persons with dementia occurring in acute care hospitals decreased from 32.6% to 24.6%, but there was an increased use of the intensive care unit in the last month of life. Hospice use at the time of death nearly doubled, from 21.6% to 42.2%. However, 28.4% used hospice for 3 or fewer days in 2009, indicating that hospice was initiated late (Teno et al, 2013). By 2012 more persons died at home than out of the home (CDC, 2013).

NURSING HOME USE

The nursing home has traditionally been used as the touchstone for LTC, but its role has changed with the changes in hospital payment under Medicare. (Nursing home care is described in more detail in Chapter 16.) The fixed-payment approach for hospitals and the consequent shortening of hospital stays have spawned a new industry of posthospital care, sometimes called subacute care or postacute care. This includes services such as dialysis, rehabilitation, management of patients on ventilators, and wound care. In effect, care that was formerly rendered in a hospital is now provided in other settings, including the nursing home and the home of the patient.

Some nursing homes have sought to increase their capacity to support such care by changing the compilation of their nursing staff and establishing separate units for short-stay postacute care versus LTC residents, whereas others provide these services to residents without making such changes. Thus, the distinction between long-stay and short-stay nursing home residents can be confusing for staff, residents, and families. Some residents are in nursing homes for chronic care, whereas others are there just for rehabilitation and to recover from an acute event such as a hip fracture.

The majority of nursing home care is paid for by Medicaid (65%) and Medicare (14%). Those who do pay privately often spend down their resources and turn to public assistance. While nursing homes have increased their Medicare business dramatically, their long-stay business has been threatened by a growing disinclination to use such facilities. New forms of care, like assisted living, personal care homes, residential care homes, or sheltered housing, have provided other options, especially for those who can pay for such care. Regardless of the name, these facilities vary greatly depending on the state in which they are in and state regulations regarding services offered, philosophy of care, and cost. Assisted living services are not covered by Medicare, although some states (approximately 38 at this time) have some coverage through Medicaid, and this may begin to increase given that it is cheaper than the cost of a long-term stay in a nursing home.

We are prone to cite an estimated 5% for the proportion of those aged 65 years and older who are in nursing homes at any moment. But such a figure is a potentially misleading generalization in two respects. Age is a very important factor. Among those aged 65 to 74 years, the rate is less than 2%. It rises to approximately 7% for those aged 75 to 84 and then jumps to 20% for those aged 85 and older. Moreover, what were formerly considered permanent stays have increasingly become short, transient visits. Thus, it is important to distinguish between these prevalence rates and the lifetime probability of entering a nursing home. Longitudinal studies suggest that persons aged 65 have a 46% chance of spending some time in a nursing home before they die. Discharge rates of residents from nursing homes to other settings (eg, assisted living, home), particularly for those who have been in the facility for less than 30 days, have increased. For those who remain in facilities for more than 90 days, however, the likelihood of being discharged continues to be low. Those who are determined to return home and have lower care needs are more likely to be discharged (Arling et al, 2010). Nursing homes are needed not only because of the presence of diseases and functional disabilities, but also as a result of a lack of social support. Often the family becomes exhausted after caring for an elderly patient for a long period. Family fatigue is especially a problem when the patient has dementia and associated behavioral symptoms that are very disruptive.

The predictors for nursing home placement include older age, functional impairment prior to nursing home admission, lower perceived health, cognitive impairment, and lack of social supports. Predictors for those diagnosed with cognitive impairment include older age, inability to independently toilet, impaired balance, and lack of social support (ie, living alone). Table 2-6 summarizes the factors associated with increased likelihood of nursing home placement for all nursing home residents as well as specifically for those with cognitive impairment (Dramé et al, 2012; Luppa et al, 2010).

The majority of admissions to nursing homes come from acute care facilities (62%–75%). To qualify for Medicare skilled nursing home services, the older individual must require daily skilled nursing (eg, wound care) or rehabilitative therapy services, generally within 30 days of a hospital stay of at least 3 days in length, and must be admitted to the nursing home due to a condition related to that hospitalization.

TABLE 2-6. Factors Affecting the Need for Nursing Home Admission

For all nursing home residents	For nursing home residents with known cognitive impairment
Age	
	Ability to use the toilet
Social supports	Balance
	Living alone
Activities of daily living	
Cognitive status and associated behavioral problems	
Clinical diagnoses including diabetes, hypertension, stroke, cancer, or having had a fall	
Ability to manage medication	
Income	
Payment eligibility	
Need for special services	
Characteristics of the support system	
Family capability	
For married respondents, age of spouse	
Presence of responsible relative (usually adult child)	
Family structure of responsible relative	
Employment status of responsible relative	
Physician availability	
Amount of care currently received from family and others	
Community resources	
Formal community resources	
Informal support systems	
Presence of long-term care institutions	
Characteristics of long-term care institutions	

Medicare offers full coverage on the first 20 days and partial coverage for days 21 to 100. Changes in the hospital environment are resulting in some situations in which older individuals are not eligible for skilled services. Increasingly, hospitals are using "observation" stays in which patients are not officially admitted to the hospital and yet remain in an "observation" bed receiving acute care services for up to 48 hours. If they do get admitted, these 2 days cannot be used toward Medicare eligibility.

Hospitalization often represents the last step in a series of steps involving the deterioration of the patient and the inability of the patient's social supports to provide the level of care needed. For others, hospitalization results from an acute event, for example, a broken hip or a stroke, that then necessitates at least a short stay for rehabilitation. Following transfers from acute care settings to nursing facilities, admissions to nursing facilities occur from home settings at a rate of 23%. A smaller, although growing, percentage of individuals in assisted living settings are transferred to nursing homes (9%), and this is particularly true if those facilities are associated with a nursing home or have one geographically close.

The care of nursing home residents is more complex than it used to be. Management of medical problems is geared toward optimizing function, physical activity, and overall quality of life. Clinical problems include such things as infections, falls, malnutrition, dehydration, incontinence, behavioral disturbances, drug side effects and interactions, and management of multiple comorbidities. Care management must be done in collaboration with the resident and family/caregiver wishes and must consider ethical issues and resource allocation.

Once in a nursing home, residents have high rates of hospitalization; approximately a quarter of all residents are likely to be transferred at least once per year to the hospital (Mor et al, 2010). Infection is the most common reason for this transfer, and it is believed that many transfers could be avoidable with appropriate systems of care and resources within the skilled facility. Interventions such as INTERACT II (http://interact2.net) are being used to decrease the rates of transfer (Ouslander et al, 2011).

With the growing number of older adults who have three or more chronic diseases, there is likely to be an increased need for the expertise of a geriatrician as well as care options to best manage not just single but multiple morbidities (Boyd and Fortin, 2011). Likewise, these individuals are going to need care that may not be best provided in a single individual home setting. Care options and choices will be important for health-care providers to understand and to share with patients and families. A more detailed guide to LTC resources is presented in Chapter 16.

REFERENCES

Anderson RN, Smith BS. Deaths: leading causes for 2002. *Natl Vital Stat Rep.* 2005. Available at: www.cdc.gov/nchs/data/nvsr/nvsr53/nvsr53_17.pdf. Accessed November 28, 2012.

Arling G, Kane RL, Cooke V, Lewis T. Targeting residents for transitions from nursing home to community. *Health Serv Res.* 2010;45:691-711.

Boult C, Wieland GD. Comprehensive primary care for older patients with multiple chronic conditions: "nobody rushes you through." *JAMA.* 2010;30:1936-1943.

Boyd C, Fortin M. Future of multimorbidity research: how should understanding of multimorbidity inform health system design? *Public Health Rev.* 2011;32:451-474.

Census Data. Resident population. National population estimates for the 2000s. Monthly postcensal resident population, by single year of age, sex, race, and Hispanic origin, July to September 2010. 2010. Available at: www.census.gov/popest/. Accessed November 28, 2012.

Centers for Disease Control and Prevention. National Ambulatory Medical Care Survey: 2008 Summary Tables. 2008. Available at: www.cdc.gov/nchs/data/ahcd/namcs_summary/2008_namcs_web_tables.pdf. Accessed November 28, 2012.

Cubanksi J, Huang J, Camico A, Jacobson G, Neuman T. *Medicare Chartbook, Fourth Edition 2010.* 2010. Available at: www.kff.org/medicare/upload/8103.pdf. Accessed November 28, 2012.

Cutler DM. Declining disability among the elderly. *Health Aff.* 2001;20(6):11-27.

Day J. *Population Projections of the United States, by Age, Sex, Race, and Hispanic Origin: 1993 to 2050, Current Population Reports.* Washington, DC: U.S. Bureau of the Census, U.S. Government Printing Office; 1993:25-1104.

Dramé M, Lang PO, Jolly D, et al. Nursing home admission in elderly subjects with dementia: predictive factors and future challenges. *J Am Med Dir Assoc.* 2012;13:17-20.

Fries JF. Aging, natural death, and the compression of morbidity. *N Engl J Med.* 1980;303:130-136.

Luppa M, Luck T, Weyerer S, König H, Brähler E, Riedel-Heller SG. Prediction of institutionalization in the elderly: a systematic review. *Age Ageing.* 2010;39:31-38.

Mor V, Intrator I, Feng V, Grabowski DC. The revolving door of rehospitalization from skilled nursing facilities. *Health Aff.* 2010;29:57-64.

Ouslander J, Lamb G, Tappen R, et al. Interventions to reduce hospitalizations from nursing homes: evaluation of the INTERACT II collaborative quality improvement project. *J Am Geriatr Soc.* 2011;59:745-753.

Preston S, Stokes A. Contribution of obesity to international differences in life expectancy. *Am J Public Health.* 2011;101:2137-2143.

Satizabal CL, Beiser AS, Chouraki V, Chene G, Dufouoil C, Shehadri S. Incidence of dementia over three decades in the Framingham Heart Study. *N Engl J Med.* 2016;374(6):523-532.

Teno JM, Gozalo PL, Bynum JP, et al. *JAMA.* 2013;309(5):470-477.

United Health Foundation. *America's Health Rankings Senior Report 2016.* Minnetonka, MN: United Health Foundation; 2016. www.americashealthrankings.org/learn/reports/2016-senior-report.

van Dieren S, Beulens JW, van der Schouw YT, Grobbee DE, Neal B. The global burden of diabetes and its complications: an emerging pandemic. *Eur J Cardiovasc Prev Rehabil.* 2010;17(Suppl 1):S3-S8.

von Bonsdorff M, Rantanen T. Benefits of formal voluntary work among older people: a review. *Aging Clin Exp Res.* 2011;23:162-169.

Zhao J, Barclay S, Farquhar M, Kinmonth AL, Brayen C, Flemming J. The oldest old in the last year of life: population based findings from Cambridge City over-75s cohort study participants aged 85 and older at death. *J Am Geriatr Soc.* 2010;38:1-11.

SUGGESTED READINGS

Arling G, Kane RL, Cooke V, Lewis T. Targeting residents for transitions from nursing home to community. *Health Serv Res.* 2010;45:691-711.

Boult C, Wieland GD. Comprehensive primary care for older patients with multiple chronic conditions: "nobody rushes you through." *JAMA.* 2010;30:1936-1943.

Boyd C, Fortin M. Future of multimorbidity research: how should understanding of multimorbidity inform health system design? *Public Health Rev.* 2011;32:451-474.

Census Data. Resident population. National population estimates for the 2000s. Monthly postcensal resident population, by single year of age, sex, race, and Hispanic origin, July to September 2010. 2010. Available at: www.census.gov/popest/. Accessed November 28, 2012.

PART I

Centers for Disease Control and Prevention. National Ambulatory Medical Care Survey: 2008 Summary Tables. 2008. Available at: www.cdc.gov/nchs/data/ahcd/namcs_summary/2008_namcs_web_tables.pdf. Accessed November 28, 2012.

Cubanksi J, Huang J, Camico A, Jacobson G, Neuman T. *Medicare Chartbook, Fourth Edition 2010*. 2010. Available at: www.kff.org/medicare/upload/8103.pdf. Accessed November 28, 2012.

Day J. *Population Projections of the United States, by Age, Sex, Race, and Hispanic Origin: 1993 to 2050, Current Population Reports*. Washington, DC: U.S. Bureau of the Census, U.S. Government Printing Office; 1993:25-1104.

Dramé M, Lang PO, Jolly D, et al. Nursing home admission in elderly subjects with dementia: predictive factors and future challenges. *J Am Med Dir Assoc*. 2012;13:17-20.

Luppa M, Luck T, Weyerer S, König H, Brähler E, Riedel-Heller SG. Prediction of institutionalization in the elderly: a systematic review. *Age Ageing*. 2010;39:31-38.

Mor V, Intrator I, Feng V, Grabowski DC. The revolving door of rehospitalization from skilled nursing facilities. *Health Aff*. 2010;29:57-64.

Ouslander J, Lamb G, Tappen R, et al. Interventions to reduce hospitalizations from nursing homes: evaluation of the INTERACT II collaborative quality improvement project. *J Am Geriatr Soc*. 2011;59:745-753.

Preston S, Stokes A. Contribution of obesity to international differences in life expectancy. *Am J Public Health*. 2011;101:2137-2143.

van Dieren S, Beulens JW, van der Schouw YT, Grobbee DE, Neal B. The global burden of diabetes and its complications: an emerging pandemic. *Eur J Cardiovasc Prev Rehabil*. 2010;17(Suppl 1):S3-S8.

von Bonsdorff M, Rantanen T. Benefits of formal voluntary work among older people: a review. *Aging Clin Exp Res*. 2011;23:162-169.

Zhao J, Barclay S, Farquhar M, Kinmonth AL, Brayen C, Flemming J. The oldest old in the last year of life: population based findings from Cambridge City over-75s cohort study participants aged 85 and older at death. *J Am Geriatr Soc*. 2010;38:1-11.

CHAPTER 3

Evaluating the Geriatric Patient

Evaluation can occur at different levels of intensity and at different stages of a disease. It can be comprehensive or more focused. Comprehensive evaluation of an older individual's health status is one of the most challenging aspects of clinical geriatrics. Geriatrics addresses multimorbidity. It involves sorting out the manifestations of multiple simultaneous problems. It requires sensitivity to the concerns of people, awareness of the many unique aspects of their medical problems, ability to interact effectively with a variety of health professionals, and often a great deal of patience. It requires a perspective different from that used to evaluate younger individuals. Not only are the a priori probabilities of diagnoses different, but one must be attuned to subtler findings. Because functioning is a key element in geriatric management, assessment must address a wider range of domains that include social function and mental health. Progress may be measured on a finer scale. Special tools are needed to ascertain relatively small improvements in chronic conditions and overall function compared with the more dramatic cures of acute illnesses often possible in younger patients. Creativity is essential to incorporate these tools efficiently in a busy clinical practice.

We have come to appreciate the implications of the range of clinical status. We typically think of the spectrum of geriatric patients in a pyramid, where those with the most disabilities are least frequent but use the most services. Figure 3-1, shows what is referred to as the Kaiser Pyramid. The topmost group, representing about 3% to 5% of the older population, accounts for a disproportionate amount of care. Another 15% to 20% need good management for a single chronic disease. By contrast, the remaining 70% to 80% need relatively little care, and much of that is directed toward health promotion. Sorting patients in this way allows for better targeting of resources. Assessment offers a means to achieve this sorting.

Assessment alone will not improve health; some action has to be taken based on the information. Assessments can be made to develop a care plan of interventions, or they can form the basis for predicting future health status. Knowing an older patient's status can help decide if he or she is a good candidate for aggressive treatment.

Comprehensive geriatric assessment, when its findings are acted on, has been shown to improve both mortality and the chances of remaining in the community (Barer, 2011; Ellis et al, 2011). The challenge is to use it efficiently. Complex patients and those facing major long-term care decisions are strong candidates, but studies have also shown benefit for persons presumably at low risk. As described in Chapter 4, home visits to basically well older persons seem to prevent nursing home admissions and functional decline.

The purpose of the evaluation and the setting in which it takes place will determine its focus and extent. Considerations important in admitting a geriatric patient with a fractured hip and pneumonia to an acute care hospital during the middle of

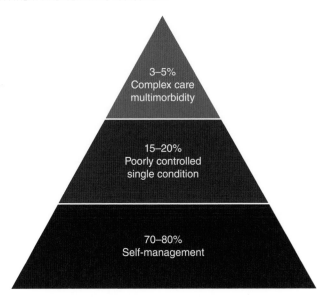

FIGURE 3-1 The Kaiser Pyramid. (*Data from National Health Services (NHS) and the University of Birmingham.*)

the night are obviously different from those in the evaluation of an older patient with dementia exhibiting disruptive behavior in a nursing home. Elements included in screening for treatable conditions in an ambulatory clinic are different from those used to assess older individuals in their own homes or in long-term care facilities.

Despite the differences dictated by the purpose and setting of the evaluation, several essential aspects of evaluating older patients are common to all purposes and settings. Figure 3-2, depicts these aspects. Several comments on addressing them are in order:

1. Physical, psychological, and socioeconomic factors interact in complex ways to influence the health and functional status of the geriatric population.
2. Comprehensive evaluation of an older individual's health status requires an assessment of each of these domains. The coordinated efforts of several different health-care professionals functioning as an interdisciplinary team are needed.
3. Functional abilities should be a central focus of the comprehensive evaluation of geriatric patients. Other more traditional measures of health status (such as diagnoses and physical and laboratory findings) are useful in dealing with underlying etiologies and detecting treatable conditions, but in the geriatric population, measures of function are often essential in determining overall health, well-being, and the need for health and social services.
4. Under person-centered care the aspects of function that are most important to the older patient should be prioritized. Thus, the assessment must also address identifying what a patient is most eager to achieve.

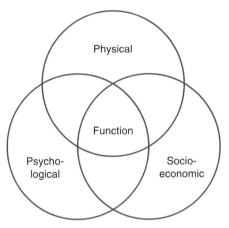

FIGURE 3-2 Components of assessment of older patients.

Just as function is the common language of geriatrics, assessment lies at the heart of its practice. Special techniques that address multiple problems and their functional consequences offer a way to structure the approach to complicated geriatric patients. The core of geriatric practice has been considered the comprehensive geriatric assessment, but its role has been actively debated. Geriatric assessment has been tested in a variety of forms. Table 3-1 summarizes the findings from a number of randomized controlled trials of different approaches to geriatric assessment. The results sometimes seem counterintuitive. Annual in-home comprehensive geriatric assessment as a preventive strategy demonstrated the potential to delay the development of disability and reduce permanent nursing home stays (Stuck et al, 2002). Controlled trials of approaches to hospitalized geriatric patients suggest comprehensive geriatric assessment by a consultation team with limited follow-up do not improve health or survival of selected geriatric patients but suggest that a special acute geriatric unit can improve function and reduce discharges to institutional care. A controlled multisite Veterans Affairs trial of inpatient geriatric evaluation and management demonstrated significant reductions in functional decline without increased costs (Cohen et al, 2002). Results of outpatient geriatric assessment have been mixed and less compelling (Cohen et al, 2002). However, a randomized trial of outpatient geriatric assessment showed that it prevented functional decline (Reuben et al, 1999).

There is considerable variation in approaches to the comprehensive assessment of geriatric patients. Various screening and targeting strategies have been used to identify appropriate patients for more comprehensive assessment. These strategies range from selection based on age to targeting patients with a certain number of impairments or specific conditions.

Sites of assessment vary as well and include the clinic, the home, the hospital, and different levels of long-term care. Geriatric assessment also varies in terms of which discipline carries out the different components of the assessment as well as

TABLE 3-1. Examples of Randomized Controlled Trials of Geriatric Assessment

Setting	Examples of assessment strategies	Selected outcomes*
Community/ outpatients	Social worker assessment and referral Nursing assessment and referral Annual in-home assessment by nurse practitioner Multidisciplinary clinic assessment	Reduced mortality Reduced hospital use Reduced permanent nursing home use Delayed development of disability
Hospital inpatient (specialized units)	Interdisciplinary teams with focus on function, geriatric syndromes, rehabilitation	Reduced mortality Improved function Reduced acute hospital and nursing home use
Hospital inpatient consultation	Geriatric consultation teams	Mixed results Some studies show improved function and lower shortterm mortality Other studies show no effects

*Not all studies show improvements in all outcomes. See text and Rubenstein et al, 1991.

in the specific assessment tools used. Despite the dramatic variation in approach to targeting, personnel used, and measures employed, a clear pattern of effectiveness has emerged. Taken together, these results are both heartening and cautioning. Systematic approaches to patient care are obviously desirable. The issue is more how formalized these assessments should be. Research suggests that the specifics of the assessment process seem to be less important than the very act of systematically approaching older people with the belief that improvement is possible.

A major concern about such assessments is efficiency. Because of the multidimensional nature of geriatric patients' problems and the frequent presence of multiple interacting medical conditions, comprehensive evaluation of the geriatric patient can be time-consuming, and thus costly. It is frequently viewed as a team effort, but teams can be very inefficient. It is important to reduce duplication of effort. It is possible to have interprofessional collaboration in determining what data should be collected, but the actual data collection is best delegated to one or, at most, a few team members. Additional expertise can be brought to bear if the initial screening uncovers an area that requires it.

The enthusiasm for teams raises some sports analogies. Should a geriatric team be more like a football team that practices all week for a single game or a baseball team that plays almost daily? In both instances teamwork relies on skilled individuals who are well trained to perform their role and who engender the confidence of their colleagues, who do not feel an obligation to duplicate that role (Kane et al, 2011).

Another crucial lesson is that assessment without follow-up is unlikely to make any difference. Thus, the term *geriatric assessment* has given way to the concept of geriatric evaluation and management. There must be strong commitment to act on the problems uncovered and to follow up long enough to be sure that they have responded to the treatment prescribed.

Strategies that can make the evaluation process more efficient include the following:

1. Developing a close-knit interdisciplinary team with minimal redundancy in the assessments performed.
2. Using carefully designed questionnaires that reliable patients and/or caregivers can complete before an appointment.
3. Incorporating screening tools that target the need for further, more in-depth assessment.
4. Using assessment forms that can be readily incorporated into a computerized relational database.
5. Integrating the evaluation process with case management activities that target services based on the results of the assessment.

This chapter focuses on the general aspects of assessing geriatric patients; sections on geriatric consultation, preoperative evaluation, and environmental assessments are included in the chapter.

Chapter 15 includes information on case management and other health services, and Chapter 16 is devoted to the assessment and management of geriatric patients in the nursing home setting.

HISTORY

Sir William Osler's aphorism "Listen to the patient, he'll give you the diagnosis" is as true in older patients as it is in younger patients, although the presentation of disease in older patients is generally atypical (as noted in Chapter 1). In the geriatric population, however, several factors make taking histories more challenging, difficult, and time-consuming.

Table 3-2 lists difficulties commonly encountered in taking histories from geriatric patients, the factors involved, and some suggestions for overcoming these difficulties. Impaired hearing and vision (despite corrective devices) are common and can interfere with effective communication.

Techniques such as eliminating extraneous noises, speaking slowly and in deep tones while facing the patient, and providing adequate lighting can be helpful. Simple and inexpensive amplification devices with earphones can be especially effective, even among those with severe hearing impairment. Patience is truly a virtue in obtaining a history; because thought and verbal processes are often slower in older than in younger individuals, patients should be allowed adequate time to answer in order to not miss potentially important information. At the same time, the cardinal rule of open-ended questions may need to be tempered to get the maximum amount of information in the time allocated.

Many older individuals underreport potentially important symptoms because of their cultural and educational backgrounds as well as their expectations of illness as a

TABLE 3-2. Potential Difficulties in Taking Geriatric Histories

Difficulty	Factors involved	Suggestions
Communication	Diminished vision Diminished hearing	Use well-lit room Eliminate extraneous noise Speak slowly in a deep tone Face patient, allowing patient to see your lips Use simple amplification device for severely hearing impaired
	Slowed psychomotor performance	If necessary, write questions in large print Leave enough time for the patient to answer
Underreporting of symptoms	Health beliefs Fear Depression Altered physical and physiological responses to disease process Cognitive impairment	Ask specific questions about potentially important symptoms (see Table 3-3) Use other sources of information (relatives, friends, other caregivers) to complete the history
Vague or nonspecific symptoms	Altered physical and physiological responses to disease process Altered presentation of specific diseases Cognitive impairment	Evaluate for treatable diseases, even if the symptoms (or signs) are not typical or specific when there has been a rapid change in function Use other sources of information to complete history
Multiple complaints	Prevalence of multiple coexisting diseases Somatization of emotions—"masked depression" (see Chap. 7)	Attend to all somatic symptoms, ruling out treatable conditions Get to know the patient's complaints; pay special attention to new or changing symptoms Interview the patient on several occasions to complete the history

normal concomitant of aging. More aggressive probing may be necessary. Fear of illness and disability or depression accompanied by a lack of self-concern may also cause less frequent reporting of symptoms. Altered physical and physiological responses to disease processes (see Chapter 1) can result in the absence of symptoms (such as painless myocardial infarction or ulcer and pneumonia without cough). Symptoms of many diseases can be vague and nonspecific because of these age-related changes. Impairments of memory and other cognitive functions can result in an imprecise or inadequate history and compound these difficulties. Asking specifically about potentially important symptoms (such as those listed in Table 3-3) and using other sources

TABLE 3-3. Important Aspects of the Geriatric History

Social history

Living arrangements
Relationships with family and friends
Expectations of family or other caregivers
Economic status
Abilities to perform activities of daily living (ADLs) (see Table 3-10)
Social activities and hobbies
Mode of transportation
Advance directives (see Chap. 17)

Past medical history

Previous surgical procedures
Major illnesses and hospitalizations
Previous transfusions
Immunization status
    Influenza, pneumococcus, tetanus, zoster
Preventive health measures
    Mammography
    Papanicolaou (Pap) smear
    Flexible sigmoidoscopy
    Antimicrobial prophylaxis
    Estrogen replacement
Tuberculosis history and testing
Medications (use the "brown bag" technique; see text)
    Previous allergies
    Knowledge of current medication regimen
    Compliance
Perceived beneficial or adverse drug effects

Systems review

Ask questions about general symptoms that may indicate treatable underlying disease
    such as fatigue, anorexia, weight loss, insomnia, recent change in functional status
Attempt to elicit key symptoms in each organ system, including the following:

System	Key symptoms
Respiratory	Increasing dyspnea
	Persistent cough
Cardiovascular	Orthopnea
	Edema
	Angina
	Claudication
	Palpitations
	Dizziness
	Syncope
Gastrointestinal	Difficulty chewing
	Dysphagia
	Abdominal pain
	Change in bowel habit

(continued)

TABLE 3-3. Important Aspects of the Geriatric History (*continued*)

System	Key symptoms
Genitourinary	Frequency
	Urgency
	Nocturia
	Hesitancy, intermittent stream, straining to void
	Incontinence
	Hematuria
	Vaginal bleeding
Musculoskeletal	Focal or diffuse pain
	Focal or diffuse weakness
Neurological	Visual disturbances (transient or progressive)
	Progressive hearing loss
	Unsteadiness and/or falls
	Transient focal symptoms
Psychological	Depression
	Anxiety and/or agitation
	Paranoia
	Forgetfulness and/or confusion

of information (such as relatives, friends, and other caregivers) can be very helpful in collecting more precise and useful information in these situations.

At the other end of the spectrum, geriatric patients with multiple complaints can frustrate the health-care professional who is trying to sort them all out. The multiplicity of complaints can relate to the prevalence of coexisting chronic and acute conditions in many geriatric patients. These complaints may, however, be deceiving. Somatic symptoms may be manifestations of underlying emotional distress rather than symptoms of a physical illness, and symptoms of physical conditions may be exaggerated by emotional distress (see Chapter 7). Getting to know patients and their complaints and paying particular attention to new or changing symptoms are helpful in detecting potentially treatable conditions.

Clinicians may become impatient with the slow pace of older patients and their tendency to wander from the subject at hand. In desperation, they shift their focus to the accompanying family members who can provide a more lucid and linear history. But this tendency to bypass the older patient can have several serious effects. Not only does it diminish the self-image of the older patient and reinforce a message of dependency, it may miss important information that the patient knows but the family member does not.

Table 3-3 lists aspects of the history that are especially important in geriatric patients. It is often not feasible to gather all information in one session; shorter interviews in a few separate sessions may prove more effective in gathering these data from some geriatric patients.

A complete systems review, focusing on potentially important and prevalent symptoms in the elderly, can help overcome many of the difficulties described earlier, but it can be overwhelming. Table 3-4 suggests some screening questions that can be used to expedite the review of systems.

General symptoms can be especially difficult to interpret. Fatigue can result from a number of common conditions such as depression, congestive heart failure, anemia, and hypothyroidism. Anorexia and weight loss can be symptoms of an underlying malignancy, depression, or poorly fitting dentures and diminished taste sensation. Age-related changes in sleep patterns, anxiety, gastroesophageal reflux, congestive heart failure with orthopnea, or nocturia can underlie complaints of insomnia. Because many frail geriatric patients limit their activity, some important symptoms may be missed. For example, such patients may deny angina and dyspnea but restrict their activity to avoid the symptoms. Questions such as "How far do you walk in a typical day?" and "What is the most common activity you carry out in a typical day?" can be helpful in patients suspected of limiting their activities to avoid certain symptoms.

Some topics that may be especially important to an older person's quality of life are often skipped over because they are embarrassing to the clinician or the patient. Issues like fecal and urinary incontinence and sexual dysfunction can be important areas to explore. Given its prevalence, vulnerability to treatment, and ability to complicate the care of other conditions, it is important to screen for depression. Chapter 7 reviews the measures available for depression screening in older patients.

Often shortchanged in medical evaluations, the social history is a critical component. This is an area where person-centered care can be emphasized. Table 3-5 offers some elements of patient-centered care. (This table also appears in Chapter 15.)

Discussing these issues sets up the important discussion about what is most salient to the older patient. What do they most want to accomplish? Understanding the patient's socioeconomic environment and ability to function within it is crucial in determining the potential impact of an illness on an individual's overall health and need for health services. Especially important is the assessment of the family's feelings and expectations. Many family caregivers of frail geriatric patients have feelings of both anger (at having to care for a dependent family member) and guilt (over not being able or willing to do enough) and have unrealistic expectations. They may also harbor strong aversions to letting the older person take risks. In many situations frail older people are labeled as vulnerable adults, who need to be protected and shielded from risk or exploitation, but older people should have the right to make informed judgments about what risks they want to take to achieve what is important to them. It is important to surface the spectrum of risk aversion in a family, including the older patient's perspective if you hope to make informed decisions about different kinds of treatment. A tool is available to help families explore this area (Kane and Ouellette, 2011). All family members complete a risk aversion test and then compare their results as the basis for understanding and hopefully resolving discrepancies.

Unrealistic expectations are often based on a lack of information and can interfere with care if not discussed. Unlike younger patients, older patients often have had multiple prior illnesses. Therefore, the past medical history is important in putting the

TABLE 3-4. Geriatric Screening Questions and Recommendations for Further Assessment

		Screening questions	Further geriatric assessment for positive responses to screening
SOCIAL	Social Support	• Do you live alone? • Are you looking for someone to help with your daily activities? • Are you a caregiver for someone?	• Consider referral to a social worker or a local Area Agency on aging if available.
	Alcohol Abuse	• Do you drink more than 2 drinks per day?	• Consider a CAGE Questionnaire.
	Elder Abuse	• Do you ever feel unsafe where you live? • Has anyone ever threatened or hurt you? • Has anyone been taking your money without your permission?	• Consider referral to a social worker and/or Adult Protective Services.
	Advance Directives	• Do you have a power of attorney for health care (DPAHC) or a living will? • Have you thought about the type of care you would want if you become seriously ill?	• Have an advance care planning discussion. • Execute a document (eg, a DPAHC or Physician Orders for Life-Sustaining Treatment [POLST] or similar form).
FUNCTIONAL	Functional Status	• Do you need assistance with shopping or finances? • Do you need assistance with bathing or taking a shower?	• Consider an instrumental ADL assessment. • Consider a basic ADL assessment.

	Driving	• Do you still drive? If yes:
		  • While driving, have you had an accident in the past 6 months?
		  • Are any family members concerned about your driving?
			• Consider vision testing.
			• Consider a formal driving evaluation.

	Vision	• Do you have trouble seeing, reading, or watching TV (with glasses, if used)?	• Consider vision testing. • Consider referral for eye exam.
	Hearing	• Do you have difficulty hearing conversation in a quiet room (with aide if used)?	• Check for cerumen in ear canals and remove if impacted. • Consider audiology referral.

GERIATRIC SYNDROMES

Polypharmacy	• Do you take 9 or more routine medications (excluding vitamins and other supplements)? • Do you understand the reason for each of your medications?	• Perform a medication reconciliation. • Consider reducing doses, stopping drugs, adherence aides, and/or consultation with a pharmacist.
Fall Risk	• Have you fallen in the past year? • Are you afraid of falling? • Do you have trouble climbing stairs? • Do you have trouble getting up from a chair?	• Take the "Get Up and Go" test. • Consider full fall assessment. • Consider physical therapy evaluation. • Consider home safety assessment.
Incontinence	• Do you have any trouble with your bladder? • Do you lose urine or stool when you do not want to? • Do you ever wear pads or adult diapers?	• If symptoms are bothersome, consider 3-IQ Questionnaire (women) or AUA 7 symptom inventory (men). • Consider continence evaluation.
Weight Loss	• Have you lost 10 or more pounds over the last 6 months without intending to do so?	• Take the Mini Nutritional Assessment. • Consider evaluation by a dietician/nutritionist.
Sleep Disturbance	• Do you often feel sleepy during the day? • Do you have difficulty falling asleep at night? • Do you know if you snore loudly?	• Consider a sleep scale (eg, Pittsburgh Sleep Index). • Consider referral for sleep evaluation.

COGNITION AND AFFECT

Pain	• Are you experiencing pain or discomfort?	• Consider pain assessment using a standard scale.
Depression	• Do you often feel sad or depressed? • Have you lost pleasure in doing things over the past few months?	• Perform PHQ-9 or Geriatric Depression Scale. • Consider screening for suicide risk. • Consider psychology or psychiatry evaluation.
Cognitive Impairment	• Do you or any family or friends think you have a problem with your memory? (In hospitalized patients the Confusion Assessment [CAM] should be used first to screen for delirium.)	• Perform Mini Cog (3-item recall and clock draw). • If failed, test with a standard tool (eg, MMSE, MOCA, SLUMS). • Consider neuropsychological testing.

TABLE 3-5. Essential Elements of Person-Centered Care

- Individualized, goal-oriented care plan based on the older person's and caregiver's preferences
- Ongoing review of the older person's and care partner's goals and care plan
- Care supported by an interprofessional team in which the older person and the caregiver are integral
- Assignment of one primary or lead point of contact on the health-care team
- Active coordination among all health-care and supportive service providers
- Continual information sharing and integrated communication
- Education and training for providers and, when appropriate, the older persons and their caregivers
- Performance measurement and quality improvement using feedback from the older person and caregivers

Data from American Geriatrics Society Expert Panel on Person-Centered Care: Person-Centered Care: A Definition and Essential Elements, *J Am Geriatr Soc.* 2016 Jan;64(1):15-18.

patient's current problems in perspective; this can also be diagnostically important. For example, vomiting in an elderly patient who has had previous intra-abdominal surgery should raise the suspicion of intestinal obstruction from adhesions; nonspecific constitutional symptoms (such as fatigue, anorexia, and weight loss) in a patient with a history of depression should prompt consideration of a relapse. Because older individuals are often treated with multiple medications, they are at increased risk of noncompliance and adverse effects (see Chapter 14).

A detailed medication history (including both prescribed and over-the-counter drugs) is essential. The brown bag technique is very helpful in this regard; have the patient or caregiver empty the patient's medicine cabinet (prescribed and over-the-counter drugs as well as nontraditional remedies) into a brown paper bag and bring it to each visit. More often than not, one or more of these medications can, at least in theory, contribute to geriatric patients' symptoms. Clinicians should not hesitate to turn to pharmacists for help in determining potential drug interactions.

PHYSICAL EXAMINATION

The common occurrence of multiple pathologic physical findings superimposed on age-related physical changes complicates interpretation of the physical examination. Table 3-6 lists common physical findings and their potential significance in the geriatric population.

An awareness of age-related physical changes is important to the interpretation of many physical findings and therefore subsequent decision making. For example, age-related changes in the skin and postural reflexes can influence the evaluation of hydration and volume status; age-related changes in the lung and lower-extremity edema secondary to venous insufficiency can complicate the evaluation of symptoms of heart failure.

TABLE 3-6. Common Physical Findings and Their Potential Significance in Geriatrics

Physical findings	Potential significance
Vital signs	
Elevated blood pressure	Increased risk for cardiovascular morbidity; therapy should be considered if repeated measurements are high (see Chap. 11)
Postural changes in blood pressure	May be asymptomatic and occur in the absence of volume depletion Aging changes, deconditioning, and drugs may play a role Can be exaggerated after meals Can be worsened and become symptomatic with antihypertensive, vasodilator, and tricyclic antidepressant therapy
Irregular pulse	Arrhythmias are relatively common in otherwise asymptomatic elderly; seldom need specific evaluation or treatment (see Chap. 11)
Tachypnea	Baseline rate should be accurately recorded to help assess future complaints (such as dyspnea) or conditions (such as pneumonia or heart failure)
Weight changes	Weight gain should prompt search for edema or ascites Gradual loss of small amounts of weight common; losses in excess of 5% of usual body weight over 12 months or less should prompt search of underlying disease
General appearance and behavior	
Poor personal grooming and hygiene (eg, poorly shaven, unkempt hair, soiled clothing)	Can be signs of poor overall function, caregiver's neglect, and/or depression; often indicates a need for intervention
Slow thought processes and speech	Usually represents an aging change; Parkinson disease and depression can also cause these signs
Ulcerations	Lower extremity vascular and neuropathic ulcers common Pressure ulcers common and easily overlooked in immobile patients
Diminished turgor	Often results from atrophy of subcutaneous tissues rather than volume depletion; when dehydration suspected, skin turgor over chest and abdomen most reliable
Ears (see Chap. 13)	
Diminished hearing	High-frequency hearing loss common; patients with difficulty hearing normal conversation or a whispered phrase next to the ear should be evaluated further Portable audioscopes can be helpful in screening for impairment

(continued)

TABLE 3-6. Common Physical Findings and Their Potential Significance in Geriatrics (*continued*)

Eyes (see Chap. 13)	
Decreased visual acuity (often despite corrective lenses)	May have multiple causes, all patients should have thorough optometric or ophthalmologic examination Hemianopsia is easily overlooked and can usually be ruled out by simple confrontation testing
Cataracts and other abnormalities	Fundoscopic examination often difficult and limited; if retinal pathology suspected, thorough ophthalmologic examination necessary

Mouth	
Missing teeth	Dentures often present; they should be removed to check for evidence of poor fit and other pathology in oral cavity Area under the tongue is a common site for early malignancies

Skin	
Multiple lesions	Actinic keratoses and basal cell carcinomas common; most other lesions benign

Chest	
Abnormal lung sounds	Crackles can be heard in the absence of pulmonary disease and heart failure; often indicate atelectasis

Cardiovascular (see Chap. 11)	
Irregular rhythms	See Vital Signs at the beginning of the table
Systolic murmurs	Common and most often benign; clinical history and bedside maneuvers can help to differentiate those needing further evaluation Carotid bruits may need further evaluation
Vascular bruits	Femoral bruits often present in patients with symptomatic peripheral vascular disease
Diminished distal pulses	Presence or absence should be recorded as this information may be diagnostically useful at a later time (eg, if symptoms of claudication or an embolism develop)

Abdomen	
Prominent aortic pulsation	Suspected abdominal aneurysms should be evaluated by ultrasound

Genitourinary (see Chap. 8)	
Atrophy	Testicular atrophy normal; atrophic vaginal tissue may cause symptoms (such as dyspareunia and dysuria) and treatment may be beneficial

Genitourinary (see Chap. 8)	
Pelvic prolapse (cystocele, rectocele)	Common and may be unrelated to symptoms; gynecologic evaluation helpful if patient has bothersome, potentially related symptoms

(*continued*)

TABLE 3-6. Common Physical Findings and Their Potential Significance in Geriatrics (*continued*)

Extremities	
Periarticular pain	Can result from a variety of causes and is not always the result of degenerative joint disease; each area of pain should be carefully evaluated and treated (see Chap. 10)
Limited range of motion	Often caused by pain resulting from active inflammation, scarring from old injury, or neurological disease; if limitations impair function, a rehabilitation therapist could be consulted
Edema	Can result from venous insufficiency and/or heart failure; mild edema often a cosmetic problem; treatment necessary if impairing ambulation, contributing to nocturia, predisposing to skin breakdown, or causing discomfort Unilateral edema should prompt search for a proximal obstructive process

Neurological	
Abnormal mental status (ie, confusion, depressed affect)	See Chaps. 6 and 7
Weakness	Arm drift may be the only sign of residual weakness from a stroke Proximal muscle weakness (eg, inability to get out of chair) should be further evaluated; physical therapy may be appropriate

Certain aspects of the physical examination are of particular importance in the geriatric population. Detection and further evaluation of impairments of vision and hearing can lead to improvements in quality of life. Walking performance can be a valuable indicator of a variety of problems. Evaluation of gait may uncover correctable causes of unsteadiness and thereby prevent potentially devastating falls (see Chapter 9). Careful palpation of the abdomen may reveal an aortic aneurysm, which, if large enough, might warrant consideration of surgical removal. The mental status examination is especially important; this aspect of the physical examination is discussed later and in Chapter 6.

LABORATORY ASSESSMENT

Abnormal laboratory findings are often attributed to "old age." While it is true that abnormal findings are common in geriatric patients, few are true aging changes. Misinterpreting an abnormal laboratory value as an aging change may result in underdiagnosis and undertreatment of conditions such as anemia.

Table 3-7 lists those laboratory parameters unchanged in older adults and those commonly abnormal. Abnormalities in the former group should prompt further evaluation;

TABLE 3-7. Laboratory Assessment of Geriatric Patients

Laboratory parameters unchanged*
Hemoglobin and hematocrit
White blood cell count
Platelet count
Electrolytes (sodium, potassium, chloride, bicarbonate)
Blood urea nitrogen
Liver function tests (transaminases, bilirubin, prothrombin time)
Free thyroxine index
Thyroid-stimulating hormone
Calcium
Phosphorus

Common abnormal laboratory parameters†	
Parameter	Clinical significance
Sedimentation rate	Mild elevations (10-20 mm) may be an age-related change
Glucose	Glucose tolerance decreases (see Chap. 12); elevations during acute illness are common
Creatinine	Because lean body mass and daily endogenous creatinine production decline, high-normal and minimally elevated values may indicate substantially reduced renal function
Albumin	Average values decline (<0.5 g/mL) with age, especially in acutely ill, but generally indicate undernutrition
Alkaline phosphatase	Mild asymptomatic elevations common; liver and Paget's disease should be considered if moderately elevated
Serum iron, iron-binding capacity, ferritin	Decreased values are not an aging change and usually indicate undernutrition and/or gastrointestinal blood loss
Prostate-specific antigen	May be elevated in patients with benign prostatic hyerplasia. Marked elevation or increasing values when followed over time should prompt consideration of further evaluation in patients for whom specific therapy for prostate cancer would be undertaken if cancer were diagnosed
Urinalysis	Asymptomatic pyuria and bacteriuria are common and rarely warrant treatment; hematuria is abnormal and needs further evaluation (see Chap. 8)
Chest radiographs	Interstitial changes are a common age-related finding; diffusely diminished bone density generally indicates advanced osteoporosis (see Chap. 12)
Electrocardiogram	ST-segment and T-wave changes, atrial and ventricular arrhythmias, and various blocks are common in asymptomatic elderly and may not need specific evaluation or treatment (see Chap. 11)

*Aging changes do not occur in these parameters; abnormal values should prompt further evaluation.
†Includes normal aging and other age-related changes.

abnormalities in the latter group should be interpreted carefully. Table 3-7 also notes important considerations in interpreting commonly abnormal laboratory values.

FUNCTIONAL ASSESSMENT

GENERAL CONCEPTS

As noted earlier, attention to function has two components: (1) functional ability and (2) functional goals. The assessment of the former may not use terms that are meaningful to the latter. The former may be couched in specific performance abilities, while the latter can refer to life activities or anticipated events activities the patient wants to be able to participate in. Ability to function should be a central focus of the evaluation of geriatric patients. Medical history, physical examination, and laboratory findings are all of obvious importance in diagnosing and managing acute and chronic medical conditions in older people, as they are in all age groups. But once the dust settles, functional abilities are just as, if not more, important to the overall health, well-being, and potential need for services of older individuals. For example, in a patient with hemiparesis, the nature, location, and extent of the lesion may be important in the management, but whether the patient is continent and can climb the steps to an apartment makes the difference between going home to live or going to a nursing home.

The concern about function as a core component of geriatrics deserves special comment. Functioning is the end result of the various efforts of the geriatric approach to care. Optimizing function necessitates integrating efforts on several fronts. It is helpful to think of functioning as an equation:

$$\text{Function} = \frac{(\text{physical capabilities} \times \text{medical management} \times \text{motivation})}{(\text{social, psychological, and physical environment})}$$

This admitted oversimplification is meant as a reminder that function can be influenced on at least three levels. The clinician's first task is to remediate the remediable. The denominator addresses these areas, including soliciting the patient's active participation in the care and the work involved in carrying out tasks. Careful medical diagnosis and appropriate treatment are essential in good geriatric care. Adequate medical management, however, is necessary but not sufficient. Once those conditions amenable to treatment have been addressed, the next step is to develop the environment that will best support the patient's autonomous function.

Environmental barriers can be both physical and psychological. It is important to recognize how physical barriers may complicate functioning for persons with various conditions (eg, stairs for a person with dyspnea, inaccessible cabinets for the wheelchair bound). Psychological barriers refer especially to the dangers of risk aversion. Those most concerned about the patient may restrict activity in the name of protecting the patient or the institution. For example, hospitals are notoriously averse to risk; older patients will be restricted to a wheelchair rather than risk them falling when walking.

This risk-averse behavior may be compounded by concerns about efficiency. Bear in mind, however, that efficiency reflects the costs of effectiveness. If you are not effective, you can never be efficient. Personal care is personnel intensive. It takes much more time and patience to work with patients to encourage them to do things for themselves than to step in and do the task. But that pseudoefficiency breeds dependence.

The third factor relates to the concept of motivation. If care providers believe that the patient cannot improve, they will likely induce despair and discouragement in their charges. The tendency toward functional decline may become a self-fulfilling prophecy. Indeed, the opposite belief—that improvement is quite likely with appropriate intervention—may account for at least part of the success of geriatric evaluation units. Belief in the possibility of improvement can play another critical role in geriatric care. Psychologists have developed a useful paradigm referred to as "the innocent victim syndrome." The basic concept holds that caregivers respond in a hostile manner to those they feel impotent to help. If given a sense of empowerment to approach the complex problems of older persons, perhaps assessment tools and intervention strategies such as the ones provided in this book, can help care providers feel more positive toward those individuals and be more willing to work with them rather than avoid them. The more an information system can provide feedback on accomplishments and progress toward improved function, the more positively the provider will feel about the older patient.

Table 3-8 summarizes several other important concepts about comprehensive functional assessment in the geriatric population, which were identified in a Consensus Development Conference at the National Institutes of Health (National Institutes of Health, 1988). They remain salient after almost 30 years. To a large extent, the purpose, setting, and timing of the assessment dictate the nature of the assessment process.

Table 3-9 lists the different purposes and objectives of functional status measures. Generally, functional assessment begins with a case-finding or screening approach in order to identify individuals for whom more in-depth and interdisciplinary assessment might be of benefit. Assessment is often carried out at points of transition, such as a threatened or actual decline in health status or impending change in living situation. Without this type of targeting, the assessment of older people may be time-consuming and not cost-effective. Numerous standardized instruments are available to assist in the assessment process.

Instruments designed for research use may not work in clinical practice, and vice versa. There are numerous potential pitfalls in the use of standardized assessment instruments (Kane and Kane, 2000) (see Table 3-8). The critical concept in using standardized instruments is that they should fit the purposes and settings for which they are intended, and there must be a solid link between the assessment process and the follow-up provision of services. In addition, the assessment process should include a clear discussion of the patient's preferences and expectations, as well as the family's expectations and willingness to provide care. The importance of functional status assessment is reflected in the ability of functional status measures to predict mortality in older hospitalized patients (Inouye et al, 1998).

TABLE 3-8. Important Concepts for Geriatric Functional Assessment

1. The nature of the assessment should be dictated by its purpose, setting, and timing (see Table 3-9)
2. Input from multiple disciplines is often helpful, but routine multidisciplinary assessment is not cost-effective
3. Assessments should be targeted
   a. Initial screening to identify disciplines needed
   b. Times of threatened or actual decline in status, impending change in living situation, and other stressful situations
4. Standard instruments are useful, but there are numerous potential pitfalls
   a. Instruments should be reliable, sensitive, and valid for the purposes and setting of the assessment
   b. How questions are asked can be critically important (eg, performance vs. capability)
   c. Discrepancies can arise between different informants (eg, self-report vs. caregiver's report)
   d. Self or caregiver's report of performance or direct observation of performance may not reflect what the individual does in everyday life
   e. Many standard instruments have not been adequately tested for reliability and sensitivity to changes over time
5. Open-ended questions are helpful in complementing information from standardized instruments
6. The family's expectations, capabilities, and willingness to provide care must be explored
7. The patient's preferences and expectations should be elicited and considered paramount in planning services
8. A strong link must exist between the assessment process and follow-up in the provision of services

TABLE 3-9. Purposes and Objectives of Functional Status Measures

Purpose	Objectives
Description	Develop normative data
	Depict geriatric population along selected parameters
	Assess needs
	Describe outcomes associated with various interventions
Screening	Identify from among population at risk those individuals who should receive further assessment and by whom
Assessment	Make diagnosis
	Assign treatment
Monitoring	Observe changes in untreated conditions
	Review progress of those receiving treatment
Prediction	Permit scientifically based clinical interventions
	Make prognostic statements of expected outcomes on the basis of given conditions

ASSESSMENT TOOLS FOR FUNCTIONAL STATUS

This chapter focuses on the assessment of physical and mental function. Mental function is also discussed in Chapter 6. Table 3-10 lists examples of measures of physical functioning. Physical functioning is measured along a spectrum. For persons with disabilities, one may focus on the ability to perform basic self-care tasks, often referred to as activities of daily living (ADLs). The patient is assessed on the ability to conduct each of a series of basic activities. Data usually come from the patient or from a caregiver (eg, a nurse or family member) who has had sufficient opportunity to observe the patient. In some cases, it may be more useful to have the patient actually demonstrate the ability to perform key tasks. Grading of performance is usually divided into three levels of dependency: (1) ability to perform the task without human assistance (one may wish to distinguish those persons who need mechanical aids like a walker but are still independent); (2) ability to perform the task with some human assistance; and (3) inability to perform the task, even with assistance. In instances like dementia, the assistance may be less physical and more cuing or reminding. Distinguishing "independent without difficulty" from "independent with difficulty" may provide complementing prognostic information (Gill, Robinson, and Tinetti, 1998).

TABLE 3-10. Examples of Measures of Physical Functioning

Basic ADLs
Feeding
Dressing
Ambulation
Toileting
Bathing
Transfer (from bed and toilet)
Continence
Grooming
Communication
IADLs
Writing
Reading
Cooking
Cleaning
Shopping
Doing laundry
Climbing stairs
Using telephone
Managing medication
Managing money
Ability to perform paid employment duties or outside work (eg, gardening)
Ability to travel (use public transportation, go out of town)

ADL, activity of daily living; IADL, instrumental ADL.

Different disciplines approach functional measurement differently. A physician, for example, may be content to ascertain whether a person can dress herself with or without assistance. By contrast, an occupational therapist might subdivide the act of getting dressed into a series of specific steps (eg, choosing appropriate clothes, getting them out of the closet or drawers, putting on different types of clothing, using various fasteners). Likewise, performance can be further assessed in terms of the time required to complete the task and the skill with which it was done.

Functioning is typically based on reports, although in some cases in may actually be demonstrated in test situations. Demonstrated function gives a better estimate of what a person can do under standardized conditions, whereas reported function reflects the role of a person's actual environment (both physical and social). For example, nursing home residents never bathe themselves, although may be capable of doing so.

There may be discrepancies between patients' or caregivers' reports and what the individuals actually do in their everyday life. Moreover, there may be differences between reported physical functional status and actual measures of physical performance. Reuben's Physical Performance Test is one example of a practical assessment that provides insights into actual performance and prognostic information (Reuben and Siu, 1990). In general, performance tests measure what occurs under standardized conditions, whereas reports address what is done under actual living conditions; hence, the latter may offer insights into the effects of the environment as well as the patient's abilities. Other performance-based assessments of gait and balance are discussed in Chapter 9.

In addition to these general geriatric measures of functional status, other functional assessment tools are commonly used in different settings. Examples include the following:

1. The Short Form-36 (SF-36)—a global measure of function and well-being that is increasingly being used in outpatient settings. This measure has a disadvantage in the frail geriatric population because of a ceiling effect—that is, it does not distinguish well between sick and very sick older people.
2. The Minimum Data Set (MDS)—a comprehensive assessment mandated on admission with quarterly updates in Medicare-/Medicaid-certified nursing facilities. The most current version is the MDS 3.0.
3. The Functional Independence Measure (FIM; now part of the Inpatient Rehabilitation Facility–Patient Assessment Instrument [IRF-PAI])—a detailed assessment tool commonly used to monitor functional status progress in rehabilitation settings.
4. The Outcome and Assessment Information Set (OASIS)—a comprehensive data collection system for use in home health care; it is mandatory for Medicare beneficiaries.

A new data system, Continuity Assessment Record and Evaluation (CARE), combines elements from MDS, OASIS, and IRF-PAI and introduces a common measurement system for all postacute care. However, it is still under development under a project called the Improving Medicare Post-Acute Care Transformation Act of 2014 (IMPACT).

A structured assessment of cognitive function should be part of every complete geriatric functional assessment. Because of the high prevalence of cognitive impairment, the potential impact of such impairment on overall function and safety and the ability of patients with early impairments to mask their deficits, clinicians must specifically attend to this aspect of functional assessment. At a minimum, assessment should include a test for orientation and memory. Although these tests do not probe the variety of intellectual functions appropriate for a more detailed assessment, they are quick, easy, scorable, and reliable. More detailed assessment of cognitive function is discussed in Chapter 6.

ENVIRONMENTAL ASSESSMENT

We emphasized earlier that patient function is the result of innate ability and environment. The clinician must, therefore, be particularly concerned with the older patient's environment. For many patients, the assessment should include an evaluation of the available and potential resources to maintain functioning. Just as physicians comfortably prescribe drugs, they should also be prepared to prescribe environmental interventions when necessary.

Rehabilitation therapists (eg, physical, occupational, speech) are especially skilled at assessing function, developing and implementing rehabilitative plans of care targeted at potentially remediable functional impairments, and making specific recommendations about environmental modifications that can enhance safety and functional ability. An environmental prescription may include alterations in the physical environment (eg, ramps, grab bars, elevated toilet seats), special services (eg, meals on wheels, homemaking, home nursing), increased social contact (eg, friendly visits, telephone reassurance, participation in recreational activities), or provision of critical elements (eg, food, money). An environmental assessment by an occupational therapist for essentially asymptomatic older persons has been shown to significantly reduce subsequent hospital use (Clark et al, 1997).

The ability to identify the environmental interventions and function supports needed to maintain in the community may be the essential difference between enabling an older person to remain at home versus transferring the person to an institution. Although identifying the need is not tantamount to providing the resource, it is an important first step.

ASSESSMENT FOR PAIN

Guidelines published by the American Geriatrics Society recommend that on initial presentation or admission of an older person to any health-care service, the patient should be assessed for evidence of persistent pain (American Geriatrics Society Panel on Persistent Pain in Older Persons, 2002). Patients with persistent pain that may affect physical function, psychosocial function, or other aspects of quality of life should undergo a comprehensive pain assessment. Tables 3-11 and 3-12 list

TABLE 3-11. Important Aspects of the History in Assessment of Pain

1. Characteristics of the pain
2. Relation of pain to impairments in physical and social function
3. Analgesic history (present, previous, prescribed, over-the-counter, alternative remedies, alcohol use, side effects)
4. Patient's attitudes and beliefs about pain and its management
5. Effectiveness of treatments
6. Satisfaction with current pain management
7. Social support and health-care accessibility

important aspects of the history and physical examination, respectively, in assessing pain. For patients who are cognitively intact, pain assessments should use direct questioning of the patient. Quantitative assessment of pain should be recorded by using a standard pain scale, such as a visual analog scale, where a patient can indicate where along the continuum their pain lies. A verbal scale of 0 to 10, with 0 meaning no pain and 10 meaning the worst pain possible, is frequently used. Other scales (pain thermometer and faces) studied in older populations are illustrated in Figure 3-3. In cognitively impaired and nonverbal patients, pain assessment should be by direct observation or history from caregivers. Patients should be observed for pain-related behaviors during movement. Unusual behavior in a patient with severe dementia should trigger assessment for pain as a potential cause.

NUTRITIONAL ASSESSMENT

Several parameters are used in assessing nutritional status in older adults. Some anthropometric variables are probably effective estimators of major aspects of body composition (Table 3-13). They cannot provide a complete description of the nutritional status of an individual and are not highly correlated with biochemical or hematologic indicators of nutritional status.

Although weight is a global measure, it can be obtained easily from adults and is useful in the absence of edema. Body mass index (BMI = kg/m^2) is best correlated with total body fat. Triceps and subscapular skin folds are highly correlated with the

TABLE 3-12. Important Aspects of the Physical Examination in Assessment of Pain

1. Careful examination of the site of pain and common sites for pain referral
2. Focus on the musculoskeletal system
3. Focus on the neurological system including weakness and dysesthesia
4. Observation of physical function
5. Psychological function
6. Cognitive function

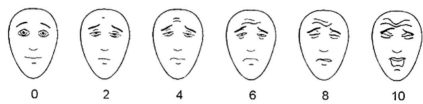

The Faces Pain Scale – Revised [1] (FPS-R) is a self-report measure of pain intensity developed for children. It was adapted from the Faces Pain Scale [2] in order to make it possible to score on the widely accepted 0-to-10 metric. It shows a close linear relationship with visual analog pain scales across the age range of 4–16 years. It is easy to administer and requires no equipment except for the photocopied faces. The absence of smiles and tears in this scale may be advantageous. It is particularly recommended for use with younger children. Numerical self-rating scales (0–10) can be used with most children over 8 years of age [3], and behavioral observation scales are required for those unable to provide a self-report.

In the following instructions, say "hurt" or "pain," whichever seems right for a particular child:

"These faces show how much something can hurt. This face *[point to left-most face]* **shows no pain. The faces show more and more pain** *[point to each from left to right]* **up to this one** *[point to right-most face]* **— it shows very much pain. Point to the face that shows how much you hurt** *[right now]* **."**

Score the chosen face 0, 2, 4, 6, 8, or 10, counting left to right, so '0' = 'no pain' and '10' = 'very much pain.' Do not use words like 'happy' and 'sad.' This scale is intended to measure how children feel inside, not how their face looks.

FIGURE 3-3 Samples of two pain intensity scales that have been studied in older persons. Directions: Patients should view the figure without numbers. After the patient indicates the best representation of his or her pain, the appropriate numerical value can be assigned to facilitate clinical documentation and follow-up. (*Reproduced with permission from Faces Pain Scale—Revised, ©2001, International Association for the Study of Pain.*)

percentage of body fat in older adults. Waist-to-hip ratio is a parameter of central adiposity. Upper arm circumference is correlated with lean body mass and may be particularly helpful in edematous patients in whom weight is misleading. The effect of the aging process on lean body mass is so great that it remains a poor reflection of nutritional status in older adults.

Serum albumin is a practical indicator of malnutrition in older adults. However, liver disease, proteinuria, and protein-losing enteropathies must be excluded. A low serum albumin may be indicative of malnutrition, but a normal or increased serum albumin concentration does not necessarily indicate normality. Thyroxine-binding prealbumin and/or retinol-binding protein are more sensitive indices than are albumin and transferrin.

In animals, dietary deprivation of protein results in anemia. Because anemia is one of the earliest manifestations of protein–calorie malnutrition, its presence should alert the physician to the possibility of malnutrition. Total lymphocyte count may be a very good marker for nutritional problems.

TABLE 3-13. Assessment of Body Composition

Assessment	Component
Weight	Global
Body mass index	Total fat
Skin fold	Percent fat
Waist-to-hip ratio	Central adiposity
Upper arm circumference	Lean body mass

TABLE 3-14. Critical Questions in Assessing a Patient for Malnutrition

Is there any reason to suspect malnutrition?
If so, of which nutrient(s) and to what extent?
What are the pathophysiological mechanisms (eg, alteration in nutrient intake, digestion and absorption, metabolism, excretion, or requirements)?
What etiology underlies the pathophysiological mechanism(s)?

Some important factors need to be considered in evaluating a given patient. Table 3-14 presents some issues that should be considered in assessing older patients at risk for malnutrition. Individuals with such problems should have an evaluation of nutritional status. Some patients may have several concurrent diseases that impair nutritional status (Table 3-15). Protein–energy malnutrition may ensue and is associated with poor prognosis.

MEDICARE ASSESSMENT VISITS

Medicare covers two levels of preventive visits. The Initial Preventive Physical Examination (IPPE) is also known as the "Welcome to Medicare Preventive Visit." The goals of the IPPE are health promotion and disease prevention and detection. Medicare pays for only one IPPE per beneficiary per lifetime for beneficiaries within the first 12 months of the effective date of the beneficiary's first Medicare Part B coverage period. Table 3-16 lists the required elements of that visit.

Medicare also covers an annual wellness visit. The required components of that visit are shown in Table 3-17.

GERIATRIC CONSULTATION

Geriatric consultation may be requested to address specific clinical issues (eg, confusion, incontinence, recurrent falling), to perform a comprehensive geriatric assessment (often in the context of determining the need for placement in a difficult living

TABLE 3-15. Factors That Place Older Adults at Risk for Malnutrition

Drugs (eg, reserpine, digoxin, antitumor agents)
Chronic disease (eg, congestive heart failure, renal insufficiency, chronic gastrointestinal disease)
Depression
Dental and periodontal disease
Decreased taste and smell
Low socioeconomic level
Physical weakness
Isolation
Food fads

TABLE 3-16. Medicare Initial Preventive Physical Examination

Required Elements
Medical and Social History
Review the beneficiary's medical and social history:
- Experiences with illnesses, hospital stays, operations
- Allergies
- Injuries
- Treatments
- Current medications and supplements (including calcium and vitamins)
- Family history (review of medical events in the beneficiary's family, including diseases that may be hereditary or place the beneficiary at risk)
- History of alcohol, tobacco, and illicit drug use
- Diet
- Physical activity

Depression Screen
Review the beneficiary's potential risk factors for depression and other mood disorders:
- Use any appropriate screening instrument for beneficiaries without a current diagnosis of depression from various available screening tests recognized by national professional medical organizations to obtain current or past experiences with depression or other mood disorders.

Functional Ability and Safety Screen
Review the beneficiary's functional ability and level of safety:
- Hearing impairment
- ADL
- Fall risk
- Home safety

Physical Examination
- Height, weight
- Body mass index
- Blood pressure
- Visual acuity screen
- Other factors deemed appropriate based on the beneficiary's medical and social history

End-of-Life Planning (on agreement of the beneficiary)
End-of-life planning is verbal or written information provided to the beneficiary about:
- The beneficiary's ability to prepare an advance directive in case an injury or illness causes the beneficiary to be unable to make health care decisions.
- Whether or not you are willing to follow the beneficiary's wishes as expressed in the advance directive.

Counseling
- Educate, counsel, and refer based on the previous five components.
- Educate, counsel, and refer for other preventive services:
  - A once-in-a-lifetime screening electrocardiogram (EKG/ECG), as appropriate
  - The appropriate screenings and other preventive services that Medicare covers

Reproduced with permission from The ABCs of the Initial Preventive Physical Examination (IPPE) Department of Health and Human Services Centers for Medicare & Medicaid Services ICN 006904 January 2015

TABLE 3-17. Medicare Annual Wellness Visit

Required Elements

Demographic Data
- Self-assessment of health status
- Psychosocial risks
- Behavioral risks
- ADLs
- IADLs

Providers and Suppliers
- List of current providers and suppliers regularly involved in providing medical care to the beneficiary

History
- Medical events in the beneficiary's parents, siblings, and children, including diseases that may be hereditary or place the beneficiary at increased risk
- Past medical and surgical history, including experiences with illnesses, hospital stays, operations, allergies, injuries, and treatments
- Use of, or exposure to, medications and supplements, including calcium and vitamins

Screening
- Depression
- Ability to successfully perform ADLs
- Fall risk
- Hearing impairment
- Home safety

Measurements
- Height
- Weight
- Body mass index (or waist circumference, if appropriate)
- Blood pressure
- Other routine measurements as deemed appropriate based on medical and family history

Cognitive Function
- Assess cognitive function by direct observation, with due consideration of information obtained via beneficiary reports and concerns raised by family members, friends, caretakers, or others

Screening Schedule
- Establish a written screening schedule for the beneficiary, such as a checklist for the next 5 to 10 years, as appropriate based on:
  - Age-appropriate preventive services that Medicare covers
  - Recommendations from the United States Preventive Services Task Force (USPSTF) and the Advisory Committee on Immunization Practices (ACIP)
  - The beneficiary's HRA, health status, and screening history

(continued)

TABLE 3-17. Medicare Annual Wellness Visit (*continued*)

Health Advice

- Furnish personalized health advice to the beneficiary and a referral, as appropriate, to health education or preventive counseling services or programs including referrals to programs aimed at:
  - Community-based lifestyle interventions to reduce health risks and promote self-management and wellness
  - Fall prevention
  - Nutrition
  - Physical activity
  - Tobacco-use cessation
  - Weight loss

Reproduced with permission from The ABCs of the Annual Wellness Visit (AWV). Department of Health and Human Services. Centers for Medicare & Medicaid Services. ICN 905706 January 2015.

setting), or to perform a preoperative evaluation of a high-risk geriatric patient. In this chapter, we discuss the latter two types of consultation.

COMPREHENSIVE GERIATRIC CONSULTATION

A comprehensive geriatric consultation includes the following:

1. A geriatric-oriented history and physical examination attending to the issues reviewed earlier in this chapter.
2. Medication review; in addition, geriatric patients should be questioned about alcohol abuse.
3. Functional assessment.
4. Environmental and social assessment, focusing especially on caregiver's support and other resources available to meet the patient's needs.
5. Discussion of advance directives.
6. A complete list of the patient's medical, functional, and psychosocial problems.
7. Specific recommendations in each domain.

A systematic screening process to identify potentially remediable geriatric problems may be a useful tool for the comprehensive consultation.

One such screening strategy is illustrated in Table 3-18 (Moore and Siu, 1996). It may also be useful, especially in capitated systems, to use a tool that identifies risk for crises and expensive health-care utilization. The Probability of Repeated Admissions (Pra) instrument is one such tool (Table 3-19) (Pacala et al, 1997). Among frail, dependent geriatric patients, screening for risk factors and elder abuse is important. Elder abuse is more common among older people who are in poor health and who are physically and cognitively impaired. Additional risk factors include shared living arrangements with a relative or friend suspected of alcohol or substance abuse,

TABLE 3-18. Example of a Screening Tool to Identify Potentially Remediable Geriatric Problems

Problem	Screening measure	Positive result
Poor vision	Ask, "Do you have difficulty driving, watching television, reading, or doing any of your daily activities because of your eyesight?" If yes, then test acuity with Snellen chart, with corrective lenses	Inability to read better than 20/40 on Snellen chart
Poor hearing	With audioscope set at 40 dB, test hearing at 1000 and 2000 Hz	Inability to hear 1000 or 2000 Hz in both ears or either frequency in one ear
Poor leg mobility	Time the patient after asking, "Rise from the chair. Walk 20 feet briskly, turn, walk back to the chair, and sit down."	Unable to complete task in 15 s
Urinary incontinence	Ask, "In the past year, have you ever lost your urine and gotten wet?" If yes, then ask, "Have you lost urine on at least 6 separate days?"	Yes to both questions
Malnutrition and weight loss	Ask, "Have you lost 10 lb over the past 6 months without trying to do so?" and then weigh the patient	Yes to the question or weight <100 lb
Memory loss	Three-item recall	Unable to remember all three items after 1 min
Depression	Ask, "Do you often feel sad or depressed?"	Yes to the question
Physical disability	Ask six questions: "Are you able to: • Do strenuous activities such as fast walking or bicycling? • Do heavy work around the house like washing windows, walls, or floors? • Go shopping for groceries or clothes? • Get to places that are out of walking distance? • Bathe: either a sponge bath, tub bath, or shower? • Dress, including putting on a shirt, buttoning and zipping, and putting on shoes?"	No to any question

Adapted with permission from Moore AA, Siu AL. Screening for common problems in ambulatory elderly: clinical confirmation of a screening instrument, *Am J Med* 1996 Apr;100(4):438-443.

TABLE 3-19. Questions on the Probability of Repeated Admissions Instrument for Identifying Geriatric Patients at Risk for Health Service Use

1. In general, would you say your health is:
   (excellent, very good, good, fair, poor)
2. In the previous 12 months, have you stayed overnight as a patient in a hospital?
   (not at all, one time, two or three times, more than three times)
3. In the previous 12 months, how many times did you visit a physician or clinic?
   (not at all, one time, two or three times, four to six times, more than six times)
4. In the previous 12 months, did you have diabetes?
   (yes, no)
5. Have you ever had: Coronary heart disease? (yes, no)
   Angina pectoris? (yes, no)
   A myocardial infarction? (yes, no)
   Any other heart attack? (yes, no)
6. Your sex?
   (male, female)
7. Is there a friend, relative, or neighbor who would take care of you for a few days if necessary?
   (yes, no)
8. Your date of birth?
   (month   , day   , year   )

Reproduced with permission from Pacala JT, Boult C, Reed RL, Aliberti E: Predictive validity of the Pra instrument among older recipients of managed care, *J Am Geriatr Soc* May 45(5):614–617, 1997.

mental illness, or a history of violence. Likewise self-neglect should be a concern, although it may engender a difficult ethical discussion about an older person's right to take risks.

Frequent emergency room visits for injury or exacerbations of chronic illness should also raise suspicion about abuse. Table 3-20 illustrates an example of an effective format for documenting the results of the consultation, listing the problems and recommendations.

PREOPERATIVE EVALUATION

Geriatricians are often called on by surgeons and anesthesiologists to assess elderly patients before surgical procedures. An important component of this evaluation is to assess the risk of postoperative delirium and suggest steps to mitigate against this untoward event. There is a movement toward co-management of complex cases, mostly commonly with hip fractures (The Agency for Clinical Innovation [ACI] Orthogeriatric Model of Care Collaborative Group, 2010). The American College of Surgeons and the American Geriatrics Society have issued joint guidelines on preoperative assessment of older patients (Chow et al, 2012). These are summarized in Table 3-21.

TABLE 3-20. Suggested Format for Summarizing the Results of a Comprehensive Geriatric Consultation

1. Identifying data, including referring physician
2. Reason(s) for consultation
3. Problems
   a. Medical problem list
   b. Functional problem list
   c. Psychosocial problem list
4. Recommendations
5. Standard documentation
   a. History, including medications, significant past medical and surgical history, system review
   b. Social and environmental information
   c. Functional assessment
   d. Advance directive status
   e. Physical examination
   f. Laboratory and other test data

Morbidity and mortality are influenced by the presence and severity of systemic illnesses and whether the procedure is elective versus emergent. Thus, evaluating a geriatric patient's preoperative status and risk for surgery necessitates a thorough assessment of cardiopulmonary and renal function as well as nutritional and hydration status. Factors that increase the risk of perioperative cardiac complications in patients undergoing noncardiac surgery include ischemic heart disease, congestive

TABLE 3-21. Preoperative Assessment Checklist

- Cognitive ability and capacity to understand the anticipated surgery
- Depression
- Risk factors for postoperative delirium
- Alcohol and substance abuse
- Preoperative cardiac evaluation according to the American College of Cardiology/American Heart Association algorithm for patients undergoing noncardiac surgery
- Risk factors for postoperative pulmonary complications and implement appropriate strategies for prevention
- Functional status and history of falls
- Frailty score
- Nutritional status
- Medication history; monitor for polypharmacy
- Treatment goals and expectations
- Family and social support system
- Other diagnostic tests as indicated

heart failure, diabetes mellitus, and renal insufficiency. Patients with a recent history of myocardial infarction, active angina, pulmonary edema, and severe aortic stenosis are at especially high risk. Preoperative pulmonary function tests and arterial blood gases are rarely of prognostic value. Assessment of exercise tolerance may be helpful, for example, the ability to climb one flight of stairs. In patients at low risk for cardiac complications, no β-blockade is necessary. In patients at increased risk for cardiac complications, modified exercise testing, dipyridamole thallium scanning, or dobutamine echocardiography may be indicated. Coronary artery bypass grafting or percutaneous coronary revascularization should be limited to patients who have a clearly defined need for the procedure that is independent of the need for noncardiac surgery.

Underlying conditions that are prevalent in the geriatric population, such as hypertension, congestive heart failure, chronic obstructive lung disease, diabetes mellitus, anemia, and undernutrition, need particularly careful management in the preoperative period. Medication regimens should be scrutinized in order to determine whether specific drugs should be continued or withheld. Patients who are already on beta blockers, particularly those with independent cardiac indications for these medications (such as arrhythmia or history of myocardial infarction), should continue them. Patients undergoing intermediate risk or vascular surgery with known coronary artery disease or with multiple clinical risk factors for ischemic heart disease should receive beta blockers.

Careful consideration should also be given to perioperative prophylactic measures for the prevention of thromboembolism and infection, many of which have documented efficacy in specific situations.

Frailty (assessed by unintentional weight loss, decreased grip strength, decreased effort and motivation, low physical activity and energy, and slow walking speed) independently predicted postoperative complications, length of stay, and discharge to a skilled or assisted living facility in older surgical patients (Makary et al, 2010). Preoperative impaired cognition, recent falls, lower albumin, greater anemia, functional dependence, and increased comorbidities were associated with higher mortality at 6 months (Robinson et al, 2009). There is growing awareness of the importance of preventing, or at least minimizing, postoperative delirium. One study found four items independently associated with delirium: prior stroke or transient ischemic attack, Mini-Mental State Examination score, abnormal serum albumin, and the Geriatric Depression Scale (Rudolph et al, 2009).

Many surgeons and anesthesiologists favor regional over general anesthesia for geriatric patients. Regional anesthesia (eg, epidural), however, may have several potential disadvantages. Patients may require added intravenous sedation and/or analgesia, thus increasing the risks of perioperative cardiovascular and mental status changes. Significant cardiovascular changes can, in fact, occur during regional anesthesia, thus invasive monitoring may be required in some patients. Neither the incidence of deep vein thrombosis nor the amount of blood loss seems to be substantially decreased compared to general anesthesia. Thus, decisions about the type of anesthesia should be carefully individualized based on patient factors, the nature of the procedure, and the preferences of the surgical team.

CAREGIVER ASSESSMENT

Supporting informal caregivers is very important in sustaining this crucial element of long-term care (LTC). Caregiver stress can lead to caregiver burnout and even elder abuse and neglect. Because caregiving is risky business, caregivers are at increased risk for bad events. Clinicians caring for persons with dementia need to be especially observant for sign of stress, depression, and deteriorating health. Clinicians should ask questions and acknowledge the stress of caregiving. Whether or not you are also the care provider for the caregiver, it is important to preserve this resource. In the former case, you need to be proactive in managing chronic diseases. In the latter case, you need to recognize early signs of problems and make effective referrals.

Concomitants of stress include:

1. High levels of stress hormones
2. Reduced immune function
3. Slow wound healing
4. Increased incidence of hypertension
5. Coronary heart disease
6. Impaired endothelial function

When the clinician is the primary care provider for the caregiver the clinician needs to be extremely vigilant for indications of stress. Clinicians should raise the subject more than they might typically do with other patients because they may be so overwhelmed that they are in denial. Caregivers often deny problems they are facing. They need to be strongly encouraged to talk about their caregiving experience and the toll it is taking. Table 3-22 lists potential topics to be discussed with caregivers.

Clinicians need to specifically inquire at each visit about whether the caregiver is facing any unmet needs in dealing with the person living with dementia. They should ask the caregiver if he or she is getting enough support from others, both in formal support from family members and more formal support from a variety of service agencies in the community. Clinicians need to be prepared to prompt for

---

TABLE 3-22. Potential Manifestations of Caregiver Stress

- Sleep (of both caregivers and person living with dementia)
- Dealing with agitated behaviors
- Caregiver eating issues (unexpected weight loss or gain)
- Fears about abuse or anger
- Comfort level with medication management
- Relationship quality
- Guilt
- Family dynamics: local and outside the area
- Feelings of competence
- How caregiver reacts to behavioral and psychological symptoms of dementia
- Anticipatory grieving

this issue because caregivers may underreport the need for additional support. They should refer to the established care plan to ask specifically about whether potential types of assistance are being received and whether there is a need for more care.

Many caregivers already have substantial physical and/or mental health problems when they enter the caregiving role. They may ignore their own health while caring for the person living with dementia. At the same time new problems may arise. In both cases each disease needs to be closely monitored to detect early changes of problems before they become crises. There is always a danger of underreporting and a need to probe more specifically into how the caregivers are faring with each of their disease problems.

Given the reluctance of some caregivers to raise issues that may be a problem, some screening efforts may be useful. One of the most important things to screen for is depression. A simple screening device for this is the PHQ-9 (discussed in Chapter 9). A basic screening test for overall caregiver stress is the REACH II Risk Appraisal. The REACH II is designed to identify a variety of domains that may create stress for caregivers (www .rosalynncarter.org/UserFiles/RAM.pdf). A number of tools are available to assess caregivers including the Zarit Burden Interview and the Parks and Novelli checklist.

REFERENCES

The Agency for Clinical Innovation (ACI) Orthogeriatric Model of Care Collaborative Group. *The Orthogeriatric Model of Care: Summary of Evidence 2010.* ACI Aged Health Care Network; 2010. www.health.nsw.gov.au/gmct.

American Geriatrics Society Panel on Persistent Pain in Older Persons. The management of persistent pain in older persons. *J Am Geriatr Soc.* 2002;50:S205-S224.

Barer D; ACP Journal Club. Review: inpatient comprehensive geriatric assessment improves the likelihood of living at home at 12 months. *Ann Intern Med.* 2011;155:JC6-2.

Chow, WB, Rosenthal, RA, Merkow, RP, Ko, CY, Esnaola, NF. *Optimal Preoperative Assessment of the Geriatric Surgical Patient: A Best Practices Guideline from the American College of Sugeons.* National Surgical Quality Improvement Program and the American Geriatrics Society. 2012. http://dx.doi.org/10.1016/j.jamcollsurg.2012.06.017.

Clark F, Azen SP, Zemke R, et al. Occupational therapy for independent-living older adults: a randomized controlled trial. *JAMA.* 1997;278:1321-1326.

Cohen HJ, Feussner JR, Weinberger M, et al. A controlled trial of inpatient and outpatient geriatric evaluation and management. *N Engl J Med.* 2002;346:905-912.

Ellis G, Whitehead MA, O'Neill D, Langhorne P, Robinson D. Comprehensive geriatric assessment for older adults admitted to hospital. *Cochrane Database Syst Rev.* 2011;7:CD006211.

Fleisher LA, Eagle KA. Clinical practice. Lowering cardiac risk in noncardiac surgery. *N Engl J Med.* 2001;345:1677-1682.

Geerts WH, Heit JA, Clagett GP, et al. Prevention of venous thromboembolism. *Chest.* 2001;119(Suppl 1):132S-175S.

Gill TM, Robinson JT, Tinetti ME. Difficulty and dependence: two components of the disability continuum among community-living older persons. *Ann Intern Med.* 1998;128:96-101.

Inouye SK, Peduzzi PN, Robinson JT, et al. Importance of functional measures in predicting mortality among older hospitalized patients. *JAMA.* 1998;279:1187-1193.

Kane RL, Kane RA, eds. *Assessing Older Persons: Measures, Meaning, and Practical Applications.* New York, NY: Oxford University Press; 2000.

Kane RL, Ouellette J. *The Good Caregiver.* New York, NY: Avery; 2011.

Kane RL, Shamliyan TA, McCarthy T. Do geriatric healthcare teams work? *Aging Health.* 2011;7(6):865-876.

Makary MA, Segev DL, Pronovost PJ, et al. Frailty as a predictor of surgical outcomes in older patients. *J Am Coll Surg.* 2010;210:901-908.

Medical Letter on Drugs and Therapeutics. Antimcrobial prophylaxis in surgery. *Med Lett.* 1999;41:75-80.

Moore AA, Siu AL. Screening for common problems in ambulatory elderly: clinical confirmation of a screening instrument. *Am J Med.* 1996;100:438-443.

National Institutes of Health. NIH Consensus Development Statement: geriatric assessment methods for clinical decision-making. *J Am Geriatr Soc.* 1988;36:342-347.

Pacala JT, Boult C, Reed RL, Aliberti E. Predictive validity of the Pra instrument among older recipients of managed care. *J Am Geriatr Soc.* 1997;45:614-617.

Reuben D, Siu A. An objective measure of physical function of elderly outpatients: The Physical Performance Test. *J Am Geriatr Soc.* 1990;38:1105-1112.

Reuben DB, Frank JC, Hirsch SH, McGuigan KA, Maly RC. A randomized clinical trial of outpatient comprehensive geriatric assessment coupled with an intervention to increase adherence to recommendations. *J Am Geriatr Soc.* 1999;47:269-276.

Robinson TN, Eiseman B, Wallace JI, et al. Redefining geriatric preoperative assessment using frailty, disability and co-morbidity. *Ann Surg.* 2009;250:449-455.

Rubenstein LZ, Harker JO, Salva A, Guigoz Y, Vellas B. Screening for undernutrition in geriatric practice: developing the Short-Form Mini-Nutritional Assessment (MNA-SF). *J Gerontol A Biol Sci Med Sci.* 2001;56:M366-M372.

Rudolph JL, Jones RN, Levkoff SE, et al. Derivation and validation of a preoperative prediction rule for delirium after cardiac surgery. *Circulation.* 2009;119:229-236.

Stuck AE, Egger M, Hammer A, Minder CE, Beck JC. Home visits to prevent nursing home admission and functional decline in elderly people: systematic review and meta-regression analysis. *JAMA.* 2002;287:1022-1028.

SUGGESTED READINGS

Applegate WB, Blass JP, Williams TF. Instruments for functional assessment of older patients. *N Engl J Med.* 1990;322:1207-1214.

Auerbach AD, Goldman L. Beta-blockers and reduction of cardiac events in noncardiac surgery: scientific review. *JAMA.* 2002;287:1435-1444.

Crum RM, Anthony SC, Bassett SS, et al. Population-based norms for the Mini-Mental State Examination by age and educational level. *JAMA.* 1993;269:2386-2391.

Feinstein AR, Josephy BR, Wells CK. Scientific and clinical problems in indexes of functional disability. *Ann Intern Med.* 1986;105:413-420.

Finch M, Kane RL, Philp I. Developing a new metric for ADLs. *J Am Geriatr Soc.* 1995;43:877-884.

Fleming KC, Evans JM, Weber DC, et al. Practical functional assessment of elderly persons: a primary-care approach. *Mayo Clin Proc.* 1995;70:890-910.

Folstein MF, Folstein S, McHuth PR. Mini-Mental State: a practical method for grading the cognitive state of patients for the clinician. *J Psychiatr Res.* 1975;12:189-198.

Gill TM, Feinstein AR. A critical appraisal of the quality of quality-of-life measurements. *JAMA*. 1994;272:619-626.

Guigoz Y, Vellas B, Garry PJ. Assessing the nutritional status of the elderly: the Mini Nutritional Assessment as part of the geriatric evaluation. *Nutr Rev*. 1996;54:S59-S65.

Katz S, Ford AB, Moskowitz RW, Jackson BA, Jaffe MW. Studies of illness in the aged. The Index of ADL: a standardized measure of biological and psychosocial function. *JAMA*. 1963;185:914-919.

Landefeld CS, Palmer RM, Kresevic DM, Fortinsky RH, Kowal J. A randomized trial of care in a hospital medical unit especially designed to improve the functional outcomes of acutely ill older patients. *N Engl J Med*. 1995;332:1338-1344.

Lee TH, Marcantonio ER, Mangione CM, et al. Derivation and prospective validation of a simple index for prediction of cardiac risk of major noncardiac surgery. *Circulation*. 1999;100:1043-1049.

Mangano DT, Goldman L. Preoperative assessment of patients with known or suspected coronary disease. *N Engl J Med*. 1995;333:1750-1756.

Palda VA, Detsky AS. Perioperative assessment and management of risk from coronary artery disease. *Ann Intern Med*. 1997;127:313-328.

Persson MD, Brismar KE, Katzarski KS, Nordenstrom J, Cederholm TE. Nutritional status using mini nutritional assessment and subjective global assessment predict mortality in geriatric patients. *J Am Geriatr Soc*. 2002;50:1996-2002.

Polanczyk CA, Marcantonio E, Goldman L, et al. Impact of age on perioperative complications and length of stay in patients undergoing noncardiac surgery. *Ann Intern Med*. 2001;134:637-643.

Reuben DB, Borok GM, Wolde-Tsadik G, et al. A randomized trial of comprehensive geriatric assessment in the care of hospital patients. *N Engl J Med*. 1995;332:1345-1350.

Reuben DB, Siu AL. An objective measure of physical function of elderly persons: the physical performance test. *J Am Geriatr Soc*. 1990;38:1105-1112.

Scheitel SM, Fleming KC, Chutka DS, et al. Geriatric health maintenance. *Mayo Clin Proc*. 1996;71:289-302.

Siu A. Screening for dementia and its causes. *Ann Intern Med*. 1991;115:122-132.

Williams ME, Hadler N, Earp JA. Manual ability as a mark of dependency in geriatric women. *J Chronic Dis*. 1987;40:481-489.

CHAPTER 4

Chronic Disease Management

Geriatrics' forte is chronic disease management (Kane et al, 2005). At a time when medical care in general is awakening to the importance of good chronic disease care, geriatrics has been doing it for years. Many of the principles of geriatrics are basically those of good chronic care. Chronic disease management has two basic components. The first aims at preventing catastrophes (ie, emergency room visits and hospitalizations) by proactively monitoring patients' conditions and intervening at the first sign of a change in the clinical course. Ideally these interventions prevent some hospitalizations, primarily by providing more effective primary care that prevents the event, but secondarily by managing crises, when they occur, without hospitalization. Figure 4-1, illustrates the paths to chronic disease catastrophe.

A growing shift in chronic disease, associated with enhanced survival and better care, is multimorbidity—the presence of multiple chronic diseases that can interact. The problems of managing chronic disease are vastly complicated by multimorbidity—a characteristic of many geriatric patients. Multimorbidity is associated with polypharmacy, which, in turn, can lead to iatrogenic complications.

Another aspect of managing chronic illness is palliative care. We tend to associate this type of care with end-of-life care, but its principles can be applied much more broadly.

Chronic disease management cannot be effectively accomplished without active central roles for patients and/or their caregivers. They live with this disease 24/7. They know its nuances. Patient-centered care has become a catchword—almost a cliché, but it lies at the heart of chronic care management.

Several models of chronic disease management have been promulgated. The popular Wagner model has spawned many variants; it envisions a productive interaction between an informed, activated patient (and caregiver) and a prepared, proactive practice team (Wagner et al, 1996). Unfortunately the current health-care system is poorly organized to facilitate such care. Fee-for-service payments, driven by in-person encounters, provide exactly the wrong climate for proactive care that uses modern communication technology to track patient status. The basic tenets of good chronic care are summarized in Table 4-1.

Elderly patients are in danger of being dismissed as hopeless or not worth the effort based on their age or their condition. Physicians faced with the question of how much time and resources to spend in searching for a diagnosis will undoubtedly consider the probability of benefit from the investment. Ironically, in some cases older patients are better investments than younger ones. This apparent paradox occurs in the case of some preventive strategies (eg, osteoporosis) when the high risk of susceptibility and the discounted benefits of future health favor older persons.

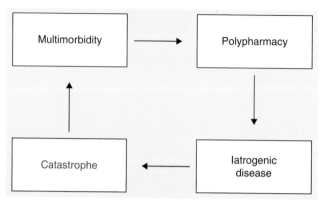

FIGURE 4-1 Paths to chronic disease catastrophe.

But it also arises in situations where small increments of change can yield dramatic differences.

Perhaps the most striking example of the latter is found in the case of nursing home patients. Ironically, very modest changes in their routine, such as introducing a pet, giving them a plant to tend, or increasing their sense of control over their environment, can produce dramatic improvements in mood and morale.

At the same time, the risk–benefit ratio is different with older patients. Treatments that might be easily tolerated in younger patients may pose a much greater risk of producing harmful effects in older patients with multiple chronic illnesses. As shown in Figure 4-2, the therapeutic window that separates benefit from harm is narrower. In effect, the dosage that will produce a positive effect more closely approaches one that can lead to a toxic effect. As noted earlier in this text, one of the hallmarks of aging is a loss of responsiveness to stress. In this context, treatment may be viewed as a stress.

Multimorbidity makes finding the sweet spot even harder. As shown in Figure 4-2, the therapeutic window becomes much smaller still in the presence of

TABLE 4-1. Chronic Care Tenets

Aggressive primary care

Proactive monitoring

Early intervention to avoid catastrophes

Patient-centeredness, meaningful patient involvement in the care process

Use of information technology to track outcomes and trigger reevaluation

Teamwork, delegation

Efficient use of time

Benefit assessment in terms of slowing decline

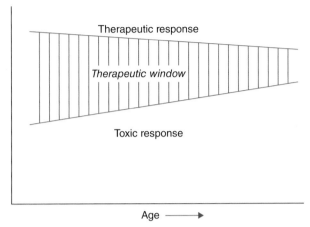

FIGURE 4-2 Narrowing of the therapeutic window. This diagram portrays in a conceptual manner how the space between a therapeutic dose and a toxic dose narrows with age.

multimorbidity because of the increased risks of disease–disease, drug–drug and drug–disease interactions.

Those who treat older patients must also consider the theory of competitive risks. Because older persons often suffer from multiple problems, treating one problem may provide an opportunity for more adverse effects from another. In essence, eliminating one cause of death increases the likelihood of death from other causes.

SYSTEM CHANGES

Professional roles need to be reexamined to look for opportunities to delegate to less expensive personnel, many tasks formerly performed by more trained professionals. For example, nurse practitioners have been shown to be capable of providing a good deal of primary care that was formerly the exclusive purview of physicians (Horrocks et al, 2002; Mundinger et al, 2000). New models of collaborative care seem promising (Callahan et al, 2006; Counsell et al, 2006).

The enthusiasm for teams needs to be tempered by an appreciation of the skills needed to work cooperatively and the willingness to delegate tasks (Kane et al, 2011).

Expectations must be recalibrated. The familiar dichotomy of care versus cure must be expanded to recognize the role of disease management. Because the natural course of chronic illness is deterioration, successful care must be defined as doing better than would be expected otherwise. This phenomenon is illustrated in Figure 4-3. The bold line represents the effects of good care. The dotted line represents the effects of the absence of such care. Both lines show decline over time. The difference between them represents the effects of good care. Most of the time, this contrast is invisible—all that is seen is decline despite the best efforts. Improving care

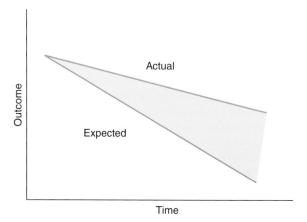

FIGURE 4-3 A conceptual model of the difference between expected and actual care. The heavier line represents what is usually observed in clinical chronic care. Despite good care, the patient's course deteriorates. The true benefit, represented by the area between the dark line and the dotted line, is invisible unless some means is found to display the expected course in the absence of good care. Such data could be developed based on clinical prognosis, or they could be derived from accumulated data once such a system is in place.

will require developing information systems that can contrast actual and expected clinical courses.

Appreciating this contrast is critical to both policy and morale. The importance of measuring success by comparing the actual clinical course to a generated expected course is central to concepts of quality in chronic disease. It is also important in maintaining the morale of workers in this field. People who see only decline despite their best efforts become discouraged (Lerner and Simmons, 1966). They need to appreciate the value of their care if they are to continue to give it in the face of so much frailty and disability. Slowing the rate of decline must be seen as positive achievement.

Likewise policymakers, and indeed the general public, are unlikely to support needed efforts to improve chronic care if they do not believe that such care can make a difference. They must be educated to appreciate and be given the information to demonstrate these differences.

A good question is where to begin. Several targets present themselves. Complex cases use up large amounts of resources and are worth the investment in better management. This is the heart of geriatrics. A particularly high-risk area is the hand-off. Any type of hand-off is associated with errors and problems, including discharge from one setting to another but even change of shift.

TRANSITIONAL CARE

Transitions from hospitals have been targeted for special attention because careful coordination and follow-up are associated with lower rates of rehospitalization and lower costs (Coleman et al, 2006; Hansen et al, 2011; Naylor et al, 1994).

Currently, discharges and other times when care is transferred represent danger zones. There is great concern about the high rate of rehospitalization, which represents signs of care failure and adds to the costs of care. Medicare provides special payment for transition activities and imposes penalties if readmission rates are high. When medical regimens are changed, the relevant information may be poorly communicated (both between clinicians and with patients and families). Transitional care consists of a set of specific actions.

1. Prior to discharge, a "coach" (who need not be a health professional) meets with the patient and her family to establish a rapport and assist with discharge planning.
2. The coach meets with the patient soon after discharge to be sure she understands the discharge plan and is comfortable with her medication regimen and any other instructions.
3. The coach stays in close contact during the ensuing period to make sure things are going well.
4. The patient's primary care physician is urged to get involved soon after discharge and gets all relevant information.

END-OF-LIFE CARE

Eliminating excessive, futile, or unnecessary care and attention to preventing iatrogenic events can improve care and save money. Two ready targets are medications and end-of-life care, including palliative care. Medication management in geriatric patients is discussed in detail in Chapter 14. In addition to the section that follows, end-of-life care is discussed in Chapters 17 and 18.

A heavily touted tool for avoiding futile care is advance directives (ADs), whereby patients indicate their preferences for care in cases where they can no longer communicate them. One may question the logic of spending so much effort assessing preferences intended to be used only if the patient is comatose. Equal or greater attention should be directed to helping those who are in a position to make these serious clinical decisions. Eliciting advance care preferences about unexperienced future states requires people to imagine what life would be like in various states of disability. Research shows that these horrible imaginings are much bleaker than the actual experience of people in those states. Since ADs may exaggerate fears of disability and are operational for only noncommunicative patients, it may be more useful to think of AD discussions as rehearsals for making actual end-of-life decisions.

The physician's concern with the patient's functioning continues throughout the course of the chronic disease. Elderly patients will die. In many cases, death is not a reflection of medical failure. The approach to the dying patient will often raise difficult dilemmas for which no simple answers suffice. Too often the dying patient is treated as an object—ignored and isolated, the patient may be discussed in the third person.

Physicians who treat elderly patients must come to terms with death. Often the patients are more comfortable with the subject than are their physicians (and their families). Fleeing from the dying patient is inexcusable; they need their doctors. At a very basic level, everything should be done to keep the patient as comfortable as possible. One simple step is to identify the pattern of discomforting symptoms and arrange the dosage schedule of palliatives to prevent rather than respond to the symptoms.

Patients need an opportunity to talk about their death. Not everyone will take advantage of that chance, but a surprising number will respond to a genuine offer made without time pressure. Such discussions are not conducted on the run. Often several invitations accompanied by appropriate behavior (eg, sitting down at the bedside) are necessary.

Some physicians are unable to confront this aspect of practice. For them, the challenge is to recognize their own behavior and get appropriate help. Such help is available at various levels: help for the physician and for the patient. Groups and therapy are readily available to assist doctors to deal with their feelings. Patients of doctors who fear death need the help of other caregivers. Often other professionals (nurses, social workers) who are working with these patients already can play the lead role in helping them work through their feelings. But the active intervention of another caregiver is not a justification to ignore the patient.

The rise of the hospice movement has created a growing cadre of persons and settings to help patients at the end of life. The lessons coming from this experience suggest that much can be done to facilitate this stage of life. Participant families express great appreciation for such care, although the formal studies done to evaluate hospice care do not show dramatic benefits. One problem that delays taking up the hospice option is essentially admitting the imminence of death. Typically hospice care is used only in the last days of life.

Patients should be encouraged to be as active as possible and as interactive as they wish. Even more than in other aspects of care, the unique condition of the dying patient necessitates that the physician be prepared to listen carefully to the patient and to share decision making about how and when to do things.

Medical care has evolved in such a way that special exemptions are made for the period at the end of life. Hospice care was created to reverse the overuse of technology and denial of dying (see Chapter 18). It can be viewed as both a success and a failure. On the one hand, it is still probably used too little and too late, only after more drastic measures have been tried. At the same time, it has led to serious reconsideration of how medicine handles the process of dying. It has spawned the concept of palliative care, an idea that many aspects of support and comfort can be applied coincident with active treatment (Morrison and Meier, 2004). It has forced a reassessment of how pain is managed, with more attention to proactive treatment in adequate doses. Palliative care is discussed in detail in Chapter 18.

SPECIAL ISSUES IN CHRONIC DISEASE MANAGEMENT

CLINICAL GLIDEPATHS

A primary goal of chronic disease management is catastrophe avoidance. Chronic care requires proactive primary care supported by better data systems. The whole approach to care needs to be rethought. Much of current practice norms are based on systems strongly influenced by payment. Doctors are paid when they have direct contact with patients, not for activities like telephone counseling. Hence, much care is delivered in person as a result of return appointments made less on knowledge of clinical trajectories than on traditional intervals. Imagine what could be accomplished if all that time were reprogrammed to encourage meaningful encounters when a change in the patient's status warranted it. The idea of scheduled revisits needs to be replaced with a system of ongoing monitoring and interventions when there is a significant change in the patient's condition. Information technology is probably the most important technological breakthrough for chronic care.

Structuring data helps focus the clinician's attention on what is most relevant. The goal of a good information system should be to present clinicians with pertinent information at the right time in the form that will capture their attention. Identifying what is salient at the moment is critical, especially in view of the brief contact times allowed. Too much information can be as dysfunctional as too little, because the pertinent facts get lost in a sea of data.

Providing effective chronic care that avoids catastrophes relies on a longitudinally oriented information system that is sensitive to change. Each clinical encounter with a chronically ill patient is essentially part of a continuing episode of care; it has a history and a future. Caring for a chronically ill patient, especially one with multiple problems, demands an enormous feat of memory as the patient's list of problems is unearthed and the history, treatments, and expectations associated with each are reviewed. Clinicians caring for such patients (often under enormous time pressures) may find themselves either overwhelmed with large volumes of data from which they must quickly extract the most salient facts or, alternatively, relying on inadequate data from which to reconstruct the patient's clinical course. Moreover, because patients live with their disease 24 hours a day, 7 days a week, they are best positioned to make regular observations about its progress. Such patient-constructive involvement responds to another principle of chronic care. These goals can be achieved using a simple information system that can focus the clinician's attention on salient parameters.

One approach to organizing clinical information and actively involving patients in their own care is the clinical glidepath. The underlying concept is based on landing an airplane. Basically, the goal is to keep the patient within the expected trajectory to avoid the need for dramatic midcourse corrections. An expected clinical course (with provision for confidence intervals) is created. Ideally this clinical trajectory would be derived from a large statistical database that shows how similar patients have done previously. However, in the absence of such a database, the expected clinical path can be based on the clinician's experience and intuition. A separate glidepath is used for each chronic problem. For each condition, the clinician selects one (or at the most two) clinical parameter(s) to track. Ideally the parameter should reflect how the problem manifests in that patient. It can be a sign or a symptom, or even a laboratory value. The data on this parameter are collected regularly, several times a week or even daily. In most cases, the patients can provide the information, having been taught to make careful, consistent observations. These are recorded on the equivalent of flow sheets, which can be entered into a computer program that produces a graphic display. The key to this monitoring is the early warning. Observations falling outside the confidence intervals prompt strong exception messages. Any pattern of deviation is the cue for action and early intervention to assess the patient's condition and to take appropriate action. These cases should be seen quickly and with enough time to evaluate the reasons for the changes in status. Figure 4-4, shows a hypothetical example of such a clinical glidepath. The patient's progress (marked with *o*'s) is within the confidence interval (which indicates a path of gradual decline) until the

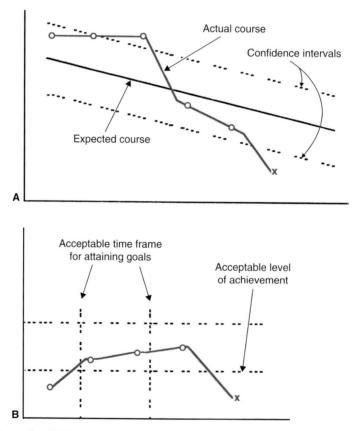

FIGURE 4-4 Clinical glidepath models. (**A**) In this model, the expected course (solid line) calls for gradual decline. The confidence intervals are shown as dotted lines. Actual measures that are within or better than the glidepath are shown as *o*'s. When the patient's course is worse than expected, the *o* changes to an *x*. The design shown uses confidence intervals with upper and lower bounds, but actually only the lower bound is pertinent. Any performance above the upper confidence interval boundary is very acceptable. (**B**) The design of the glidepath can also take another form. It may be preferable to think in terms of reaching a threshold level within a given time window (eg, in recuperating from an illness) and then maintaining that level.

last observation (noted with an x, which falls outside the confidence interval and hence should trigger a warning).

Patients (or their caregivers) can be trained to make systematic observations about salient clinical parameters and to report meaningful changes (determined by established protocols) to their clinicians. Even better, they can enter such observations into a simple computerized data system that has been programmed to notify clinicians when the patterns exceed predetermined algorithms. Devices are available that automatically enter the data (such as self-reporting scales and sphygmomanometers), but patient involvement can be maximized by having them enter the data. In most instances nothing is done at data entry; routine data (which indicate the patient is staying on the trajectory) are not actionable, only meaningful changes.

The clinician's task is then to evaluate the meaning of such a change, when it occurs. The patient should be seen quickly (either by a physician or another clinician) to have the findings analyzed. The basic approach addresses three questions:

1. Are the data accurate? Has there been a real change?
2. Has the patient adhered to his or her prescribed regimen?
3. Has there been an intervening event (eg, infection, change in diet)?

The change really occurred; if the patient was following her regimen, and there is no obvious explanation for the change, then a full assessment is warranted to determine the reason for the deviation.

The glidepath approach meets several needs for chronic care. (1) It helps focus physicians' attention on salient parameters. It provides an indication of early problems in time to make midcourse corrections. (2) It provides a means to involve patients more actively in their care. They learn about what is important and assume greater responsibility. (3) It is a basis for reapportioning time and effort to focus attention where an intervention is likely to produce a greater impact. Ideally, clinicians would stop making blanket return appointments, and instead track conditions and intervene when the circumstances change.

It is important to distinguish the clinical glidepath approach from clinical pathways approach. The latter specifies an expected course with specific milestones and dictate what care should be provided at specific junctures. It can be useful for both clinicians and families by indicating what to expect and when it is necessary to address exceptions. This approach works well in very predictable situations such as postoperative recovery and even some instances of rehabilitation, but most of chronic care management is not as predictable. The glidepath method specifies what data should be collected, not what actions should be taken. Its underlying premise holds that when clinicians can be aided in focusing their attention on a patient's salient parameters, they will be able to manage the chronic problems better.

TARGETING AND TRACKING

Case management, which is used to target interventions and monitor outcomes, has received a lot of attention, although its efficacy has yet to be established. One of the problems in assessing the benefits of case management has been the multiple ways the term has been used. (For a discussion of case management, see Chapter 15.) The effectiveness of care management (by whatever name) depends on its level of integration with ongoing primary care. It is not effective when it is simply grafted on.

Focusing attention on the management of specific problems has become a consistent theme in the effort to improve the management of chronic illness. *Disease management* is most commonly used by health plans, which use the available administrative data from encounters, drug records, and laboratory tests to identify all enrollees with a given condition. Protocols can then be applied to look for errors of both omission and commission. In some cases, potential complications can be flagged and checks built in to try to avoid untoward events such as drug interactions.

A more active approach to disease management uses *case managers* for patients who are determined to need special attention, either because they have a diagnosis that suggests high risk of subsequent use or their history indicates problems in controlling their disease(s). These case managers work with the patients to be sure that they understand their regimens. They encourage the patients to raise any questions early. They telephonically monitor the course of the illness using parameters like those described earlier. They may make home visits to ascertain how the patients are doing and to ensure that they can function effectively in their natural habitats. The positive reports from trials of this approach have encouraged many replications.

Another variation on disease management being practiced in a few managed care organizations is *group care*. Here patients with a given disease (sometimes a more heterogeneous cluster of patients is assembled) are brought together for periodic sessions that include health education and group support, as well as individual clinical attention. It has proven more efficient to use groups in this way. The same sessions can draw upon specialists to see problematic cases more efficiently.

Particularly in the context of managed care, there is a strong incentive to try to identify high-risk patients in order to attend to them before they develop into high-cost cases. Various predictive models have been developed to identify such cases. One widely used model is the Probability of Repeated Admissions (Pra). (See Chapter 3.) This tool uses an eight-item questionnaire to flag older patients who are most likely to have two or more hospital admissions in the next several years (Boult et al, 1993). A modification of this method has been developed to use administrative databases as well. A similar approach is being developed to identify those at high risk for needing long-term care (LTC). Once these patients have been targeted, an intervention is needed to change the predicted course. The Pra model does not specify what actions should be taken; it was initially developed as a method for identifying those in need of a comprehensive geriatric examination.

Other efforts have sought to target high-risk groups (Yourman et al, 2012). An analysis of the Medicare Current Beneficiary Survey identified the Vulnerable Elders-13 tool that can identify older persons at risk of death or functional decline (Min et al, 2009). Another index can identify older adults who have an increased risk of death 1 year after hospitalization (Walter et al, 2001). Changes in Medicare reimbursement have focused attention on 30-day hospital readmissions. Identifying predictors of 30-day readmissions other than a recent hospitalization has proven challenging (Kansagara et al, 2011). A team at the University of California, San Francisco has developed a simple tool to inform clinicians about mortality outcomes—ePrognosis (http://eprognosis.ucsf.edu/about.php).

Interventions have also been developed to address those at highest risk. Compressive geriatric assessment has been shown to improve survival and prolong living at home (Barer, 2011; Ellis et al, 2011). Some interventions seem surprisingly effective. Home visits to basically well older persons can prevent nursing home admissions and functional decline (Stuck et al, 2002). Likewise an in-home visit by an occupational therapist was associated with improved health, function, and quality of life (Clark et al, 1997). No single intervention has strong evidence for its effectiveness in reducing 30-day hospital readmissions (Hansen et al, 2011). Given the complexity of patients with multiple chronic diseases and the multiple factors that contribute to the decision to hospitalize them, multicomponent interventions will be needed to reduce preventable hospital admissions and readmissions in this population. Addressing underlying depression can reduce hospitalization rates for older adults receiving home health care (Bruce et al, 2016).

Major investments in coordinated care have shown an ability to alter clinical trajectories, although the economic case for such approaches is not yet clear (Counsell et al, 2006). Function has proven to be an important predictive risk factor for both subsequent use of expensive services and outcomes in general. Poor functional status in hospital patients predicts later mortality over and above the effects of burden-of-illness measures. The concept of functional deficit has been extended to frailty, a condition defined by fatigue, slow walking, sarcopenia, decreased muscle strength, and low physical activity (Fried et al, 2001); it is associated with high susceptibility to disease. (Frailty is addressed in more detail in Chapter 1.)

CAREGIVING

Informal (unpaid) caregivers are central to chronic disease management (Kane and Ouellette, 2011). Clinicians should recognize that caregivers are important allies. In essence they are the boots on the ground of the caregiving movement. They are closest to the person receiving care and are in a position to make useful observations about what is happening to make sure that medical instructions are carried out as intended. Family caregivers' knowledge, well-being, and sustained engagement with health-care providers are critical. Clinicians need to meaningfully involve them and address their questions. Caregiving is discussed at greater length in Chapter 15.

TEAMS

Talk of comprehensive care inevitably turns to teams. Different disciplines can bring to bear specific skills and knowledge, but to be effective and efficient this feat must be accomplished in a coordinated fashion. While team care has been hailed as a central element in managing chronic diseases, the evidence to buttress that enthusiasm is less clear than many believe.

Team care is inherently expensive and its effectiveness, to say nothing of its efficiency, is not yet well established. Nor is it always clear what people mean when they talk about team care. What does it take to be a team? What makes a successful team? Enthusiasts agree that creating good teamwork takes work. Most suggest training and regular practice are prerequisites for success. Many favor regular meetings to discuss cases and exchange perspectives, but such a high level of preparation and maintenance can be very expensive. The question is whether the product of team care justifies such a large investment.

Health-care teams vary widely in their composition and function. In some cases, a second discipline is added to an existing practice to complement the physician, usually on the premise that the best way to change physician behavior is to give the task to someone else. The most common pairings have been with case managers, who assume responsibility for managing a specific problem, and pharmacists, who review and improve drug management. In other cases there is a full commitment to integrating care across an interdisciplinary group. Discussions of team effectiveness must recognize this variation.

Likewise, team care will have different levels of effectiveness on different types of problems. The best success story of case management has been around care for depression. Several models have evolved to combine mental health and medical care in this area (Kane, Shamliyan, McCarthy, 2011). All have in common a case manager who undertakes active care of persons with depression. Although numerous studies suggest improvements in clinical depression, emerging evidence also suggests improvements in managing medical conditions among patients with depression. Other aspects of the team process may vary. An analysis of the effects of varying team attributes for treating depression suggests that the intensity of these other components is not associated with better outcomes (Kane, Shamliyan, McCarthy, 2011). Given the centrality of drug therapy and the multiple opportunities for mischief, it is hardly surprising that adding a pharmacist to a physician's practice or in other settings is generally associated with improved care and fewer adverse consequences (Bruce, Lohman, Greenberg, 2016).

The structure of teams varies. Table 4-2 offers a taxonomy of team types. As shown, team members may simply work in parallel, staying within their professional roles, or they may create an integrated workgroup where hierarchies have been eliminated, with many stops in between. Some observers have tried to distinguish collaboration from coordination, although the distinction may be subtle and in some instances the actual name applied reflects the opposite approach. Much is made of the distinction between multidisciplinary and interdisciplinary; it seems to come down to the extent to which the specific disciplinary roles are preserved, as opposed to allowing various team members to perform similar functions depending on circumstances.

In the end, the key issue is whether team members can accept having some of their traditional tasks performed by others. In practice it is not often easy to discern precisely what level of coordination is in play or how much of the traditional medical hierarchy has been suspended.

TABLE 4-2. Team Models

Team Characteristic	Definition
Parallel	Practitioners work in the same setting, but independently. Roles are formally defined within one's clinical scope of practice.
Consultative	Expert advice is shared between practitioners via personal contact, letter, or referral note.
Collaborative	Patient is seen independently by each practitioner. Practitioners informally share information concerning the treatment of a particular patient on a case-by-case basis.
Coordinated	Administrative structure stimulates collaboration. Patients' files are shared among practitioners. Liaison among practitioners is ensured by a manager/coordinator.
Multidisciplinary	A leader is in charge of the planning of patient care. Each practitioner carries out treatment independently, according to his or her expertise. Formalized extension of the coordinated model.
Interdisciplinary	Planning of patient care is decided by a group of practitioners, via regular face-to-face meetings. It is an extension of the multidisciplinary model.
Integrative	Involves nonhierarchical holistic collaboration of practitioners. Practitioners and patient contribute to patient care. It is an extension of the interdisciplinary model.

Modified with permission from Gaboury I, Boon H, Verhoef M, et al: Practitioners' validation of framework of team-oriented practice models in integrative health care: a mixed methods study, *BMC Health Serv Res.* 2010 Oct 14;10:289.

As shown in Table-4-3, teams come in various types. The composition is more modal than mandatory.

The enthusiasm for team care will continue to grow as the number of primary care physicians declines. If teams are to survive, they need to be both more effective and more efficient. Communication cannot be done through expensive, time-consuming meetings; ways to facilitate better communication among team members are essential. Structured information systems may offer a vehicle for more efficient communication. Increasing efficiency will also depend on clear roles and responsibilities. Duplication of effort must be avoided. It is important to distinguish what is done from who does it. For example, in the case of assessments, many disciplines can contribute items, but a single person should be able to collect the data, at least in the initial evaluation phase. The emerging electronic medical records systems could play a role in facilitating communication if they are properly designed, but too many are structured to reproduce traditional modes of data recording.

TABLE 4-3. Team Composition

Target	Composition
Disability, frailty, geriatric conditions	Primary care physician and geriatrician, geriatric nurse, clinical psychologist, psychiatrist, social worker, caregiver, dietitian.
Chronic diseases/ multimorbidity	Primary care physician, geriatrician, nurse, clinical pharmacist, physiotherapist, occupational therapist, social worker, rehabilitation physician.
Depression	Case manager, mental health consultant added to primary care; may include training for primary care.
Medication management	Pharmacist added to primary care role.
Stroke	Physical therapist, occupational therapist, speech pathologist, nurse, dietitian, physician (specialist and/or primary care).
Blood pressure	Pharmacist, primary care physician, sometimes a nurse.
Congestive heart failure	Team composition varies. Cardiologist and nurse team is the most common; may also include primary care physician, physical therapist, dietitian or pharmacist.
Diabetes	Team composition varies. A physician (primary or specialist) and nurse are core; dietitian or community worker may be added or substituted for the nurse.

Data from Kane RL and Ouellette J. The Good Caregiver. New York: Avery; 2011.

DECISION MAKING

Chronic care implies making a variety of decisions along the course of the disease. As the situations change these decisions will need to be reevaluated. Some of the decisions will be made every day such as the following: Is the treatment working? Which treatment is best? Is it time to try a new treatment? Other decisions will be made in times of crisis like when leaving the hospital; these questions may include: Where should the person living with dementia go when they are discharged from the hospital? Can the family continue to keep the person living with dementia at home? Should they try to do this? Some decisions will address plans and preferences for care at the end of life and include: Is this what the older person wants? How does the caregiver feel about this?

There are a few principles of decision making to bear in mind. Decisions about medical care should be made by the older person, his or her caregivers, and other relevant parties including primary care providers working together to consider all options and decide on the preferred option. The doctor provides information about the pros and cons of possible treatments and the family and the older person choose a course of action, taking into account that information and the values and preferences of the person living with dementia. Whenever possible the older person should play a central role in making decisions. As the disease progresses, decisions need to be continuously reassessed and possibly changed. This process should not be hurried. It may take several days, and in some cases even weeks, to make each decision.

A widely favored approach to such decision making is shared decision making. Shared decision making is a collaborative process that allows older persons, their caregivers and family, and their doctors to make health-care decisions together, taking into account the best scientific evidence available as well as the values and preferences of the older person. This process provides older persons with the support they need to make the best individualized care decisions, while allowing the clinicians to feel confident in the care they prescribe. For more information see www.informed-medicaldecisions.org/what-is-shared-decision-making/.

Hospitalization of an older person is never easy. Planning for discharge from that hospital can truly be a crisis. Hospital discharge is complicated, not the least because caregivers and families are often required to make complex, emotionally laden decisions about future care and placement very quickly. One way to help reduce this time pressure is to start discussions about postdischarge care as early as possible in the hospital stay. Getting discharge planners to start discussions early on can help, but it is important to appreciate that such planners are hospital employees responsible first to the institution. They are not necessarily advocates of the patients or their families. Medicaid clients typically have some kind of case manager assigned to them. For those paying privately, it may be worth the cost to consider hiring a knowledgeable case manager who can serve as an advocate.

The event that led to the hospitalization and the treatment in the hospital may have changed the health status of the older person. Hospital discharge planners, who are typically tasked with discharging the patient as quickly as possible, may not be the best source for good discharge decisions.

Clinicians may find themselves in an uncomfortable situation. They are both part of the hospital and at the same time advocates for the patients and their families. If they feel they cannot fully represent the patient, they should take active steps to be sure the patients and their families have a competent advocate. That person is not the discharge planner, who has a strong loyalty to the hospital.

We propose a two-stage decision-making process. Each stage involves a different aspect and uses different criteria. The process is summarized in Table 4-4.

Determining the type of care that will match the overarching goals of the older adult and the family may not happen quickly. Time must be found to bring the family

---

TABLE 4-4. The Two-Step Discharge Decision-Making Process
- Step 1: Determining the type of care that will meet goals of the older person and family
  - Bringing everyone together to determine care
- Step 2: Identifying the best vendor for the new services
  - Visiting potential vendors
  - Putting services into place

Data from Kane RL and Ouellette J: *The Good Caregiver.* New York: Avery; 2011.

together to resolve conflicts. The best type of care for the older person may differ from what is the best type of care for the family. An important but rarely discussed factor is the question of risk aversion. When they think about options, different family members may have very different levels of tolerance for the risks they are comfortable seeing the person living with dementia take. Some options for care (such as living alone) may be considered unsafe by some parties, and hence prematurely removed from consideration. One way to make these differences more explicit (as the first step in addressing them) is to ask each participant (family members and the older person) to complete a simple assessment of their tolerance of older people taking risks. The questions are designed to provoke discussion. Family members should compare their answers and use the differences as the basis for discussing this important but generally neglected issue. They should talk about why each person feels the way he or she does. Although family members may never agree altogether, at least they will understand each other's positions better. More detailed information about decision making and tools to help can be found in the book *The Good Caregiver* (Kane and Ouellette, 2011).

Once the type of care is agreed on, it is necessary to identify who can best provide that service. Those criteria may involve looking at the quality of the services provided but will also be heavily influenced by the availability of the service. If the older person is returning home, new services may need to be put in place in the home. If the choice is for placement in a nursing home or assisted living facility, having an open bed when it is needed will be critical. In choosing the best vendor, families need to visit potential providers to see firsthand what the care looks like. All of this takes time. It may be useful to think of the discharge planning decision process as having two distinct steps. The first step involves deciding what type of care is most likely to achieve the goals that have been set. Only then would you go to the second step of deciding who is the best vendor to provide the desired service. Separating the decision making in this way allows for applying different criteria for each step.

The following aspects of good decision making should be kept in mind:

- Good decision making is crucial for chronic disease management.
- Decisions cannot always be predicted or prepared for.
- Decisions need to be revisited as the older person's condition changes or the caregiving circumstances change.
- Using a shared decision approach can reduce stress.
- Proper decision making requires sharing information about goals, options, and consequences.
- Families should seek outside help in making the most informed decisions.
- Making good decisions often takes substantial time.

CULTURAL COMPETENCE

Caregivers come from an array of cultures. Their heritage and language preferences can affect their help-seeking behaviors and access to care. More is known about African Americans, Hispanics, and Chinese Americans than about subgroups like the LGBT (lesbian, gay, bisexual, and transgender) community, American Indians, and Hawaiian native populations. Cultural tailoring requires substantial insight into a culture. If you feel unprepared to deal with people from another culture, try to find someone from that culture to help you avoid major gaffes.

ROLE OF OUTCOMES IN ENSURING QUALITY OF CHRONIC CARE

Quality of care remains a critical, if elusive, goal for chronic care. As we consider steps for resource allocation, we might first address the question of whether we are spending our current funds most wisely. There is at once a growing demand for more creativity and more accountability in care. It may be possible to reduce the regulatory burden, increase the meaningful accountability, and make the incentives within the system more rational. Progress in chronic care will require not only more innovation and creativity, but also accountability. Outcome monitoring (and ultimately outcome-based rewards) allows both to coexist.

Before we can talk about how to package care or how to buy it cheaper, we need a better understanding of what we are really buying. One hears more and more about the value of shifting attention from the process of care to the actual outcomes achieved in chronic care.

Two basic concepts must be kept in mind when discussing outcomes:

1. The term *outcomes* is used to mean the relationship between what is achieved and what is expected.
2. Because outcomes rely on probabilities, it is inappropriate to base assessments of outcomes on an individual case. Outcomes are averages and are always judged on the basis of group data.

Table 4-5 summarizes the reasons for looking toward outcomes as the way to assess and ensure quality.

Nonetheless, clinicians frequently balk at being judged based on outcomes. This discomfort can be traced to several issues.

1. Virtually all of clinical training addresses the process of care. Clinicians are schooled in what to do for whom. They reasonably believe, therefore, that if they do the right thing well, they have provided a quality service. They do not like to discuss clusters of patients, preferring to review their care one patient at a time.
2. Many factors can affect the outcomes of care that are out of the clinicians' control. They have difficulty with the concept of probability and prefer to either be responsible or not.
3. Outcomes are by their nature post hoc. Often, a long period can elapse between the time the action occurs and the report of its success. It is thus too late to intervene in that case.
4. Outcomes indicate a problem but offer no solution. Outcomes do not often point to specific actions that must be taken to correct the problems.

Hence, introducing outcomes, however rational, has not been easy. Making clinicians comfortable with the outcomes philosophy will require substantial training and new incentives. Physicians need to be trained to think in terms of both condition-specific and generic outcomes. They need access to data systems that can display the outcomes

TABLE 4-5. Rationale for Using Outcomes

1. Outcomes encourage creativity by avoiding domination by current professional orthodoxies or powerful constituencies.
2. Outcomes permit flexibility in the modality of care.
3. Outcomes permit comparisons of efficacy across modalities of care.
4. Outcomes permit more flexible responses to different levels of performance, and thus avoid the "all-or-none" difficulties of many sanctions. At the same time, outcomes have some limitations.
5. Outcomes necessitate a single point of accountability; all the actors—facility operators, agencies, staff, physicians, patients, and family—contribute to them. Under this approach the role of the provider includes motivating others.
6. Outcomes are largely influenced by the patient's status at the beginning of treatment. The easiest and most direct way to address this issue is to think of the relationship between achieved and expected outcomes as the measure of success.
7. Outcomes must also be cognizant of case mix. Predicting outcomes necessitates information about disease characteristics (eg, diagnosis, severity, comorbidity) and patient characteristics (eg, demographic factors, prior history, social support).

of their care for clinically relevant groups of patients under their care and compare them with what are reasonable outcomes for comparable patients receiving good care. Table 4-6 summarizes the key issues in outcomes measurement and its applications.

Outcomes should be used as the basis for quality assurance in LTC. The outcomes approach can be used in several ways.

1. Outcome measures can be substituted for most of the current structure and process measures. It is appropriate to continue regulation in areas such as life safety. Concomitant with an outcomes emphasis would be the reduction of regulatory burden. It is important to recognize, however, that it is not appropriate to dictate structure, process, and outcome at the same time. Such a policy removes all degrees of freedom and stifles creativity at the point when we want to encourage it. Under an outcome-regulated approach, providers whose patients do better than expected are rewarded and are less worried about their style of caregiving, whereas those whose patients do relatively poorly are investigated more closely.

2. Outcomes can be incorporated into the payment structure to link payment with effects of care, but the outcomes must be adjusted to recognize differences in case mix. Payments, either in the form of bonuses and penalties or as a more fundamental part of the payment structure, can be used to reward and penalize good and bad outcomes, respectively (eg, an outcomes approach might use a factor reflecting the overall achieved–expected ratio for a patient as a multiplier against the costs of care to develop a total price paid for that period of time; or one might use a similar ratio to weigh the amount of money going to a given provider from a fixed pool of dollars committed to such care). Such an approach must be viewed carefully within the context of our present case-mix reimbursement (such as that used in nursing homes), because the latter

TABLE 4-6. Outcomes Measurement Issues

Issue	Comments
Need outcome measures that are both clinically meaningful and psychometrically sound	Use combination of condition-specific and generic measures. Usually better to adapt extant measures than to develop measures de novo.
Outcomes are always post hoc	Expand outcomes information systems to include data on risk factors. These data should be useful in guiding clinicians to collect information that will identify potential problems. Use these data to create risk warnings to flag high-risk cases.
Every physician has all the tough cases	Need to include a wide variety of case-mix adjusters for severity and comorbidity. Ask clinicians in advance to identify potential risk adjusters. Collect almost any item that a clinician might want to see. Test the ability of the potential risk factor to predict outcomes and discard if it has little predictive power.
Because no two clinicians see the same cases, comparisons are unfair	Use risk adjustment to create clinically homogeneous subgroups; use risk propensities to create groups of patients with same a priori likelihood of developing the outcome.
Cannot control for selection bias; patients may receive different treatments because of subtle differences	Adjust for all clinically identifiable differences. Use statistical methods (eg, instrumental variables) to adjust for unmeasured differences.

indirectly rewards deterioration in function. An outcomes approach to payment is compatible with a case-mix approach that is used at intake.

3. An outcomes approach can be incorporated into the basic caring process. Where the information base used in assessing patients and developing care plans is structured, the emphasis on outcomes can become a proactive force to guide care. Optimally, the information used to assess outcomes will come from the clinical records and will be the same information used to guide care. Using available computer technology, it is now feasible to collect such data, translate them into care plans, and aggregate these data for quality assurance at minimal additional cost. The great advantage of such a scheme is its potential both to provide a better information base with which to plan care and to reinforce the creative use of such information to achieve improvements in function. Much of the current efforts going into more traditional regulatory activities might be redirected to this effort, with assessors used to validate the assessment and to focus more intense efforts on the miscreants.

TABLE 4-7. Geriatric Outcome Categories

- Physiological function (eg, blood pressure control, lack of decubitus)
- Functional status (usually a measure of activities of daily living [ADLs])
- Pain and discomfort
- Cognition (intellectual activity)
- Affect (emotional activity)
- Social participation (based on preferences)
- Social relations (at least one person who can act as a confidant)
- Satisfaction (with care and living environment)
- Global outcomes, such as death and admission to hospital

We have generally good consensus on the components of outcomes, which include elements of both quality of care and quality of life, but we are less clear about how to sum them to produce composite scores. Outcome categories are listed in Table 4-7.

Current work has shown reasonable consensus across a variety of constituencies about the relative weights to be placed on them for different kinds of patients (eg, different levels of physical and cognitive function at baseline).

The outcomes approach offers significant assistance with a recurrent problem in regulation—the development of standards. This approach may avoid many of these difficulties by relying on empirical standards. Rather than arguing about what is a reasonable expectation, the standard can be empirically determined. Expectations can be derived from the actual outcomes associated with real care given by those felt to represent a reasonable level of practice. This could include the entire field or a designated subset. Under this arrangement, providers would be comparing their achievements to each other's past records, with the possibility that everyone can do better.

TECHNOLOGY FOR QUALITY IMPROVEMENT

Ideally, one would like to see a measurement approach that:

- Can cover the spectrum of performance
- Is easy and rapid to administer
- Is sensitive to meaningful change in performance
- Is stable within the same patient over time when the patient has been clinically stable
- Performs consistently in different hands
- Cannot be manipulated to meet the needs of either the provider or the patient

The solution to this challenge is to create an assessment approach that incorporates the features designed to maximize these elements. To cover the broad spectrum sought and still be relatively quickly administered, an instrument should have multiple branch points. These permit the user to focus on the area along the continuum where the patient is most likely to function and to expand that part of the scale to measure meaningful levels of performance. Branching can also ensure that the assessment is comprehensive but not burdensome.

By using key questions to screen an area, interviewers can ascertain whether to obtain more detailed information in each relevant domain. Where the initial response is negative, they can go on to the next branch point. Reliability is more likely to be achieved when the items are expressed in a standardized fashion tied closely to explicit behaviors. Whenever possible, performance is preferred over reports of behavior.

One cannot expect to totally avoid the gaming of an assessment. If the patient knows that poor performance is needed to ensure eligibility, he or she may be motivated to achieve the requisite low level. One can use some test of reporting bias, such as measures of social desirability, but they will not prevent gaming the system or detect all cheating.

VARIATION

One way to think about quality is to start by recognizing the geographic variation in practice. Geographic variation has been shown to be particularly prevalent for health services that can be considered *discretionary* because there is no consensus and, hence, more than one medically reasonable option (Wennberg, 2011). Variation reflects how clinicians view what they do.

- *Effective care* is defined as interventions for which the benefits far outweigh the risks; in this case the "right" rate of treatment is 100% of patients defined by evidence-based guidelines to be in need, and unwarranted variation is generally a matter of underuse.
- *Preference-sensitive care* is when more than one generally accepted treatment option is available, such as elective surgery; here, the right rate should depend on informed patient choice, but treatment rates can vary extensively because of differences in professional opinion.
- *Supply-sensitive care* comprises clinical activities such as doctor visits, diagnostic tests, and hospital admissions, for which the frequency of use relates to the capacity of the local health-care system.

In an effort to address this variation, medical societies have identified aspects of practice that are considered poor care. These practices have been identified under a program called *Choosing Wisely*. Table 4-8 summarizes the recommendations from the American Geriatrics Society and the American College of Physicians (which represents internal medicine).

COMPUTER TECHNOLOGY

Clinical medicine is becoming reliant on electronic medical records. This transition has met with mixed enthusiasm. The idea of being able to access a great deal of data and share them widely is offset by the effort to record all these data. An increasing number of patients see caregivers only on the other side of a computer screen. Better information could represent a major advance in the care of older people, if the opportunity is properly harnessed. Clinicians would benefit from more focused information that directs their attention to the most salient aspects of a given problem.

Computer technology can dramatically reduce redundancy. Properly mobilized, computers can provide the structure needed to ensure a comprehensive assessment with no duplication of effort. Because they are interactive, they can carry out much

---

TABLE 4-8. *Choosing Wisely* Recommendations

American Geriatrics Society
1. Don't recommend percutaneous feeding tubes in patients with advanced dementia; instead offer oral assisted feeding.
2. Don't use antipsychotics as first choice to treat behavioral and psychological symptoms of dementia.
3. Avoid using medications to achieve hemoglobin A1c <7.5% in most adults age 65 and older; moderate control is generally better.
4. Don't use benzodiazepines or other sedative-hypnotics in older adults as the first choice for insomnia, agitation, or delirium.
5. Don't use antimicrobials to treat bacteriuria in older adults unless specific urinary tract symptoms are present.
6. Don't prescribe cholinesterase inhibitors for dementia without periodic assessment for perceived cognitive benefits and adverse gastrointestinal effects.
7. Don't recommend screening for breast or colorectal cancer, nor prostate cancer (with the PSA test) without considering life expectancy and the risks of testing, overdiagnosis, and overtreatment.
8. Avoid using prescription appetite stimulants or high-calorie supplements for treatment of anorexia or cachexia in older adults; instead, optimize social supports, provide feeding assistance, and clarify patient goals and expectations.
9. Don't prescribe a medication without conducting a drug regimen review.
10. Avoid physical restraints to manage behavioral symptoms of hospitalized older adults with delirium.

American College of Physicians
1. Don't obtain screening exercise electrocardiogram testing in individuals who are asymptomatic and at low risk for coronary heart disease.
2. Don't obtain imaging studies in patients with nonspecific low back pain.
3. In the evaluation of simple syncope and a normal neurological examination, don't obtain brain imaging studies (CT or MRI).
4. In patients with low pretest probability of venous thromboembolism (VTE), obtain a high-sensitive D-dimer measurement as the initial diagnostic test; don't obtain imaging studies as the initial diagnostic test.
5. Don't obtain preoperative chest radiography in the absence of a clinical suspicion for intrathoracic pathology.

Data from Choosingwisely.org

of the desired branching and can even use simple algorithms to clarify areas of ambiguity and retest areas where some unreliability is suspected. Similar algorithms can look for inconsistency to screen for cheating.

Data stored on computers can be aggregated to display performance across patients by provider (eg, physician, nursing home, or agency). Data on a patient can be traced across time to look at changes in function and, in turn, can be aggregated.

The next important step in the progression is to move the focus from a single point of care to the linking of related elements of care. In an ideal system, patient information would be linked to permit tracing changes in status for that individual as he or she moves from one treatment modality to another. Linking data does not mean that everyone should have access to all information. Leaving aside the concerns about confidentiality built into the Health Insurance Portability and Accountability Act (HIPAA), being bombarded with a data deluge or largely extraneous information may be counterproductive. Instead, providers need a small amount of salient information (eg, diagnoses, medications and other therapies, goals of care, prior utilization, and perhaps advance directives). Thus, hospital admission and discharge information, LTC information, and primary care information would be merged into a common computer-linked record that allows one to trace the patient's movements and status. Finally, it would be desirable to have data on the process of care as well as the outcomes. This combination would permit analysis of what elements of care made a difference for which patients.

Computerized records greatly facilitate the task of monitoring the outcomes of care. Ideally, such a record system should be proactive, directing the collection of clinical information to encourage adequate coverage of relevant material. LTC is actually ahead of acute care in this regard, with the federal requirement for computerized versions of the Minimum Data Set. Unfortunately, most of the systems in use are simply inputting mechanisms. They do not begin to tap the real potential of a computerized information system. Because LTC depends heavily on poorly educated personnel for so much of its core services, the availability of an information support system, which can provide feedback and direction, is especially appropriate.

The computer's ability to compare observed and expected outcomes extends beyond its role as a regulatory device. It could be a major source of assistance to caregivers. One of the great frustrations in LTC, especially in the trenches, is the difficulty in sensing whether the caregiver is making a difference. Because so many patients enter care when they are already declining, the benefits of care are often best expressed as a slowing of that decline curve. Without some measure of expected course in the absence of good care, those who render care daily may not appreciate how much they are accomplishing and thereby may forgo one of the important rewards of their labors.

Displaying information about the change in patient's condition over time, which is a simple task for a computer, will assist the long-term caregiver to think more in terms of the overall picture, rather than a series of separate snapshots in time. Given the computer's ability to translate data into graphics, it is a simple procedure to develop pictorial representations of the changes occurring for a given patient or group of patients and to contrast those with what might be reasonably expected.

Again the effort is directed toward changing perceptions about older persons, especially those in LTC. For too long, LTC has worked in a negative spiral—a self-fulfilling prophecy that expected patients to deteriorate—serving to discourage both care providers and patients. Such an attitude is hardly likely to attract the best and the brightest in any of the health professions. As noted earlier in this chapter, nursing home patients are among the most responsive to almost any form of intervention. Any information system that can reinforce a prospective view of LTC, especially one that can display patient progress, represents an important adjunct to such care.

ACOVE

One frequently used source of quality measures for treating older patients is Assessing Care of Vulnerable Elders (ACOVE), which provides a number of recommendations about steps in providing better care. Although they make good clinical sense, none is supported by strong evidence (Wenger and Shekelle, 2007). The most recent version, ACOVE-3, includes 392 quality indicators (QIs), covering 26 conditions, across 14 different types of care processes, including screening and prevention (31% of QIs), diagnosis (20%), treatment (35%), and follow-up and continuity (14%) (www.rand.org/health/projects/acove/acove3.html). These recommendations are summarized in Table 4-9.

TABLE 4-9. ACOVE Recommendations

- All patients should be able to identify a physician or clinic to call for medical care and know how to reach them.
- After a new medication is prescribed for a chronic illness, the following should be noted at follow-up:
  - Medication is being taken as prescribed.
  - Patient was asked about the medication (eg, side effects, adherence, availability).
  - Medication was not started because it was not needed or changed.
- If a patient is seen by two or more physicians and a new medication is prescribed by one, the other(s) should be aware of the change.
- If a patient is referred to a consultant, the referring physician should show evidence of the consultant's findings and recommendations.
- If a diagnostic test is ordered, the following should be documented at the next visit:
  - Result of the test specifically acknowledged.
  - Note that the test was not needed or not performed and why.
  - Note that the test is pending.
- If a patient misses a scheduled preventive visit, there should be a reminder.
- When patients are seen in an emergency department (ED) or admitted to hospital, the continuity physician should be notified within 2 days.
- Patients discharged from hospital and who survive 6 weeks should have some contact with their continuity physician who should be aware of the hospitalization.
- When a patient is discharged to home from hospital and receives new chronic disease medication, the continuity physician should document the change in medication within 6 weeks.
- When a patient is discharged to home or to a nursing home from hospital and tests are pending, the results should be available within 6 weeks.
- When a patient is discharged to home or to a nursing home from hospital, there should be a discharge summary in the continuity physician's records.
- If a patient does not speak English, an interpreter or translated materials should be used.

NEXT STEPS

It has long been recognized that fee-for-service payment is a major barrier to good chronic disease management. Several developments in the organization and financing of care, stimulated by the Patient Protection and Affordable Care Act of 2010, will have implications for changing that arrangement. As discussed in Chapter 15, the Accountable Care Organization concept calls for developing a framework where clinicians would be paid in a manner that reflects, at least in part, their contribution to saving money by more efficient care. Likewise, medical/health-care homes will at least promote more comprehensive approaches to care, including some variant of case management (albeit many such programs do not focus on patients with chronic disease). Bundling payments for hospital and posthospital care will encourage transitional care and better choice of posthospital venues.

SUMMARY

In many respects, geriatrics is the epitome of chronic disease care. New paradigms are needed that recognize the changing role of patients in their own care, the need to think differently about the payoff horizons for investments in care, and the tracking of the course of disease to identify when intervention is needed. With geriatrics and chronic disease in general, the benefits of good care may be hard to discern because they represent a slowing of decline. This effect is invisible unless there is some basis for forming an expected clinical course against which to compare the actual course.

Physicians caring for older patients need to think in prospective terms. They will enjoy their practices more if they can learn to set reasonable goals for patients, to record progress toward these goals, and to use the failure to achieve progress as an important clinical sign of the need for reevaluation.

REFERENCES

Barer D; ACP Journal Club. Review: inpatient comprehensive geriatric assessment improves the likelihood of living at home at 12 months. *Ann Intern Med.* 2011;155:JC6-2.

Boult C, Dowd B, McCaffrey D, Boult L, Hernandez R, Krulewitch H. Screening elders for risk of hospital admission. *J Am Geriatr Soc.* 1993;41:811-817.

Bruce ML, Lohman, MC, Greenberg RL, et al. Integrating depression care management into Medicare home health reduces risk of 30- and 60-day hospitalization: the Depression Care for Patients at Home Cluster-Randomized Trial. *J Am Geriatr Soc.* 2016;64(11):1196-2203.

Callahan CM, Boustani MA, Unverzagt FW, et al. Effectiveness of collaborative care for older adults with Alzheimer disease in primary care: a randomized controlled trial. *JAMA.* 2006;295:2148-2157.

Clark F, Azen SP, Zemke R, et al. Occupational therapy for independent-living older adults: a randomized controlled trial. *JAMA.* 1997;278:1321-1326.

Coleman EA, Parry C, Chalmers S, Min SJ. The care transitions intervention: results of a randomized controlled trial. *Arch Intern Med.* 2006;166:1822-1828.

Counsell SR, Callahan CM, Buttar AB, Clark DO, Frank KI. Geriatric Resources for Assessment and Care of Elders (GRACE): a new model of primary care for low-income seniors. *J Am Geriatr Soc.* 2006;54:1136-1141.

Ellis G, Whitehead MA, O'Neill D, Langhorne P, Robinson D. Comprehensive geriatric assessment for older adults admitted to hospital. *Cochrane Database Syst Rev.* 2011;7:CD006211.

Fried LP, Tangen CM, Walston J, Newman AB, Hirsch C, et al. Frailty in older adults: evidence for phenotype. *J Gerontol A Biol Sci Med Sci.* 2001;56(5);M146-M156.

Hansen LO, Young RS, Hinami K, Leung A, Williams MV. Interventions to reduce 30-day rehospitalization: a systematic review. *Ann Intern Med.* 2011;155:520-528.

Horrocks S, Anderson E, Salisbury C. Systematic review of whether nurse practitioners working in primary care can provide equivalent care to doctors. *BMJ.* 2002;324:819-823.

Kane RL, Ouellette J. *The Good Caregiver.* New York, NY: Avery; 2011.

Kane RL, Priester R, Totten AM. *Meeting the Challenge of Chronic Illness.* Baltimore, MD: Johns Hopkins University Press; 2005.

Kane RL, Shamliyan T, McCarthy T. Do geriatric healthcare teams work? *Aging Health.* 2011;7:865-876.

Kansagara D, Englander H, Salanitro A, et al. Risk prediction models for hospital readmission: a systematic review. *JAMA.* 2011;306:1688-1698.

Lerner MJ, Simmons CH. Observer's reaction to the "innocent victim": compassion or rejection. *J Pers Soc Psychol.* 1966;4:203-210.

Min L, Yoon W, Wenger NS, et al. The vulnerable elders-13 survey predicts 5-year functional decline and mortality outcomes in older ambulatory care patients. *J Am Geriatr Soc.* 2009;57(11)2070-2076.

Morrison RS, Meier DC. Clinical practice. Palliative care. *N Engl J Med.* 2004;350:2582-2590.

Mundinger M, Kane R, Lenz E, et al. Primary care outcomes in patients treated by nurse practitioners or physicians: a randomized trial. *JAMA.* 2000;283:59-68.

Naylor M, Brooten D, Jones R, Lavizzo-Mourey R, Mezey M, Pauly M. Comprehensive discharge planning for the hospitalized elderly: a randomized clinical trial. *Ann Intern Med.* 1994;120:999-1006.

Stuck AE, Egger M, Hammer A, Minder CE, Beck JC. Home visits to prevent nursing home admission and functional decline in elderly people: systematic review and meta-regression analysis. *JAMA.* 2002;287:1022-1028.

Wagner EH, Austin BT, Von Korff M. Organizing care for patients with chronic illness. *Milbank Q.* 1996;74:511-543.

Walter LC, Brand RJ, Counsell SR, et al. Development and validation of a prognostic index for 1-year mortality in older adults after hospitalization. *JAMA.* 2001;285:2987-2994.

Wenger NS, Shekelle PG. Measuring medical care provided to vulnerable elders: the Assessing Care of Vulnerable Elders-3 (ACOVE-3) quality indicators. *J Am Geriatr Soc.* 2007;55(Suppl 2):S247-S487.

Wennberg JE. Time to tackle unwarranted variations in practice. *BMJ.* 2011;342:d513.

Yourman LC, Lee SJ, Schonberg MA, Widera EW, Smith AK. Prognostic indices for older adults: a systematic review. *JAMA.* 2012;307(2):182-192.

PART II

DIFFERENTIAL DIAGNOSIS AND MANAGEMENT

CHAPTER 5

Prevention

GENERAL PRINCIPLES

Today's older adults are increasingly interested in promoting healthy aging. The terms *health promotion* and *prevention* are used almost interchangeably. Prevention runs a gamut. For the most part, we think of prevention in terms of warding off disease or delaying its onset, but prevention can also involve simply avoiding bad events or complications of care. As noted in Chapter 4, in the context of chronic disease management, proactive primary care represents a form of prevention (tertiary prevention, as defined later). Prevention is typically targeted at specific diseases or conditions, but among older adults prevention of syndromes such as falls, dizziness, and functional decline are more important. Moreover, some preventive efforts, like stopping smoking and exercising, can affect many diseases.

Ageism may lead people to discount the value of prevention in caring for older persons, but the evidence suggests that many preventive strategies are effective in this age group. Ironically, the effects of prevention may be the greatest in older people because the benefit of preventive activities depends on two basic factors: the prevalence of the problem and the likelihood of an effective intervention. Thus, flu and pneumonia shots, for example, have the advantage of preventing not only the risk of disease but also may result in a shorter period of illness and less of a need for hospitalization and risk of functional decline. Likewise, osteoporosis prevention is more cost-effective in older adults than in younger individuals because the baseline levels of the problem, and of falling, are high. Plans for prevention in older people should consider the issues delineated in Table 5-1. Perhaps the most preventable problem connected with caring for older persons is iatrogenic disease.

The major thesis here, as with much covered elsewhere in this book, is that age alone should not be a predominant factor in choosing an approach to a patient. Preventive strategies for older adults should be based on immediate and future benefits with a focus on morbidity and quality of life rather than on mortality.

Preventive activities can be divided into three types. *Primary prevention* refers to action taken to render the patient more resistant or the environment less harmful. It is basically a reduction in risk. The term *secondary prevention* is used in two ways. One implies screening or early detection for asymptomatic disease or early disease. The idea here is that finding a problem early allows more effective treatment. In geriatrics however, the goal is really not to screen for diseases that will be identified but those that might never become problematic to the individual with regard to either mortality or morbidity (eg, screening for breast cancer in a 90-year-old woman). The second

TABLE 5-1. Considerations in Assessing Prevention in Older Patients

1. Baseline risk
   - The higher the baseline risk, the greater is the likelihood that an effective preventive intervention will have an impact. Hence, some preventive strategies may be paradoxically more effective with older patients.
2. Competing risks/limited life expectancy
   - Multimorbidity means that reducing the risk of one disease may leave older people vulnerable to others.
   - Limited life expectancy influences judgments about the expected course of benefits.
3. Time to achieve an effect
   - Interventions related to prevention should focus on immediate/early benefits and focus less on extending length of life.
4. Vulnerability/risk of harms
   - Older people have a narrower therapeutic window (see Chap. 4).
   - They may be susceptible to the side effects of prevention and thus risk benefits should be carefully considered.
5. Response to intervention
   - The preventive intervention may not work as well in older patients.
   - Some older patients may have difficulty following the preventive regimen and thus regimens should be simplified.
6. The value of the health gained
   - Other problems may reduce the benefit.
7. The cost of the preventive activity
   - Direct costs
   - Indirect costs, such as anxiety, impact on quality of life, restricted lifestyle, and false-positive results

meaning of secondary prevention may be of greater value in care of older adults as it involves using the techniques of prevention on people who already have the disease in an effort to delay progression and more importantly morbidity; for example, getting people who have arterial insufficiency to stop smoking. That behavior may help prevent disease progression and reduce the risks of increased pain and tissue death. *Tertiary prevention* involves efforts to improve care to avoid later complications and rehabilitation to optimize function; proactive chronic disease management is a good example of this approach. In essence, chronic disease management is effectively catastrophe prevention. As noted in Chapter 4, tertiary prevention is the central part of good geriatric care, which strives to minimize the progression of disease to disability. It requires a comprehensive effort to address the physiological, psychological, and environmental factors that can create dependency. All three types of prevention are relevant to geriatric care. Table 5-2 offers examples of activities in each category.

The federal government has set new Healthy People 2020 goals for various population groups, including older people. Table 5-3 shows those that are noted specifically for older persons or are particularly relevant for these individuals.

TABLE 5-2. Preventive Strategies for Older Persons

Primary	Secondary: screenings	Tertiary
Immunizations		Proactive primary care
Influenza		Comprehensive geriatric assessment
Pneumococcus		Foot care
Tetanus	Mammography (< age 75)	Dental care
Herpes zoster		
Blood pressure	Fecal blood, colonoscopy (< age 79)	Toileting efforts Rehabilitation/exercise Dietary protein
Smoking	Hypothyroidism	
Exercise	Depression	
Heart-healthy diet: chol/salt	Vision	
Weight management		
Cholesterol	Hearing	
Sodium restriction	Oral cavity	
Social support	Tuberculosis	
Home environmental improvements	Skin care: hygiene/growths	
Seat belts		
Medication review		
Oral care		

The U.S. Preventive Services Task Force (USPSTF, 2014) is charged with reviewing the evidence on prevention and making recommendations. Tables 5-4 and 5-5 provide the current recommendations from the USPSTF for preventive care that may be relevant to older persons. Clinicians have an opportunity to address preventive health behaviors and interventions when working with older adults during a Welcome to Medicare Visit and Annual Wellness Visit (Department of Health and Human Services, Centers for Medicare & Medicaid Services, 2015). These visits focus exclusively on the review and evaluation of preventive behavior among older adults. Details of these visits are described in Table 5-6. This allows for time to interact with older individuals who may not follow these guidelines and believe they still need, for example, to go for annual mammograms and Pap tests. The annual wellness visit can be used to help prevent such futile testing.

Primary prevention is generally the most desirable approach to preventive care, although challenges in implementation of primary prevention vary. Giving a one-time immunization is much easier to achieve than the more challenging ongoing behavior change required for adherence to heart-healthy diets or exercise.

TABLE 5-3. Healthy People 2020 Report Card Items Most Relevant for Older Adults

Health status (minimize the following)

    Reduce the proportion of older adults who have moderate to severe functional limitations.

    Increase the proportion of adults aged 65 years and older with diagnosed Alzheimer's disease and other dementias, or their caregiver, who are aware of the diagnosis.

    Increase the number of days older adults report feeling well or very well.

    Reduce the number of individuals with untreated coronal caries, root surface caries, who have periodontitis or who have lost all their teeth.

    Reduce the number of people with new, invasive or antibiotic resistant pneumonia.

Health behaviors

    Increase the proportion of older adults with reduced physical or cognitive function who engage in light, moderate or vigorous leisure time physical activities.

    Increase the number of older adults with healthy weights.

Preventive care and screening

    Increase the proportion of older adults who use the Welcome to Medicare benefit.

    Increase the proportion of older adults who are up to date on core set of clinical preventive services (eg, immunizations; appropriate screening tests).

    Increase the proportion of older adults with one or more chronic health conditions who report confidence in managing their symptoms.

    Increase the proportion of older adults who receive Diabetes Self-Management benefits.

Injuries

    Reduce the rate of hip fracture hospitalizations.

    Reduce the rate of emergency department visits following falls.

Reproduced with permission from Healthy People 2020. U.S. Department of Health and Human Services.

Health promotion is a subset of primary prevention; it is the science and art of helping people change their lifestyle to move toward a state of optimal health, defined as a balance of physical, emotional, social, spiritual, and intellectual health. The purpose of health promotion and disease prevention, therefore, as noted previously, is to reduce the potential years of life lost in premature mortality and to ensure better quality of remaining life. Thus, health promotion activities should be cost-effective.

CHALLENGES TO PREVENTIVE CARE AMONG OLDER ADULTS

Many of the health behaviors that need to change to prevent disease require giving up lifelong habits that are pleasurable. In the case of older persons, it is important to weigh quality of life benefits against the impact on the individual and society. Putting a 90-year-old diabetic on a strict diet and making that individual forgo the craved sweets will adversely affect his quality of life without substantially improving his health. Conversely, if he was symptomatic from hyperglycemia, then pharmacological options might improve his quality of life.

TABLE 5-4. U.S. Preventive Services Task Force (USPSTF) Recommendations for Screening Older Adults

Services	USPSTF recommendation	
	Summary of recommendation	Grade
Abdominal aortic aneurysm screening	The USPSTF recommends one-time screening for abdominal aortic aneurysm (AAA) by ultrasonography in men aged 65 to 75 who have ever smoked.	B
	The USPSTF makes no recommendation for or against screening for AAA in men aged 65 to 75 who have never smoked.	C
	The USPSTF recommends against routine screening for AAA in women.	D
Breast cancer screening	The USPSTF recommends biennial screening mammography for women aged 50 to 74 years.	B
	The USPSTF concludes that the current evidence is insufficient to assess the additional benefits and harms of screening mammography in women 75 years or older.	C
	The USPSTF recommends against teaching breast self-examination (BSE).	I
	The USPSTF concludes that the current evidence is insufficient to assess the additional benefits and harms of clinical breast examination (CBE) beyond screening mammography in women 40 years or older.	D
	The USPSTF concludes that the current evidence is insufficient to assess the additional benefits and harms of either digital mammography or magnetic resonance imaging (MRI) instead of film mammography as screening modalities for breast cancer.	I
Carotid artery stenosis screening	The USPSTF recommends against screening for asymptomatic carotid artery stenosis (CAS) in the general adult population.	D

(continued)

TABLE 5-4. U.S. Preventive Services Task Force (USPSTF) Recommendations for Screening Older Adults (continued)

Services	USPSTF recommendation	
	Summary of recommendation	Grade
Cervical cancer screening	The USPSTF recommends screening for cervical cancer in women aged 21 to 65 years with cytology (Pap smear) every 3 years or, for women aged 30 to 65 years screen every 3 years with a combination of cytology and human papillomavirus (HPV) testing every 5 years.	A
	The USPSTF recommends against screening for cervical cancer in women older than age 65 years who have had adequate prior screening and are not otherwise at high risk for cervical cancer.	D
	The USPSTF recommends against screening for cervical cancer in women who have had a hysterectomy with removal of the cervix and who do not have a history of a high-grade precancerous lesion (ie, cervical intraepithelial neoplasia [CIN] grade 2 or 3) or cervical cancer.	D
Colorectal cancer screening	The USPSTF recommends screening for colorectal cancer (CRC) using fecal occult blood testing, sigmoidoscopy, or colonoscopy in adults, beginning at age 50 years and continuing until age 75 years.	A
	The USPSTF recommends against routine screening for colorectal cancer in adults aged 76 to 85 years. There may be considerations that support colorectal cancer screening in an individual patient.	C
	The USPSTF recommends against screening for colorectal cancer in adults older than age 85 years.	D
	The USPSTF concludes that the evidence is insufficient to assess the benefits and harms of computed tomographic colonography and fecal DNA testing as screening modalities for colorectal cancer.	I
Coronary heart disease screening	The USPSTF recommends against routine screening with resting electrocardiography (ECG), exercise treadmill test (ETT).	D
	The USPSTF found insufficient evidence to recommend for or against routine screening with ECG, ETT, at increased risk for CHD events.	I
Dementia screening	The USPSTF concludes that the evidence is insufficient to recommend for or against routine screening for dementia in older adults.	I

Hormone replacement therapy	The USPSTF recommends against the routine use of combined estrogen and progestin for the prevention of chronic conditions in postmenopausal women.	D
	The USPSTF recommends against the routine use of unopposed estrogen for the prevention of chronic conditions in postmenopausal women who have had a hysterectomy.	D
Osteoporosis screening	The USPSTF recommends screening for osteoporosis in women aged 65 years or older without previous fracture or secondary cause of osteoporosis.	B
	The USPSTF concludes that the current evidence is insufficient to assess the balance of benefits and harms of screening for osteoporosis in men.	I
Ovarian cancer screening	The USPSTF recommends against routine screening for ovarian cancer among asymptomatic women without known genetic risk.	I
Peripheral arterial disease screening	The USPSTF recommends against routine screening for peripheral arterial disease (PAD) in asymptomatic adults.	I
Prostate cancer screening	The USPSTF recommends against screening for prostate cancer in men age 75 years or older with prostatic-specific-antigen (PSA).	D
Thyroid disease screening	The USPSTF concludes the evidence is insufficient to recommend for or against routine screening for thyroid disease in adults.	I
Vision screening in older adults	The USPSTF concludes that the current evidence is insufficient to assess the balance of benefits and harms of screening for visual acuity for the improvement of outcomes in older adults.	I

USPSTF recommendation codes:

A = strongly recommends in favor

B = recommends in favor

C = recommends against

D = strongly recommends against

I = evidence is insufficient

Data from U.S. Preventive Services Task Force. Recommendations. Available at: http://www.uspreventiveservicestaskforce.org/recommendations.htm; Medicare.gov. Preventive and screening services. Available at: http://www.medicare.gov/navigation/manage-your-health/preventive-services/preventive-service-overview.aspx; Centers for Disease Control and Prevention. Immunization schedules. Available at: http://www.cdc.gov/vaccines/schedules/index.htm. Accessed February, 2016.

TABLE 5-5. Additional Preventive Services From U.S. Preventive Services Task Force (USPSTF) (May Be Suitable for Older Adults)

Services	Summary of recommendation	Grade
	USPSTF recommendation	
Alcohol misuse screening and counseling	The USPSTF recommends screening and behavioral counseling interventions to reduce alcohol misuse by adults, including pregnant women, in primary care settings.	B
Aspirin/NSAIDs for prevention of colorectal cancer	The USPSTF recommends against the routine use of aspirin and nonsteroidal anti-inflammatory drugs (NSAIDs) to prevent colorectal cancer in individuals at average risk for colorectal cancer.	D
Cardiovascular disease (behavioral therapy)	The USPSTF recommends the use of aspirin for men aged 45 to 79 years when the potential benefit due to a reduction in myocardial infarctions outweighs the potential harm due to an increase in gastrointestinal hemorrhage.	A
Aspirin for the prevention of cardiovascular disease	The USPSTF recommends the use of aspirin for women aged 55 to 79 years when the potential benefit of a reduction in ischemic strokes outweighs the potential harm of an increase in gastrointestinal hemorrhage.	A
	The USPSTF concludes that the current evidence is insufficient to assess the balance of benefits and harms of aspirin for cardiovascular disease prevention in men and women aged 80 years or older.	I
	The USPSTF recommends against the use of aspirin for stroke prevention in women younger than 55 years and for myocardial infarction prevention in men younger than 45 years.	D
Cholesterol abnormalities in adults (dyslipidemia, lipid disorders)	The USPSTF strongly recommends screening men aged 35 and older for lipid disorders.	A
	The USPSTF strongly recommends screening women aged 45 and older for lipid disorders if they are at increased risk for coronary heart disease.	A
	The USPSTF makes no recommendation for or against routine screening for lipid disorders in men aged 20 to 35 or in women aged 20 and older who are not at increased risk for coronary heart disease.	C
Back pain, low (low back pain)	The USPSTF concludes that the evidence is insufficient to recommend for or against the routine use of interventions to prevent low back pain in adults in primary care settings.	I
Bacteriuria	The USPSTF recommends against screening for asymptomatic bacteriuria in men and nonpregnant women.	D

Bladder cancer	The USPSTF concludes that the current evidence is insufficient to assess the balance of benefits and harms of screening for bladder cancer in asymptomatic adults.	I
Blood pressure in adults (hypertension)	The USPSTF recommends screening for high blood pressure in adults aged 18 and older.	A
Breast cancer, BRCA testing (ovarian cancer)	The USPSTF recommends against routine referral for genetic counseling or routine breast cancer susceptibility gene (BRCA) testing for women whose family history is not associated with an increased risk for deleterious mutations in breast cancer susceptibility gene 1 (BRCA1) or breast cancer susceptibility gene 2 (BRCA2).	D
	The USPSTF recommends that women whose family history is associated with an increased risk for deleterious mutations in BRCA1 or BRCA2 genes be referred for genetic counseling and evaluation for BRCA testing.	B
Breast cancer	The USPSTF recommends against routine use of risk reducing medications for those ≥35 years of age for the primary prevention of breast cancer.	D
Lipid disorders	The USPSTF strongly recommends screening women aged 45 and older for lipid disorders if they are at increased risk for coronary heart disease.	A
	The USPSTF makes no recommendation for or against routine screening for lipid disorders in men aged 20 to 35 or in women aged 20 and older who are not at increased risk for coronary heart disease.	C
Chronic obstructive pulmonary disease	The USPSTF recommends against screening adults for chronic obstructive pulmonary disease (COPD) using spirometry.	D
Depression in adults	The USPSTF recommends screening adults for depression when staff-assisted depression care supports are in place to ensure accurate diagnosis, effective treatment, and follow-up.	B
	The USPTF recommends against routinely screening adults for depression when staff-assisted depression care supports are not in place. There may be considerations that support screening for depression in an individual patient.	C

(continued)

PART II

TABLE 5-5. Additional Preventive Services From U.S. Preventive Services Task Force (USPSTF) (May Be Suitable for Older Adults) *(continued)*

Services	USPSTF recommendation	
	Summary of recommendation	Grade
Diabetes mellitus	The USPSTF recommends screening for type 2 diabetes in asymptomatic adults with sustained blood pressure (either treated or untreated) greater than 135/80 mm Hg.	B
	The USPSTF concludes that the current evidence is insufficient to assess the balance of benefits and harms of screening for type 2 diabetes in asymptomatic adults with blood pressure of 135/80 mm Hg or lower.	I
Healthy diet and physical activity	The USPSTF concludes that the evidence is insufficient to recommend for or against routine behavioral counseling to promote a healthy diet in unselected patients in primary care settings. Selective counseling is recommended.	I
Falls	The USPSTF recommends that a falls intervention be provided for community dwelling older adults aged 65 or older at risk for falls.	B
	The USPSTF recommends against routine risk assessment for falls among older adults who are not at risk.	C
Elder abuse	The USPSTF found insufficient evidence to recommend for or against routine screening of older adults or their caregivers for elder abuse.	I
Glaucoma	The USPSTF found insufficient evidence to recommend for or against screening adults for glaucoma.	I
Gonorrhea	The USPSTF recommends that clinicians screen all sexually active women, including those who are pregnant, for gonorrhea infection if they are at increased risk for infection.	B
	The USPSTF found insufficient evidence to recommend for or against routine screening for gonorrhea infection in men at increased risk for infection.	I
	The USPSTF recommends against routine screening for gonorrhea infection in men and women who are at low risk for infection.	D
Hearing loss, older adults	The USPSTF found insufficient evidence to recommend for or against screening adults aged 50 or older for hearing loss.	I
Hepatitis B virus infection	The USPSTF recommends against routinely screening the general asymptomatic population for chronic hepatitis B virus infection.	D

Hepatitis C virus infection	The USPSTF recommends screening in individuals at high risk who were born between 1945 and 1965.	B
Herpes simplex, genital	The USPSTF recommends against routine serological screening for herpes simplex virus in asymptomatic adolescents and adults.	D
Human immunodeficiency virus (HIV) infection	The USPSTF strongly recommends that clinicians screen for HIV in all adolescents and adults at increased risk for HIV infection.	A
Lung cancer	The USPSTF recommends screening for adults aged 50 to 80 with computed tomography annually if they have a history of a 30-pack per year of smoking and/or have quit smoking with in the past 15 years.	B
Obesity in adults	The USPSTF recommends that clinicians screen all adult patients for obesity and offer intensive counseling and behavioral interventions to promote sustained weight loss for obese adults for those with a BMI $\geq 30 \text{kg/m}^2$	B
Oral cancer	The USPSTF concludes that the evidence is insufficient to recommend for or against routinely screening adults for oral cancer.	I
Pancreatic cancer	The USPSTF recommends against routine screening for pancreatic cancer in asymptomatic adults using abdominal palpation, ultrasonography, or serological markers.	D
Sexually transmitted infections	The USPSTF recommends high-intensity behavioral counseling to prevent sexually transmitted infections (STIs) for all sexually active adolescents and for adults at increased risk for STIs.	B
	The USPSTF concludes that the current evidence is insufficient to assess the balance of benefits and harms of behavioral counseling to prevent STIs in non–sexually active adolescents and in adults not at increased risk for STIs.	I
Skin cancer	The USPSTF concludes that the current evidence is insufficient to assess the balance of benefits and harms of using a whole-body skin examination by a primary care clinician or patient skin self-examination for the early detection of cutaneous melanoma, basal cell cancer, or squamous cell skin cancer in the adult general population.	I
	The USPSTF concludes that the evidence is insufficient to recommend for or against routine counseling by primary care clinicians to prevent skin cancer in adults aged 24 or older.	I

(continued)

TABLE 5-5. Additional Preventive Services From U.S. Preventive Services Task Force (USPSTF) (May Be Suitable for Older Adults) (*continued*)

Services	USPSTF recommendation	
	Summary of recommendation	Grade
Smoking (tobacco use)	The USPSTF recommends that clinicians ask all adults about tobacco use and provide tobacco cessation interventions for those who use tobacco products.	A
Suicide risk	The USPSTF concludes that the evidence is insufficient to recommend for or against routine screening by primary care clinicians to detect suicide risk in the general population.	I
Syphilis	The USPSTF strongly recommends that clinicians screen persons at increased risk for syphilis infection.	A
	The USPSTF recommends against routine screening of asymptomatic persons who are not at increased risk for syphilis infection.	D
Vitamin D supplementation to prevent cancer and fractures	The USPSTF concludes that the evidence is insufficient to recommend for or against use of vitamin D for prevention of cancer or fractures.	I
Vitamin supplementation to prevent cancer and coronary heart disease	The USPSTF concludes that the evidence is insufficient to recommend for or against the use of multivitamins or single or paired vitamins or vitamin E for the prevention of cancer or cardiovascular disease.	I
	The USPSTF recommends against the use of beta-carotene supplements, either alone or in combination, for the prevention of cancer or cardiovascular disease.	D

TABLE 5-6. Requirements for the Welcome to Medicare Visit and Annual Wellness Visit

Welcome to Medicare Visit	Annual Wellness Visit
• Record and evaluate your patient's medical and family history, current health conditions, and prescriptions. • Check your patient's blood pressure, vision, weight, and height to get a baseline for your care. • Make sure your patient is up-to-date with preventive screenings and services, such as cancer screenings and shots. • Order further tests, depending on your patient's general health and medical history. • Following the visit, give your patient or caregiver a plan or checklist with Medicare-covered screenings and preventive services that he or she currently needs.	• Complete a health risk assessment (psychosocial risks, behavioral risks, and functional risks). • Review list of providers. • Review family and medical history. • Review risk factors for depression, functional changes, safety. • Obtain height, weight and body mass, blood pressure, and cognitive status. • Establish a written screening schedule. • Establish a list of potential health risks (eg, depression). • Provide health education and/or refer.

Data from United states Preventive Health Services Task Force. The guide to Clinical Preventive Services. Available at: http://wwwahrqgov/professionals/clinicians-providers/guidelines-recommendations/guide/indexhtml 2014. Last accessed April, 2016; Department of Health and Human Services Centers for Medicare & Medicaid Services. The ABCs of the Annual Wellness Visit. Availabe at: https://wwwcmsgov/Outreach-and-Education/Medicare-Learning-Network-MLN/MLNProducts/downloads/AWV_chart_ICN905706pdf 2015. Last accessed April, 2016.

EFFECTIVENESS OF PREVENTION IN OLDER PEOPLE

While older persons traditionally have been excluded from prevention trials, that situation is changing. Research studies increasingly focus on the impact of certain health-promoting activities such as immunizations and exercise among older adults. Unfortunately, inclusion is often limited to those who are healthy and relatively young (eg, less than 90 years of age and free of multiple comorbidities commonly found in older adults), and enrollees are typically volunteers who may be more likely to follow the prescribed regimens. Consequently, it is still challenging to know for sure the impact of preventive care on the growing group of individuals greater than 90 years of age.

Appropriate treatment may help keep older adults functional and medically stable. It is important, therefore, to carefully consider those areas in which prevention across any of the three levels (primary, secondary, or tertiary) is most likely to be beneficial. Specifically, these include things such as the benefits of immunizations, prevention of infections, benefits of exercise and physical activity and high-protein diets in the prevention of sarcopenia, fall prevention, the use of preventive pharmacotherapy, and prevention of iatrogenesis by protecting older adults from polypharmacy and futile care.

IMMUNIZATIONS

No immunization is 100% effective in preventing the relevant disease. Evidence suggests, however, that immunizations can be effective in prevention of disease and most importantly can reduce the length and severity of the illness should it occur and possibly prevent a hospitalization. The benefit of preventing a zoster infection with a vaccination for herpes zoster can have an even more direct impact on older adults than that received by influenza and pneumonia vaccinations. The prevalence of zoster infection is approximately 50% for those who are 85 years of age and older. The incidence of postherpetic neuralgia and chronic pain is present in at least 15% of those 80 years of age and older. Fortunately, the vaccine against herpes zoster results in a 50% reduction in cases of herpes zoster and 66% reduction in the risk of having long-term postherpetic neuralgia. Aside from the obvious negative impact of pain from a zoster infection, either acute or chronic, immunization will decrease the risk of having to isolate older adults from friends and family when actively infected with zoster. This is particularly true for those who live in institutional or communal settings. Likewise, there is benefit to immunizing older adults with Prevnar-13 for pneumococcal infection as this can decrease the risk of episodes of vaccine-type community-acquired pneumonia and decrease the rate of vaccine-type invasive pneumococcal disease in the vaccinated group.

Despite potential benefits, the immunization adherence rates among older adults range from 8% to 60%. In 2012 the rate of influenza and pneumococcal vaccine among older adults across all races and ethnicities was approximately 60%. For tetanus the rate was similarly 55%, although for tetanus with pertussis the rate was only 8%. Last, the rate for herpes zoster vaccination was 20%. This is in contrast to the Healthy People 2020 adult goal of achieving immunization rates of 90%.

CANCER SCREENING AND OLDER ADULTS

The value of screening for cancer depends on the availability of an effective intervention and the likelihood that the intervention will change the clinical course. Some cancers may behave differently in older persons. Although the incidence (and certainly the prevalence) of many cancers increases with age, the rate of growth may be slower. As noted earlier, the USPSTF provides a comprehensive review of what is currently known about the risks and benefits of screening for cancers among all groups of individuals. At intervals these reviews are updated. Currently, updates are ongoing with regard to recommendations for skin and ovarian and prostate cancer screening. As of 2016, the recommendations from the USPSTF are noted in Table 5-4. Generally, the recommendations discourage cancer screening in older persons. They recommend not to screen women over the age of 74 for breast cancer, to not screen men at all for prostate cancer, to not screen women for cervical cancer unless the woman is at high risk, to not screen for lung cancer unless the individual is at high risk, and to stop screening for bowel cancer at the age of 79.

In contrast to the recommendations by the USPSTF, the American Cancer Society promotes more liberal screening in older adults. Its guidelines suggest that women 55 and older should get mammograms every 2 years or continue yearly screening and that screening should continue as long as a woman is in good health and is expected to live 10 years or more. Similarly there is no stop date for colon cancer screening. For prostate cancer screening the recommendation is for men aged 50 and above to talk with a health-care provider about the pros and cons of testing to decide if testing is the right choice.

Screening for skin lesions is not recommended by the USPSTF as there is no evidence that skin examination by clinicians results in decreased morbidity or mortality for malignant melanoma. Other skin lesions generally do not cause death or significant morbidity and thus have not been the focus of reviews by USPSTF. Moreover, with regard to skin screenings, there is evidence that screenings result in harm due to misdiagnosis and overdiagnosis and resulting cosmetic and even functional adverse effects due to biopsies and overtreatment (eg, aggressive removals of lesions) (Waldmann et al, 2012).

When recommending cancer screening for older patients, consider the patient's anticipated life expectation and discuss with the individual and/or his or her proxy the risks and benefits of screenings. The likelihood of surviving for a year can be calculated using a program referred to as ePrognosis. The information on ePrognosis is intended to be a rough guide to inform clinicians about mortality outcomes. When talking with a patient or caregiver about screening opportunities it is particularly helpful to ask the question: What will he or she do with the information? Would the individual want to undergo treatment? If the older adult is not interested in further treatment, then screening may be psychologically harmful and of no clinical value.

Once a cancer is identified in an older individual there are questions about whether or not to treat and how to treat. At this point in time there are insufficient data to guide providers in terms of the impact of chemotherapy or surgical interventions, particularly among the old-old (Hurria et al, 2015). Management, for example, of the toxicities associated with targeted anticancer therapies may be particularly challenging in older adults. Due to normal skin changes, skin reactions associated with some treatments may increase the morbidity associated with this side effect when these drugs are used in older adults. Palliative treatment, or tertiary prevention, for a noted malignancy should be considered. There is some evidence, however, that palliative treatment may cause more morbidity and mortality than conservative comfort measures.

SCREENING FOR IDENTIFICATION OF PSYCHOSOCIAL PROBLEMS

Early identification and management of some of the psychosocial problems associated with aging may be of greater value to the older patient than a focus on medical diagnoses. For example, as part of the Medicare Annual Wellness Visit an assessment for depression and signs and symptoms of depression can and should be done. Further, assessments for depression and associated symptoms should be integrated into every patient encounter. Early treatment can then be initiated as appropriate. Other psychosocial factors to consider are alcohol use and abuse, drug use and abuse, loneliness, and apathy. Screening tools are provided in Table 5-7.

Screening for cognitive impairment among older adults continues to be controversial. Some groups like the Alzheimer's Association advocate strongly for early identification. On the Alzheimer's Association web page the message to older adults and their caregivers is to monitor for the 10 early signs of memory loss and if evident

PART II

TABLE 5-7. Measurement of Psychosocial Factors Among Older Adults

Measures	Focus and description	Access
Patient Health Questionnaire-9 (PHQ-9)	A 9-item depression scale; each item is scored from 0 to 3, providing a 0 to 27 severity score.	http://lphi.org/LPHIadmin/ uploads/.PHQ-9-Review-Kroenke-63754.PDF
Beck Depression Inventory (BDI) or the Beck Depression Inventory-II (BDI-II)	21-question symptom-rating scales for depression providing a 0 to 63 severity score.	www.all-on-depression-help.com/ depression-scale.html
Hamilton Depression Rating Scale	A 17-item questionnaire designed for adults and used to rate the severity of their depression by probing mood, feelings of guilt, suicide ideation, insomnia, agitation or retardation, anxiety, weight loss, and somatic symptoms.	http://img.medscape.com/pi/ emed/ckb/psychiatry/79926-1889862-1859039-2124408.pdf
Major Depression Inventory	Addresses 12 symptoms of depression.	http://img.medscape.com/pi/ emed/ckb/psychiatry/79926-1889862-1859039-2129923.pdf
Center for Epidemiologic Studies Depression Scale (CES-D)	A 20-item instrument that allows patients to evaluate their feelings, behavior, and outlook from the previous week.	http://img.medscape.com/pi/ emed/ckb/psychiatry/285911-1335297-1859039-1859099.pdf
Zung Depression Scale	A 20-item survey.	http://img.medscape.com/pi/ emed/ckb/psychiatry/79926-1889862-1859039-2129979.pdf
Geriatric Depression Scale Short Version	A 15-item measure of commonly noted symptoms of depression among older adults.	http://img.medscape.com/pi/ emed/ckb/psychiatry/285911-1335297-1859039-1859095.pdf
Cornell Scale for Depression in Dementia	A 19-item measure that asks about depressive symptoms and signs and can be completed by a caregiver.	www.scalesandmeasures.net/files/ files/The%20Cornell%20Scale% 20for%20Depression%20in% 20Dementia.pdf
A Short Scale to Measure Loneliness	A 20-item measure that reflects symptoms of loneliness.	http://psychology.uchicago.edu/ people/faculty/cacioppo/ jtcreprints/hwhc04.pdf A Short Scale for Measuring Loneliness in Large Surveys[3]

TABLE 5-7. Measurement of Psychosocial Factors Among Older Adults (*continued*)

Measures	Focus and description	Access
Apathy	A 7-item short version of the Apathy Evaluation Scale which has patients or providers rate factors associated with the individual's personality that reflect apathy.	The Apathy Evaluation Scale [4]

Data from [3]A short scale for measuring loneliness: https://www.ncbi.nlm.nih.gov/pmc/articles/PMC2394670/pdf/nihms47842.pdf
[4]The apathy evaluation scale http://www.tbims.org/combi/aes/AES.PDF

set up a visit with a health-care provider to diagnose cognitive impairment. Early detection is encouraged so that patients can get "maximum benefit from available treatments" and live independently for as long as possible. Unfortunately, there is little evidence to support the benefit of early diagnosis in terms of starting treatment with currently available medication management such as cholinesterase inhibitors. A recent meta-analysis of 17 studies concluded that there was no benefit to using medications, vitamins, or nutritional supplements when compared to controls in terms of memory (Fitzpatrick-Lewis et al, 2015). Findings within the same analysis suggested that there may be some benefit to behavioral interventions involving exercise interventions or cognitive training. The findings from behavioral interventions such as exercise are, however, inconsistent and challenging to interpret. The interventions tested vary in terms of type and intensity of the exercise program and across the studies cognition is measured differently (Hoffmann et al, 2015; Poulin et al, 2016; Sink et al, 2015). Despite these inconsistencies across studies, the findings are helpful in terms of guiding providers in care management and decision making regarding treatments.

Another reason that it may not be worthwhile to screen for dementia is that only a small proportion of dementia cases have reversible etiologies. Screening for dementia does not, therefore, pass the first test of screening. Further, screening for cognitive impairment and early disease identification can have a devastating impact psychologically for some individuals and may make them ineligible for long-term care insurance. The advantage to screening from the perspective of providers and families/caregivers is to understand the level of cognitive function present so that they can help the individual optimize function and independence for as long as possible and remain safe in the least restrictive setting. Increasingly there are Information and Communication Technologies including robotics, telemedicine, sensor technology, medication management applications, and video games that have been used to optimize independence and help individuals remain safe (Khosravi and Ghapanchi, 2016). Ongoing research is needed to establish the efficacy of these interventions.

ROUTINE COMPREHENSIVE HISTORY AND PHYSICAL

A yearly comprehensive history and physical has traditionally been considered important to maintain health and even believed to be preventive in nature. Recent reviews have raised questions about this belief. A 2012 review from the Cochrane Collaboration concluded that annual medical checkups had no effect on hospital admission rates, absences from work, disability, specialist referrals, additional doctor visits, or even patient anxiety. They didn't improve patient health or reduce mortality, and overall it was concluded that such checks were "unlikely to be beneficial." In contrast, the use of the Medicare Annual Wellness Visit may be a better way in which to encourage participation in and adherence to preventive health care.

PRIORITIZING PREVENTIVE BEHAVIORS AND BEHAVIOR CHANGE

Behavior change represents at once the most promising and the most frustrating component of prevention. While some may argue that you "can't teach an old dog new tricks" or that ingrained habit patterns are hard to break, there is no evidence to support such pessimism. To the contrary, there is evidence that older adults can and will change behavior if the activities result in beneficial outcomes. Behavior change may be helpful with regard to physical activity, healthy diets, and smoking cessation. Older adults tend to have lower rates of smoking than other age groups but continue to smoke at a rate of about 8.5%, and only a small percentage of older adults engage in recommended levels of physical activity (21%). Thus there are opportunities to improve these behaviors. The first step in changing behavior in working with older adults is to know what to recommend across a variety of health behaviors and help older adults believe that these behaviors are safe and have the potential to be beneficial with regard to providing immediate positive benefits.

PHYSICAL ACTIVITY RECOMMENDATIONS

A substantial body of scientific evidence indicates that regular physical activity can provide some health benefits to older adults (**Table 5-8**). Specifically benefits include improvement and maintenance of function and strength, and decreased risk of falls. Physical activity allows older individuals to increase the likelihood that they will extend years of active independent life, reduce disability, optimize mental health, and improve their quality of life in midlife and beyond. The exact amount and type

TABLE 5-8. Types of Exercises	
Type	**Purpose/expected benefit**
Aerobic/anaerobic	Cardiovascular conditioning
Resistance/weights	Strength, tone, muscle mass
Antigravity	Prevent osteoporosis
Balance	Prevent falls
Stretching	Flexibility

PART II

of activities across all these studies varied, making it difficult to recommend any individual approach. In some studies, combined aerobic and resistance exercise was implemented while in others high- versus low-intensity programs were provided. Thus the best approach when working with older adults is to make recommendations consistent with current physical activity guidelines, to focus on activities that the individual will enjoy and adhere to, and to encourage working at the highest intensity possible for the individual.

The current recommendation is that older adults need to engage in both aerobic and resistive exercise weekly to optimize health. In addition, balance exercise should be added if the individual is at risk of falling. A total of 150 minutes of moderate-intensity physical activity weekly should be recommended, although individuals should start at levels that they can successfully complete and try to maintain some intensity of activity for at least 10-minute periods. Ultimately, the 10-minute periods can be spread throughout the day and over the course of the week. Moderate intensity of activity is defined as physical activity that is done at 3.0 to 5.9 times the intensity of rest. On a scale relative to an individual's personal capacity, moderate-intensity physical activity is usually a 5 or 6 on a scale of 0 to 10. Moderate-intensity activities generally include brisk walking, dancing, swimming, or biking. Resistance training or muscle strengthening should be done 2 days a week and include all the major muscle groups (legs, hips, back, abdomen, chest, shoulders, and arms). The National Institute of Aging has an easy-to-follow guideline for older adults. For strengthening exercises generally eight repetitions of each exercise are recommended and the amount of resistance will vary for each individual. The individual should use a weight that can be comfortably lifted for eight repetitions of the exercise. Balance exercises, such as backward walking, sideways walking, heel walking, toe walking, and standing from a sitting position should be done at least 3 days a week.

GUIDELINES FOR SCREENING BEFORE EXERCISE

Initiation of a moderate-intensity exercise program is safe for all older adults. If the clinician feels that it will be helpful to the older adult to go through some type of screening, the Exercise and Screening for You (EASY) screening tool can be completed. This interactive web-based tool can be done by the older individual or the clinician and provides assurance that, given underlying clinical problems, the individual is safe to exercise. In addition, the tool provides guidance for what type of exercises to do given underlying health concerns.

PREVENTION THROUGH OPTIMAL NUTRITIONAL INTAKE

Nutritional health is an important component of health promotion and disease prevention among older adults as nutritional status contributes to frailty. A low body mass index (BMI) (kg/m^2 < 20) or an unintentional weight loss of > 10 pounds in 6 months suggests poor nutrition and should be evaluated. With age there is a general decline in calorie needs due to a slowing of metabolism and a decrease in physical activity. Nutritional requirements, however, generally remain the same. MyPlate for older adults addresses the needs of older adults based on the 2010 Dietary Guidelines

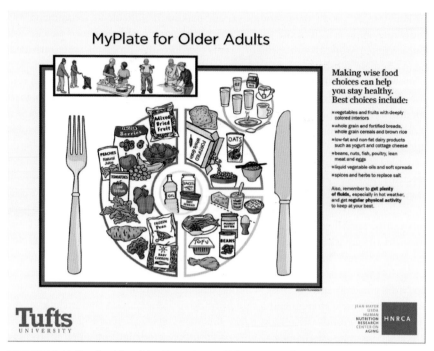

FIGURE 5-1 MyPlate for older adults. (*Copyright 2016 Tufts University, all rights reserved. "My Plate for Older Adults" graphic and accompanying website were developed with support from the AARP Foundation. "Tufts University" and "AARP Foundation" are registered trademarks and may not be reproduced apart from their inclusion in the "My Plate for Older Adults" graphic without express permission from their respective owners.*)

for Americans (Tufts University, 2016). Figure 5-1, provides a picture of MyPlate to help guide older individuals in daily dietary intake. Most importantly, to prevent sarcopenia, defined as the age-associated loss of skeletal muscle mass and function, consideration should be given to protein intake. Protein intake facilitates higher levels of insulin-like growth factor (IGF-1), resulting in direct and positive effects on muscle mass. Current protein intake recommendations for older adults are 0.2 to 1.4 g/kg to maintain muscle mass. Spreading the daily protein requirement equally throughout the day at a dose of 30 grams with each meal is beneficial and even greater value in terms of building muscle can be achieved if this is combined with exercise.

Assessment of nutritional status can be done by having the individual complete a Mini Nutritional Assessment (MNA). This assessment can help identify individuals who are at risk for being malnourished. Obesity, defined as a BMI >30, is a growing problem among older adults and BMI assessment is also one of the items on the MNA. Obesity puts older adults at risk for decreased physical activity and may actually be indicative of poor diet quality.

PROPHYLACTIC MEDICATION USE

Prevention of Cardiovascular Disease

In 2013, the American College of Cardiology and the American Heart Association released guidelines stating that every adult should have their cardiovascular risk calculated at least every 5 years (Meschia et al, 2015). This is done by evaluating age, race, blood pressure, smoking history, history of diabetes, and cholesterol levels. An estimate of risk of developing heart disease in the next 10 years is calculated and recommendations can then be made about aspirin use or other type of anticoagulation for prophylaxis of cardiovascular events. Aspirin, 81 mg daily, has been noted to be effective for prevention of a first stroke among women, including those with diabetes mellitus, whose risk is sufficiently high for the benefits to outweigh risk associated with treatment. See Chapter 11 for more details on prophylactic anticoagulation in cardiovascular disease.

Beta-blocker use has been recommended to prevent first events of nonfatal myocardial infarction in patients with high blood pressure since 1989. The most recent American Heart Association (AHA)/American College of Cardiology (ACC) guidelines for secondary prevention and risk reduction in patients with atherosclerotic vascular disease (eg, left ventricular systolic dysfunction, a prior myocardial infarction or have heart failure) continue to recommend beta-blocker therapy. There is some controversy, however, about the risk benefit of widespread use of these medications (Calhoun et al, 2013). Specifically, the risks include orthostatic hypotension and bradycardia, particularly among older adults who have a sinus bradycardia and partial atrioventricular block and are also receiving diltiazem, verapamil, or digoxin. Bronchoconstriction can also occur, especially when nonselective beta-blockers are administered to asthmatic patients. Therefore, nonselective beta-blockers are contraindicated in patients with asthma or chronic obstructive pulmonary disease. Last, abrupt withdrawal of a beta-blocker may precipitate rebound tachycardia or a myocardial infarction. With regard to statins, a meta-analysis by the Cholesterol Treatment Trialists Collaboration concluded that statins prevented 18 major cardiovascular events for every 1000 patients without preexisting coronary heart disease treated. A Cochrane review similarly reported that statin therapy for primary prevention was safe and effective in terms of preventing major vascular events (Taylor et al, 2013). The decisions to treat older adults, however, particularly those older than 85 years of age, must be carefully considered as the studies did not generally include individuals in this age group and there are associated risks with treatment that may not outweigh the benefits. Discussions with patients and/or their caregivers should review the associated risks when taking statins. These risks include diabetes, muscle pain, cognitive impairment, drug–drug interactions, and possible liver damage. Further, there is some evidence that among older individuals high cholesterol may actually be associated with better survival.

PREVENTION OF OSTEOPOROSIS AND DEGENERATIVE JOINT DISEASE

It is never too late to initiate bone health behaviors to help prevent the development or progression of osteoporosis and degenerative joint disease. Osteoporosis is defined as a bone density that is 2.5 or more standard deviations below the young-adult peak bone density. Osteopenia is defined as 1 to 2.5 standard deviations below the young-adult peak bone density and will progress to osteoporosis with time if not treated. Bone health includes both pharmacological and nonpharmacological treatments, specifically exercise and diet. Based on a systematic review of exercise programs and prevention of osteoporosis, walking was noted to provide a modest increase in skeleton load and thus has limited benefit for osteoporosis prevention. Conversely, strength training is effective in improving and maintaining bone mass. Exercise programs that combine strength training, aerobic activity, high-impact or weight-bearing training as well as whole-body vibration were noted to help increase bone mass or prevent further decline in older individuals.

Medication management for bone health includes the use of calcium, vitamin D, and other pharmacological interventions such as biphosphonates. When calcium from diet is inadequate, supplements spread out through the day for a total intake of 1200 to 1500 mg are recommended. No more than 500 mg should be consumed at one time to optimize absorption. The upper limit for calcium supplementation is 2500 mg per day. Calcium is difficult to absorb, and foods such as spinach, green beans, peanuts, and summer squash inhibit calcium absorption. In addition, high levels of protein, sodium, or caffeine increase excretion of calcium and should be avoided. Calcium citrate is better absorbed than is calcium carbonate and does not need to be taken with food.

There is some controversy about the benefits of vitamin D supplementation for the prevention of osteoporosis or associated fractures. Currently the USPSTF has concluded that there is insufficient evidence to assess the balance of the benefits and harms of combined vitamin D and calcium supplementation for the primary prevention of fractures in premenopausal women or men or of daily supplementation (400 IU or less of vitamin D_3 and greater than 1000 mg of calcium) for the primary prevention of fractures in postmenopausal women. The American Geriatrics Society recommends that the minimum daily vitamin D supplementation dose be 1000 IU as this is safe for most patients (Sanderson, 2015). Excess vitamin D intake can pose the risk of hypervitaminosis D, which is associated with hypercalcemia, hypercalciuria, acute renal failure, and increased resorption of bone. Pharmacological treatment for management of osteoporosis includes mainly the use of bisphosphonates. As with other pharmacological prevention interventions, decisions regarding use should be based on the individual's comorbidities, lifestyle, cognition, and personal preferences as there are associated risks and controversies over benefits. Risks of taking a biphosphonate include gastrointestinal irritation, osteonecrosis of the jaw, muscle pain, and atypical fractures, and the drugs need to be used cautiously in individuals with renal impairment and immunosuppression. Table 5-9 provides an overview of the effectiveness of biphosphonates on fracture prevention.

Prevention or progression of degenerative joint disease is generally best done with nonpharmacological interventions, specifically exercise (Humphreys et al, 2014). There is little evidence to support the efficacy of glucosamine and chondroitin as a way to manage pain and prevent progression of degenerative joint disease. There are some patients, however, who may find these treatments helpful for pain management. Since these drugs have a low-risk profile, supporting continued use in those who find them beneficial is appropriate.

TABLE 5-9. Efficacy of Common Biphosphonates for the Prevention of Fractures

	Wrist	Nonvertebral	Vertebra	Hip
Alendronate (70 mg)	√	√	√	√
Risedronate (35 mg)	√	√	√	√
Ibandronate (150 mg)	NT	√	√	NT
Ibandronate IV (3 mg)	NT	√	√	NT
Zoledronate IV (5 mg)	NT	√	√	√
Raloxifene (60 mg)	NE	√	√	NE
Denosumab	NT	√	√	√
Teriparatide	NT	√	√	NT

NT, not tested; NE, not effective.

INTERVENTIONS TO PREVENT COGNITIVE IMPAIRMENT

Although there continues to be much hope for prevention, there is currently no evidence to support the value of pharmacological or nonpharmacological interventions for the prevention of Alzheimer disease. The Alzheimer's Association among other organizations recommends an overall healthy lifestyle to optimize health and well-being and in so doing prevent the development of cardiovascular disease which can contribute to vascular dementias. A healthy lifestyle generally includes eating a healthy diet, adhering to regular exercise, maintaining a goal weight, getting regular and adequate amounts of sleep, and not smoking.

There has been a focus on the use of technology, specifically computerized cognitive training, on primary and secondary prevention of dementia. A review of computerized cognitive training interventions concluded that the evidence is mixed in terms of even moderate evidence of efficacy to improve cognitive performance in healthy older adults.

With regard to the use of complementary medicine there is no strong benefit for treatments for primary or secondary prevention of dementia. Examples of treatments used include ginkgo biloba, acetyl-L-carnitine, lecithin, piracetam, curcumin, vinpocetine, phosphatidylserine, and alpha tocopherol, among others. A recent study of vitamin E, alpha tocopherol, suggested that there may be benefit among patients with mild to moderate Alzheimer disease to taking 2000 IU per day of alpha tocopherol in terms of slowing functional decline. Ongoing research is still needed.

PREVENTING DISABILITY

Although discussions of prevention tend to focus on the prevention of disease, in geriatrics the emphasis is on function and thus we take a much broader approach to the idea of prevention. When caring for older patients, it is critical to focus on physical activity and the prevention of functional decline. Keeping individuals as active as possible and not taking over activities that the individual can and should perform are important aspects of preventive care. While little may be done to prevent the occurrence of a disease in older adults, much can be done to minimize the impact of that disease. Impairments should not be allowed to become disabilities. Recent work in studying disability has raised new questions about the possible differences between transient and persistent disabled states. Studies that followed older people closely showed that many of them move in and out of transient states of disability. Hence, measures of disability over long periods may contain elements of both permanent and transient disability. This distinction is important because efforts to prevent disability may be falsely positive if they reflect transient conditions that would have improved on their own.

The overarching goal of geriatric practice is to improve, or at least preserve, function. Function is influenced by many factors including intrapersonal factors such as genetics, the individual's health status and comorbidities, mood, motivation, cognition, and beliefs; interpersonal factors and whether she or he is encouraged to engage in functional and physical activities or if the caregiver simply provides care to the individual; the environment and whether the chair height is such that the when sitting, the older individual's feet are flat on the floor so that she or he can lean forward and stand and if areas are clear of clutter and safe for ambulation; and last, policy and the impact of rules and regulations, particularly in institutional settings, on function and opportunities to access pleasant outdoor walking paths. Some hospitals, for example, have regulations that every patient who is at risk for falling gets a bed alarm on his or her bed and is unable to ambulate in the room. This increases fear among older patients and results in deconditioning and functional decline when hospitalized.

Much of the discussion in this book deals with ways to maximize the patient's health status by proper diagnosis and treatment. Such steps are necessary, but not sufficient, for good geriatric care. It is essential to appreciate that a person's environment and his or her caregivers can play a critical role in affecting functioning. Simple interventions such as providing verbal encouragement to bathe, dress, and go for a walk or simply walking with an older adult rather than pushing him or her in a wheelchair can make a major difference in the individual's ability to maintain function over time.

Environmental safety is also an important area of prevention. This includes both physical as well as psychological safety for the individual. Environmental safety hazards include things such as narrow doorways, poor lighting, clutter, slippery surfaces, and unsafe hand rails on stairs. It is important, however, to carefully consider if the risk factor identified is problematic for the older adult because disrupting the individual's known environment may serve no benefit and can be psychologically upsetting. Occupational therapists can be especially helpful in assessing the patient's environment to suggest modifications and adaptive equipment. Special efforts may be necessary to deal with the older adult's family members as their concerns about potentially dangerous accidents may lead them to become overprotective and thereby create or exacerbate dependency.

The psychological health and motivation of older adults are particularly important to consider when it comes to engaging individuals in physical activity and ensuring maintenance of function. There is a tendency for caregivers to perform tasks for the older individual due to frustration about the length of time it might otherwise take the individual to complete the task at hand. This sends a message to the older individual that he or she is not able to perform the task or not safe to do so, and creates dependency and results in contractures and functional decline. This might be as simple as dressing the individual or combing his or her hair. Completing these tasks eliminates the opportunity to maintain range of motion in joints that are used to bathe, dress, and perform personal hygiene.

Conversely, many things can be done to help motivate older adults to engage in physical activity and perform daily functional tasks. Approaches include verbally encouraging the individual to perform a certain task, providing role modeling by showing the individual what to do, eliminating any unpleasant sensations around the completion of the task (eg, provide pain medication before going for a walk), and helping him or her successfully complete the task. Identifying goals and setting rewards for goal achievement are also helpful techniques. The rewards may be as simple as spending some time talking with the individual, giving a hug and positive accolades, or engaging in more concrete rewards such as going out for a visit to family. When working with cognitively impaired individuals, modeling the behavior you want them to do is particularly helpful—using less talk and less touch and simply demonstrating the activity. Getting to know the individual and "what makes them tick" is also very helpful. For example, if an older gentleman was a television repairperson, he may be willing to go for a walk with you if you tell him he needs to "help deliver repaired televisions." Likewise, a retired nurse may walk with you to "do her rounds" or a retired police officer may "walk the beat."

Other types of social support can also be helpful to encourage participation in physical activity. Using self-help groups, technology-based social supports such as emailing friends and relatives or using chat rooms around health promotion activities, and taking care of pets or plants are also effective tools for optimizing physical activity.

IATROGENESIS

Probably the most important preventable problems encountered by older adults are those associated with iatrogenesis. Iatrogenesis is derived from Greek and refers to problems "brought forth by the healer." Specifically, iatrogenic events are those resulting from any activity by a health-care professional that has an unintended negative impact on the individual and is not consistent with his or her goals. Table 5-10 lists some of the iatrogenic problems older adults commonly experience. While the risk of exposure may be higher in acute care settings due to easier access and patient willingness to undergo testing and treatments, the risk of iatrogenesis is high in long-term care settings as well. In some cases, these iatrogenic problems can be traced to oversights and omissions. In other cases, overzealous care can be blamed. Some of the

PART II

TABLE 5-10. Common Iatrogenic Problems of Older Persons

Underdiagnosis
Bed rest
Polypharmacy
Enforced dependency
Environmental hazards
Transfer trauma
Oversedation
Overtreatment of pain/undertreatment of pain
Delirium
Fluid overload
Dehydration
Overuse of antibiotics
Overevaluation (excessive testing)
Learned dependence

problems are attributable to lack of expertise in managing older persons, but a substantial portion is caused by simply doing too much too quickly and not using one of the best philosophies of geriatric care, "a tincture of time." Generally, the more aggressive the treatment is the greater the chance that it will produce adverse effects. Moreover, older adults are less resilient and less able to tolerate the dose of the intervention, particularly with regard to medications, that is provided. Figure 5-2, portrays in a conceptual manner this narrowing of the therapeutic window (ie, the space between a therapeutic dose and a toxic dose) with age. As the response to therapy decreases, the susceptibility to toxic side effects increases. These changes are attributable to many

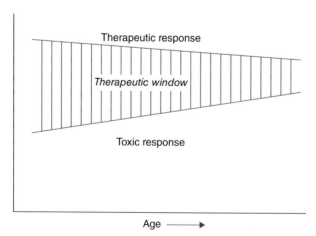

FIGURE 5-2 Narrowing of the therapeutic window. This diagram portrays in a conceptual manner how the space between a therapeutic dose and a toxic dose narrows with age.

factors, including the ability to metabolize drugs, changes in receptor behavior, and an altered chemical environment produced by other simultaneous drugs.

In the face of reduced capacity for metabolizing and excreting many drugs, the older patient can develop high blood levels on "normal" dosages. Changes in receptors may alter sensitivity to chemicals in either direction. Common examples where medications result in iatrogenic problems include bleeding associated with anticoagulants when used for prevention of cardiovascular events, secondary infections such as *Clostridium difficile* from antibiotics for a urinary tract infection in which treatment was not critical, and overzealous treatment of hypertension with subsequent orthostatic hypotension and a fall.

Across all settings of care approximately 15% of older adults are at risk for adverse events from medications. At least half of these events are anticipated to be preventable. Common problems associated with iatrogenic impact of medications include falls, orthostatic hypotension, bleeding, congestive heart failure, renal impairment, and delirium.

SPECIAL RISKS OF HOSPITALS

Hospitals are particularly dangerous places for any older adult. The risks of iatrogenic events are exacerbated in these settings as the providers may not be familiar with the patient and his or her baseline function (cognitive or physical) and prior responses to medications and treatments. Moreover, the easier access to treatments and tests in the acute care setting further increases the risk of exposure to procedures such as colonoscopies, endoscopies, or the placement of central lines. Clinicians tend to be risk aversive and order tests and procedures to avoid missing a diagnosis rather than taking the time to speak with the patient and/or caregiver to discuss the pros and cons of testing or treatment, how the test results will inform (or will not inform) or change treatment, and what the anticipated benefits and risks of the treatment are, and engage the patient and caregiver in the decision to test or treat.

As noted earlier, the risks in older adults are exacerbated because of multimorbidity and diminished reserves in cognitive, renal, and hepatic function. This culminates in the risk for what has been labeled as cascade iatrogenesis, defined as the serial development of multiple medical complications that can be set in motion by a seemingly innocuous first event. Elective surgery, for example, can result in postoperative oversedation with pain medication, a subsequent decline in respiratory function, a need for mechanical ventilation, subsequent ventilator-associated pneumonia, and ultimately even sepsis and death. A medical admission for a pneumonia or acute exacerbation of congestive heart failure can result in immobility, a subsequent urinary tract infection due to the insertion of an indwelling Foley catheter to monitor urinary output, and deconditioning, delirium, and sepsis.

The hospital environment also presents physical challenges for older adults. Specifically, this includes such things as not knowing where the bathroom is, not being able to visualize the signs and cues within the environment such as clocks and calendars that are too small, not being around familiar objects, excessive clutter increasing the risk of falls, and inappropriate bed and chair height. Last, the routine in the hospital

TABLE 5-11. Potential Complications of Bed Rest in Older Adults

Pressure sores
Bone resorption
Hypercalcemia
Postural hypotension
Atelectasis and pneumonia
Thrombophlebitis and thromboembolism
Urinary and fecal incontinence
Constipation and fecal impaction
Decreased muscle strength/deconditioning
Decreased cardiac output/aerobic capacity
Contractures
Depression and anxiety
Sensory deprivation

will be foreign to the older adult and thus he or she may miss meals by not knowing how to order a meal or ask for help with this. In a strange environment the older adult may hallucinate and become delirious. He or she may attempt to get up out of bed in the unfamiliar area and trip and fall. Not getting out of bed, a major risk factor for older adults who are hospitalized, will result in numerous consequences each of which contributes to iatrogenic episodes. Complications of bed rest are summarized in Table 5-11 and detailed in Chapter 10.

SPECIAL RISKS IN LONG-TERM CARE FACILITIES

A major iatrogenic event that is common in long-term care facilities is learned dependency. Regardless of the underlying physical capability of the older individual, caregivers across settings of care perform functional tasks for the individual rather than have them engage in the given activity. Typically this is done based on a false sense of improving efficiency—the belief that it is faster to do a task than to help the patient do it. This includes such things as pulling the older adult up in bed or turning him or her rather than having the individual perform or at least participate in the activity. When care is provided for, rather than with, residents in long-term care settings the opportunity for optimizing function is lost to the individual. Older individuals interpret this as meaning they are unable to perform the activity or that it might put them at risk. Despite extensive evidence supporting the benefit of physical activity and mobility, many caregivers continue to believe that keeping older adults in bed or immobilized in wheelchairs will decrease the risk of falls. This support of limited activity results in a vicious cycle of continued deconditioning, risk of falls and contractures, and progressive dependence.

Fortunately, there are ways to prevent iatrogenic events regardless of setting. Strategies to prevent adverse drug events include discontinuing medications if they are not needed, prescribing new medications only when needed, taking a "start low and go slow" philosophy with regard to medication management, and using the Beers Criteria, the Screening Tool of Older Persons' Potentially Inappropriate Prescriptions (STOPP), and the Screening Tool to Alert Doctors to Right Treatment (START) as guidance during care interactions. Likewise, taking the time to explain to patients and/or their caregivers that certain tests and treatments hold greater risk than benefit for the older individual may help prevent exposure and thereby prevent iatrogenic events.

Maintaining a philosophy of care that focuses on optimizing function and physical activity regardless of setting can help prevent the iatrogenic events due to immobility. This philosophy, referred to as function-focused care and involving engaging patients in functional tasks during all care interactions and encourages physical activity, has been shown to have positive outcomes in terms of optimizing and maintaining function, increasing physical activity, and preventing rehospitalizations (Boltz et al, 2014; Resnick et al, 2013; Resnick et al, 2014).

Altering environments to facilitate function and physical activity and engage older adults in stimulating and meaningful activities can also help prevent iatrogenic events. Hospital rooms often have no place to sit and so bed rest is the only option. Moreover, hallways are cluttered with equipment and there are no pleasant destination areas. For children who are hospitalized there are playrooms and attempts are made to entertain them in meaningful ways during their hospital stays. Unfortunately we do not do the same thing for older adults. Making adult activity rooms can help not only prevent deconditioning, but it also can serve as a source of orientation to prevent delirium and prevent falls by allowing for supervision of a group of patients rather than leaving patients alone in a room. Long-term care facilities are required to have activities available for older adults in these settings and while the activities may not always be meaningful to all, they provide an important first step in prevention of iatrogensis.

Special units for managing geriatric patients are beginning to emerge. Staffed by an interdisciplinary team, which may include a social worker, physician, physical or occupational therapist, and nurses, these units apply techniques of multidimensional functional evaluation to assess the needs and capacity of geriatric patients and develop treatment plans to address them.

HOSPITAL AND LONG-TERM CARE DISCHARGE PLANNING

Prevention of clinical problems and syndromes does not stop at the time of discharge from hospitals or long-term care settings. The first step in the discharge process should be ensuring that the patient is going to the most appropriate setting to optimize his or her continued recovery. The following factors should be considered:

1. The patient truly needs care in such a setting and cannot reasonably get such care elsewhere.
2. The institution is capable of providing the needed care.
3. The patient is prepared for the transfer to a nursing home, assisted living, or other type of community-based setting.

PART II

There is often pressure to get a patient discharged and insufficient time to discuss and plan the discharge with the patient and his or her caregivers. In addition, these decisions are often based on reimbursement and the resources (financial and social) of the patient. Good discharge decision making should separate two major classes of decisions: (1) What types of care are most likely to achieve the primary goals for this patient? (2) Having chosen the modality, what vendor can best provide those services? These two components require quite different sets of information. The former requires goal clarification and agreement with the patient and caregiver. Then one needs to know about the relative risks and benefits of each type of posthospital care. The choice of a vendor may involve quite different factors. Here, location, quality, and policies may be salient.

Making a good discharge decision includes at least six critical steps:

1. Adequate identification of those at risk of needing special arrangements on discharge
2. Assessment to identify problems and strengths
3. Clarification of what goals should be maximized
4. Determination of the risks and benefits associated with alternative modalities of care
5. Determination of the most suitable vendor among the modality of care selected
6. Transmission of adequate information to ensure a successful transition

Adequate information about the risks and benefits of alternative modalities may not be presented (it may not be known). Encouragement or assistance may not be provided to help patients and families determine precisely what outcomes they seek to maximize. Too often, insufficient time is allowed to weigh the complexities of the choice. When it comes to choosing among vendors of a given service, real choices may not exist because of the constraints of payment arrangements, including managed care.

As discussed in Chapter 16, the nature of nursing home care is changing. The pressure for earlier discharges from hospitals has created a new demand for what has been termed subacute care—in essence, care that was formerly provided in hospitals.

SUMMARY

Many useful steps can improve and protect the health of older adults and these should be carefully considered and encouraged. The older individual represents a different risk–benefit ratio than the younger patient. Actions well tolerated in others may produce serious consequences in the older adult and thus testing and treatments should be carefully considered. A simple preventive measure that is well supported across all settings of care involves engaging older adults in physical activity (including basic activities of daily living). This philosophy and approach to care is critical to preventive care; the bed is a dangerous place for the older patient and confinement to bed rest should be avoided whenever possible. Clinicians must guard against several potential iatrogenic problems when working with older adults. Discussing the risks and benefits of all testing and treatments and avoiding the tendency to create dependency through well-intentioned care are central to prevention of iatrogenesis.

REFERENCES

Boltz M, Resnick B, Chippendale T, Galvin J. Testing a family-centered intervention to promote functional and cognitive recovery in hospitalized older adults. *J Am Geriatr Soc.* 2014;62:2398-2407.

Calhoun M, Cross L, Cooper-DeHoff R. Clinical utility of β-blockers for primary and secondary prevention of coronary artery disease. *Expert Rev Cardiovas Ther.* 2013;11:289-291.

Department of Health and Human Services, Centers for Medicare & Medicaid Services. The ABCs of the Annual Wellness Visit. 2015. www.cms.gov/Outreach-and-Education/Medicare-Learning-Network-MLN/MLNProducts/downloads/AWV_chart_ICN905706pdf. Accessed April 2016.

Fitzpatrick-Lewis D, Warren R, Ali MU, Sherifali D, Raina P. Treatment for mild cognitive impairment: a systematic review and meta-analysis. *Can Med Assoc J Open.* 2015;3:E419-E427.

Hoffmann K, Sobol NA, Frederiksen KS, et al. Moderate-to-high intensity physical exercise in patients with Alzheimer's disease: a randomized controlled trial. *J Alzheimer's Dis.* 2015;50:443-453.

Humphreys B, McLeod L, Ruseski J. Physical activity and health outcomes: evidence from Canada. *Health Econ.* 2014;23:33-54.

Hurria A, Levit LA, Dale W, et al; American Society of Clinical Oncology. Improving the evidence base for treating older adults with cancer: American Society of Clinical Oncology statement. *J Clin Oncol.* 2015;33:3826-3833.

Khosravi P, Ghapanchi AH. Investigating the effectiveness of technologies applied to assist seniors: a systematic literature review. *Int J Med Inform.* 2016;85:17-26.

Meschia J, Bushnell C, Boden-Albala B, et al. Guidelines for the primary prevention of stroke. *Stroke.* 2015;45:3754-3832.

Poulin M, Eskes G, Hill M. Physical activity vs health education for cognition in sedentary older adults. *JAMA.* 2016;315:415.

Resnick B, Galik E, Boltz M. Function focused care approaches: progress and future possibilities. *J Am Med Dir Assoc.* 2013;14:313-318.

Resnick B, Galik E, Vigne E, Payne A. Testing the feasibility of implementing FFC-AL to 100 AL facilities in Maryland. *Fam Comm Health.* 2014;37:155-165.

Sanderson J. Clinical effectiveness of bisphosphonates for prevention of fragility fractures: a systematic review and network meta-analysis. *Value in Health.* 2015;18:A634-A638.

Sink KM, Espeland MA, Castro CM; LIFE Study Investigators. Effect of a 24-month physical activity intervention vs health education on cognitive outcomes in sedentary older adults: the LIFE randomized trial. *JAMA.* 2015;314:781-790.

Taylor F, Huffman M, Macedo A, et al. Statins for the primary prevention of cardiovascular disease. *Cochrane Database Syst Rev.* 2013;1.

Tufts University. Mayer J. MyPlate for Older Adults. 2016. http://hnrca.tufts.edu/myplate/. Accessed April 2016.

United States Preventive Services Task Force. The guide to clinical preventive services, 2014. www.ahrq.gov/professionals/clinicians-providers/guidelines-recommendations/guide/index.html. Accessed April 2016.

Waldmann A, Nolte S, Weinstock M, et al. Skin cancer screening participation and impact on melanoma incidence in Germany—an observational study on incidence trends in regions with and without population-based screening. *Br J Cancer.* 2012;106:970-974.

SELECTED READINGS

American Cancer Society. Screening guidelines. 2016. www.cancer.org/healthy/find-cancer-early/cancer-screening-guidelines/american-cancer-society-guidelines-for-the-early-detection-of-cancer.

American Heart Association. 2015–2016 clinical practice guideline for cardiovascular disease. www.bcbsil.com/pdf/clinical/cardiovascular_cpg.pdf.

Centers for Disease Control and Prevention. Surveillance for certain health behaviors among states and selected local areas—Behavioral Risk Factor Surveillance System, United States. *MMWR Surveill Summ.* www.cdc.gov/mmwr/preview/mmwrhtml/ss6309a1.htm.

Centers for Disease Control and Prevention. 2008 physical activity guidelines for Americans fact sheet for health professionals on physical activity guidelines for older adults. www.cdc.gov/physicalactivity/downloads/pa_fact_sheet_olderadults.pdf.

Department of Health and Human Services, Centers for Medicare & Medicaid Services. The ABCs of the Annual Wellness Visit. www.cms.gov/Outreach-and-Education/Medicare-Learning-Network-MLN/MLNProducts/downloads/AWV_chart_ICN905706pdf. Accessed February 2016.

Estimating Prognosis in Older Adults. ePrognosis. 2016. http://eprognosis.ucsf.edu/about.php.

National Institute of Aging. Exercise: a guide from the National Institute of Aging. 2016. www.google.com/search?q=National+Institute+of+Aging+Exercise%3A+A+guide+from+the+National+Institute+of+Aging&oq=National+Institute+of+Aging+Exercise%3A+A+guide+from+the+National+Institute+of+Aging&aqs=chrome69i573542j0j4&sourceid=chrome&es_sm=93&ie=UTF-8 2016.

Nestlé Nutritional Institute. Mini Nutritional Assessment. 2016. www.mna-elderly.com/forms/mini/mna_mini_english.pdf.

Tufts University. Mayer J. MyPlate for Older Adults. 2016. http://hnrcatuftsedu/my-plate-for-older-adults/.

United States Preventive Services Task Force. The guide to clinical preventive services, 2014. www.ahrq.gov/professionals/clinicians-providers/guidelines-recommendations/guide/index.html.

CHAPTER 6

Delirium and Dementia

Diagnosis and management of geriatric patients exhibiting symptoms and signs of impaired cognitive functioning can make a critical difference to their overall health and their ability to function independently. Impaired cognitive function can be acute in onset, or it can be slowly progressive. The major causes of impaired cognition in the geriatric population are delirium and dementia. As more people live into the tenth decade of life, the chance that they will develop some form of dementia increases substantially. Community-based studies report a prevalence of dementia as high as 47% among those 85 years of age and older. Recent evidence suggests that the incidence of dementia is decreasing in more recent cohorts of people studied (Larson et al, 2013; Satizabal et al, 2016). Between 25% and 40% of older patients admitted to acute care medical and surgical services are delirious on admission or develop delirium during their hospital stay. In nursing homes, 50% to 80% of those older than 65 years of age have some degree of cognitive impairment which can range from mild cognitive deficits to end-stage dementia. Dementia is a major risk factor for delirium, and delirium is often superimposed on dementia in both hospital and community settings, can persist for days to weeks after discharge from an acute hospital, and is a risk factor for functional decline and mortality. Both dementia and delirium are associated with high health-care costs (Amjad et al, 2016; Okie, 2011).

Misdiagnosis, overdiagnosis, or underdiagnosis and resulting inappropriate management of conditions associated with cognitive impairment in geriatric patients can cause substantial morbidity among the patients, hardship for their families and caregivers, and excessive health-care expenditures. This chapter provides a practical framework for diagnosing and managing geriatric patients who demonstrate "confusion" or signs of cognitive impairment. We focus on the most common causes of confusion in the geriatric population—delirium and dementia—although a variety of other disorders can cause the same or similar signs.

Imprecise definition of the abnormalities of cognitive function in older patients labeled as "confused" has led to problems in diagnosis and management. Descriptions such as impairment of cognitive function or cognitive impairment coupled with careful documentation of the timing and nature of specific abnormalities provide more precise and clinically useful information. Screening for dementia is controversial and is not recommended by the U.S. Preventive Services Task Force (Moyer, 2014). The best method of evaluating a patient suspected of cognitive impairment or dementia is a thorough mental status examination.

MENTAL STATUS EXAMINATION

In acutely ill older patients, identification of delirium can be accomplished with the confusion assessment method (CAM). There are many cognitive tests that can be used to identify patients with dementia (Tsoi et al, 2015). The Mini-Cog is useful

PART II

in screening for cognitive impairment and dementia. These tests are discussed later in the chapter.

A thorough mental status examination has several basic components that are essential in diagnosing dementia, delirium, or other syndromes (Table 6-1). The examiner should focus on each of these components in a systematic manner. Recording observations in each area facilitates recognizing and evaluating changes over time. Standardized and validated measures of cognitive function should be used in diagnosis for patients who have a positive Mini-Cog, and for subsequent monitoring. Several factors may, however, influence performance and interpretation of standard mental status tests, such as prior educational level, primary language other than English, severely impaired hearing, or poor baseline intellectual function. Thus, scores on these tests should not be used to replace a more comprehensive examination such as that in Table 6 -1.

Important information can be gleaned unobtrusively from simply observing and interacting with the patient during the history. Is the patient alert and attentive? Does the patient respond appropriately to questions? How is the patient dressed and groomed? Does the patient repeat herself or give an imprecise social or medical history, suggesting memory impairment? Orientation, insight, and judgment can sometimes be assessed during the history as well.

Questions relating to specific areas of cognitive functioning should be introduced in a nonthreatening manner, because many patients with early deficits respond defensively. Each of the three basic components of memory should be tested: immediate recall (eg, repeating digits), recent memory (eg, recalling three objects after a few minutes), and remote memory (eg, ability to give details of early life). Language and other cognitive functions should be carefully evaluated. Is the patient's speech clear? Can the patient read (and understand) and write? Does there seem to be a good general fund of knowledge (eg, current events)? Other cognitive functions that can be tested easily include the ability to perform simple calculations (eg, one that relates to making change while shopping) and to copy diagrams. The ability to

---

TABLE 6-1. Key Aspects of Mental Status Examination

State of consciousness
General appearance and behavior
Orientation
Memory (short- and long-term)
Language
Visuospatial function
Executive control function (eg, planning and sequencing of tasks)
Other cognitive functions (eg, calculations, proverb interpretation)
Insight and judgment
Thought content
Mood and affect

interpret proverbs abstractly and to list the names of animals (listing 12 names in 1 minute is normal) is a sensitive indicator of cognitive function and is easy to test.

Judgment and insight can usually be assessed during the examination without asking specific questions, although input from family members or other caregivers can be helpful, and is sometimes necessary. Any abnormal thought content should also be noted during the examination; bizarre ideas, mood-incongruent thoughts, and delusions (especially paranoid delusions) may be present in older patients with cognitive impairment and are important both diagnostically and therapeutically. Observations during the examination may also detect abnormalities of executive control. Executive function involves the planning, sequencing, and execution of goal-directed activities. These functions are critical to the ability to perform instrumental activities of daily living (IADLs). Screening tests for executive dysfunction include a clock-drawing test, which is a component of the Mini-Cog (see later in this chapter).

Throughout the examination, the patient's mood and affect should be assessed. Depression, apathy, emotional liability, agitation, and aggression are common in older patients with cognitive impairment, and failure to recognize these abnormalities can lead to improper diagnosis and management. In some patients—such as those who are poorly educated or have low intelligence, as well as those in whom depression is suspected—more detailed neuropsychological testing by an experienced neuro (i.e. neuropsychologist) psychologist is helpful in precisely defining abnormalities in cognitive function and in differentiating between the many and often interacting underlying causes.

DIFFERENTIAL DIAGNOSIS

The causes of impaired cognitive function in the geriatric population are myriad. The differential diagnosis in an older patient who presents with confusion includes disorders of the brain (eg, stroke, dementia), a systemic illness presenting atypically (eg, infection, metabolic disturbance, myocardial infarction, congestive heart failure), sensory impairment (eg, hearing loss), and adverse effects of a variety of drugs or alcohol.

Like many other disorders in geriatric patients, cognitive impairment often results from multiple interacting processes rather than a single causative factor. Accurate diagnosis depends on specifically defining abnormalities in mental status and cognitive function and on consistent definitions for clinical syndromes. Disorders causing cognitive impairment in the geriatric population can be broadly categorized into three groups:

1. Acute disorders usually associated with acute illness, drugs, and environmental factors (ie, delirium)
2. More slowly progressive impairment of cognitive function as seen in most dementia syndromes
3. Impaired cognitive function associated with affective disorders and psychoses

Age-associated disorders such as impaired hearing and Parkinson's disease can lead to mislabeling an older patient as "confused" or "senile." Old age alone does not cause impairment of cognitive function of sufficient severity to render an individual dysfunctional. Slowed thinking and reaction time, mild recent memory loss, and impaired executive function can occur with increasing age and may or may not progress to dementia. *Mild cognitive impairment (MCI)* and *cognitive impairment, not dementia (CIND)* have been used to describe these deficits. MCI is defined in Table 6-2. Just over 20% of people aged 71 and older in the United States have cognitive impairment without dementia (Plassman et al, 2008). Data suggest that up to 15% to 20% of those diagnosed with MCI will progress to dementia over the course of a year; thus most people with MCI will progress to dementia within 5 years (Petersen, 2011; Sachdev et al, 2012). The therapeutic implications of MCI are subjects of intensive research. No nonpharmacological or pharmacological intervention has been shown to prevent progression to dementia.

Three questions are helpful in making an accurate diagnosis of the underlying cause(s) of cognitive impairment:

1. Has the onset of abnormalities been acute (ie, over a few hours or a few days)?
2. Are there physical factors (eg, medical illness, sensory deprivation, drugs) that may contribute to the abnormalities?
3. Are psychological factors (ie, depression and/or psychosis) contributing to or complicating the impairments in cognitive function?

TABLE 6-2. NIA–AA Core Clinical Diagnostic Criteria for Mild Cognitive Impairment

Mild cognitive impairment*
The patient, an informant who knows the patient well, or a clinician observing the patient notes a concern regarding a change in cognition in comparison to the patient's previous level.
There is evidence of lower performance in one or more cognitive domains (memory, executive function, attention, language, and/or visuospatial skills) that is greater than would be expected for the patient's age and educational background.
The patient maintains preserved independence in functional abilities, although they may take more time, be less efficient, and make more errors at performing such activities than in the past.
The patient does *not* meet criteria for dementia.

*DSM-5 "mild neurocognitive disorder" criteria also states that these deficits do not occur exclusively in the context of a delirium or other mental disorder (eg, major depressive disorder, schizophrenia). Identification and exclusion of other neurologic, psychiatric, and medical disorders is implied in the text of the NIA–AA MCI diagnostic criteria.

Data from Albert MS, DeKosky ST, Dickson D, et al. The diagnosis of mild cognitive impairment due to Alzheimer's disease: recommendations from the National Institute on Aging-Alzheimer's Association workgroups on diagnostic guidelines for Alzheimer's disease, *Alzheimers Dement.* 2011 May;7(3):270-279.

These questions focus on identifying treatable conditions, which, when diagnosed and treated, might result in substantially improved cognitive function and better individualized care planning.

DELIRIUM

Delirium is an acute or subacute alteration in mental status especially common in the geriatric population (Table 6-3). Although most clinicians recognize hyperactive delirium with agitation, many fail to appreciate the hypoactive form. The prevalence of delirium in hospitalized geriatric patients is approximately 15% on admission, and the incidence in this setting may be up to one-third. Delirium may persist for days or weeks and is, therefore, common in postacute care settings. Many factors predispose geriatric patients to the development of delirium, including impaired sensory functioning and sensory deprivation, sleep deprivation, immobilization, and transfer to an unfamiliar environment.

The key features of this disorder include the following:

- Disturbance of consciousness (including hyperactivity and agitation, or hypoactive presentations such as lethargy and apathy)
- Change in cognition not better accounted for by dementia
- Symptoms and signs developing over a short period of time (hours to days)
- Fluctuation of the symptoms and signs
- Evidence that the disturbances are caused by the physiological consequences of a medical condition

The disturbances of consciousness and attention, with sudden onset and fluctuating cognitive status, are the major features that distinguish delirium from other

---

TABLE 6-3. Diagnostic Criteria for Delirium

A. A disturbance in attention (ie, reduced ability to direct, focus, sustain, and shift attention) and awareness (reduced orientation to the environment).

B. The disturbance develops over a short period of time (usually hours to a few days), represents a change from baseline attention and awareness, and tends to fluctuate in severity during the course of a day.

C. An additional disturbance in cognition (eg, memory deficit, disorientation, language, visuospatial ability, or perception).

D. The disturbances in Criteria A and C are not better explained by another preexisting, established, or evolving neurocognitive disorder and do not occur in the context of a severely reduced level of arousal, such as coma.

E. There is evidence from the history, physical examination, or laboratory findings that the disturbance is a direct physiological consequence of another medical condition, substance intoxication or withdrawal (ie, due to a drug of abuse or to a medication), or exposure to a toxin, or is due to multiple etiologies.

Data from American Psychiatric Association: *Diagnostic and statistical manual of mental disorders*, 5th edition. Arlington: American Psychiatric Association; 2013.

causes of impaired cognitive function. Delirium is characterized by difficulty in sustaining attention to external and internal stimuli, sensory misperceptions (eg, illusions), and a fragmented or disordered stream of thought. Disturbances of psychomotor activity (eg, restlessness, picking at bedclothes, attempting to get out of bed, sluggishness, drowsiness, and generally decreased psychomotor activity) and emotional disturbances (eg, anxiety, fear, irritability, anger, apathy) are common in delirious patients. Neurological signs (except asterixis) are uncommon in delirium.

Several predisposing factors are associated with the development of delirium, and there are multiple factors that can precipitate delirium (Table 6-4).

Rapid recognition of delirium is critical because it is often related to other reversible conditions and its development may be a poor prognostic sign for adverse

---

TABLE 6-4. Predisposing and Precipitating Factors for Delirium From Validated Predictive Models

Predisposing factors

- Dementia or underlying cognitive impairment
- Severe illness
- Comorbidity
- Depression
- Vision and/or hearing impairment
- Functional impairment
- History of transient ischemia or stroke
- History of alcohol abuse
- History of delirium
- Advanced age (>70 years)

Precipitating factors

- Medications, including polypharmacy, psychoactive, sedative–hypnotic
- Use of physical restraints
- Indwelling bladder catheters
- Dehydration
- Poor nutritional status, abnormal serum albumin
- Iatrogenic complications
- Major surgical procedure (eg, aortic aneurysm repair, noncardiac thoracic surgery, neurosurgery)
- Metabolic derangements (electrolytes, glucose, metabolic acidosis)
- Infection
- Trauma admission
- Urgent admission

Reproduced with permission from Halter JB, Ouslander JG, Studenski S, et al: *Hazzard's Geriatric Medicine and Gerontology*, 7th ed. New York: McGraw-Hill Education; 2016.

outcomes including nursing home placement and death. The CAM is a validated tool to identify delirium (Table 6-5; Inouye et al, 1990). The diagnosis of delirium by the CAM requires the presence of:

- Acute onset and fluctuating course *and*
- Inattention *and*
- Disorganized thinking *or*
- Altered level of consciousness

Differentiating delirium from dementia and other conditions such as depression and acute psychosis is important, because inappropriately labeling a delirious patient as demented or depressed may delay the diagnosis of serious and treatable underlying medical conditions. It is not possible to make the diagnosis of dementia when delirium is present in a patient with previously normal or unknown cognitive function. The diagnosis of dementia must await the treatment of the potentially reversible causes of delirium. Table 6-6 shows some of the key clinical features that are helpful in differentiating delirium from dementia, depression, and acute psychosis.

TABLE 6-5. The Confusion Assessment Method Diagnostic Algorithm*

Feature 1. Acute onset and fluctuating course

This feature is usually obtained from a reliable reporter, such as a family member, caregiver, or nurse, and is shown by positive responses to these questions: Is there evidence of an acute change in mental status from the patient's baseline? Did the (abnormal) behavior fluctuate during the day, that is, tend to come and go, or did it increase and decrease in severity?

Feature 2. Inattention

This feature is shown by a positive response to this question: Did the patient have difficulty focusing attention, for example, being easily distractible, or have difficulty keeping track of what was being said?

Feature 3. Disorganized thinking

This feature is shown by a positive response to this question: Was the patient's thinking disorganized or incoherent, such as rambling or irrelevant conversation, unclear or illogical flow of ideas, or unpredictable switching from subject to subject?

Feature 4. Altered level of consciousness

This feature is shown by any answer other than "alert" to this question: Overall, how would you rate this patient's level of consciousness (alert [normal], vigilant [hyperalert], lethargic [drowsy, easily aroused], stupor [difficult to arouse], or coma [unarousable])?

*The diagnosis of delirium by CAM requires the presence of features 1 and 2 and of either 3 or 4. Data from Inouye SK, vanDyck CH, Alessi CA, et al. Clarifying confusion: the confusion assessment method. A new method for detection of delirium, *Ann Intern Med*. 1990 Dec 15;113(12):941-948.

TABLE 6-6. Differentiating Delirium, Dementia, Depression, and Acute Psychosis

Characteristic	Delirium	Dementia	Depression	Acute psychosis
Onset	Acute (hours to days)	Progressive, insidious (weeks to months)	Either acute or insidious	Acute
Course over time	Waxing and waning	Unrelenting	Variable	Episodic
Attention	Impaired, a hallmark of delirium	Usually intact, until end-stage disease	Decreased concentration and attention to detail	Variable
Level of consciousness	Altered, from lethargic to hyperalert	Normal, until end-stage disease	Normal	Normal
Memory	Impaired commonly	Prominent short- and/or long-term memory impairment	Normal, some short-term forgetfulness	Usually normal
Orientation	Disoriented	Normal, until end-stage disease	Usually normal	Usually normal
Speech	Disorganized, incoherent, illogical	Notable for parsimony, aphasia, anomia	Normal, but often slowing of speech (psychomotor retardation)	Variable, often disorganized
Delusions	Common	Common	Uncommon	Common, often complex
Hallucinations	Usually visual	Sometimes	Rare	Usually auditory and more complex
Organic etiology	Yes	Yes	No	No

Reproduced with permission from Halter JB, Ouslander JG, Studenski S, et al: *Hazzard's Geriatric Medicine and Gerontology*, 7th ed. New York: McGraw-Hill Education; 2016.

Sundowning is a term that describes an increase in confusion that commonly occurs in geriatric patients, especially those with preexisting dementia, at night. This condition is probably related to sensory deprivation in unfamiliar surroundings (such as the acute care hospital), and patients who sundown may meet the criteria for delirium.

A complete list of conditions that can cause delirium is too long to be useful in a clinical setting. Table 6-7 lists some of the common causes of this disorder. Several of them deserve further attention. Each geriatric patient who becomes acutely confused should be evaluated to rule out treatable conditions such as metabolic disorders, infections, and causes for decreased cardiac output (ie, dehydration, acute blood loss, heart failure). The evaluation should include vital signs (including pulse oximetry and a finger-stick glucose determination in diabetics), a careful physical examination, a complete blood count and basic metabolic panel, and other diagnostic tests as indicated by the findings and the patient's comorbidities.

Sometimes this evaluation is unrevealing. Small cortical strokes, which do not produce focal symptoms or signs or obvious changes on brain imaging, can cause delirium. These events may be difficult or impossible to diagnose with certainty, but there should be a high index of suspicion for this diagnosis in certain subgroups of patients—especially those with a history of hypertension, previous strokes, transient ischemic attacks, or cardiac arrhythmias. If delirium recurs, a source of emboli should be sought, and associated conditions (such as hypertension) should be treated

PART II

TABLE 6-7. Common Causes of Delirium in Geriatric Patients

Metabolic disorders
   Hypoxia
   Hypercarbia
   Hypo- or hyperglycemia
   Hyponatremia
   Azotemia
Infections
Decreased cardiac output
   Dehydration
   Acute blood loss
   Acute myocardial infarction
   Congestive heart failure
Stroke (small cortical)
Drugs (see Table 6-8)
Intoxication (alcohol, other)
Hypo- or hyperthermia
Acute psychoses
Sensory impairment
Transfer to unfamiliar surroundings (especially when sensory input is diminished)
Other
   Fecal impaction
   Urinary retention

optimally. Fecal impaction and urinary retention, as well as urinary tract infections, common in geriatric patients in acute care hospitals, can have dramatic effects on cognitive function and may be causes of acute confusion. The response to relief from these conditions can be just as impressive.

Medications are a major cause of acute and chronic impairment of cognitive function in older patients. Anesthesia poses a special risk, and thus preoperative assessment of cognitive function in older adults is important. Table 6-8 lists selected drugs that can cause or contribute to delirium. Every attempt should be made to avoid or discontinue any medication that may be worsening cognitive function in a delirious geriatric patient. This may not be possible, and in some patients, psychotropic drugs may be needed to treat delirium. If the patient is a danger to themselves or others low dose haloperidol (0.25–0.5 mg) is generally recommended; more sedating antipsychotics and benzodiazepines should be avoided unless the goal is to put the patient to sleep for a short time. If a benzodiazepine is used, it should be short-acting and in a low dose.

Environmental factors, especially rapid changes in location (such as being hospitalized, going on vacation, or entering a nursing home) and sensory deprivation, can precipitate delirium. This is especially true of those with early forms of dementia (see next section). Measures such as preparing older patients for changes in location; placing familiar objects in the surroundings; and maximizing sensory input with lighting, clocks, and calendars may help prevent or manage delirium in some patients. A Hospital Elder Life Program has been described that may help prevent delirium and cognitive and functional decline among high-risk older patients in acute hospitals (Inouye et al, 1999; Inouye et al, 2000; see http://hospitalelderlifeprogram. org/public/public-main.php [accessed November 20, 2016]). This program incorporates several strategies for identifying risk factors and causes of delirium and medical behavioral and environmental interventions for patients who develop delirium and has been shown to be sustainable in a community hospital setting (Table 6-9).

TABLE 6-8. Drugs That Can Cause or Contribute to Delirium and Dementia[*]

Analgesics	Cardiovascular
Narcotic	Antiarrhythmics
Nonnarcotic	Digoxin
Nonsteroidal anti-inflammatory agents	H_2 receptor antagonists
Anticholinergics/antihistamines	Psychotropic drugs
Anticonvulsants	Antianxiety drugs
Antidepressant drugs	Sedative–hypnotics
Antipsychotics	
Antiparkinsonism drugs	
Alcohol	
	Skeletal muscle relaxants
	Steroids

[*]Other drugs may contribute but are less common.

TABLE 6-9. Interventions for Risk Factors for Delirium

Risk factor	Intervention protocol
Cognitive impairment	• Oriented communication, including orientation board • Therapeutic activities program
Immobilization	• Early mobilization (eg, ambulation or bedside exercises) • Minimization of immobilizing equipment whenever possible (eg, restraints, bladder catheters oxygen, intravenous lines)
Psychoactive medications	• Restricted use of PRN sleep and psychoactive medications (eg, sedative–hypnotics, narcotics, anticholinergic drugs) • Nonpharmacological protocols for management of sleep and anxiety
Sleep deprivation	• Noise-reduction strategies • Scheduling of nighttime medications, procedures, and nursing activities to allow uninterrupted period of sleep
Vision impairment	• Provision of vision aids (eg, magnifiers, special lighting) • Provision of adaptive equipment (eg, illuminated phone dials, large-print books)
Hearing impairment	• Provision of amplifying devices; repair hearing aids • Staff instruction in communication methods
Dehydration	• Early recognition and volume repletion

Data from Inouye SK, Bogardus ST Jr, Charpentier PA, et al. A clinical trial of a multicomponent intervention to prevent delirium in hospitalized older patients, *N Engl J Med.* 1999 Mar 4;340(9):669-676.

DEMENTIA

Dementia is a clinical syndrome involving a sustained loss of cognitive function of sufficient severity to cause dysfunction in daily living. Loss of functional ability due to impaired cognition is the key feature that distinguishes dementia from mild cognitive impairment (MCI). Its key features include:

• A gradually progressing course (usually over months to years)
• No disturbance of consciousness

Table 6-10 lists the clinical diagnostic criteria for all-cause dementia and for dementia due to Alzheimer disease.

While it is important to rule out treatable and potentially reversible causes of dementia in individual patients, these dementias account for a very small proportion of dementias. Moreover, finding a reversible cause does not guarantee that the dementia will improve after the putative cause has been treated. Table 6-11 lists potentially reversible causes of cognitive impairment that can mimic or contribute to dementia. Total reversal of cognitive impairment is uncommon.

TABLE 6-10. NIA-AA Core Clinical Diagnostic Criteria for All-Cause Dementia and Dementia Due to Alzheimer Disease

Dementia

The patient has cognitive or behavioral symptoms that:
- Interfere with the ability to function at work or at usual activities;
- Represent a decline from previous levels of functioning and performing; and
- Are not explained by delirium or major psychiatric disorder.

Cognitive impairment is detected and diagnosed through a combination of:
- History-taking from the patient and a knowledgeable informant; and
- An objective cognitive assessment, either a "bedside" mental status examination or neuropsychological testing.

The cognitive or behavioral impairment involves a minimum of two of the following domains:*
- Impaired ability to acquire and remember new information;
- Impaired reasoning, judgment, and handling of complex tasks;
- Impaired visuospatial abilities;
- Impaired language functions; and/or
- Changes in personality, behavior, or comportment.

Probable dementia due to Alzheimer disease[†]

The patient meets criteria for dementia *and* has the following characteristics:
- Insidious onset over months to years, not sudden over hours or days;
- Clear-cut history of worsening cognition by report or observation; and
- Initial and most prominent cognitive deficits that are evident on history and examination in one of the following categories:

Amnestic presentation (most common presentation)—Deficits should include impairment in learning and recall of recently learned information, plus cognitive dysfunction in at least one other cognitive domain.

Non-amnestic presentations:[‡]

Language presentation —The most prominent deficits are in word-finding, but deficits in other cognitive domains should be present.

Visuospatial presentation—The most prominent deficits are in spatial cognition, but deficits in other cognitive domains should be present.

Executive dysfunction—The most prominent deficits are impaired reasoning, judgment, and problem solving, but deficits in other cognitive domains should be present.

The diagnosis of probable AD dementia *should not* be applied when there is evidence of:
- Substantial concomitant cerebrovascular disease (defined by a history of a stroke temporally related to onset or worsening of cognitive impairment or presence of multiple or extensive infarcts or severe white matter hyperintensity burden); or
- Core features of dementia with Lewy bodies.

(continued)

TABLE 6-10. NIA-AA Core Clinical Diagnostic Criteria for All-Cause Dementia and Dementia Due to Alzheimer Disease (*continued*)

Probable dementia due to Alzheimer disease[†]

- Prominent features of behavioral variant frontotemporal dementia; or
- Prominent features of primary progressive aphasia; or
- Active neurological disease or a medical comorbidity or use of medication that could have a substantial effect on cognition.

*Diagnostic criteria for DSM-5 "major neurocognitive disorder" require a significant cognitive decline in *one* or more cognitive domains (complex attention, executive function, learning and memory, language, perceptual-motor, or social cognition).

[†]The diagnosis of "probable AD dementia with increased level of certainty" is made when there is a documented cognitive decline and/or evidence of a causative genetic mutation (*APP, PSEN1,* or *PSEN2; not APOE4*) in addition to the above diagnostic criteria.

[‡]Diagnostic criteria for DSM-5 "major neurocognitive disorder due to Alzheimer's disease" require that one of the affected cognitive domains be memory and learning.

Data from Albert MS, DeKosky ST, Dickson D, et al. The diagnosis of mild cognitive impairment due to Alzheimer's disease: recommendations from the National Institute on Aging-Alzheimer's Association workgroups on diagnostic guidelines for Alzheimer's disease, *Alzheimers Dement.* 2011 May;7(3):270-279.

These disorders can be detected by careful history, physical examination, and selected laboratory studies. Medications known to cause abnormalities in cognitive function (see Table 6-8) should be discontinued whenever feasible. There should be a high index of suspicion regarding excessive alcohol intake in older patients. The incidence of alcohol consumption varies considerably in different populations but is easily missed and can cause dementia as well as delirium, depression, falls, and other medical complications.

Depressive pseudodementia is a term that has been used to refer to patients who have reversible or partially reversible impairments of cognitive function caused by depression. Depression may coexist with dementia in more than one-third of out-patients with dementia and in an even greater proportion in nursing home patients. The interrelationship between depression and dementia is complex. Many patients with early forms of dementia become depressed, and depression may be diagnosed in many patients before they become demented. Sorting out how much of the cognitive impairment is caused by depression and how much by an organic factor (or factors) can be difficult. Some clinical characteristics can be helpful in diagnosis including prominent complaints of memory loss, patchy and inconsistent cognitive deficits on examination, and frequent "don't know" answers. Detailed neuropsychological testing, performed by a psychologist or other health-care professional skilled in the use of these tools, can be helpful in many patients. At times, even after a complete assessment, uncertainty still exists regarding the role of depression in producing intellectual deficits. Under these circumstances, a careful trial of an antidepressant is justified to facilitate the diagnosis and may help improve overall functioning and quality of

TABLE 6-11. Potentially Reversible Conditions That Can Contribute to Cognitive Impairment and Dementia

Depression

Adverse medication effects

Delirium

Acute alcohol intoxication

Substance use disorders

Obstructive sleep apnea

Other sleep disorders

Chronic hypoxia and/or hypercapnia

Recurrent hypoglycemia

Thyroid diseases

Other metabolic-endocrine disorders

Vitamins B_1 (thiamine), B_{12}, and/or D deficiencies

Uremia

Hepatic encephalopathy

Environmental toxicity (lead, mercury, polychlorinated biphenyls [PCBs], dioxins, etc)

Lyme disease

HIV-associated neurocognitive disorders (HAND)

Chronic meningitis/encephalitis

Neurosyphilis

Adapted with permission from Halter JB, Ouslander JG, Studenski S, et al: *Hazzard's Geriatric Medicine and Gerontology*, 7th ed. New York: McGraw-Hill Education; 2016.

life. Older patients who develop reversible cognitive impairment while depressed appear at relatively high risk for developing dementia over the following few years, and their cognitive function should be followed closely over time.

TYPES OF DEMENTIA

Table 6-12 lists various types or causes of dementias and Table 6-13 compares common clinical features of four of the most prevalent forms of dementia.

Alzheimer disease (AD) and multi-infarct dementia account for the majority of dementias in the geriatric population. They frequently coexist in the same patient (Langa et al, 2004; Snowden et al, 1997). Dementia with Lewy bodies (DLB) accounts for up to 25% of dementias in some series, and the symptoms may overlap with Alzheimer and Parkinson dementias. Cardiac scintigraphy may be helpful in distinguishing DLB from AD, but this is not generally performed in clinical practice. In addition to the characteristic pathologic findings, DLB is characterized by:

- Visual hallucinations
- Parkinsonian signs
- Alterations of alertness and attention

TABLE 6-12. Causes of Dementia

Alzheimer disease

Lewy body dementia

Vascular dementia/vascular cognitive impairment

Frontotemporal dementia

Parkinson disease dementia

Progressive supranuclear palsy

Corticobasal degeneration

Prion-related diseases (Creutzfeldt-Jakob, bovine spongiform encephalopathy)

Normal pressure hydrocephalus (NPH)

Huntington's disease

Alcohol-related dementia

Wernicke-Korsakoff syndrome

Traumatic brain injury

Chronic traumatic encephalopathy (CTE)

Mass lesions (neoplasms, benign tumors, hematomas)

Central nervous system rheumatologic/autoimmune disorders (systemic lupus erythematosus, sarcoidosis, vasculitis, multiple sclerosis, etc)

Paraneoplastic syndromes

CADASIL (cerebral autosomal dominant arteriopathy with subcortical infarcts and leukoencephalopathy)

Carotid artery disease

Postoperative cognitive dysfunction

Seizure disorder

Adapted with permission from Halter JB, Ouslander JG, Studenski S, et al: *Hazzard's Geriatric Medicine and Gerontology*, 7th ed. New York: McGraw-Hill Education; 2016.

Patients with DLB can be very sensitive to the extrapyramidal effects of antipsychotic medication and they must be used cautiously in this patient population.

Table 6-10 lists the diagnostic criteria for AD dementia. Family history and increasing age are its primary risk factors. Approximately 6% to 8% of persons older than age 65 have AD. The prevalence doubles every 5 years, so that nearly 30% of the population older than age 85 has AD. By the age of 90, almost 50% of persons with a first-degree relative living with AD might develop the disease themselves. Rare genetic mutations on chromosomes 1, 14, and 21 cause early-onset familial forms of AD, and some forms of late-onset AD are linked to chromosome 12. The strongest genetic linkage with late-onset AD identified thus far is the apolipoprotein E epsilon 4 (apo E-E4) allele on chromosome 19. The relative risk of AD associated with one or more copies of this allele in whites is approximately 2.5. However, apo E-E4 does not appear to confer increased risk for AD among African Americans or Hispanics. Because the presence of one or more apo E-E4 alleles is neither sensitive nor specific,

TABLE 6-13. Clinical Features of Common Dementias

Type of dementia	Alzheimer disease	Vascular dementia	Dementia with Lewy bodies	Frontotemporal dementia
Must first meet diagnostic criteria for dementia (see Table 6-1)				
Typical course	Insidious onset and gradually progressive	Acute onset of cognitive impairment with some stabilization (if only one vascular event) and/or stepwise deterioration (if multiple infarcts)	Progressive cognitive decline with fluctuating cognition, attention, and alertness	Insidious onset and gradually progressive
Cognitive symptoms	Memory is the most commonly affected cognitive domain. May also have impairments in executive function, language, and/or visuospatial skills	Various cognitive domains may be affected depending on the location of the clinical stroke(s) and/or severe subcortical cerebrovascular disease	Cognitive symptoms may fluctuate. May have prominent impairment in visuospatial ability, attention, and/or executive function	Will have early behavioral disinhibition and apathy (frontal lobe predominance) or early prominent language abnormalities (temporal lobe predominance). Deficits are chiefly noted in executive tasks with relative sparing of memory and visuospatial skills
Other associated symptoms/signs	Some patients may have agitation and/or behavioral changes	May or may not have focal neurologic signs on exam. Should have evidence of relevant cerebrovascular disease by brain imaging	May have recurrent well-formed visual hallucinations (usually people or animals), parkinsonism (including tremor, rigidity, and postural instability), recurrent falls and syncope, rapid eye movement (REM) sleep behavior disorder, neuroleptic sensitivity, and/or delusions	In behavioral variant frontotemporal dementia, may have early behavioral disinhibition, apathy, loss of empathy, perseverative behaviors, and hyperorality

Reproduced with permission from Halter JB, Ouslander JG, Studenski S, et al: *Hazzard's Geriatric Medicine and Gerontology*, 7th ed. New York: McGraw-Hill Education; 2016.

there is no agreement on recommending it as a screening test for AD. Thus, routine screening, even among high-risk populations, is generally not recommended.

Other possible risk factors for AD include previous head injury, female sex, lower education level, and other yet-to-be-identified susceptibility genes. Studies on the protective effects of antihypertensive medications, omega-3 fatty acids, physical activity, and cognitive engagement are ongoing; these factors may help prevent or delay cognitive decline or AD, but no firm conclusions can be drawn from the growing data available (National Institutes of Health, 2010).

Vascular Dementia

Vascular dementia predominately caused by multiple infarcts (multi-infarct dementia) and other vascular changes is common in the geriatric population. Vascular dementia can occur alone or in combination with other disorders that cause dementia (Zekry et al, 2002). Autopsy studies suggest that cerebrovascular disease may play an important role in the presence and severity of symptoms of AD (Snowden et al, 1997). Multi-infarct dementia results when a patient has sustained recurrent cortical or subcortical strokes. Many of these strokes are too small to cause permanent or residual focal neurological deficits or evidence of strokes on computed tomography (CT). Magnetic resonance imaging (MRI) may be more sensitive in detecting small infarcts. Table 6-13 contrasts characteristics of patients likely to have vascular versus AD. A key feature of multi-infarct dementia is the stepwise deterioration in cognitive functioning compared to the generally more slowly progressive decline in AD, as illustrated in Figure 6-1.

EVALUATION

The first step in diagnosing dementia is to recognize clues that dementia may be present. The Mini-Cog assessment is a useful screening tool in identifying patients who should undergo further assessment. It screens both memory (three-item recall) and executive function (clock drawing) (Borson et al, 2003). The value of screening for cognitive impairment has been debated. Despite the lack of specific therapies, screening can identify impairments that should be followed over time, which in turn will help guide support and education of the patient and family as well as planning for the future.

Table 6-14 lists symptoms that should suggest further evaluation. Patients exhibiting one or more of these symptoms should be considered for the following evaluation:

- Focused history and physical examination, including assessment for delirium and depression and identification of comorbid conditions (eg, sensory impairment)
- A functional status assessment (see Chapter 3)
- A mental status examination (see Table 6-1)
- Selected laboratory studies to rule out reversible dementia and delirium

PART II

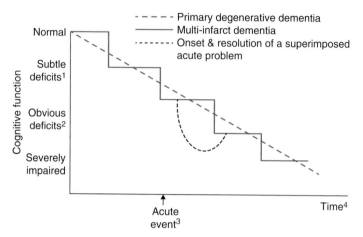

FIGURE 6-1 Primary degenerative dementia versus multi-infarct dementia: comparison of time courses. (1) Recognized by patient, but detectable only on detailed testing. (2) Deficits recognized by family and friends. (3) See text for explanation. (4) Exact time courses are variable; see text.

Table 6-15 outlines key aspects of the history. Because many physical illnesses and drugs can cause cognitive dysfunction, active medical problems and use of prescription and nonprescription drugs (including alcohol) should be reviewed. The nature and severity of the symptoms should be characterized. What are the deficits? Does the patient admit to them, or is the family member describing them? How is the patient reacting to the problems? The responses to these questions can be helpful in differentiating between dementia, depressive, and mixed condition. The onset of symptoms and the rate of progression are particularly important. The sudden onset

---

TABLE 6-14. Symptoms That May Indicate Dementia

- Difficulty learning and retaining new information and/or handling complex tasks (eg, managing finances, driving)
- Repetition
- Trouble remembering recent conversations, events, or appointments
- Frequently misplaces objects
- Difficulty with abstract thinking
- Difficulty following a complex train of thought or performing tasks that require many steps, such as balancing a checkbook or cooking a meal (ie, executive function)
- Impaired reasoning or judgment
- Impaired spatial ability
- Impaired orientation
- Difficulty with finding the words or following conversations
- Behavioral or personality changes (eg, appears more passive with less initiative, is more irritable or suspicious than usual; misinterprets visual or auditory stimuli)

TABLE 6-15. Evaluating Dementia: The History

Summarize active medical problems and current physical complaints
List medications (including over-the-counter preparations and alcohol)
Cardiovascular and neurological history
Characterize the symptoms
  Nature of deficits (memory vs other cognitive functions)
  Onset and rate of progression
  Impaired function (eg, managing money or medications)
  Associated psychological symptoms
    Depression
    Anxiety or agitation
    Paranoid ideation
    Psychotic thought processes (delusions and/or hallucinations)
Ask about
  Driving and car accidents
  Wandering and/or getting lost
  Dangerous driving and car crashes
  Disruptive or self-endangering behaviors
  Verbal agitation
  Physical aggression
  Insomnia
  Poor hygiene
  Malnutrition
  Incontinence
Assess the social situation
  Living arrangements
  Social supports
Availability of relatives and other caregivers
Employment and health of caregivers

of cognitive impairment (over a few days) should prompt a search for one of the underlying causes of delirium listed in Table 6-4. Irregular, stepwise decrements in cognitive function (as opposed to a more even and gradual loss) favor a diagnosis of vascular or multi-infarct dementia (see Table 6-13 and Fig. 6-1). Patients with dementia are often brought for evaluation at a time of sudden worsening of cognitive function (as illustrated by the broken line in Fig. 6-1) and may even meet the criteria for delirium. These sudden changes may be triggered by acute events (a small stroke without focal signs, acute physical illness, drugs, changes in environment, or personal loss such as the death or departure of a relative). Only a careful history (or familiarity with the patient) will help determine when an acute event has been superimposed on a preexisting dementia. Appropriate management of the acute event may result in improvement in cognitive function (see Fig. 6-1, broken line).

The history should also include specific questions about common problems requiring special attention in patients with dementia. These problems may include wandering, dangerous driving and car crashes, disruptive behavior (eg, verbal agitation, physical aggression, and nighttime agitation), delusions or hallucinations, insomnia, poor hygiene, malnutrition, and incontinence. They require careful management and most often substantial involvement of family or other caregivers.

A social history is especially important in patients with dementia. Living arrangements and social supports should be assessed. Along with functional status, these factors play a major role in the management of patients with dementia and are of critical importance in determining the possible necessity for institutionalization. A patient with dementia and weak social supports may require institutionalization at a higher level of function than a patient with strong social supports. In addition to the lack of availability of a spouse, child, or other relative who can serve as a caregiver, the caregiver's employment and/or poor health can play an important role in determining the need for institutional care.

A general physical examination should focus particularly on cardiovascular and neurological assessment. Hypertension and other cardiovascular findings and focal neurological signs (eg, unilateral weakness or sensory deficit, hemianopia, Babinski reflex) favor a diagnosis of multi-infarct dementia. Pathologic reflexes (eg, the glabellar and palmomental reflexes) are nonspecific and occur in many forms of dementia as well as in a small proportion of normal-aged persons. These frontal lobe release signs—as well as impaired stereognosis or graphesthesia, gait disorder, and abnormalities on cerebellar testing—are significantly more common in patients with AD than in age-matched controls. Parkinsonian signs (tremor, bradykinesia, muscle rigidity) should be sought because they may indicate either DLB or frank Parkinson disease.

A careful mental status examination (see Table 6-1) and a standardized mental status test should be performed. Neuropsychological testing can be helpful when there is a normal mental status score but also functional and/or behavioral changes (this can occur in patients with high baseline intelligence) or when there is a low score without functional deficits (this can occur in patients with lower educational levels). Neuropsychological testing can also be helpful in differentiating depression and dementia and in pinpointing specific cognitive strengths and weaknesses for patients, families, and health-care providers.

Selected diagnostic studies are useful in ruling out reversible forms of dementia (Table 6-16). Although CT and MRI scans of the head are expensive, they are generally readily available and one of these imaging tests should be done to exclude unsuspected correctable structural lesions for patients with dementia of recent onset in whom no other clinical findings explain the dementia and in those with focal neurological signs or symptoms. Cerebral atrophy on one of these scans does not establish the diagnosis of AD; it can occur with normal aging as well as with several specific disease processes. The scan is thus recommended to rule out treatable causes (eg, subdural hematoma, tumors, normal-pressure hydrocephalus). CT and MRI each have advantages and disadvantages. They are roughly equivalent in the detection of most remediable structural lesions. MRI will demonstrate more lesions than CT in patients with multi-infarct dementia, but will also demonstrate white matter changes of uncertain clinical significance. Position emission tomography (PET) scan

TABLE 6-16. Evaluating Dementia: Recommended Diagnostic Studies

Blood studies
   Complete blood count
   Glucose
   Urea nitrogen
   Electrolytes
   Calcium and phosphorous
   Liver function tests
   Thyroid-stimulating hormone
   Vitamin B_{12}
   Serologic test for syphilis (if suspected)
   Human immunodeficiency virus antibodies (if suspected)
Radiographic studies
   Computed tomography (or magnetic resonance imaging) of the head
Other studies
   Neuropsychological testing (selected patients; see text)

abnormalities of glucose metabolism can precede the development of clinical deficits by several years in patients at risk for AD. However, PET scanning using glucose metabolism or the presence of amyloid-containing plaques remains a research tool rather than a clinical practice one. The blood tests recommended are directed at finding common comorbidities as opposed to identifying the cause of the underlying dementia. For example, thyroid hormone and/or vitamin B_{12} replacement may be important for a patient's health but have not been shown to reverse cognitive deficits (Balk et al, 2007; Clarfield, 2003).

MANAGEMENT OF DEMENTIA

GENERAL PRINCIPLES

Diagnosing dementia is just the first step. The patient and his or her family must be involved in developing a care plan to address the condition and its implications. That plan will be revised as the condition and circumstances change. Table 6-17 outlines key principles for the management of dementia. Optimizing therapy for comorbid conditions in the context of dementia, counseling families about the stages of dementia and avoidance of certain drugs and excessive alcohol, discussing strategies to manage behavioral symptoms if they arise and advance directives, and planning for the future are critical early steps in management. Optimal management can provide improvements in the ability of patients with dementia to function with a minimum of behavioral symptoms, and improve their overall well-being and that of their families and other caregivers. An important component of such a plan is protecting the caregiver. Caregiving is critical, but dangerous, work. Provisions for respite and support are essential.

TABLE 6-17. Key Principles in the Management of Dementia

Optimize the patient's physical and mental function through physical activity and mind plasticity principals and activities

    Treatment of underlying medical and other conditions (eg, hypertension, Parkinson disease, depression [Chap. 7])

    Avoid use of drugs with central nervous system side effects (unless required for management of psychological or behavioral disturbances—see Chap. 14)

    Assess the environment and suggest alterations, if necessary

    Encourage physical and mental activity

    Avoid situations stressing intellectual capabilities; use memory aids whenever possible

    Prepare the patient for changes in location

    Emphasize good nutrition

Identify and manage behavioral symptoms and complications

    Driving (consider a formal driving evaluation)

    Wandering

    Dangerous driving

    Behavioral disorders

    Depression (see Chap. 7)

    Agitation or aggressiveness

    Psychosis (delusions, hallucinations)

    Malnutrition

    Incontinence (see Chap. 8)

Provide ongoing care

    Reassessment of cognitive and physical function

    Treatment of medical conditions

Provide information to patient and family

    Nature of the disease

    Extent of impairment

    Prognosis

Provide social service information to patient and family/caregivers

    Local Alzheimer's Association

    Community health-care resources (day centers, homemakers, home health aides)

    Legal and financial counseling

    Use of advance directives

    Provide family counseling for:

        Setting realistic goals and expectations

        Identifying and resolving family conflicts

        Handling anger and guilt

        Making decisions on respite or institutional care

        Taking care of legal concerns

        Dealing with ethical concerns (see Chap. 17)

        Considering palliative and hospice care (see Chap. 18)

Protect the caregiver from effects of caregiver stress and burnout

If causes of reversible or partially reversible forms of dementia are identified (see Table 6-11), they should be specifically treated. Small strokes (lacunar infarcts), which can cause further deterioration of cognitive function in patients with AD, as well as those with vascular dementia, may be prevented by controlling hypertension; thus, hypertension should be treated in patients with dementia if side effects, such as postural hypotension and falls, can be avoided. Other specific diseases such as Parkinson disease and diabetes should be optimally managed. The treatment of these and other medical conditions is especially challenging because drug side effects may adversely affect cognitive function.

PHARMACOLOGICAL TREATMENT OF DEMENTIA

There are four basic approaches to the pharmacological treatment of dementia; they involve:

1. Avoiding medications that can worsen cognitive function, mainly those with strong anticholinergic activity
2. Agents that enhance cognition and function
3. Drug treatment of coexisting depression
4. Pharmacological treatment of complications such as paranoia, delusions, psychosis, and behavioral symptoms such as agitation (verbal and physical)

Drug treatment of depression may provide substantial benefits in patients with dementia (Lyketsos et al, 2003) and is discussed in Chapter 7. The use of antipsychotics to treat the neuropsychiatric symptoms of dementia is highly controversial (Maher et al, 2011). Most experts and guidelines recommend avoiding these drugs and using nonpharmacological strategies unless patients are a danger to themselves and others or if nonpharmacological interventions have failed. Atypical antipsychotics are associated with weight gain and now have black box warnings from the U.S. Food and Drug Administration because of the increased risk of death associated with their use. Moreover, the U.S. Centers for Medicare & Medicaid Services has an ongoing campaign to improve the appropriateness and reduce the use of these drugs in nursing homes. Patients with new or worsening behavioral symptoms associated with dementia should have a medical evaluation to identify potentially treatable precipitating conditions. Pain may be especially hard to detect. For severely demented patients who develop physical or verbal agitation without an obvious underlying cause, empiric treatment with acetaminophen has shown some efficacy (Husebo et al, 2011). Nonpharmacological approaches should be used before psychotropic drugs are prescribed, unless patients are clearly psychotic and/or an immediate danger to themselves or others around them. Pharmacological treatments, including antipsychotics, are discussed further in Chapter 14.

The primary pharmacological approach to the treatment of AD has been the use of cholinesterase inhibitors. Their effectiveness in improving function and quality of life in patients with AD, vascular dementia, Lewy body dementia and dementia in Parkinson disease is controversial, and the potential benefits of these drugs versus their risks and costs must be weighed carefully in individual patients. The best evidence for effectiveness is in delaying progression of AD and increasing the time before institutional placement is needed (Birks, 2012; Raina et al, 2008; Rolinski et al, 2012). The three most commonly used drugs in this class are donepezil, rivastigmine, and galantamine. Simultaneous treatment with drugs that have anticholinergic activity can diminish the effectiveness of these drugs. Gastrointestinal side effects can be problematic and include nausea, vomiting, and diarrhea; nightmares can be bothersome as well. In addition to these bothersome side effects, cholinesterase inhibitors can cause bradycardia, and have been associated with syncope, injurious falls, and pacemaker placement (Gill et al, 2009). However, the benefits of these drugs include slight improvements in cognitive function and up to a several-month delay in the progression of cognitive impairment and the development of related behavioral symptoms. Memantine is an NMDA receptor antagonist that has also been used to treat dementia, usually in combination with a cholinesterase inhibitor. The efficacy of memantine is controversial and it can cause dizziness, headache, confusion, and constipation. In one study vitamin E was more effective than memantine in preventing functional decline in patients with AD (Dysken et al, 2014). These drugs have been used to help manage behavioral symptoms associated with dementia, but at least one controlled study of one of them (donepezil) failed to demonstrate efficacy for this purpose (Howard et al, 2007).

Other drugs, including estrogen (in women), vitamin E, ginkgo biloba, and nonsteroidal anti-inflammatory drugs, have been used to prevent and/or treat dementia. There is, however, no evidence that these drugs are effective in preventing or treating dementia (most evidence suggests they are not). There is also no evidence that vitamin B_{12}, vitamin B_6, or folic acid supplementation improves cognitive function (Balk et al, 2007).

NONPHARMACOLOGICAL MANAGEMENT

A variety of supportive measures and other nonpharmacological management strategies are useful in improving the overall function and well-being of patients with dementia and their families and caregivers (see Table 6-17). These interventions range from specific recommendations for caregivers, such as alterations in the physical environment, the use of memory aids, the avoidance of stressful tasks, and preparation for the patient's move to another living setting with a higher level of care, to more general techniques, such as providing information and counseling services. Resources are available through the Alzheimer's Association and the Rosalynn Carter Institute's Savvy Caregiver Program to assist caregivers (see websites at end of chapter). Many nursing homes have developed special care units for dementia patients, but there is little evidence that such units improve outcomes. Assisted-living facilities have also developed specialized dementia units, with specially designed environments, trained staff, and intensive activities programming, and without the more hospital-like environment typical of many nursing homes. The effectiveness of such units and whether people with advanced dementia can optimally be cared for in them have not been well studied.

Symptoms commonly associated with moderate to severe cognitive impairment, such as memory loss, aphasia, motor apraxia, visual agnosia, and apathy, make it challenging for caregivers to interact, motivate, and implement restorative care interventions. In addition to functional and motivational challenges, problematic behavioral symptoms, such as verbal and physical aggression, sleep disturbance, depression, delusions, hallucinations, and resistance to care, occur in at least 50% to 80% of individuals diagnosed with dementia at some time during the course of their illness. Caregivers in home settings commonly suffer from severe stress, and caregiving for people with dementia can impair the caregiver's quality of life and health. Thus, recommending and assisting in locating resources to reduce caregiver burden are essential aspects of managing dementia. Nursing assistants, who provide the majority of hands-on care in long-term care settings, are frequently challenged by the agitated and uncooperative behaviors of cognitively impaired residents. Many different types of nonpharmacological interventions have been described that have been used to treat these disruptive symptoms, but none have strong evidence of effectiveness (Brasure et al, 2016). There are, however, a variety of strategies that may be effective in engaging these individuals in functional activities while managing behavioral problems. These include getting to know individuals and drawing on their past experiences and patterns (eg, memory boxes outside rooms in dementia units, giving a housewife household activities to do), using humor, providing simple repetitive activities, encouraging mimicking by demonstrating the behavior/activity that you want the individual to perform, communicating face-to-face, and using multiple sources of input (eg, verbal and written).

Providing ongoing care is especially important in the management of dementia patients. Reassessment of the patient's cognitive abilities can be helpful in identifying potentially reversible causes for deteriorating function and in making specific recommendations to family and other caregivers about remaining capabilities. The family is the primary target of strategies to help manage dementia patients in noninstitutional settings. Caring for relatives with dementia is physically, emotionally, and financially stressful. Information on the disease itself and the extent of impairment and on community resources helpful in managing these patients can be of critical importance to family and caregivers. The local chapter of the Alzheimer's Association and the Area Agency on Aging are examples of community resources that can provide education and linkages with appropriate services. Anticipating and teaching family members, strategies to cope with common behavioral problems associated with dementia—such as wandering, incontinence, day–night reversal, and nighttime agitation—can be of critical importance. Hazardous driving can result in car crashes and is an especially troublesome problem. Better validated screening methods for identifying individuals who may be unable to drive safely are now available (Carr et al, 2011). Several states require reporting patients with dementia who maintain driver's licenses. Wandering may be especially hazardous for the dementia patient's safety and is associated with falls. Incontinence is common and often very difficult for families to manage (see Chapter 8). Books providing information and suggestions for family management techniques are very useful (see Suggested Readings). Support groups for families of patients with AD through the Alzheimer's Association are available in most large cities. Family counseling can be helpful in dealing with a variety of issues such as anger, guilt, decisions on institutionalization, handling the patient's assets, and terminal care. Dementia patients and their families should also be encouraged to discuss and document their wishes, using a durable power of attorney for health care or an equivalent mechanism early in the course of the illness (see Chapter 17). Family members should be encouraged to seek respite care periodically to provide time for themselves. Some communities have formal respite care programs available. In the absence of such programs, informal arrangements can often be made to relieve the primary family caregivers for short periods of time at regular intervals. Such relief will help the caregiver cope with what is generally a very stressful situation. Often a multidisciplinary group of health professionals—made up of a physician, a nurse, a social worker, and, when needed, rehabilitation therapists, a lawyer, and a clergy member—must coordinate efforts to manage these patients and provide support to family and caregivers.

Dementia is now recognized as a terminal illness. Many diagnostic and therapeutic interventions have been shown to be burdensome without benefits on quality of life and function in patients with end-stage dementia; some persons with dementia are enrolled in hospice care. Advanced care planning and establishing advance directives with designated surrogate decision makers is a critical aspect of managing this patient population. Advanced dementia is the subject of a recent review by several experts in this area (Mitchell et al, 2012), and management of these patients is addressed in Chapters 16, 17, and 18.

Evidence Summary

Do's

- Assess for correctable underlying causes of delirium, dementia, and new or worsening behavioral symptoms associated with dementia.
- Carefully review medication regimens to determine if one or more medication can affect cognitive function and try to eliminate potential offenders.
- Screen for behaviors and symptoms that put patients with dementia at risk (eg, trying to cook unattended, hazardous driving, wandering at night).
- Screen older patients with dementia for depression, which can exacerbate cognitive impairment.
- Pay attention to the health and emotional status of caregivers.
- Discuss advance care planning and set realistic goals and expectations for patients and caregivers.

Don'ts

- Automatically do brain imaging in every patient with cognitive impairment.
- Use psychoactive drugs if they can be avoided in patients with cognitive impairment.
- Prescribe antipsychotics for behavioral symptoms associated with dementia unless underlying treatable conditions have been excluded and nonpharmacological interventions have failed or unless patients are an immediate danger to themselves or others around them.
- Use physical restraints in hospitalized older patients with delirium or dementia unless essential for their safety and medical care.

Consider

- Formal neuropsychological testing if the diagnosis is uncertain, or if the patient or family wants to better understand cognitive capabilities.
- A trial of a cholinesterase inhibitor for older patients with dementia.
- Judicious use of antidepressants for dementia patients with concomitant depression.
- Referring family members for support groups, in-home help, and respite programs when appropriate.

REFERENCES

Amjad H, Carmichael D, Austin AM, et al. Continuity of care and health care utilization in older adults with dementia in fee-for-service Medicare. *JAMA Intern Med.* doi:10.1001/jamainternmed.2016.3553.

Balk EM, Raman G, Tatsioni A, et al. Vitamin B_6, B_{12}, and folic acid supplementation and cognitive function. *Arch Intern Med.* 2007;167:21-30.

Birks, JS. Cholinesterase inhibitors for Alzheimer's disease. *Cochrane Database Syst Rev.* 2012. doi:10.1002/14651858.CD005593.

Borson S, Scanlan JM, Chen P, et al. The Mini-Cog as a screen for dementia: validation in a population-based sample. *J Am Geriatr Soc.* 2003;51:1451-1454.

Brasure M, Jutkowitz E, Fuchs E, et al. Nonpharmacologic interventions for agitation and aggression in dementia. *Comparative Effectiveness Review* No. 177. (Prepared by the Minnesota Evidence-Based Practice Center under Contract No. 290-2012-00016-I.) AHRQ Publication No. 16-EHC019-EF. Rockville, MD: Agency for Healthcare Research and Quality; February 2016. www.effectivehealthcare.ahrq.gov/reports/final.cfm.

Carr DB, Barco PP, Wallendorf MJ, et al. Predicting road test performance in drivers with dementia. *J Am Geriatr Soc.* 2011;59:2112-2117.

Clarfield AM. The decreasing prevalence of reversible dementias: an updated meta-analysis. *Arch Intern Med.* 2003;163:2219-2229.

Gill SS, Anderson GM, Fischer HD, et al. Syncope and its consequences in patients with dementia receiving cholinesterase inhibitors: a population-based cohort study. *Arch Intern Med.* 2009;169:867-873.

Howard RJ, Juszczak E, Ballard CG, et al. Donepezil for the treatment of agitation in Alzheimer's disease. *N Engl J Med.* 2007;357:1382-1392.

Husebo BS, Ballard C, Sandvik R, Nilsen OB, Aarsland D. Efficacy or treating pain to reduce behavioural disturbances in residents of nursing homes with dementia: cluster randomized trial. *BMJ.* 2011;343:d4065.

Inouye SK, Bogardus ST, Baker DI, et al. The hospital elder life program: a model of care to prevent cognitive and functional decline in older hospitalized patients. *J Am Geriatr Soc.* 2000;48:1697-1706.

Inouye SK, Bogardus ST Jr, Charpentier PA, et al. A multicomponent intervention to prevent delirium in hospitalized older patients. *N Engl J Med.* 1999;340:669-676.

Inouye SK, van Dyck CH, Alessi CA, et al. Clarifying confusion: the confusion assessment method: a new method for detection of delirium. *Ann Intern Med.* 1990;113:941-948.

Katzman R, Lasker B, Bernstein N. Advances in the diagnosis of dementia: accuracy of diagnosis and consequences of misdiagnosis of disorders causing dementia. In: Terry RD, ed. *Aging and the Brain.* New York, NY: Raven Press; 1988:17-62.

Langa KM, Foster NL, Larson EB. Mixed dementia: emerging concepts and therapeutic implications. *JAMA.* 2004;292:2901-2908.

Larson EB, Yaffe K, Langa KM. New insights into the dementia epidemic. *N Engl J Med.* 2013;369:2275-2277.

Lyketsos CG, DelCampo L, Steinberg M, et al. Treating depression in Alzheimer disease: efficacy and safety of sertraline therapy, and the benefits of depression reduction: the DIADS. *Arch Gen Psychiatry.* 2003;60:737-746.

Maher M, Maglione M, Bagley S, et al. Efficacy and comparative effectiveness of atypical antipsychotic medications for off-label uses in adults. *JAMA.* 2011;306:1359-1369.

Mitchell SL, Black BS, Ersek M, et al. Advanced dementia: state of the art and priorities in the next decade. *Ann Intern Med.* 2012;156:45-51.

Moyer, VA on behalf of the U.S. Preventive Services Task Force. Screening for cognitive impairment in older adults: U.S. Preventive Services Task Force Recommendation Statement. *Ann Intern Med.* 2014;160:791-797.

National Institutes of Health. Preventing Alzheimer's disease and cognitive decline. http://consensus.nih.gov/2010/alzstatement.htm. Accessed December 4, 2012.

Okie S. Confronting Alzheimer's disease. *N Engl J Med.* 2011;365;1069-1072.

Petersen, RC. Mild cognitive impairment. *N Engl J Med.* 2011;364:2227-2234.

Plassman BL, Langa KM, Fisher GG, et al. Prevalence of cognitive impairment without dementia in the United States. *Ann Intern Med.* 2008;148:427-434.

Raina P, Santaguida P, Ismaila A, et al. Effectiveness of cholinesterase inhibitors and memantine for treating dementia: evidence review for clinical practice guideline. *Ann Intern Med.* 2008;148:379-397.

Rolinski M, Fox C, Maidment I, et al. Cholinesterase inhibitors for dementia with Lewy bodies, Parkinson's disease dementia and cognitive impairment in Parkinson's disease. *Cochrane Database Syst Rev.* 2012. doi:10.1002/14651858.CD006504.pub2.

Sachdev PS, Lipnicki DM, Crawford J, et al. Risk profiles of subtypes of mild cognitive impairment: the Sydney memory and ageing study. *J Am Geriatr Soc.* 2012;60:24-33.

Satizabal CL, Beiser AS, Chouraki V, et al. Incidence of dementia over three decades in the Framingham Heart Study. *N Engl J Med.* 2016;374:523-532.

Snowden DA, Greiner LH, Mortimer JA, et al. Brain infarction and the clinical expression of Alzheimer's disease: the nun study. *JAMA.* 1997;277:813-817.

Tsoi KKF, Chan JYC, Hirai HW, et al. Cognitive tests to detect dementia: a systematic review and meta-analysis. *JAMA Intern Med.* doi:10.1001/jamainternmed.2015.2152.

Zekry D, Hauw JJ, Gold G. Mixed dementia: epidemiology, diagnosis, and treatment. *J Am Geriatr Soc.* 2002;50:1431-1438.

SUGGESTED READINGS

Adelman RD; Tmanova LL; Delgado D, et al. Caregiver burden: a clinical review. *JAMA.* 2014;311:1052-1059.

American Geriatrics Society; American Association for Geriatric Psychiatry. Consensus statement on improving the quality of mental health care in U.S. nursing homes: management of depression and behavioral symptoms associated with dementia. *J Am Geriatr Soc.* 2003;51:1287-1298.

AGS/NIA Delirium Conference Writing Group, Planning Committee and Faculty. The American Geriatrics Society/National Institute on Aging Bedside-to-Bench Conference: Research Agenda on Delirium in Older Adults. *J Am Geriatr Soc.* 2015;63:843–852.

Cummings JL. Alzheimer's disease. *N Engl J Med.* 2004;351:56-67.

Dysken MW, Sano M, Asthana S, et al. Effect of vitamin E and memantine on functional decline in Alzheimer disease: the TEAM-AD VA Cooperative Randomized Trial. *JAMA.* 2014;311(1):33-44. doi:10.1001/jama.2013.282834.

Holsinger T, Deveau J, Boustani M, et al. Does this patient have dementia? *JAMA.* 2007;297:2391-2404.

Inouye SK. Delirium in older persons. *N Engl J Med.* 2006;354:1157-1165.

Kane RL, Ouellette J. *The Good Caregiver.* New York, NY: Avery; 2011.

Lyketsos G, Colenda CC, Beck C, et al. Position statement of the American Association for Geriatric Psychiatry regarding principles of care for patients with dementia resulting from Alzheimer disease. *Am J Geriatr Psychiatry.* 2006;14:561-573.

Mitchell SL. A 93-year-old man with advanced dementia and eating problems. *JAMA.* 2007;298:2527-2536.

Rabins P, Lyketsos C, Steele C. *Practical Dementia Care.* New York, NY: Oxford University Press; 2006.

Wenger NS, Solomon DH, Roth CP, et al. Application of assessing care of vulnerable elders-3 quality indicators to patients with advanced dementia and poor prognosis. *J Am Geriatr Soc.* 2007;55:S457-S463.

SELECTED WEBSITES (ACCESSED 2017)

Alzheimer's Association, www.alz.org
Alzheimer's Society, http://alzheimers.org.uk/
ConsultGeri, a clinical website of The Hartford Institute for Geriatric Nursing, http://consultgerirn.org/
National Institute on Aging, www.nia.nih.gov/alzheimers
Rosalynn Carter Institute for Caregiving, www.rosalynncarter.org

TOOLS (ACCESSED 2017)

Confusion Assessment Method, www.hospitalelderlifeprogram.org/
Mini-Cog, www.hospitalmedicine.org/geriresource/toolbox/mini_cog.htm
Montreal Cognitive Assessment, www.mocatest.org/
Saint Louis University Mental Status Examination (SLUMS), http://aging.slu.edu/index.php?page=saint-louis-university-mental-status-slums-exam

CHAPTER 7

Diagnosis and Management of Depression

Depression in older adults is a persistent or recurrent disorder resulting from psychosocial stress or the physiological effects of disease and is commonly referred to as late-life depression. This psychological problem is more common than dementia and can lead to disability, cognitive impairment, exacerbation of medical problems, increased use of health-care services, and increased risk of falls and suicide. The presence of depression complicates the treatment of other physiological problems. Unlike dementia, depression is treatable and thus diagnosis is very important. Unfortunately, depression is severely underrecognized and undertreated. This lack of identification and treatment can be traced to providers assuming that the signs and symptoms of depression are normal age changes and/or normal responses to life events or medical problems.

Old age can be a time of loss and those losses can trigger depressive symptoms. It is challenging to be able to separate out true depression from sadness. Generally, sadness in response to losses should not be sustained for longer than 6 months. For example, an older adult may lose a spouse, a home, and a pet all within a short period of time. Time is needed to adjust to these losses and grieve. When the individual continues to experience feelings of sadness and other associated symptoms of depression, concerns should be raised about depression.

Older individuals may not present with the typical symptoms of depression, such as depressed mood or sadness. Conversely, they may have these symptoms but not complain about them or admit they exist. They may, however, respond to focused questions about whether or not they feel depressed. Thus, it is important to ask older individuals directly about depression using brief screening tools or even by just asking if they feel depressed. The signs and symptoms indicative of depression (eg, change in appetite or sleep), which are part of the tools commonly used to screen for depression in younger adults, may not work as well with older people because they are related to symptoms of physical illness. Although it may be a slow and difficult diagnostic process, it is critical to rule out medical problems (acute or chronic) prior to a definitive diagnosis of depression. Even once it is identified, depression is often not treated due to concerns about drug side effects associated with antidepressants and polypharmacy and beliefs that psychotherapy and other nonpharmacological interventions will not be effective for older individuals. Although it is appropriate to be concerned about drug side effects, it is important to appreciate that treating depression can dramatically improve the quality of life of older adults.

Sorting out the complex interrelationships between symptoms and signs of depression caused by physical illnesses and those caused primarily by an affective disorder or related psychiatric diagnosis is challenging for clinicians. New guidelines from the *Diagnostic and Statistical Manual of Mental Disorders* version 5 (DSM-5) recommend that individuals be screened for substance abuse, other psychiatric disorders (eg, schizophrenia), or bereavement that lasts greater than 2 months in addition to medical problems that may be causing depression. This chapter addresses depression from the perspective of the nonpsychiatrist, highlighting diagnostic techniques and initial management options. However, managing depression may be best done by using an interdisciplinary approach that includes psychiatrists and psychologists, among others.

AGING AND DEPRESSION

Major depression, or what is referred to in the DSM-5 as persistent depressive disorder, is defined as clinically significant distress or impairment in social, occupational, or other important areas of life that lasts for more than 2 weeks. Associated symptoms include change in appetite, sleep, activity, loss of energy, feelings of guilt or worthlessness, decreased concentration, and thoughts of suicide. The prevalence of major depression among older adults actually decreases with age. Approximately 5% to 10% of older persons living in the community have major depression. The rate of major depression is higher among those living in the community who require home health care and higher yet among those in assisted living facilities, nursing homes, or acute care settings (range is from 16% to 50% in these settings). The prevalence of subsyndromal depression (ie, symptoms of depression that last for more than 2 weeks but do not meet standard criteria for major depression), however, steadily increases with age and ranges from 10% to 25% among community-dwelling adults and increases to 50% among those in nursing homes or acute care settings.

The implications of depression include increased mortality and morbidity, including incidence of metabolic syndrome, weight changes, declines in function, and impaired cognition. When depression is associated with other medical problems (eg, hip fracture or osteoarthritis), there is often an exacerbation of associated pain, poor motivation and adherence to rehabilitation, and impaired recovery of function. Depression also increases the risk of suicide. Individuals aged 65 and over account for 18% of all suicides, and the majority of the older adults who commit suicide suffer from depression. Approximately 3% of community-dwelling older adults report serious thoughts about suicide, and 0.6% have made a plan to commit suicide. Several factors are associated with suicide in the geriatric population (Table 7-1).

Lifelong bipolar affective disorder is not uncommon in older persons; these disorders account for 10% to 25% of all geriatric patients with mood disorders and 5% of patients admitted to geropsychiatric inpatient units (Sajatovic et al, 2015). The incidence of late-onset bipolar disease, however, decreases with age and presents differently than it does in younger individuals. The most important age-related differences in presentation are that older adults tend to present with better psychosocial function, less severe psychopathology, and a higher frequency of neurological etiologies than younger individuals. Older adults with bipolar disease generally have extensive medical comorbidities including cognitive impairment. With regard to presentation, older adults with bipolar disorder are more likely to have a mixture of

TABLE 7-1. Factors Associated With Suicide in the Geriatric Population

Factor	High risk	Low risk
Sex	Male	Female
Religion	Protestant	Catholic or Jewish
Race	White	Nonwhite
Marital status	Widowed or divorced Recent death of a spouse	Married
Occupational background	Blue-collar low-paying job	Professional or white-collar job
Current employment status	Retired or unemployed	Employed full- or part-time
Living environment	Urban Living alone Isolated Recent move	Rural Living with spouse or other relatives Living in close-knit neighborhood
Physical health	Poor health Terminal illness Pain and suffering Multiple comorbid conditions	Good health
Mental health	Depression (current or previous) Alcoholism Low self-esteem Loneliness Feeling rejected, unloved Poor quality of life	Happy and well adjusted Positive self-concept and outlook Sense of personal control over life
Personal background	Broken home Dependent personality History of poor interpersonal relationships Family history of mental illness Poor marital history Poor work record	Intact family of origin Independent, assertive, flexible personality History of close friendships No family history of mental illness No previous suicide attempts No history of suicide in family Good marital history Good work record

PART II

depression and marked irritability. Pressured speech that tends to go off on tangents is common, although the severity of thinking disturbance is less pronounced than in young adults and flight of ideas is less common. Hypersexuality and grandiosity may be present but also tend to be less prominent in older adults. Manic-like syndromes in late life are distinguished by a greater likelihood of confusion, often a reflection of an underlying cognitive disturbance, such as an incipient dementia.

Depression is caused by a combination of factors including neurobiological changes, psychological factors, biochemical changes, and environmental and social factors as well as genetic predisposition. A listing of these factors is provided in Table 7-2. Age changes in the central nervous system, such as changes in neurotransmitter concentrations (especially catecholaminergic neurotransmitters), may play a role in the development of geriatric depression. Other physical problems such as impaired vision and chronic pain and mild cognitive impairment are similarly associated with depression. There are several medical diagnoses that increase the risk for depression in older adults. These include cardiovascular disease, cancer, Parkinson disease, stroke, lung disease, arthritis, loss of hearing, and dementia.

Vascular depression, commonly seen in about 30% of stroke survivors, is linked to white-matter hyperintensities, which are bright regions seen in the brain parenchyma on T2-weighted magnetic resonance imaging (MRI). Inflammatory markers such as interleukin 6 (IL-6) and vitamin D deficiency have likewise been associated with depression. Individuals with vascular depression tend to be aggressive and have

TABLE 7-2. Factors Predisposing Older People to Depression

Biological
   Family history (genetic predisposition)
   Prior episode(s) of depression or suicide attempt
   Aging changes in neurotransmission
Physical
   Specific diseases (see Table 7-5)
   Chronic medical conditions (especially loss of function)
   Exposure to drugs (see Table 7-6)
   Sensory deprivation (loss of vision or hearing)
   Loss of physical function
   Acute or chronic pain
   Damage to body image from amputation or organ failure
Psychological
   Unresolved conflicts (eg, anger, guilt)
   Memory loss and dementia
   Personality disorders
   Fear of death
   Substance abuse
Social
   Losses of family and friends (bereavement)
   Isolation
   Loss of job
   Loss of income
   Lack of social supports
   Stressful life events
   Living alone
   Being single, unmarried, divorced, or widowed

increased alexithymia (the inability to identify and describe one's emotions). The causes of vascular depression are multifactorial including physiological changes as well as psychosocial factors (Turk et al, 2015).

Many psychosocial factors increase the likely occurrence of depression in older adults. These factors include being unmarried, living alone, having limited or no social support, recent loss and prolonged bereavement, being a caregiver, and having a low socioeconomic status (Freitas et al, 2016). Risk for depression is further increased if there is a family history of depression, current or past substance abuse, or the individual had a prior depressive episode or suicide attempt. Losses, whether real or perceived, are common in the geriatric population and can be a contributory factor to depression. Loss of job, income, and social supports (especially the death of family members and friends) increase with age and can result in social isolation and subsequent abnormally prolonged grief and frank depression. Loss of independence, which occurs with the loss of a driver's license or acute decline in function, can further cause depression. The inability to be resilient against these many losses and accept them and optimize remaining abilities and explore alternative resources (eg, different methods of transportation) can result in prolonged bereavement and grief and depression. Other psychosocial factors such as impaired spiritual well-being and a perceived sense of unmet needs have similarly been noted to contribute to depression.

SYMPTOMS AND SIGNS OF DEPRESSION

It is critical to continually assess older adults for possible signs and symptoms of depression, especially during periods of loss or transition (eg, a move into a retirement community, assisted living facility, or nursing home). Anticipating depression and recognizing these signs and symptoms early in the presentation period will allow for immediate intervention with appropriate treatments.

As noted, major depression typically is diagnosed by evidence of depressed mood and/or loss of interest or pleasure. There may also be an associated appetite change, particularly a loss of appetite, insomnia or hypersomnia, psychomotor agitation or retardation, loss of energy and fatigue, feelings of worthlessness, difficulties with concentration, and/or recurrent thoughts of death or suicide. These typical signs and symptoms are often not observed in older adults or assumed to be due to normal aging or other comorbidities. Older depressed patients are more likely to present with a preoccupation with somatic and cognitive symptoms and will less frequently report depressed mood and guilty preoccupations, have crying spells, feel sadness or fear, or have feelings that their life has been a failure. They commonly report poor self-perception of health and complain repeatedly about constipation or urinary frequency. These individuals may not acknowledge sustained feelings of sadness. They will, however, report a persistent loss of pleasure and interest in previously enjoyable activities (anhedonia).

The diagnosis of depression, whether major or minor, in older persons is complicated by the overlap of physical illnesses and normal age changes (Jones et al, 2016). The physical appearance of older patients suspected of being depressed should be interpreted cautiously. Normal age changes such as pale, thin, or wrinkled skin, loss of teeth, kyphosis, and a wide-based slow gait, alone or in addition to the presence of diseases such as anemia or Parkinson disease, may make the older individual look depressed. Parkinson disease, which manifests by masked facies, bradykinesia, and stooped posture, can be misinterpreted as depression. Patients with sensory changes resulting in impaired vision and hearing may appear withdrawn and disinterested simply because they cannot see or hear you or others and, therefore, withdraw from social interactions. The psychomotor retardation of hypothyroidism may offer the physical appearance of depression. Systemic illnesses such as malignancy, dehydration, malnutrition, or chronic obstructive pulmonary disease can produce a depressed appearance with a flat affect or decreased energy. It is possible that the older individual will present with both medical problems and associated depression (Jones et al, 2016).

Patients with serious medical illness and those at the end of life may be preoccupied, for example, with thoughts about death or worthlessness because of concomitant disability. Older adults with depression also tend to have a higher rate of anxiety, nervousness, and irritability than their younger counterparts. They may engage in somatization, seek regular visits with health professions, and put themselves at risk for iatrogenic disease due to unnecessary tests and treatments. As noted earlier, before making a diagnosis of depression it is important to make sure that medical problems alone are not causing the signs and symptoms of what might otherwise be depression. These include:

- Nonspecific physical symptoms (eg, fatigue, weakness, anorexia, diffuse pain) commonly associated with comorbid conditions.
- Specific physical symptoms, relating to every major organ system, that are indicative of depression as well as physical illness in geriatric patients.
- Symptoms of coexisting physical illnesses such as exacerbation of memory changes or pain associated with arthritis.
- Pharmacologically induced depressive symptoms from substance use, particularly alcohol, and abuse of prescribed or over-the-counter medications or as a side effect of prescribed medications for the treatment of diseases such as hypertension.

When there is evidence of medical problems that could be causing depressive symptoms, management for each of the underlying problems in addition to treating the depression is critical. Table 7-3 provides an overview of some common examples of somatic symptoms that may actually represent, or be exacerbated by, depression in older patients.

INSOMNIA

Insomnia deserves special mention because it is a very common symptom in the older population and is associated with depression. Older adults with undiagnosed depression or anxiety may in fact initially present with complaints of sleep disorders. Those with underlying shortness of breath, paroxysmal nocturnal dyspnea, anxiety and restlessness, and gastroesophageal reflux disease are likely to suffer from

TABLE 7-3. Examples of Physical Symptoms That Can Represent Depression

System	Symptom
General	Fatigue
	Weakness
	Anorexia
	Weight loss
	Anxiety
	Insomnia (see Table 7-4)
	"Pain all over"
	Apathy
Cardiopulmonary	Chest pain
	Shortness of breath
	Palpitations
	Dizziness
Gastrointestinal	Abdominal pain
	Constipation
	Diarrhea
	Nausea
	Anorexia
Genitourinary	Frequency
	Urgency
	Incontinence
	Pain/discomfort associated with prolapse
Musculoskeletal	Diffuse pain
	Back pain
	Functional impairment
Neurological	Headache
	Memory disturbance
	Dizziness
	Paresthesias

insomnia because these medical problems are exacerbated by a recumbent posture and may interfere with falling or staying asleep. Although it is a key symptom in diagnosing different forms of depression, a variety of factors may underlie insomnia (Table 7-4). Insomnia can also be caused by the effects of (or withdrawal from) several medications or use of alcohol or late-night caffeine.

In addition to depression as a contributing factor, sleep problems among older adults may be caused by underlying physiological or psychological problems such as pain, anxiety, shortness of breath, gastritis, urinary frequency, or unrealistic sleep expectations (eg, belief in the need to sleep for a straight 8 hours). In addition, a number of specific sleep disorders are known to present more frequently in older individuals. Obstructive sleep apnea (OSA), which results in abnormal breathing, is the most common sleep-related problem. The development of OSA seems to be

TABLE 7-4. Key Factors in Evaluating the Complaint of Insomnia

Sleep disturbance should be carefully characterized
  Delayed sleep onset
  Frequent awakenings
  Early morning awakenings
Physical symptoms can underlie insomnia (from patient and bed partner)
  Symptoms of physical illnesses
    Pain from musculoskeletal disorders
    Orthopnea, paroxysmal nocturnal dyspnea, or cough
    Nocturia
    Gastroesophageal reflux
  Symptoms suggestive of periodic leg movements
  Uncomfortable sensations in legs with a desire to move the legs
  Symptoms suggestive of sleep apnea
    Loud or irregular snoring
    Awakening sweating, anxious, tachycardiac
    Excessive movement
    Morning drowsiness
Aging changes occurring in sleep patterns
  Increased sleep latency
  Decreased time in deeper stages of sleep
  Increased awakenings
Behavioral factors can affect sleep patterns
  Daytime naps >30 min
  Earlier bedtime
  Increased time spent in bed not sleeping
Medications can affect sleep
  Hypnotic withdrawal
  Caffeine
  Alcohol (causes sleep fragmentation)
  Certain antidepressants
  Diuretics
  Steroids

more common in older adults and men. The incidence is also higher in individuals who are obese and have enlarged neck circumferences. The risks associated with untreated OSA include nighttime hypoxia with associated risks for cardiac arrhythmias and myocardial and cerebral infarction. Specific signs such as loud snoring, which are often elicited from the bed partner, and daytime napping should prompt the provider to refer the older individual to a sleep center for further workup. Once diagnosed, the treatment for OSA includes weight loss and exercise, continuous positive airway pressure, dental appliances, and uvulopalatopharyngoplasty.

Another common sleep disorder that can cause insomnia is restless leg syndrome (RLS). RLS is a neurological disorder that can be diagnosed based on a patient's description of symptoms and additional clinical history. The incidence of RLS increases to approximately 10% to 28% of those over the age of 65 and is more prevalent in females than males. Additional risk factors include a family history, iron deficiency, use of alcohol or caffeine, smoking, and depression. Patients with RLS have uncomfortable sensations in the lower extremities that they attempt to relieve by moving their legs during sleep or by rising and walking around. Older adults with cognitive impairment may not be able to express those symptoms and should be observed for restlessness during the night and rubbing of the legs or slapping of the legs against the mattress, difficulty sitting still, and excessive fidgeting. Managing RLS is challenging but can be achieved with nonpharmacological interventions and pharmacological treatment as needed. In addition to treating the underlying contributing causes of RLS such as iron deficiency, nonpharmacological interventions should be tried including avoiding excessive fatigue; limiting caffeine, tobacco, and alcohol use; losing weight (if overweight); massaging the leg; engaging in mild-to-moderate physical activity and stretching lower extremities before bedtime; taking warm baths; and doing mentally stimulating activities prior to bedtime. Non-ergot dopamine agonists are considered the best pharmacological approach for restless leg syndrome.

Even without disease, aging is associated with changes in sleep patterns, such as daytime naps, early bedtime, increased time until onset of sleep, decreases in the absolute and relative amounts of the deeper stages of sleep, and increased periods of wakefulness, all of which contribute to the complaint of insomnia. Insomnia is a good example of how a primary symptom of depression must be evaluated to first determine that there is not a treatable underlying cause. It is important to avoid assuming or blaming the symptom on age or depression before a comprehensive medical workup has been completed.

DEPRESSIVE SYMPTOMS ASSOCIATED WITH MEDICAL CONDITIONS

Medical disorders that may imitate depressive symptoms are particularly important to consider in older patients because of the increased vulnerability of this population to physical illnesses. Hypothyroidism, for example, may present with apathy and diminished energy that mimics depression. Cardiovascular and nervous system diseases can also mimic or precipitate depression. Because these diseases are life threatening and potentially disabling, they can bring on symptoms of depression. Overall, being functionally dependent and medically ill with shorter life expectancy significantly increases the likelihood that the older individual will be depressed. The relationship between depression and medical outcomes is reciprocal with poor health resulting in symptoms of depression and the depression resulting in worsening of disease states. For example, myocardial infarction, with attendant fear of shortened life span and restricted lifestyle, commonly precipitates depression. Stroke is often accompanied by depression, although the depression may not always correlate with the extent of physical disability. Stroke patients who are substantially disabled (eg, hemiparesis, aphasia) can become depressed in response to their loss of function; others may become depressed because of vascular depression after stroke. Complicated by depression, recovery may not be optimal following these acute events. It is therefore particularly important to treat depression among these individuals using behavioral interventions and medications to not only manage mood but also to optimize disease-related outcomes.

Other causes of brain damage (eg, tumors and subdural hematomas), especially when the damage is in the frontal lobes, can likewise be associated with depression. Older individuals with dementia, both Alzheimer and multi-infarct dementia, may have prominent symptoms of depression (see Chap. 6). Patients with Parkinson disease also have a high incidence of clinically diagnosed depression.

Overall, a wide variety of physical illnesses can present with or be accompanied by symptoms and signs of depression (Table 7-5). Any medical condition associated with systemic involvement and metabolic disturbances can have profound effects on mental function and affect. The most common among these are fever, dehydration, decreased cardiac output, electrolyte disturbances, and hypoxia. Hyponatremia (whether from a disease process or drugs) and hypercalcemia (associated with malignancy) may also cause older patients to appear depressed. Systemic diseases, especially malignancies and endocrine disorders such as diabetes, are often associated with symptoms of depression. Depression is commonly present in patients with cancer of the pancreas and is often accompanied by the symptoms of anorexia, weight loss, and back pain. Among the endocrine disorders, thyroid and parathyroid conditions are most commonly accompanied by symptoms of depression. Most hypothyroid patients manifest psychomotor retardation, irritability, or depression. Hyperthyroidism may also present as withdrawal and depression in older patients—so-called apathetic thyrotoxicosis. Hyperparathyroidism with attendant hypercalcemia can simulate depression and is often manifested by apathy, fatigue, bone pain, and constipation. Other systemic physical conditions, such as infectious diseases, anemia, and nutritional deficiencies, can also have prominent manifestations of depression in the geriatric population.

Symptoms of depression associated with medical problems may simply be a response to the treatment. For example, institutionalization (placement in nursing homes or hospitalizations) associated with medical illnesses can result in feelings of isolation, sensory deprivation, and immobilization and contribute or cause depressive symptoms. Likewise, iatrogenic complications associated with bedrest once institutionalized such as functional impairment, constipation and fecal impaction, a urinary tract infection, or urinary retention that causes new-onset incontinence or pressure ulcers with subsequent pain can also cause depression. Drugs are the most common cause of treatment-induced depression and a wide variety of pharmacological agents can produce symptoms of depression (Table 7-6). These drugs include antihypertensive agents, antilipids, antiepilepsy medications, selective estrogen receptor modulators, H_2-receptor antagonists, corticosteroids, nonsteroidal anti-inflammatory drugs, and sedative–hypnotics. The true impact of medications on the development of depression is inconsistent, however, and it has been suggested that genetic differences among individuals may impact the side effects of these medications. Given the individual impact of medications, whenever possible, drugs that can potentially exacerbate depression should be discontinued.

TABLE 7-5. Medical Illnesses Associated With Depression

Metabolic disturbances
  Dehydration
  Azotemia, uremia
  Acid–base disturbances
  Hypoxia
  Hypo- and hypernatremia
  Hypo- and hyperglycemia
  Hypo- and hypercalcemia
Endocrine
  Hypo- and hyperthyroidism
  Hyperparathyroidism
  Diabetes mellitus
  Cushing disease
  Addison disease
Infections
Cardiovascular
  Congestive heart failure
  Myocardial infarction
  Atrial fibrillation
Pulmonary
  Chronic obstructive lung disease
  Malignancy
Gastrointestinal
  Malignancy (especially pancreatic)
  Irritable bowel
Genitourinary
  Urinary incontinence
Musculoskeletal
  Degenerative arthritis
  Osteoporosis with vertebral compression or hip fracture
  Polymyalgia rheumatica
  Paget disease
Neurological
  Dementia (all types)
  Parkinson disease
  Stroke
  Tumors
Other
  Anemia (of any cause)
  Vitamin deficiencies
  Hematological or other systemic malignancy

Adapted with permission from Levenson AJ, Hall RCW: *Neuropsychiatric Manifestations of Physical Disease in the Elderly.* New York: Raven Press; 1981.

TABLE 7-6. Drugs That Can Cause Symptoms of Depression

Antihypertensives	Antipsychotics
Angiotensin-converting enzyme	Chlorpromazine
inhibitors	Haloperidol
Calcium channel blockers (verapamil)	Thiothixene
Clonidine	Hypnotics
Hydralazine	Chloral hydrate
β-Blockers (eg, propranolol)	Benzodiazepines
Reserpine	Steroids
Analgesics	Corticosteroids
Narcotics	Estrogens
Antiparkinsonism drugs	Anticonvulsants
Levodopa	Celontin
Bromocriptine	Zarontin
Antimicrobials	Antiviral
Sulfonamides	Zovirax
Isoniazid	Antibiotics
Cardiovascular preparations	Ciprofloxacin
Digitalis	Statins
Diuretics	Pravachol
Lidocaine	Others
Hypoglycemic agents	Alcohol
Psychotropic agents	Cancer chemotherapeutic agents
Sedatives	Cimetidine
Barbiturates	
Benzodiazepines	
Meprobamate	

Data from Kotlyar M, Dysken M, Adson DE: Update on drug-induced depression in the elderly, *Am J Geriatr Pharmacother.* 2005 Dec;3(4):288-300.

DIAGNOSING DEPRESSION

The interrelationship between the signs and symptoms of depression, medical illnesses, and treatment effects makes diagnosing depression particularly challenging. As noted previously, it is important to continually assess for depression among older adults. The following general guidelines can help with the differential diagnosis between depression and other causes of the associated signs and symptoms reported by older adults:

- Screening tools that screen for depressive symptoms may be helpful in identifying depressed geriatric patients. Tools developed specifically for older adults, such as the Geriatric Depression Scale, are more useful than measures developed for all adults because the tools developed for older adults do not focus as much on somatic symptoms.
- Consider using a simple, brief screening question(s) to help identify those who might be at risk for depression (see later discussion of the Patient Health

Questionnaire). A more comprehensive tool can then be used to provide additional information to confirm or refute a diagnosis.

- Nonspecific or multiple somatic symptoms that suggest depression should not be diagnosed as such until physical illnesses have been excluded.
- Somatic symptoms unexplained by physical findings or diagnostic studies, especially those of relatively sudden onset in an older person who is not usually hypochondriacal, should raise the suspicion of depression.
- Drugs used to treat medical illnesses (see Table 7-6), sedative-hypnotics, and excessive alcohol use should be considered as potential causes for symptoms and signs of depression.
- Standard diagnostic criteria should form the basis for diagnosing various forms of depression in the geriatric population, but several differences may distinguish depression in older, as opposed to younger, patients. Older adults with depression tend to have more agitation and express more somatic symptoms (particularly gastrointestinal symptoms such as constipation) and hypochondriasis than younger individuals. In contrast, younger individuals tend to report more guilt associated with depression and loss of sexual interest than older adults.
- Major depressive episodes should be differentiated from other diagnoses such as uncomplicated bereavement, bipolar disorder, dysthymic disorder, minor depression, and adjustment disorders with a depressed mood.
- Consultation with experienced geriatric psychiatrists, psychologists, or psychiatric nurse practitioners may be helpful when there is no response to appropriate nonpharmacological and pharmacological interventions.
- Whenever there is uncertainty about the diagnosis, or while medical workup is being initiated, the depression and associated symptoms should be treated with a judicious (but adequate) therapeutic trial of behavioral interventions and an antidepressant if behavioral interventions are not effective.

Several differences in the presentation of depression can make the diagnosis much more challenging and difficult in older people, as compared to younger people (Table 7-7). The most common clinical problem is differentiating major depressive

TABLE 7-7. Some Differences in the Presentation of Depression in the Older Population, as Compared With the Younger Population

1. Somatic complaints, rather than psychological symptoms, often predominate in the clinical picture.
2. Older patients often deny having a dysphoric mood.
3. Apathy and withdrawal are common.
4. Feelings of guilt are less common.
5. Loss of self-esteem is prominent.
6. Inability to concentrate with resultant impairment of memory and other cognitive functions is common (see Chap. 6).

TABLE 7-8. Summary Criteria for Major Depressive Episode

A. If the patient experiences either depressed mood or decreased interest or pleasure in usual activities and meets at least four (or more) of the following symptoms. The symptoms must be present nearly every day during the same 2-week period and represent a change from previous functioning. Symptoms that are caused by substance abuse or a general medical condition should not be counted.

1. Significant weight loss when not dieting, or weight gain, or decrease or increase in appetite
2. Insomnia or hypersomnia
3. Psychomotor agitation or retardation
4. Fatigue or loss of energy
5. Feelings of worthlessness or excessive or inappropriate guilt (which may be delusional)
6. Diminished ability to think or concentrate, or indecisiveness
7. Recurrent thoughts of suicide

Data from American Psychiatric Association: *Diagnostic and Statistical Manual of Mental Disorders,* 5th Ed. Arlington: American Psychiatric Association; 2013.

episodes from other forms of depression. Table 7-8 outlines the criteria for major depression based on the DSM-5 (American Psychiatric Association, 2013). The DSM-5 criteria suggests that an older individual meets the criteria for major depressive disorder if he or she experiences either depressed mood or decreased interest or pleasure in usual activities and meets at least four of the following criteria: significant appetite and weight changes, increased agitation or motor retardation, loss of energy, changes in sleep, feelings of guilt or worthlessness, problems with memory or concentration, or thoughts of suicide. Symptoms must exist almost daily for at least 2 weeks, lead to functional impairment, and not be the result of substance abuse or other medical conditions. Table 7-9 lists some of the key features that can aid in distinguishing major depression from other conditions.

As noted, there are several valid and reliable measures to screen older adults for depression. Table 7-10 lists these measures. Most commonly used is the Patient Health Questionnaire, either the 2- or 9-item measure, and the Geriatric Depression Scale, which is available in 30-item, 15-item, 5-item, and 2-item versions. While all of these measures have cut scores indicating depression, they should be considered screening tools and further diagnostic workup should be considered.

As shown in Table 7-10, some measures were specifically developed to help identify depression among individuals with common geriatric syndromes and disease such as cognitive impairment and stroke. For example, the Cornell Depression Scale (Alexopoulos et al, 1988) was developed to screen for depression in older adults with dementia and the Stroke Aphasic Depression Questionnaire (Bennett et al, 2007) was developed to assess for depression in older adults with stroke. Brief measures of depression such as the Visual Analogue Scale or the 2- or 9-item Patient Health Questionnaire (Kroenke et al, 2001) are commonly used in primary care settings

TABLE 7-9. Major Depression Versus Other Forms of Depression

Diagnostic classification	Key features distinguishing from major depression
Bipolar disorder	The patient may meet, or have met in the past, criteria for major depression but is having or has had one or more manic episode; the latter are characterized by distinct periods of a relatively persistent elevated or irritable mood and other symptoms such as increased activity, restlessness, talkativeness, flight of ideas, inflated self-esteem, and distractibility.
Cyclothymic disorder	There are numerous periods during which symptoms of depression and mania are present but not of sufficient severity or duration to meet the criteria for a major depressive or manic episode; in addition to a loss of interest and pleasure in most activities, the periods of depression are accompanied by other symptoms such as fatigue, insomnia or hypersomnia, social withdrawal, pessimism, and tearfulness.
Dysthymic disorder	Patient usually exhibits a prominently depressed mood, marked loss of interest or pleasure in most activities, and other symptoms of depression; the symptoms are not of sufficient severity or duration to meet the criteria for a major depressive episode, and the periods of depression may be separated by up to a few months of normal mood.
Adjustment disorder with depressed mood	The patient exhibits a depressed mood, tearfulness, hopelessness, or other symptoms in excess of a normal response to an identifiable psychosocial or physical stressor; the response is not an exacerbation of another psychiatric condition, occurs within 3 months of the onset of the stressor, eventually remits after the stressor ceases (or the patient adapts to the stressor), and does not meet the criteria for other forms of depression or uncomplicated bereavement.
Uncomplicated bereavement	This is a depressive syndrome that arises in response to the death of a loved one—its onset is not more than 2–3 months after the death, and the symptoms last for variable periods of time; the patient generally regards the depression as a normal response—guilt and thoughts of death refer directly to the loved one; morbid preoccupation with worthlessness, marked or prolonged functional impairment, and marked psychomotor retardation are uncommon and suggest the development of major depression.

TABLE 7-10. Examples of Screening Tools for Depression

Measures	Number of items	Time to complete	Scoring	Reference
Patient Health Questionnaire (PHQ-2)	2	1 minute	≥3 suggests depression	www.cqaimh.org/pdf/ tool_phq2.pdf
Geriatric Depression Scale	15	5 minutes	>5 suggests depression	www.healthcare.uiowa .edu/igec/tools/ depression/GDS.pdf
Center for Epidemiologic Studies Depression Scale	20	5 minutes	≥16 suggests depression	www.actonmedical.com/ documents/cesd_long .pdf
Beck Depression Inventory	4	5 minutes	If there is a yes on 2 or more questions, do full 21-item inventory	http://mhinnovation .net/sites/default/files/ downloads/innovation/ research/BDI%20with%20 interpretation.pdf
Zung Self-Rating Depression Scale	20		≥50 suggests depression	http://healthnet .umassmed .edu/mhealth/Zung SelfRatedDepressionScale .pdf
Patient Health Questionnaire (PHQ-9)	9	5 minutes	1–4 Minimal depression 5–9 Mild depression 10–14 Moderate depression 15–19 Moderately severe depression 20–27 Severe depression	www.integration.samhsa .gov/images/res/PHQ%20 -%20Questions.pdf
Cornell Scale for Depression in Dementia	19	5 minutes with input from caregiver	≥12 indicates depression	www.amda.com/ resources/2005_updates_ ltc_teaching_kits/ dementia.pdf

(continued)

TABLE 7-10. Examples of Screening Tools for Depression (*continued*)

Measures	Number of items	Time to complete	Scoring	Reference
Stroke Aphasic Depression Questionnaire	10	5 minutes	≥ 6 indicates depression	www.google.com/search?q=stroke+aphasic+depression+questionnaire&oq=Stroke+Aphasic+Depression+Questionnaire&aqs=chrome.0.0l6.3480j0j4&sourceid=chrome&es_sm=93&ie=UTF-8
Visual Analogue Scale	1	<5 minutes	Range from 0 to 10	www4.parinc.com/Products/Product.aspx?ProductID=VAMS
Yale Single Item Depression Screening Tool	1	<5 minutes	Yes or no	www.scalesandmeasures.net/files/files/Single%20Question%20Depression%20Screening%20Scale%20(1994).pdf

to screen for depression among those who may have these and/or other comorbid conditions.

Because of the overlap of symptoms and signs of depression and physical illness and the close association between many medical conditions and depression, older patients presenting with what appears to be depression should have physical illnesses carefully excluded. This evaluation can usually be accomplished by a thorough history, physical examination, and basic laboratory studies (Table 7-11). Complaints of fatigue, for example, should be explored to rule out hypothyroidism or anemia. Sometimes the assurance that there are no acute problems or exacerbations in chronic medical illnesses will help the individual recognize that the symptoms may be caused by mood and focused depression treatment can be initiated. In other situations the individual may be disappointed that there are no serious medical problems and may continue to believe that if the clinical problem (eg, constipation) could be resolved then he or she would be fine. Other diagnostic studies can provide helpful objective data for particularly difficult to distinguish persistent somatic symptoms/complaints such as shortness of breath, changes in appetite, or fatigue. For example, echocardiography and radionuclide cardiac scans can help rule out organic heart disease as a basis for these symptoms. It is particularly common to have a combination of depression and executive dysfunction. These individuals commonly present with apathy rather than anhedonia, psychomotor slowing, and lack of insight into their depression.

TABLE 7-11. Diagnostic Studies Helpful in Evaluating Depressed Geriatric Patients With Somatic Symptoms

Basic evaluation
History
Physical examination
Complete blood count
Erythrocyte sedimentation rate
Serum electrolytes, glucose, and calcium
Renal function tests
Liver function tests
Thyroid function tests
Calcium and vitamin D
Serum B_{12} or methylmalonic acid
Folate
Syphilis serology
Urinalysis

Examples of other potentially helpful studies	
Symptom or sign	Diagnostic study
Pain	Evaluation for underlying cause (eg, appropriate radiological procedure such as bone film, bone scan, GI series)
Chest pain	ECG, noninvasive cardiovascular studies (eg, exercise stress test, echocardiography, radionuclide scans)
Shortness of breath	Chest films, pulmonary function tests, pulse oximetry arterial blood gases
Constipation	Test for occult blood in stool, colonoscopy, abdominal X-ray, thyroid function tests
Focal neurological signs or symptoms	CT or MRI scan, EEG

CT, computed tomography; ECG, electrocardiography; EEG, electroencephalography; GI, gastrointestinal; MRI, magnetic resonance imaging.

MANAGEMENT

GENERAL CONSIDERATIONS

Several treatment modalities are available to manage depression in older persons (Table 7-12). Pharmacological and behavioral interventions and psychotherapy have all been effective in treating depression (Arean and Niu, 2014). Specifically, effective treatments include cognitive behavioral therapy, problem-solving therapy, interpersonal therapy, antidepressant medications, and electroconvulsive therapy (ECT) for those who do not respond to the other treatment approaches. There continues to be debate about which treatment, or combination of treatments, results in the most beneficial results. Antidepressants and cognitive behavioral therapy seem to be more

TABLE 7-12. Evidence-Based Treatment Modalities for Depression

Treatment	Evidence level	Description of the intervention
Psychotherapy	A	Active time-limited therapy that aims to change the thinking and behavior of individuals that influences their depression; effective when compared to no treatment.
Medication	A	Tricyclic antidepressants. Selective serotonin reuptake inhibitors. Monoamine oxidase inhibitors can all effectively treat depression.
Hormone therapy	C	Estrogen use in females given as a patch, cream, injection, implant, or suppository. Effective only in women posthysterectomy. Use of testosterone in men orally, by injection, as skin patches, or as a gel. Single group study showed decrease in depression among a small group of older men.
Exercise	A	A wide variety of exercise interventions have been shown to decrease depression among older adults.
ECT	A	Involves delivering a brief electric current to the brain to produce a cerebral seizure. ECT was better than placebo (sham ECT).
Complementary and alternative medicine (CAM)	B	Select CAM and integrative interventions add to established conventional treatment of depression and may be considered when formulating a treatment plan.

A, supported by one or more high-quality randomized trials; B, supported by one or more high-quality nonrandomized cohort studies or low-quality RCTs; C, supported by one or more case series and/or poor-quality cohort and/or case-control studies; D, supported by expert opinion and/or extrapolation from studies in other populations or settings; X, evidence supports the treatment being ineffective or harmful.

There is insufficient evidence to support multiple herbal remedies (with the exception of St. John's wort), acupuncture, music therapy, or vitamins.

ECT, electroconvulsive therapy.

effective than interpersonal therapy for late-life depression. Behavioral interventions often need to be adapted to the special needs of older adults and adjusted to different sites of care and living situations. For example, information may need to be repeated or provided at a slower pace.

Additional alternative treatments for depression include exercise, psychoeducation (ie, education for patients and family to help empower them to manage their depression), and supportive care. Exercise interventions that have been shown to decrease depressive symptoms include tai chi, relaxation exercises, and aerobic exercise (Arean and Niu, 2014; Klainin-Yobas et al, 2015; Tully et al, 2015). It is possible that the benefits of exercise are better when the exercise is done in a group versus individual exercise program. While exercise is certainly beneficial, there may be a need for persistent motivational interventions to engage individuals in these activities (eg, verbal encouragement and positive reinforcement for participation).

Overall treatment using pharmacotherapy and psychotherapy renders similar, moderate to large effect sizes in the treatment of late-life depression. Unfortunately, although treatment is quite effective in reducing the symptoms of depression, we have been less successful in maintaining remission of depression for those who are older, and relapse rates tend to be higher in older individuals. The choice of treatment(s) for an individual patient depends on many factors, including the primary disorder causing the depression, the severity of symptoms, the availability and practicality of the various treatment modalities, and underlying conditions that might contraindicate a specific form of treatment (eg, cognitive issues that may make psychotherapy more difficult, underlying medical problems that increase the risk of medication management). The first step in any treatment approach is to remove the underlying factors that may be contributing to depression, whether these are medical or situational. For example, if a specific pharmacological treatment is being given that may cause depression, attempts should be made to remove this agent. While difficult to achieve, strategies to alleviate or cope with multiple losses (such as death of loved ones and pets or change in living locations) can be considered. Likewise, attempts to resolve acute illness, or exacerbations of chronic illness, are needed to ensure that the individual is at his or her optimal state of health. These interventions should be implemented before other therapies are initiated unless the depression is severe enough to warrant immediate treatment (eg, the patient is delusional or suicidal).

When selecting the treatment for depression, consider the individual's age, executive function, and socioeconomic status. Because there is less likelihood that pharmacological interventions will be effective with increasing age, behavioral interventions should be considered. Those with lower socioeconomic status may benefit from the addition of case management and those with impaired executive function may respond better to scheduled activities and problem-solving therapy than medications (Arean and Niu, 2014).

The course of treatment for depression, particularly major depression, should proceed as follows: initial treatment to reverse the current episode, continuation of treatment to prevent relapse for 6 months and then an attempt to wean off the medication, and maintenance evaluation to prevent or manage recurrence of depression.

There are risks to some long-term pharmacological interventions for depression (Dinz and Reynolds, 2014). Ongoing treatment with serotonin reuptake inhibitors (SSRIs) can result in osteoporosis, drug interactions, and bleeding. Long-term treatment of tricyclic antidepressants can result in orthostatic hypotension, arrhythmias, cognitive impairment, and anticholinergic side effects. Monitoring for these problems and reviewing the risks and benefits of treatment should be considered throughout the treatment course.

NONPHARMACOLOGICAL MANAGEMENT

Exercise, psychotherapy and other behavioral interventions, electroconvulsive therapy (ECT), transcranial magnetic stimulation, deep brain stimulation, vagus nerve stimulation, and magnetic seizure therapy are all treatment options for depression, with varying amounts of support for efficacy as shown in Table 7-12.

Psychotherapy

Most guidelines encourage using psychotherapy as adjunctive treatment to pharmacotherapy, but this can be tried as first-line therapy as well, especially when there are concerns about risk of drug side effects. The most common and most effective psychotherapies include cognitive behavior therapy (CBT); the Program to Encourage Active, Rewarding Lives for Seniors (PEARLS); and problem-solving therapy (PST). The aim of CBT, which is usually 14 to 16 weeks, is to help patients change patterns of behavior that come from dysfunctional thinking by eliminating or reducing negative thoughts and behaviors. PEARLS was designed for use in the community and involves four to six home sessions that incorporate the use of a care manager to help the individual develop problem-solving skills and engage in pleasant activities. Overall participants were noted to have a 50% reduction in depressive symptoms. PST involves working with the patient to identify practical life difficulties that are causing distress and provide guidance to help the patient identify solutions. The treatment is delivered generally in six to eight meetings spaced 1 to 2 weeks apart. PST is often combined with behavioral activation and involves encouraging older adults to select and solve daily problems as a way of increasing confidence and decreasing the sense of helplessness that are common symptoms of depression. There is also consistent evidence that psychotherapy is effective in decreasing depressive symptoms among older adults (Leea et al, 2012).

Exercise

A systematic review of current research shows evidence that exercise interventions and ongoing physical activity can improve depression in older adults (Park et al, 2014). The studies reviewed used a variety of different types of exercise programs to effectively decrease depression in individuals. In some cases the exercise program was combined with counseling and effects of treatment were seen by 3 months. The reason for the decrease in depression following exercise is not known specifically. It may be a result of the benefits older adults experience in terms of weight loss or improvement in physical and functional health and performance or simply a result of the sense of overall well-being that occurs with regular physical activity.

Electroconvulsive Therapy

Electroconvulsive therapy (ECT) was first used in 1938 and has evolved to be an effective and safe treatment option for older adults with major depressive disorder who do not respond to other treatments. ECT is now done under general anesthesia, with oxygenation, muscle relaxants, and physiological monitoring. The frequency and length of initial treatment will vary based on response and in many individuals long-term maintenance therapy is needed.

PHARMACOLOGICAL TREATMENT

When symptoms and signs of depression are of sufficient severity and duration to meet the criteria for major depression (see Table 7-8), if the depression is producing marked functional disability or interfering with recovery from other illnesses (eg, not participating in rehabilitation services), or when the patient is not responding to nonpharmacological interventions alone, drug treatment should be considered. Treatment should be initiated using subtherapeutic dosages of medications initially and increasing these until therapeutic at 4-week intervals. Treatment should continue for 4 to 9 months and then attempts to wean off the medication should be tried. If symptoms of depression reoccur, then maintenance treatment may be needed.

There are numerous classes of pharmacological agents for treatment of depression including heterocyclic antidepressants (which include tricyclic antidepressants), monoamine oxidase inhibitors (MAOIs), SSRIs, serotonin norepinephrine reuptake inhibitors (SNRIs), and serotonin antagonist/reuptake inhibitors. Single agents include noradrenergic and specific serotonergic antidepressants, norepinephrine and dopamine reuptake inhibitors, norepinephrine reuptake inhibitors, and serotonin reuptake enhancers. Last, stimulants have also been used to treat depression. Examples of drugs that fall within these groups are shown in Table 7-13. The choice of agent depends on the patient's comorbid medical conditions, signs and symptoms of the depression, the side effect profile of the antidepressant, and the individual patient's sensitivity to these effects. General guidelines for treatment approaches are shown in Table 7-14 (Mulsant et al, 2014).

Potential interactions with other medications and prior use of antidepressant medications also should be considered. Current complaints of sleep disturbance, anxiety, poor appetite or weight changes, or psychomotor retardation help to further direct the practitioner's choice of a therapeutic agent. For individuals who do not sleep well, for example, a drug that is more sedating such as mirtazapine would be appropriate. There is evidence to support that treatment using either TCAs or SSRIs is effective in older adults, although TCAs are well known to have more side effects.

Common side effects of concern associated with antidepressants when used with older adults include anticholinergic effects which can worsen cognitive function, postural hypotension, and sedation. The risk of hyponatremia induced by all SSRIs increases with age and is associated with being female, having low body weight, renal failure, and when combined with other drugs and treatments that cause hyponatremia. The SSRIs can also result in delayed ejaculation in men and failure to achieve orgasm in women, changes in appetite and sleep patterns, fatigue, and altered bowel function. Use of SSRIs has also been associated with gastrointestinal bleeding. Citalopram, mirtazapine, bupropion, escitalopram, paroxetine, sertraline, venlafaxine, and duloxetine have been described as preferred agents for older adults based on efficacy and side effect profiles. Citalopram, escitalopram, and sertraline are the safest with regard to drug–drug interactions and impact on the cytochrome P450 enzymes.

TABLE 7-13. Antidepressants for Geriatric Patients

Drug group generic name (brand name)	Drug group side effects	Special concerns with older adults
Tricyclic antidepressants		
Amitriptyline (Elavil) Amoxapine (Asendin) Clomipramine (Anafranil) Desipramine (Norpramin or Pertofrane) Doxepin (Sinequan or Adapin) Imipramine (Tofranil) Maprotiline (Ludiomil) Nortriptyline (Pamelor or Aventyl) Protriptyline (Vivactil) Trimipramine (Surmontil)	Dry mouth Blurred vision Constipation Difficulty urinating Increased heart rate Loss of sex drive and erectile failure Increased sensitivity to the sun Weight gain Drowsiness Dizziness and nausea	These drugs are best avoided because of the side effects Amoxapine can cause extrapyramidal effects
MAOIs		
Phenelzine (Nardil) Tranylcypromine (Parnate) Isocarboxazid (Marplan) Selegiline (Emsam)	Light-headedness upon standing Dizziness Insomnia Weight gain Headaches Insomnia Sexual problems such as impotence Sleepiness	All foods and drinks containing tyramine must be avoided, or the patient may experience a hypertensive crisis, stroke, or myocardial infarction
SSRIs		
Fluoxetine (Prozac) Fluvoxamine (Luvox) Sertraline (Zoloft) Paroxetine (Paxil) Escitalopram (Lexapro) Citalopram (Celexa) Vortioxetine	Nausea Insomnia Anxiety and restlessness Decreased sex drive Dizziness Weight gain or weight loss Tremors Sweating Drowsiness or fatigue	SSRIs can cause an increase in suicidal thoughts and behaviors SSRIs also carry a risk for increased hostility, agitation, and anxiety SSRIs should not be taken at the same time as MAOIs Taking an SSRI within 2 weeks of an MAOI can cause a fatal reaction In adults aged 65 and older, SSRIs increase the risk for falls, fractures, and bone loss

(continued)

TABLE 7-13. Antidepressants for Geriatric Patients (*continued*)

Drug group generic name (brand name)	Drug group side effects	Special concerns with older adults
Duloxetine (Cymbalta) Mirtazapine (Remeron)	Dry mouth Diarrhea or constipation Headaches Nausea Nervousness	Duloxetine may be effective in those suffering from both depression and pain Mirtazapine causes significant sedation and weight gain so is effective for those with sleep disorders and weight loss
Bupropion (Wellbutrin) Trazodone (Desyrel) Venlafaxine (Effexor)	Sexual dysfunction Dry mouth Fatigue	Venlafaxine should not be used in those with hypertension Monitor for side effects Hyponatremia is also possible
Desvenlafaxine	Elevated blood pressure Abnormal bleeding Nausea Dizziness Sexual function disorders Headache Irritability Weight loss Hot flashes Abnormal dreams Lipid Abnormalities	
Adjunctive therapy: antipsychotics		
Aripiprazole	Akathisia Restlessness Insomnia Constipation Fatigue Blurred vision Anxiety/jittery Weight gain Sedation Myalgia Extrapyramidal disorders Impaired attention	At risk for cerebrovascular adverse events Tardive dyskinesia Hypotension

(*continued*)

TABLE 7-13. Antidepressants for Geriatric Patients (*continued*)

Drug group generic name (brand name)	Drug group side effects	Special concerns with older adults
Quetiapine XR	Vertigo Blurred vision Dry mouth Constipation Nausea/vomiting Fatigue Irritability Upper respiratory infection Extrapyramidal symptoms Hypersomnia Dysarthria Abnormal dreams Restlessness Decreased libido Depression	Cardiovascular events Hyperglycemia/hyperlipidemia Weight gain Tardive dyskinesia Hypotension

MAOIs, monoamine oxidase inhibitors; SSRIs, selective serotonin reuptake inhibitors.

TABLE 7-14. General Treatment Approaches for Use of Antidepressants

Recommended drug treatment	Selective serotonin reuptake inhibitors (SSRIs) or venlafaxine XR are preferred as first line of treatment along with psychotherapy
Starting dose	Begin at lower dosages than in younger patients—generally at half the dose recommended
Dose increases	After 2–4 weeks increase the dose if there is little or no response
Discontinuing one drug and starting another	May consider changing drugs when the patient is at a therapeutic dose for 3–6 weeks with little or no response
Treatment options when there is no response	Switch to venlafaxine or bupropion, or try nortriptyline, mirtazapine, or another SSRI If drugs are not effective consider adding a mood stabilizer if appropriate, psychotherapy, or electroconvulsive therapy
Combination therapy options	Bupropion, lithium, or nortriptyline Mirtazapine, bupropion, or lithium

Data from Mulsant BH, Blumberger DM, Ismail Z, et al: A systematic approach to pharmacotherapy for geriatric major depression, *Clin Geriatr Med.* 2014 Aug;30(3):517-534.

PART II

Table 7-15 provides a detailed summary of dosing, formulations, precautions, and advantages of the individual antidepressants. Although SSRIs are generally free of severe side effects, as noted a proportion of older adults develop hyponatremia because of the syndrome of inappropriate antidiuretic hormone secretion, and some experience anxiety, sleep disturbance, or agitation. Sexual side effects and weight gain or loss occur commonly with all SSRIs and may be a reason for poor treatment adherence. The SNRIs can cause a rise in blood pressure, and overdose can be dangerous or fatal. In addition, some SNRIs may cause nausea, dry mouth, and constipation. Atypical antidepressants cause fewer sexual side effects than other antidepressants do. They may, however, cause sedation and weight gain.

SSRIs inhibit the hepatic isoenzyme *CYP2D6*, which can interfere with the oxidative metabolism of many drugs. The most frequent interactions involving the *CYP2D6* system involve fluoxetine and fluvoxamine, whereas drug interactions are less common with citalopram. SSRIs may increase the anticoagulant effects of medications such as warfarin, potentially through cytochrome isoenzyme inhibition or the inhibition of platelet activity. Careful monitoring of blood clotting is indicated following the introduction of a SSRI to patients being treated with warfarin. Fluoxetine causes substantial inhibition of *CYP2C19* and consequently inhibits the metabolism of alprazolam, quinidine, calcium channel blockers, TCAs, and carbamazepine via the cytochrome P450 (CYP) 3A4 subsystem.

Serotonin syndrome is a potentially life-threatening adverse reaction to use of SSRIs. Symptoms include mental status changes, agitation, myoclonus, hyperreflexia, tachycardia, sweating, shivering, tremor, diarrhea, lack of coordination, fever, and even death. The risk of serotonin syndrome is increased in individuals with deficits in peripheral 5-hydroxytryptamine (5-HT) metabolism from cardiovascular, liver, or pulmonary diseases; with tobacco use; or when SSRIs are used with nefazodone, venlafaxine, mirtazapine, and MAOIs, TCAs, SSRIs, meperidine, opioids, St. John's wort, or tramadol. Following the discontinuation of an SSRI, there have been reports of a serotonergic withdrawal syndrome. This may last for 2 to 3 weeks and is characterized by light-headedness, insomnia, agitation, nausea, headache, and sensory disturbances. Mood disturbance may also occur. The shorter-acting SSRIs (ie, sertraline, paroxetine) appear to induce this syndrome, but venlafaxine and other SSRIs have also been implicated. Therefore, these agents should be tapered rather than stopped abruptly.

Tricyclic Antidepressants

Tricyclic antidepressants (TCAs) have substantial and often quite bothersome anticholinergic side effects including dry mouth, confusion, constipation, difficulty urinating, sedation, weight gain, and changes in sexual ability. In addition to anticholinergic side effects, TCAs have a quinidine-like effect that delays ventricular conduction. This group of drugs should not be used with individuals who already have cognitive impairment. If TCAs are considered, nortriptyline and desipramine are the most appropriate because of evidence of efficacy and side effect profiles when used with older persons. Table 7-15 provides a detailed summary of drug names, side effects, and special issues concerning usage in older adults. Therapeutic response to TCAs is associated with blood levels between 50 and 150 ng/mL for nortriptyline and levels above 120 ng/mL for desipramine. Over 60% of patients with nonpsychotic major depression or with depression that is not associated with dementia respond within 6 weeks to levels in these ranges. Although 5% of the population requires lower dosing because of the absence of the enzyme required to metabolize secondary amine tricyclics, most patients achieve target concentrations at dosages of 50 to 75 mg/day of nortriptyline and 100 to 150 mg/day of desipramine.

Other Antidepressants

Table 7-15 provides a summary of dosing, formulations, precautions, and advantages of other common pharmacological agents used to treat depression. MAOIs are not commonly used because they also have unpleasant side effects and can be potentially dangerous. The side effects include dizziness, dry mouth, upset stomach, difficulty with urination, twitching muscles, sexual side effects, drowsiness, and sleep problems. MAOIs can cause potentially fatal high blood pressure when combined with certain foods and beverages and certain other medications. Antipsychotics are used as adjunctive therapy in management of depression and have significant side effects including restlessness, insomnia, constipation, fatigue among others and put individuals at risk for cardiovascular events.

Bupropion is generally safe, free of sexual side effects, and well tolerated when used at recommended doses. Bupropion can be activating in some individuals and has been associated with a 0.4% risk of seizures, which is much higher when recommended doses are exceeded. Bupropion, therefore, is contraindicated in persons with a seizure disorder. Bupropion appears to act by increasing the activity of dopamine and norepinephrine and therefore the stimulant-like qualities. Venlafaxine acts as an SSRI at lower doses, while also inhibiting the reuptake of norepinephrine at the high end of the therapeutic range of 75 to 225 mg/day. Venlafaxine is effective for both generalized anxiety and major depression. Blood pressure should be monitored in individuals receiving high dosages of this drug. Venlafaxine should be discontinued by gradual tapering to avoid the risk of flu-like discontinuation symptoms.

Duloxetine was approved for the treatment of both depression and neuropathic pain secondary to diabetes mellitus and has been noted to improve depression and well as to decrease pain. Duloxetine is a serotonin and norepinephrine reuptake inhibitor; its pharmacodynamic characteristics are generally like those of venlafaxine, although it is structurally unique. Duloxetine should not be used in patients with hepatic impairment. Mirtazapine is a norepinephrine, $5\text{-}HT_2$, and $5\text{-}HT_3$ antagonist and consistently has the side effects of sedation and weight gain. Therefore, this drug is often used to treat depression among individuals who have anorexia and sleep disturbance.

Management of Bipolar Disorders

Most persons with bipolar disorders have a history of episodes in early adulthood and often receive chronic treatment with mood stabilizers versus antidepressants.

TABLE 7-15. Characteristics of Selected Antidepressants for Geriatric Patients

Drug*	Recommended starting daily dosage	Daily dosage range	Level of sedation	Elimination half-life†	Comments
Selective serotonin reuptake inhibitors					
Citalopram (Celexa)	10–20 mg	20–30 mg	Very low	Very long	Less inhibition of hepatic cytochrome P450 May cause somnolence, insomnia, anorexia
Escitalopram (Lexapro)	10 mg	10 mg	Very low	Very long	Side effects as for citalopram
Fluoxetine (Prozac)	5–10 mg	20–60 mg	Very low	Very long	Inhibits hepatic cytochrome P450‡ Must be discontinued 6 weeks before initiating monoamine oxidase inhibitor
Paroxetine (Paxil)	10 mg	10–50 mg	Very low	Long	Inhibits hepatic cytochrome P450‡ Has anticholinergic side effects
Sertraline (Zoloft)	25 mg	50-200 mg	Very low	Very long	Less inhibition of cytochrome P450
Serotonin–norepinephrine reuptake blockers					
Venlafaxine (Effexor)	25 mg	75–225 mg	Very low	Intermediate	Reduced clearance with renal or hepatic impairment Can cause dose-related hypertension Must be tapered over 1–2 weeks when discontinuing

PART II

Tricyclic antidepressants					
Nortriptyline (Pamelor, others)	10–30 mg	25–150 mg	Mild	Long	Lower but still substantial anticholinergic effects[§] Blood levels can be monitored
Other agents[†]					
Bupropion (Wellbutrin)	50–100 mg	150–450 mg	Mild	Intermediate	Divided doses necessary
Mirtazapine (Remeron)	15 mg	15–45 mg	Mild	Long	Reduced clearance with renal impairment May cause or exacerbate hypertension
Trazodone (Desyrel)	25–50 mg	75–400 mg	Moderate–high	Short	Can cause hypotension May be useful in low doses as a hypnotic

*Other less commonly used antidepressants are discussed in the text.

[†] Short = <8 h; intermediate = 8–20 h; long = 20–30 h; very long = >30 h. Half-lives may vary in older patients, and some drugs have active metabolites.

[‡]See text for drug interactions.

[§]See text for anticholinergic side effects.

Older adult bipolar disease is generally defined as bipolar disease that occurs in individuals aged ≥50 years (Sajatovic et al, 2015). Treatment of bipolar disorders in older adults is most effective when lithium, divalproex sodium, carbamazepine, lamotrigine, and atypical antipsychotics and antidepressants are used. Prior to starting treatment with an antidepressant, however, careful evaluation of patients for evidence of motor activation, pressured speech, and racing thoughts is recommended to avoid possible exacerbation of manias. Although there are no specific guidelines for the treatment of these patients, monotherapy followed by combination therapy of the various classes of drugs may help with the resolution of symptoms. ECT and psychotherapy may be useful in the treatment of refractory disease.

Summary of Evidence-Based Recommendations for Depression Interventions

Do's

- Identify and treat aggressively.
- Provide individual cognitive behavioral therapy, particularly problem-solving therapy.
- Consider depression care management with medications when behavioral interventions alone are not effective, with treatment decisions based on side effect profile of drugs.
- Routinely screen older adults for depression using a brief questionnaire such as the 2-item patient health questionnaire and then followed by a longer screening tool if there is an indication that the patient is depressed.
- Carefully differentiate physical symptoms caused primarily by medical illness versus physical symptoms caused by depression.
- Try nonpharmacological treatments first.

Don'ts

- Prescribe physical rehabilitation and occupational therapy unless indicated for specific functional impairments.
- Use nutrition interventions.
- Encourage peer support.

Consider

- Exercise interventions.
- Combining exercise with medications when either is ineffective alone.
- Suicide prevention.
- Psychoeducation (ie, psychotherapy with the patient and family to empower them in managing the symptoms of depression) and supportive interventions.
- Bereavement therapy.

REFERENCES

Sajatovic M, Strejilevich SA, Gildengers AG, et al. A report on older-age bipolar disorder from the International Society for Bipolar Disorders Task Force. *Bipolar Disord.* 2015;17(7):689-704.

Turk B, Gschwandtner M, Mauerhofer M, Löffler-Stastka H. Can we clinically recognize a vascular depression?: the role of personality in an expanded threshold model. *Medicine* 2015;94(18):e743.

Freitas C, Deschênes S, Au B, Smith K, Schmitz N. Evaluating lifestyle and health-related characteristics of older adults with co-occurring depressive symptoms and cardiometabolic abnormalities. *Int J Geriatr Psychol* 2016;31(1):66-75.

Jones SMW, Dagmar Amtmann D, Gell NM. A psychometric examination of multimorbidity and mental health in older adults. *Aging Ment Health* 2016;20(3):309-317.

American Psychiatric Association. *Diagnostic and Statistical Manual of Mental Disorders.* 5th ed. Arlington, VA: APA; 2013.

Alexopoulos G, Abrams R, Young R, Shamoian C. Cornell scale for depression in dementia. *Biol Psychol.* 1988;23:271-284.

Bennett H, Thomas S, Austen R, Morris A, Lincoln N. Validation of screening measures for assessing mood in stroke patients. *Br J Clin Psychol.* 2007;46(3):367-376.

Kroenke K, Spitzer RL, Williams JB. The PHQ-9: validity of a brief depression severity measure. *J Gen Intern Med.* 2001;16(9):606-613.

Arean PA, Niu G. Choosing treatment for depression in older adults and evaluating response. *Clin Geriatr Med.* 2014;30:535-551.

Klainin-Yobas P, Oo WN, Yew S, Ying P, Lau Y. Effects of relaxation interventions on depression and anxiety among older adults: a systematic review. *Aging Ment Health.* 2015;19(12):1043-1055.

Tully PJ, Selkow T, Bengel J, Rafanelli C. A dynamic view of comorbid depression and generalized anxiety disorder symptom change in chronic heart failure: the discrete effects of cognitive behavioral therapy, exercise, and psychotropic medication. *Disability Rehabil.* 2015;37(7):585-592.

Dinz BS, Reynolds CF. Major depressive disorder in older adults: benefits and hazards of prolonged treatment. *Drugs and Aging.* 2014;31:661-669.

Leea SY, Franchettia MK, Imanbayeva A, Galloa JJ, Spiraa AP, Leeb HB. Non-pharmacological prevention of major depression among community-dwelling older adults: a systematic review of the efficacy of psychotherapy interventions. *Arch Gerontol Geriatr.* 2012;55(3):522–529.

Park SH, Han KS, Kang CB. Effects of exercise programs on depressive symptoms, quality of life, and self-esteem in older people: a systematic review of randomized controlled trials. *App Nurs Res.* 2014;27(4):219-226.

Mulsant BH, Blumberger DM, Ismail Z, Rabheru K, Rapoport MJ. A systematic approach to pharmacotherapy for geriatric major depression. *Clin Geriatr Med.* 2014;30:517-534.

SUGGESTED READINGS

Arean PA, Niu G. Choosing treatment for depression in older adults and evaluating response. *Clin Geriatr Med.* 2014;30:535-551.

Coggins MD. Poststroke depression. *Today's Geriatr Med.* 2015;8(5). www.todaysgeriatricmedicine.com/archive/0915p0916.shtml. Accessed March 2016.

Jones SMW, Amtmann D, Gell NM. A psychometric examination of multimorbidity and mental health in older adults. *Aging Ment Health.* 2016;20(3):309-317.

PART II

SELECTED WEBSITES (ACCESSED 2017)

American Psychological Association, Depression and Suicide in Older Adults Resource Guide, www.apa.org/pi/aging/resources/guides/depression.aspx

Centers for Disease Control and Prevention, Prevention Research Centers Healthy Aging Research Network-Depression, www.cdc.gov/aging/mentalhealth/depression.htm

The Community Guide, Mental Health Recommendations, www.thecommunityguide.org/mentalhealth/index.html

Geriatric Mental Health Foundation, www.gmhfonline.org/

National Council on Aging, Center for Healthy Aging Mental Health Resources, www.ncoa.org/center-for-healthy-aging/behavioral-health/older-americans-behavioral-health-series/

National Institute of Mental Health, Depression, www.nimh.nih.gov/health/topics/depression/index.shtml

CHAPTER 8

Incontinence

Incontinence is a common, bothersome, and potentially disabling condition in the geriatric population. It is defined as the involuntary loss of urine or stool in sufficient amount or frequency to constitute a social and/or health problem. Figure 8-1, illustrates the prevalence of urinary incontinence across various settings. The prevalence depends on the definition used. Incontinence ranges in severity from occasional episodes of dribbling small amounts of urine to continuous urinary incontinence with concomitant fecal incontinence.

Approximately one in three women and 15% to 20% of men older than age 65 years have some degree of urinary incontinence. Between 5% and 10% of community-dwelling older adults have incontinence more often than weekly and/or use a pad for protection from urinary accidents. The prevalence is as high as 60% to 80% in many nursing homes, where residents often have both urinary and fecal incontinence. In community and institutional settings, incontinence is associated with both impaired mobility and poor cognition.

Physical health, psychological well-being, social status, and the costs of health care can all be adversely affected by incontinence (Table 8-1). It can be a precipitating factor in the decision to seek nursing home care. Urinary incontinence is curable or controllable in many geriatric patients, especially those who have adequate mobility and mental functioning. Even when it is not curable, incontinence can always be managed in a manner that keeps people comfortable, makes life easier for caregivers, and minimizes the costs of caring for the condition and its complications.

Many older people are embarrassed and frustrated by their incontinence and either deny it or do not discuss it with a health professional. It is therefore essential that specific questions about incontinence be included in periodic assessments and that incontinence be noted as a problem when it is detected in institutional settings. Examples of such questions include the following:

"Do you have trouble with your bladder?"
"Do you ever lose urine when you don't want to?"
"Do you ever wear padding to protect yourself in case you lose urine?"

This chapter briefly reviews the pathophysiology of geriatric incontinence and provides detailed information on the evaluation and management of this condition. Although most of the chapter focuses on urinary incontinence, some of the pathophysiology also applies to fecal incontinence, which is briefly addressed at the end of the chapter.

PART II

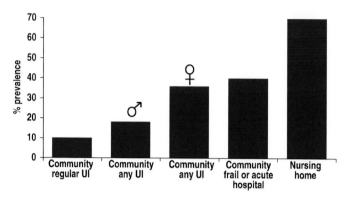

FIGURE 8-1 Prevalence of urinary incontinence (UI) in the geriatric population. "Regular UI" is more often than weekly and/or the use of a pad. (Percentages range in various studies; those shown reflect approximate averages from multiple sources.)

NORMAL URINATION

Continence requires effective functioning of the lower urinary tract, adequate cognitive and physical functioning, motivation, and an appropriate environment (Table 8-2). Thus, the pathophysiology of geriatric incontinence can relate to the anatomy and physiology of the lower urinary tract as well as to functional, psychological, and environmental factors. Several anatomic components participate in normal urination (Fig. 8-2). Urination is influenced by the brain as well as by reflexes centered in the sacral micturition center. Afferent pathways (via somatic and autonomic nerves) carry information on bladder volume to the spinal cord as the

---

TABLE 8-1. Potential Adverse Effects of Urinary Incontinence

Physical health
   Skin irritation and breakdown
   Recurrent urinary tract infections
   Falls (especially with nighttime incontinence)
Psychological health
   Isolation
   Depression
   Dependency
Social consequences
   Stress on family, friends, and caregivers
   Predisposition to institutionalization
Economic costs
   Supplies (padding, catheters, etc)
   Laundry
   Labor (nurses, housekeepers)
   Management of complications

TABLE 8-2. Requirements for Continence

Effective lower urinary tract function
  Storage
    Accommodation by bladder of increasing volumes of urine under low pressure
      Closed bladder outlet
      Appropriate sensation of bladder fullness
      Absence of involuntary bladder contractions
  Emptying
    Bladder capable of contraction
    Lack of anatomic obstruction to urine flow
    Coordinated lowering of outlet resistance with bladder contractions
Adequate mobility and dexterity to use toilet or toilet substitute and to manage clothing
Adequate cognitive function to recognize toileting needs and to find a toilet or toilet
  substitute
Motivation to be continent
Absence of environmental and iatrogenic barriers such as inaccessible toilets or toilet
  substitutes, unavailable caregivers, or drug side effects

bladder fills. Motor output is adjusted accordingly (Fig. 8-3). Thus, as the bladder fills, sympathetic tone closes the bladder neck, relaxes the dome of the bladder, and inhibits parasympathetic tone; somatic innervation maintains tone in the pelvic floor musculature (including striated muscle around the urethra). When urination occurs, sympathetic and somatic tones diminish, and parasympathetic cholinergically mediated impulses cause the bladder to contract. All of these processes are under the influence of higher centers in the brain stem, cerebral cortex, and cerebellum.

This is a simplified description of a very complex process, and the neurophysiology of urination remains incompletely understood. The cerebral cortex exerts a predominantly inhibitory influence, and the brain stem facilitates urination. Thus, loss of the central cortical inhibiting influences over the sacral micturition center from diseases such as dementia, stroke, and parkinsonism can cause incontinence. Disorders of the brain stem and suprasacral spinal cord can interfere with the coordination of bladder contractions and lowering of urethral resistance, and interruptions of the sacral innervation can cause impaired bladder contraction and problems with continence.

Normal urination is a dynamic process, requiring the coordination of several physiological processes. Figure 8-4, depicts a simplified schematic diagram of the pressure–volume relationships in the lower urinary tract, similar to measurements made in urodynamic studies. Under normal circumstances, as the bladder fills, bladder pressure remains low (eg, <15 cm H_2O). The first urge to void is variable but generally occurs between 150 and 300 mL, and normal bladder capacity is 300 to 600 mL. Many older people have the sensation to urge at low bladder volumes, which can cause urinary frequency and nocturia. When normal urination is initiated, true detrusor pressure (bladder pressure minus intra-abdominal pressure) increases, urethral resistance decreases, and urine flow occurs when detrusor pressure exceeds urethral resistance. If at any time

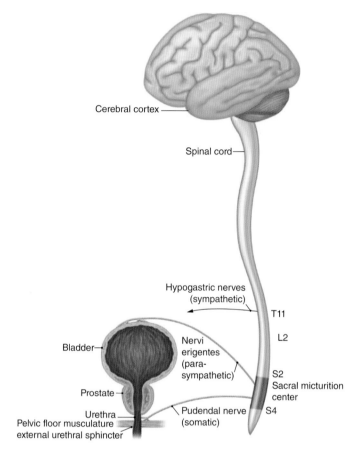

FIGURE 8-2 Structural components of normal micturition.

during bladder filling total intravesicular pressure (which includes intra-abdominal pressure) exceeds outlet resistance, urinary leakage will occur. This will happen if, for example, intra-abdominal pressure rises without a rise in true detrusor pressure when someone with low outlet or urethral sphincter weakness coughs or sneezes. This would be defined as genuine stress incontinence in urodynamic terminology. Alternatively, the bladder can contract involuntarily and cause urinary leakage.

CAUSES AND TYPES OF INCONTINENCE

BASIC CAUSES

Determining the cause(s) of urinary incontinence is essential to proper management. It is important to distinguish between urological and neurological disorders that cause incontinence and other problems (such as diminished mobility and/or mental

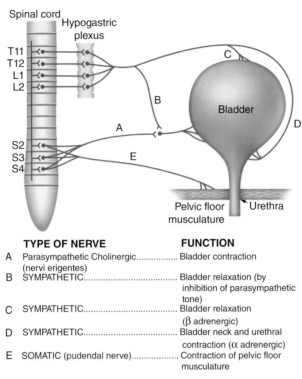

Spinal cord

Hypogastric plexus

T11
T12
L1
L2

S2
S3
S4

A

B

C

Bladder

D

E

Pelvic floor musculature

Urethra

	TYPE OF NERVE	FUNCTION
A	Parasympathetic Cholinergic (nervi erigentes)	Bladder contraction
B	SYMPATHETIC	Bladder relaxation (by inhibition of parasympathetic tone)
C	SYMPATHETIC	Bladder relaxation (β adrenergic)
D	SYMPATHETIC	Bladder neck and urethral contraction (α adrenergic)
E	SOMATIC (pudendal nerve)	Contraction of pelvic floor musculature

FIGURE 8-3 Peripheral nerves involved in micturition.

function, inaccessible toilets, and psychological problems) that can cause or contribute to the condition. As is the case for a number of other common geriatric problems discussed in this text, multiple disorders often interact to cause urinary incontinence.

Aging alone does not cause urinary incontinence. Several age-related changes can, however, contribute to its development. In general, with age, bladder capacity declines, residual urine increases, and involuntary bladder contractions become more common. Aging is also associated with a decline in bladder outlet and urethral resistance pressure in women. This decline is related to diminished estrogen influence and laxity of pelvic floor structures associated with prior childbirths, surgeries, and deconditioned muscles, which predisposes to the development of stress incontinence (Fig. 8-5). Decreased estrogen can also cause atrophic vaginitis and urethritis, which can, in turn, cause symptoms of dysuria and urgency and predispose to the development of urinary infection and urgency incontinence. In men, prostatic enlargement is associated with decreased urine flow rates and involuntary bladder contractions and can lead to overactive bladder symptoms, urge incontinence, and incontinence associated with incomplete bladder emptying (discussed later). Aging is also associated with abnormalities of arginine vasopressin (AVP) and atrial natriuretic peptide

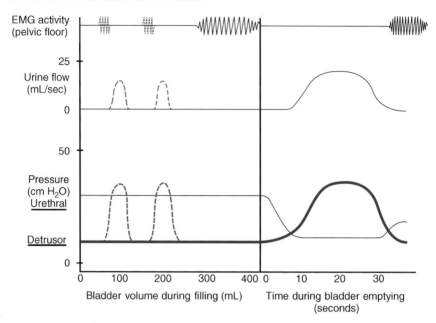

FIGURE 8-4 Simplified schematic of the dynamic function of the lower urinary tract during bladder filling (*left*) and emptying (*right*). As the bladder fills, true detrusor pressure (*thick line at bottom*) remains low (<15 cm H_2O) and does not exceed urethral resistance pressure (*thin line at bottom*). As the bladder fills to capacity (generally 300–600 mL), pelvic floor and sphincter activity increase as measured by electromyography (EMG). Involuntary detrusor contractions (illustrated by *dashed lines*) occur commonly among incontinent geriatric patients (see text). They may be accompanied by increased EMG activity in attempts to prevent leakage (*dashed lines at top*). If detrusor pressure exceeds urethral pressure during an involuntary contraction, as shown, urine will flow. During bladder emptying, detrusor pressure rises, urethral pressure falls, and EMG activity ceases in order for normal urine flow to occur (*right side of figure*).

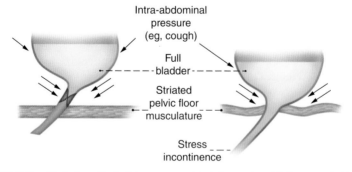

FIGURE 8-5 Simplified schematic depicting age-associated changes in pelvic floor muscle, bladder, and urethra–vesicle position, predisposing to stress incontinence. Normally (*left*), the bladder and outlet remain anatomically inside the intra-abdominal cavity, and rises in pressure contribute to bladder outlet closure. Age-associated changes (eg, estrogen deficiency, surgeries, childbirth) can weaken the structures maintaining bladder position (*right*); in this situation, increases in intra-abdominal pressure can cause urine loss (stress incontinence).

(ANP) levels. Lack of the normal diurnal rhythm of AVP secretion and increased levels of ANP associated with sleep apnea may contribute to nocturnal polyuria and predispose many older people to nighttime incontinence.

REVERSIBLE FACTORS CAUSING OR CONTRIBUTING TO INCONTINENCE

Numerous potentially reversible conditions and medications may cause or contribute to geriatric incontinence (Tables 8-3 and 8-4). The term *acute incontinence* refers to those situations when the incontinence is of sudden onset, usually related to an acute illness or an iatrogenic problem, and subsides once the illness or medication problem has been resolved (this has also been termed *transient incontinence*). Persistent incontinence refers to incontinence that is unrelated to an acute illness and persists over time.

Potentially reversible conditions can play a role in both acute and persistent incontinence. A search for these factors should be undertaken in all incontinent geriatric patients. The causes of acute and reversible forms of urinary incontinence can be remembered by the mnemonic DRIP (Table 8-5).

Many older persons, because of urinary frequency and urgency, especially when they are limited in mobility, carefully arrange their schedules (and may even limit social activities) in order to be close to a toilet. Thus, any acute illness can precipitate incontinence by disrupting this delicate balance. Hospitalization with its attendant environmental barriers (eg, bed rails, poorly lit rooms) and the immobility that often accompanies acute illnesses can precipitate acute incontinence. Incontinence in these situations is likely to resolve with resolution of the underlying acute illness and hospitalization. Hospital-acquired urinary incontinence can often be prevented. Unless an indwelling or external catheter is necessary during an acute illness to record urine output accurately, this type of incontinence should be managed by environmental manipulation, scheduled toileting, appropriate use of toilet substitutes (eg, urinals, bedside commodes, pads), and careful attention to skin care. Fecal impaction is a common problem in both acutely and chronically ill geriatric patients. Large impactions may cause mechanical obstruction of the bladder outlet in women and may stimulate involuntary bladder contractions induced by sensory input related to rectal distention. Relief of fecal impaction can improve and sometimes resolve the urinary incontinence.

Urinary retention with "overflow" incontinence should be considered in any patient who suddenly develops urinary incontinence. Immobility, anticholinergic and narcotic drugs, and fecal impaction can all precipitate urinary retention and overflow incontinence in geriatric patients. In addition, this condition may be a manifestation of an underlying acute process causing spinal cord compression.

Any acute inflammatory condition in the lower urinary tract that causes frequency and urgency can precipitate incontinence. Treatment of acute cystitis, atrophic vaginitis, or urethritis can restore continence.

Conditions that cause polyuria, including hyperglycemia and hypercalcemia, as well as diuretics (especially the rapid-acting loop diuretics), can precipitate acute incontinence. Some older people drink excessive amounts of fluids, and others ingest

TABLE 8-3. Reversible Conditions That Cause or Contribute to Geriatric Urinary Incontinence

Condition	Management
Conditions affecting the lower urinary tract	
Urinary tract infection (symptomatic with frequency, urgency, dysuria, etc)	Antimicrobial therapy
Atrophic vaginitis/urethritis	Topical estrogen
Stool impaction	Disimpaction; appropriate use of stool softeners, bulk-forming agents, and laxatives if necessary; implement high fiber intake, adequate mobility, and fluid intake (see Table 8-21)
Medication side effect (see Table 8-4)	Discontinue or change therapy if clinically appropriate. Dosage reduction or modification (eg, flexible scheduling of rapid-acting diuretics) may also help
Increased urine production	
Metabolic (hyperglycemia, hypercalcemia)	Better control of diabetes mellitus Therapy for hypercalcemia depends on underlying cause
Excess fluid intake	Reduction in intake of diuretic fluids (eg, caffeinated beverages)
Volume overload with increased urine production at night	Support stockings
Venous insufficiency with edema	Leg elevation Sodium restriction Diuretic therapy
Congestive heart failure	Medical therapy
Impaired ability or willingness to reach a toilet	
Delirium	Diagnosis and treatment of underlying cause(s)
Chronic illness, injury, or restraint that interferes with mobility	Regular toileting Use of toilet substitutes Environmental alterations (eg, bedside commode, urinal) Remove restraints if possible
Psychological	Appropriate nonpharmacological and/or pharmacological treatment

TABLE 8-4. Medications That Can Cause or Contribute to Urinary Incontinence

Type of medication	Potential effects on incontinence
Diuretics	Polyuria, frequency, urgency
Anticholinergics	Urinary retention with "overflow" incontinence, stool impaction
Psychotropics	
Tricyclic antidepressants	Anticholinergic actions, sedation
Antipsychotics	Anticholinergic actions, sedation, immobility
Sedative–hypnotics	Sedation, delirium, immobility, muscle relaxation
Narcotic analgesics	Urinary retention with "overflow" incontinence, fecal impaction, sedation, delirium
α-Adrenergic blockers	Urethral relaxation
α-Adrenergic agonists	Urinary retention with "overflow" incontinence
Cholinesterase inhibitors	Urinary frequency, urgency
Angiotensin-converting enzyme inhibitors	Cough precipitating stress incontinence
Calcium channel blockers	Urinary retention with "overflow" incontinence, edema (nocturia)
Gabapentin, pregabalin, glitazones	Edema (nocturia)
Alcohol	Polyuria, frequency, urgency, sedation, delirium, immobility
Caffeine	Polyuria, bladder irritation

a large amount of caffeine without understanding the effects it can have on the bladder. Patients with volume-expanded states, such as congestive heart failure and lower extremity venous insufficiency, may have polyuria at night, which can contribute to nocturia and nocturnal incontinence.

As in the case of many other conditions discussed throughout this text, a wide variety of medications can play a role in the development of incontinence in older patients via several different mechanisms (see Table 8-4). Whether the incontinence is acute or persistent, the potential role of these medications in causing or contributing to patients'

TABLE 8-5. Mnemonic for Potentially Reversible Conditions*

D	Delirium
R	Restricted mobility, retention
I	Infection, inflammation, impaction
P	Polyuria, pharmaceuticals

*See Tables 8-3 and 8-4.

incontinence should be considered. When feasible, stopping the medication, switching to an alternative, or modifying the dosage schedule can be helpful in restoring continence.

PERSISTENT INCONTINENCE

Persistent forms of incontinence can be classified clinically into four basic types.

An individual patient may have more than one type simultaneously. Although this classification does not include all the neurophysiological abnormalities associated with incontinence, it is helpful in approaching the clinical assessment and treatment of incontinence in the geriatric population.

Incontinence can result from one or a combination of the two basic abnormalities in lower genitourinary tract function: (1) failure to store urine, caused by an overactive or poorly compliant bladder or by diminished outflow resistance; and/or (2) failure to empty the bladder, caused by a poorly contractile bladder or by increased outflow resistance. Table 8-6 shows the clinical definitions and common causes of persistent urinary incontinence.

Stress incontinence is common in older women, especially in ambulatory settings. It may be infrequent and involve very small amounts of urine and need no specific treatment in women who are not bothered by it. On the other hand, it may be so severe and bothersome that it necessitates surgical correction. It is most often associated with weakened supporting tissues of the pelvic floor and consequent hypermobility of the bladder outlet and urethra caused by lack of estrogen and/or previous vaginal deliveries or surgery (see Fig. 8-5). Obesity and chronic coughing can exacerbate this condition. Women who have had previous vaginal repair and/or surgical bladder neck suspension may develop a weak urethra (intrinsic sphincter deficiency [ISD]). These women generally present with severe incontinence and symptoms of urinary loss with any activity. This condition should be suspected during office evaluation if a woman loses urine involuntarily with coughing in the supine position during a pelvic examination when her bladder is relatively empty. In general, women with ISD are less responsive to nonsurgical treatment but may benefit from periurethral injections or a surgical sling procedure. Stress incontinence is unusual in men but can occur after transurethral surgery and/or radiation therapy for lower urinary tract malignancy when the anatomic sphincters are damaged.

Urgency incontinence can be caused by a variety of lower genitourinary and neurological disorders (see Table 8-6). Patients with urgency incontinence typically present with symptoms of an overactive bladder, including frequency (voiding more than every 2 hours), urgency, and nocturia (two or more voids during usual sleeping hours). Urgency incontinence is most often, but not always, associated with involuntary bladder contractions on urodynamic testing (see Fig. 8-4). Some patients have a poorly compliant bladder without involuntary contractions (eg, as a result of radiation or interstitial cystitis, both relatively unusual conditions).

Other patients have symptoms of urgency incontinence but do not exhibit involuntary bladder contractions on urodynamic testing. Some patients with neurological disorders have involuntary bladder contractions on urodynamic testing but do not have urgency and are incontinent without any warning symptoms. These patients

TABLE 8-6. Basic Types and Causes of Persistent Urinary Incontinence

Types	Definition	Common causes
Stress	Involuntary loss of urine (usually small amounts) with increases in intra-abdominal pressure (eg, cough, laugh, exercise)	Weakness of pelvic floor musculature and urethral hypermobility Bladder outlet or urethral sphincter weakness
Urge	Leakage of urine (variable but often larger volumes) because of inability to delay voiding after sensation of bladder fullness is perceived	Detrusor overactivity, isolated or associated with one or more of the following: Local genitourinary condition such as tumors, stones, diverticula, or outflow obstruction Central nervous system disorders such as stroke, dementia, parkinsonism, spinal cord injury
Incontinence associated with incomplete bladder emptying ("overflow incontinence")	Symptoms are variable and nonspecific Classic "overflow" incontinence involves leakage of urine (usually small amounts) resulting from mechanical forces on an overdistended bladder with little or no sensation of urinary urgency	Anatomic obstruction by prostate, stricture, cystocele A contractile bladder associated with diabetes mellitus or spinal cord injury Neurogenic (detrusor-sphincter dyssynergy), associated with multiple sclerosis and other suprasacral spinal cord lesions
Functional	Urinary incontinence associated with inability to toilet because of impairment of cognitive and/or physical functioning, psychological unwillingness, or environmental barriers	Severe dementia and other neurological disorders Psychological factors such as depression and hostility

are generally treated as if they had urgency incontinence if they empty their bladders and do not have other correctable genitourinary pathology. A subgroup of older incontinent patients with an overactive bladder also have impaired bladder contractility—emptying less than one-third of their bladder volume with involuntary contractions on urodynamic testing. This condition has been termed *detrusor hyperactivity with impaired contractility (DHIC)* (Elbadawi et al, 1993; Resnick and Yalla, 1987). Patients with DHIC may present with symptoms that are not typical of urge incontinence and may strain to complete voiding. These patients may be challenging to manage because of their incomplete bladder emptying (Taylor and Kuchel, 2006).

Some older patients suffer from an overactive bladder but are not incontinent. The hallmark symptom of overactive bladder is urinary urgency. Patients with overactive bladder usually also complain of urinary frequency (more than eight voids in 24 hours) and nocturia (awakening from sleep to void). Overactive bladder symptoms are common in older adults; approximately 30% of women and 40% of men aged 75 and older admit to these symptoms, most of whom also have urgency incontinence. The conditions that contribute to symptoms of overactive bladder as well as the diagnostic evaluation and management of this symptom complex are essentially the same as for urgency incontinence (Ouslander, 2004).

Incontinence associated with incomplete bladder emptying (which in the past has been termed "overflow incontinence") can result from anatomic or neurogenic outflow obstruction, a hypotonic or acontractile bladder, or both. The most common causes include prostatic enlargement, diabetic neuropathic bladder, and urethral stricture. Low spinal cord injury and anatomic obstruction in females (caused by pelvic prolapse and urethral distortion) are less common causes of overflow incontinence. Several types of drugs can also contribute to this type of persistent incontinence (see Table 8-4). Some patients with suprasacral spinal cord lesions (eg, multiple sclerosis) develop detrusor-sphincter dyssynergy and consequent urinary retention, which must be treated in a similar manner as overflow incontinence; in some instances, a sphincterotomy is necessary. The symptoms of this type of incontinence are nonspecific, and urinary retention is easily missed on physical examination. Thus, a postvoid residual determination must be performed to exclude this condition in patients at risk for urinary retention who present with incontinence.

The term *functional incontinence* refers to incontinence associated with the inability or lack of motivation to reach a toilet on time. Factors that contribute to functional incontinence (such as inaccessible toilets and psychological disorders, especially dementia) can also exacerbate other types of persistent incontinence. Patients with incontinence that appears to be predominantly related to functional factors may also have abnormalities of the lower genitourinary tract. In some patients, it can be very difficult to determine whether the functional factors or the genitourinary factors predominate without a trial of specific types of treatment. However, no matter what specific treatments are prescribed, patients with functional incontinence require systematic toileting assistance as a component of their management plan.

These basic types of incontinence may occur in combination in an individual patient. Older women commonly have a combination of stress and urgency incontinence (generally referred to as mixed incontinence). Geriatric patients with dementia and/or mobility disorders often have urgency incontinence as well as functional disabilities that contribute to their incontinence.

EVALUATION

BASIC EVALUATION

In patients with the sudden onset of incontinence (especially when associated with an acute medical condition and hospitalization), the common reversible factors that can cause acute incontinence (see Tables 8-3, 8-4, and 8-5) can be ruled out by a brief history, physical examination, postvoid residual determination, and basic laboratory studies (urinalysis, culture, and serum glucose).

Table 8-7 shows the components of the basic evaluation of persistent urinary incontinence. The basic evaluation should include a focused history, targeted physical examination, urinalysis, and postvoiding residual (PVR) determination in most patients (American Medical Directors Association, 2006; Fung et al, 2007). The history should focus on the characteristics of the incontinence, current medical problems and medications, the most bothersome symptom(s), and the impact of the incontinence on the patient and caregivers (Table 8-8). Bladder records or voiding diaries such as those shown in Figure 8-6 (for outpatients) and Figure 8-7

TABLE 8-7. Components of the Diagnostic Evaluation of Persistent Urinary Incontinence

Basic evaluation in all patients
    History, including bladder record or voiding diary if necessary to clarify symptoms
    Physical examination
    Urinalysis
    Postvoid residual determination[*]
Selected patients[†]
    Laboratory studies
        Urine culture
        Urine cytology
        Blood glucose, calcium
        Renal function tests
        Renal ultrasonography
    Gynecological evaluation
    Urological evaluation
    Cystourethroscopy
    Urodynamic tests
        Simple
            Observation of voiding
            Cough test for stress incontinence
        Complex
            Urine flowmetry[‡]
            Multichannel cystometrogram
            Pressure-flow study
            Leak-point pressure
            Urethral pressure profilometry
            Sphincter electromyography
            Video urodynamics

[*]Postvoid residual determination may not be necessary in carefully selected patients (see text).
[†]See text and Table 8-9.
[‡]Urine flowmetry is a useful screening test in older men (see text).

TABLE 8-8. Key Aspects of an Incontinent Patient's History

Active medical conditions, especially neurological disorders, diabetes mellitus, congestive heart failure, venous insufficiency

Medication review for drugs that can contribute (see Table 8-4)

Fluid intake pattern

   Type and amount of fluid (especially caffeine and fluids before bedtime)

Past genitourinary history, especially childbirth, surgery, dilatations, urinary retention, recurrent urinary tract infections

Symptoms of incontinence

   Onset and duration

   Type—stress vs urge vs mixed vs other

   Frequency, timing, and amount of incontinence episodes and of continent voids (see Figs. 8-8 and 8-9)

Other lower urinary tract symptoms

   Irritative—dysuria, frequency, urgency, nocturia

   Voiding difficulty—hesitancy, slow or interrupted stream, straining, incomplete emptying

   Other—hematuria, suprapubic discomfort

Other symptoms

   Neurological (indicative of stroke, dementia, parkinsonism, normal-pressure hydrocephalus, spinal cord compression, multiple sclerosis)

   Psychological (depression)

   Bowel (constipation, stool incontinence)

   Symptoms suggestive of volume-expanded state (eg, lower extremity edema, shortness of breath while horizontal or with exertion)

Environmental factors

   Location of bathroom

   Availability of toilet substitutes (eg urinal, bedside commode)

Perceptions of incontinence

   Patient's concerns or ideas about underlying cause(s)

   Most bothersome symptom(s)

   Interference with daily life

   Severity (eg, "Is it enough of a problem for you to consider surgery?")

(for institutionalized patients) can be helpful in initially characterizing symptoms as well as in following the response to treatment.

Physical examination should focus on abdominal, rectal, and genital examinations and an evaluation of lumbosacral innervation (Table 8-9). During the history and physical examination, special attention should be given to factors such as mobility, mental status, medications, and accessibility of toilets that may either be causing the incontinence or interacting with urological and neurological disorders to worsen the condition. The pelvic examination in women should include careful inspections of the labia, vulva, and vagina for signs of inflammation suggestive of atrophic vaginitis and for pelvic prolapse. Most older women have some degree of pelvic prolapse

BLADDER RECORD

Day:_____   Date:_____/_____.
                                                      month   day

1NSTRUCTIONS:

(1) In the 1st column make a mark every time during the 2-hour period you urinate into the toilet

(2) Use the 2nd column to record the amount you urinate (if you are measuring amounts)

(3) In the 3rd or 4th column, make a mark every time you accidentally leak urine

Time interval	Urinated in toilet	Amount	Leaking accident	or	Large accident	Reason for accident *
6–8 AM						
8–10 AM						
2–4 PM						
4–6 PM						
6–8 PM						
8–10 PM						
10–12 PM						
Overnight						

Number of pads used today:_____

* For example, if you coughed and have a leaking accident, write "cough".
  If you had a large accident after a strong urge to urinate, write "urge".

FIGURE 8-6 Example of a bladder record for ambulatory care settings.

(eg, grade 1 or 2 cystocele as depicted in Fig. 8-8). Not all incontinent older women with these degrees of prolapse need gynecological evaluation (see later discussion).

A clean urine sample should be collected for urinalysis. For men who are frequently incontinent, making a "clean-catch" specimen difficult to obtain, a clean specimen can be obtained using a condom catheter after cleaning the penis. For cognitively and functionally impaired women, a clean specimen can be obtained by cleaning the urethral and perineal area and having the patient void into a disinfected bedpan as an alternative to in-and-out catheterization. Persistent microscopic hematuria (>5 red blood cells per high-power field) in the absence of infection is a potential indication for further evaluation with cytology and/or cystoscopy to exclude a tumor or other urinary tract pathology.

Because the prevalence of "asymptomatic bacteriuria" roughly parallels the prevalence of incontinence, incontinent geriatric patients commonly have significant bacteriuria.

INCONTINENCE MONITORING RECORD

INSTRUCTIONS: EACH TIME THE PATIENT IS CHECKED:
1) Mark *one* of the circles in the BLADDER section at the hour closest to the time the patient is checked.
2) Make an X in the BOWEL section if the patient has had an incontinent or normal bowel movement.

= Incontinent, small amount	= Dry	X = Incontinent BOWEL
= Incontinent, large amount	= Voided correctly	X = Normal BOWEL

PATIENT NAME _____ ROOM # _____ DATE _____

	BLADDER			BOWEL			
	INCONTINENT OF URINE	DRY	VOIDED CORRECTLY	INCONTINENT X	NORMAL X	INITIALS	COMMENTS
12 AM	● ●	○	△ cc ___				
1	● ●	○	△ cc ___				
2	● ●	○	△ cc ___				
3	● ●	○	△ cc ___				
4	● ●	○	△ cc ___				
5	● ●	○	△ cc ___				
6	● ●	○	△ cc ___				
7	● ●	○	△ cc ___				
8	● ●	○	△ cc ___				
9	● ●	○	△ cc ___				
10	● ●	○	△ cc ___				
11	● ●	○	△ cc ___				
12 PM	● ●	○	△ cc ___				
1	● ●	○	△ cc ___				
2	● ●	○	△ cc ___				
3	● ●	○	△ cc ___				
4	● ●	○	△ cc ___				
5	● ●	○	△ cc ___				
6	● ●	○	△ cc ___				
7	● ●	○	△ cc ___				
8	● ●	○	△ cc ___				
9	● ●	○	△ cc ___				
10	● ●	○	△ cc ___				
11	● ●	○	△ cc ___				
TOTALS:							

FIGURE 8-7 Example of a record to monitor bladder and bowel functions in institutional settings. This type of record is especially useful for implementing and following the results of various training procedures and other treatment protocols. (*Reproduced with permission from Ouslander JG, Uman GC, Urman HN. Development and testing of an incontinence monitoring record,* J Am Geriatr Soc. *1986 Feb;34(2):83-90.*)

In the initial evaluation of incontinent noninstitutionalized patients, especially those in whom the incontinence is new or worsening, bacteriuria should be treated before further evaluation is undertaken. In the nursing home population, eradicating bacteriuria does not affect the severity of chronic, stable incontinence (Ouslander et al, 1995).

TABLE 8-9. Key Aspects of an Incontinent Patient's Physical Examination

Mobility and dexterity
  Functional status compatible with ability to self-toilet
  Gait disturbance (eg that may suggest parkinsonism, normal-pressure hydrocephalus)
Mental status
  Cognitive function compatible with ability to self-toilet
  Motivation
  Mood and effect
Neurological
  Focal signs (especially in lower extremities) that could suggest a central nervous
    system condition
  Signs of parkinsonism
  Sacral arc reflexes (eg loss of perianal sensation or an anal wink in response to
    perianal stimulation)
Abdominal
  Bladder distension
  Suprapubic tenderness
  Lower abdominal mass
Rectal
  Perianal sensation
  Sphincter tone (resting and active)
  Impaction
  Masses
  Size and contour of prostate (neither is diagnostic of urethral obstruction)
Pelvic
  Perineal skin condition
  Perineal sensation
  Atrophic vaginitis (friability, inflammation, bleeding)
  Pelvic prolapse (ie, cystocele, rectocele; see Fig. 8-8)
  Pelvic mass
  Other anatomic abnormality
Other
  Lower extremity edema or signs of congestive heart failure (if nocturia is a
    prominent complaint)

PART II

However, new onset of incontinence, worsening incontinence, unexplained fever, and decline in mental and/or functional status may be the manifestations of a urinary tract infection in this population.

A PVR determination can be done either by catheterization or using a portable ultrasound to detect urinary retention, which cannot always be detected by physical examination. Although the symptoms of incontinence associated with urinary retention can be nonspecific and significant residual urine can be easily missed on physical examination, some older incontinent patients may not need a PVR before a trial of treatment. Examples of such patients include those with pure symptoms of stress

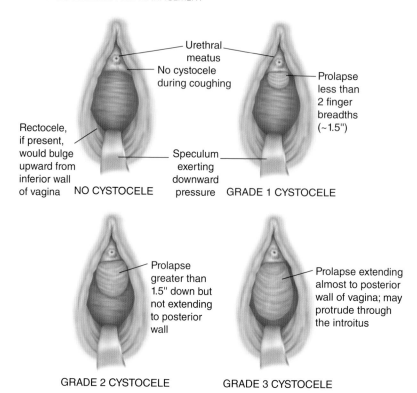

FIGURE 8-8 Example of a simplified grading system for cystoceles.

incontinence, urgency incontinence, or overactive bladder who have no symptoms of voiding difficulty and have no risk factors or urinary retention (eg, diabetes, spinal cord disease).

Patients with residual volumes of more than 200 mL should be considered for further evaluation. The need for further evaluation in patients with lesser degrees of retention should be determined on an individual basis, considering the patient's symptoms, whether they have had recurrent symptomatic urinary tract infections, and the degree to which they complain of straining or are observed to strain with voiding.

In older men, a noninvasive flow rate determination can be very helpful in screening for impaired bladder contractility or obstruction. Very low peak urinary flow rates (eg, <10 m/s) after an adequate void (eg, >150 mL) are suggestive of one of these conditions. Uroflowmeters are relatively inexpensive but are rare in physicians' offices (except for urologists).

FURTHER EVALUATION

The need for further evaluation and the specific diagnostic procedures listed in Table 8-7 should be determined on an individual basis. Clinical practice guidelines state that not all incontinent geriatric patients require further evaluation. Patients who have unexplained polyuria should have their blood glucose and calcium levels determined because both hyperglycemia and hypercalcemia can contribute to increased urine production and precipitate or exacerbate symptoms of incontinence or overactive bladder. Patients with significant urinary retention should have renal function tests and be considered for renal ultrasound and urodynamic testing to determine whether obstruction, impaired bladder contractility, or both are present. Persistent microscopic hematuria in the absence of infection is an indication for urine cytology and urological evaluation, including cystoscopy. Even in the absence of hematuria, patients with recent and sudden onset of irritative urinary symptoms who have risk factors for bladder cancer (heavy smoking, industrial exposure to aniline dyes) should be considered for these evaluations. Women with marked pelvic prolapse (see Fig. 8-8) should be referred for gynecological evaluation.

Complex urodynamic testing is helpful in guiding treatment in selected patients and is essential to determine the cause(s) of urinary retention and for any older patient for whom surgical intervention is being considered. Table 8-10 summarizes criteria for referral for further evaluation, and Figure 8-9 summarizes the overall approach to the evaluation of geriatric urinary incontinence.

MANAGEMENT

GENERAL PRINCIPLES

Several therapeutic modalities can be used in managing incontinent geriatric patients (Table 8-11). Treatment can be especially helpful if specific diagnoses are made and attention is paid to all factors that may be contributing to the incontinence in a given patient. Even when cure is not possible, risks of complications can be reduced, and the comfort, satisfaction and quality of life of both patients and caregivers can almost always be enhanced.

Acute incontinence may be transient if managed appropriately. All of the potential reversible factors that can cause or contribute to incontinence (see Tables 8-3, 8-4, and 8-5) should be attended to in order to maximize the potential for regaining continence. A common approach to incontinent geriatric patients in acute care hospitals is indwelling catheterization. In some instances, this is justified by the need for accurate measurement of urine output during the acute phase of an illness. In many instances, however, it is unnecessary and poses a substantial and unwarranted risk of catheter-associated infection. Catheter-associated infections that arise in hospitals are not reimbursed by Medicare, and most hospitals now have protocols on when to use catheters and how to minimize duration of use. Making toilets and toilet substitutes accessible and combining this with some form of scheduled toileting and appropriate use of absorbent pads and undergarments are appropriate approaches in patients who do not require indwelling catheterization. Supportive measures are critical in managing all forms of incontinence and should be used in conjunction with other, more specific treatment modalities.

Education (available in many booklets and on many websites), environmental manipulation, appropriate use of toilet substitutes, avoidance of iatrogenic contributions to

TABLE 8-10. Criteria for Considering Referral of Incontinent Patients for Urological, Gynecological, or Urodynamic Evaluation

Criteria	Definition	Rationale
History		
Recent history of lower urinary tract or pelvic surgery or irradiation	Surgery or irradiation involving the pelvic area or lower urinary tract within the past 6–12 months	A structural abnormality relating to the recent procedure should be sought
Recurrent symptomatic urinary tract infections	Two or more symptomatic episodes in a 12-month period	A structural abnormality or pathologic condition in the urinary tract predisposing to infection should be excluded
Risk factors for bladder cancer	Recent or sudden onset of irritative symptoms, history of heavy smoking, or exposure to aniline dyes	Urine for cytology and cystoscopy to exclude bladder cancer should be considered
Physical examination		
Marked pelvic prolapse	A prominent cystocele that descends the entire height of the vaginal vault with coughing during speculum examination	Anatomic abnormality may underlie the pathophysiology of the incontinence (and recurrent infections), and selected patients may benefit from a pessary or surgical repair
Marked prostatic enlargement and/or suspicion of cancer	Gross enlargement of the prostate on digital examination; prominent induration or asymmetry of the lobes	An evaluation to exclude prostate cancer may be appropriate and have therapeutic implications
Postvoid residual (PVR)		
Difficulty passing a 14-F straight catheter	Impossible catheter passage, or passage requiring considerable force, or a larger, more rigid catheter	Anatomic blockage of the urethra or bladder neck may be present
Postvoid residual volume >200	Volume of urine remaining in the bladder within a few minutes after the patient voids spontaneously in as normal a fashion as possible	Anatomic or neurogenic obstruction or poor bladder contractility may be present

(continued)

TABLE 8-10. Criteria for Considering Referral of Incontinent Patients for Urological, Gynecological, or Urodynamic Evaluation (*continued*)

Criteria	Definition	Rationale
Urinalysis		
Hematuria	>5 red blood cells per high-power field on repeated microscopic examinations in the absence of infection	A pathologic condition in the urinary tract should be excluded
Therapeutic trial		
Failure to respond	Persistent symptoms that are bothersome to the patient after adequate trials of behavioral and/or drug therapy	Urodynamic evaluation may help guide specific therapy

incontinence, modifications of diuretic and fluid intake patterns, and good skin care are all important. For example, encouraging patients with nocturia to use a urinal or bedside commode may both promote continence and prevent falls. Specially designed incontinence undergarments and pads can be very helpful to many patients but must be used appropriately. Although they can be effective, several caveats should be noted:

1. Garments and pads are a nonspecific treatment. They should not be used as the first response to incontinence or before some type of diagnostic evaluation is done.
2. Many patients are curable if treated with specific therapies, and some have potentially serious factors underlying their incontinence that must be diagnosed and treated.
3. Underpants and pads can interfere with attempts at behavioral intervention and thereby foster dependency.
4. Many disposable products are relatively expensive and are not covered by Medicare or other insurance.

To a large extent, the optimal treatment of persistent incontinence depends on identifying the type(s). Table 8-12 outlines the primary treatments for the basic types of persistent incontinence in the geriatric population. Each treatment modality is briefly discussed in the following sections. Behavioral interventions have been well studied in the geriatric population. These interventions are generally recommended by guidelines as an initial approach to therapy in many patients because they are generally noninvasive and nonspecific (ie, patients with stress and/or urgency incontinence respond equally well).

BEHAVIORAL INTERVENTIONS

Many types of behavioral interventions are effective in the management of urinary incontinence (Shamliyan et al, 2008). The term *bladder training* has been used to

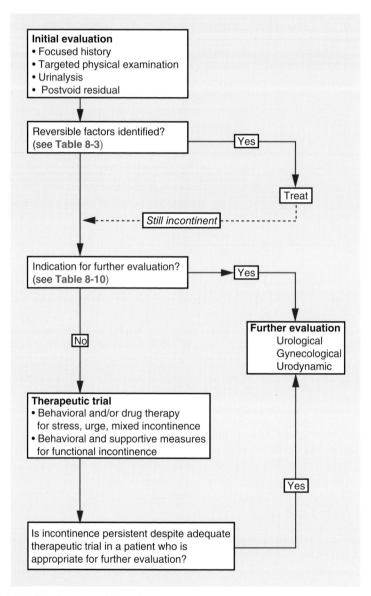

FIGURE 8-9 Algorithm protocol for evaluating incontinence.

encompass a wide variety of techniques. It is, however, important to distinguish between procedures that are patient dependent (ie, necessitate adequate function, learning capability, and motivation of the patient), in which the goal is to restore a normal pattern of voiding and continence, and procedures that are caregiver dependent that can be used for functionally disabled patients, in which the goal is to

TABLE 8-11. Treatment Options for Geriatric Urinary Incontinence

Nonspecific supportive measures
   Education
   Modifications of fluid (eg, caffeine) and medication intake
   Use of toilet substitutes
   Environmental manipulations
   Garments and pads
Behavioral interventions (see Table 8-13)
   Patient dependent
      Pelvic muscle exercises
      Bladder training
      Bladder retraining (see Table 8-14)
   Caregiver dependent
      Scheduled toileting
      Habit training
      Prompted voiding (see Table 8-15)
Drugs (see Table 8-16)
   Antimuscarinics (bladder relaxants)
   α-Antagonists
   α-Agonists
   Estrogen
Periurethral injections
Surgery
   Bladder neck suspension or sling
   Removal of obstruction or pathologic lesion
Mechanical devices
   Penile clamps
   Artificial sphincters
   Sacral nerve stimulators
Catheters
   External
   Intermittent
   Indwelling

keep the patient and their surrounding environment dry. Table 8-13 summarizes behavioral interventions. All of the patient-dependent procedures generally involve the patient's continuous self-monitoring, using a record such as the one depicted in Figure 8-6; the caregiver-dependent procedures usually involve a record such as the one shown in Figure 8-7.

Pelvic floor muscle (Kegel) exercises are an essential component of patient-dependent behavioral interventions. They have been shown to produce the greatest benefit in treating urinary incontinence (Shamliyan et al, 2008). The exercises consist of repetitive contractions and relaxations of the pelvic floor muscles. The exercises may be taught by having the patient interrupt voiding to get a sense of

TABLE 8-12. Primary Treatments for Different Types of Geriatric Urinary Incontinence

Type of incontinence	Primary treatments
Stress	Pelvic muscle (Kegel) exercises
	Other behavioral interventions (see Table 8-13)
	α-Adrenergic agonists
	Topical estrogen (not alone)
	Periurethral injections
	Surgical bladder neck suspension or sling
Urge	Bladder relaxants
	Topical estrogen (if atrophic vaginitis present)
	Bladder training (including pelvic muscle exercises)
Overflow	Surgical removal of obstruction
	Bladder retraining (see Table 8-14)
	Intermittent catheterization
	Indwelling catheterization
Functional	Behavioral interventions (caregiver dependent; see Tables 8-13 and 8-15)
	Environmental manipulations
	Incontinence undergarments and pads

the muscles being used or by having women squeeze the examiner's fingers during a vaginal examination (without doing a Valsalva maneuver, which is the opposite of the intended effect). A randomized trial has documented that many young-old women (mean age in the mid to upper 60s) can be taught these exercises during an in-office examination and derive significant reductions in incontinence (Burgio et al, 2002). Many women, however, especially those older than age 75, require biofeedback to help them identify the muscles and practice the exercises. One full exercise is a 10-second squeeze and a 10-second relaxation. Most older women will have to build endurance gradually to this level. Once learned, the exercises should be practiced many times throughout the day (up to 40 exercises per day) and, importantly, should be used in everyday life during situations (eg, coughing, standing up, hearing running water) that might precipitate incontinence. Older men respond to pelvic muscle and bladder training techniques as well, and it should be considered as an alternative or adjunctive therapy for overactive bladder and urgency incontinence in the male population (Burgio et al, 2011). Biofeedback can be very effective for teaching pelvic floor muscle exercises. It generally involves the use of vaginal (or rectal) pressure or electromyography (EMG) with or without abdominal muscle EMG recordings to train patients to contract pelvic floor muscles and relax the abdomen. Studies show that these techniques improve management of both stress and urgency incontinence in the geriatric population. Numerous software packages are available to assist with biofeedback training.

TABLE 8-13. Examples of Behavioral Interventions for Urinary Incontinence

Procedure	Definition	Types of incontinence	Comments
Patient dependent			
Pelvic muscle (Kegel) exercises	Repetitive contraction and relaxation of pelvic floor muscles	Stress and urge	Requires adequate function and motivation and ability to learn Biofeedback often helpful in teaching the exercise
Bladder training	Use of education, bladder records, pelvic muscle, and other behavioral techniques	Stress and urge	Requires trained therapist, adequate cognitive and physical functioning, and motivation
Bladder retraining	Progressive lengthening or shortening of intervoiding interval, with intermittent catheterization used in patients recovering from overdistention injuries with persistent retention (see Table 8-14)	Acute (eg, postcatheterization with urge or overflow, poststroke)	Goal is to restore normal pattern of voiding and continence Requires adequate cognitive and physical function and motivation
Caregiver dependent			
Scheduled toileting	Routine toileting at regular intervals (scheduled toileting)	Urge and functional	Goal is to prevent wetting episodes Can be used in patients with impaired cognitive or physical functioning Requires staff or caregiver availability and motivation

(continued)

TABLE 8-13. Examples of Behavioral Interventions for Urinary Incontinence (*continued*)

Procedure	Definition	Types of incontinence	Comments
Habit training	Variable toileting schedule based on patient's voiding patterns	Urge and functional	Goal is to prevent wetting episodes Can be used in patients with impaired cognitive or physical functioning Requires staff or caregiver availability and motivation
Prompted voiding	Offer opportunity to toilet every 2 hours during the day; toilet only on request; social reinforcement; routine offering of fluids (see Table 8-15); individualize toileting at night based on patient preferences and degree of bother and risk for falls	Urge, stress, mixed, functional	Same as above 25%–40% of nursing home residents respond well during the day and can be identified during a 3-day trial (see text and Table 8-15)

Other forms of patient-dependent interventions include bladder training and bladder retraining. Bladder training involves education, pelvic muscle exercises (with or without biofeedback), strategies to manage urgency, and the regular use of bladder records (see Fig. 8-6). Bladder training is highly effective in selected community-dwelling patients, especially those who are motivated and functional. A major challenge is sustaining the effectiveness of patient-dependent interventions because they require continuous practice by the patient over an extended period of time.

Table 8-14 provides an example of a bladder retraining protocol. This protocol is applicable to patients who have had indwelling catheterization for monitoring of urinary output during a period of acute illness or for treatment of urinary retention with overflow incontinence. Such catheters should be removed as soon as possible, and this type of bladder retraining protocol should enable most indwelling catheters to be removed from patients in acute care hospitals as well as some in long-term

TABLE 8-14. Example of a Bladder Retraining Protocol

Objective: To restore a normal pattern of voiding and continence after the removal of an indwelling catheter.

1. Remove the indwelling catheter (clamping the catheter before removal is not necessary).
2. Treat urinary tract infection if present.
3. Initiate a toileting schedule. Begin by toileting the patient:
   a. Upon awakening
   b. Every 2 hours during the day and evening
   c. Before getting into bed
   d. Every 4 hours at night
4. Monitor the patient's voiding and continence pattern with a record that allows for the recording of:
   a. Frequency, timing, and amount of continent voids
   b. Frequency, timing, and amount of incontinence episodes
   c. Fluid intake pattern
   d. Postvoid catheter volume
5. If the patient is having difficulty voiding (complete urinary retention or very low urine outputs, eg, 240 mL in an 8-hour period while fluid intake is adequate):
   a. Perform bladder ultrasound or in-and-out catheterization, recording volume obtained, every 6–8 hours until residual values are 200 mL.
   b. Instruct the patient on techniques to trigger voiding (eg, running water, stroking inner thigh, suprapubic tapping) and to help completely empty bladder (eg, bending forward, suprapubic pressure, double voiding).
   c. If the patient continues to have high residual volumes after 1–2 weeks, consider urodynamic evaluation.
6. If the patient is voiding frequently (ie, more often than every 2 hours):
   a. Perform postvoid residual determination to ensure the patient is completely emptying the bladder.
   b. Encourage the patient to delay voiding as long as possible, and instruct the patient to use techniques to help completely empty bladder and pelvic muscle exercises.
   c. If the patient continues to have frequency and nocturia with or without urgency and incontinence:
      1. Rule out other reversible causes (eg, urinary tract infection, medication effects, hyperglycemia, and congestive heart failure).
      2. Consider further evaluation to rule out other pathology.

PART II

care settings. A patient who continues to have difficulty voiding after 1 to 2 weeks of bladder retraining should be examined for other potentially reversible causes of voiding difficulties, such as those mentioned in the preceding discussion of acute incontinence. When difficulties persist, a urological referral should be considered to rule out correctable lower genitourinary pathology.

The goal of caregiver–dependent interventions is to prevent incontinence episodes rather than to restore normal patterns of voiding and complete continence. Such procedures are effective in reducing incontinence in selected nursing home residents and functionally and cognitively impaired patients in home and other settings. In its simplest form, scheduled toileting involves toileting the patient at regular intervals, usually every 2 hours during the day and every 4 hours during the evening and night. Habit training involves a schedule of toiletings or prompted voidings that is modified according to the patient's pattern of continent voids and incontinence episodes as demonstrated by a monitoring record such as that shown in Figure 8-7. Adjunctive techniques to prompt voiding (eg, running tap water, stroking the inner thigh, or suprapubic tapping) and to facilitate complete emptying of the bladder (eg, bending forward after completion of voiding) may be helpful in some patients. Prompted voiding has been the best studied of these procedures. Table 8-15 provides an example of a prompted voiding protocol. Up to 40% of incontinent nursing home residents may be essentially dry during the day with a consistent prompted voiding program. The success of these interventions is largely dependent on the knowledge and motivation of the caregivers who are implementing them, rather than on the physical, functional and mental status of the incontinent patient. Targeting of prompted voiding to selected patients after a 3-day trial may enhance its cost-effectiveness (see Table 8-15). Quality improvement methods, based on principles of industrial statistical quality control, have been shown to be helpful in maintaining the effectiveness of prompted voiding in nursing homes (Ouslander, 2007). However, unless adequate staffing, training, and administrative support for the program persist, the effectiveness of prompted voiding will not be maintained in an institutional setting.

Toileting at night should be individualized because prompted voiding and other similar interventions can disrupt sleep. Many functionally dependent patients are appropriately managed supportively at night with pads and adult diapers. This type of supportive management is appropriate for incontinent patients whose sleep is not disrupted and whose skin is not irritated.

DRUG TREATMENT

Table 8-16 lists the drugs used to treat various types of incontinence. Several clinical trials show that the efficacy of drug treatment in the geriatric population is similar to that in younger populations (Shamliyan et al, 2012). One trial demonstrated efficacy in older patients who met selected criteria for "vulnerability" (DuBeau et al, 2013). Drug treatment can be prescribed in conjunction with various behavioral interventions. Treatment decisions should be individualized and will depend in large on the characteristics and preferences of the patient (including risks and costs) and the preference of the health-care professional.

For urgency incontinence, antimuscarinic drugs with anticholinergic and relaxant effects on the bladder smooth muscle are used. All of them have proven efficacy in older patients, but they can have bothersome systemic anticholinergic side effects, especially dry mouth and constipation. Dry mouth can be relieved by small sips of water, hard candy, or over-the-counter oral lubricants. Constipation can be managed proactively (see "Fecal Incontinence" section). Patients should be warned about exacerbation of gastroesophageal reflux and glaucoma. Although open-angle glaucoma is not an absolute contraindication, patients being treated for glaucoma should be instructed to consult their ophthalmologist before initiating treatment.

TABLE 8-15. Example of a Prompted Voiding Protocol for a Nursing Home

Assessment period (3–5 days)

1. Contact resident every hour from 7 AM to 7 PM for 2–3 days, then every 2 hours for 2–3 days.
2. Focus attention on voiding by asking resident whether he or she is wet or dry.
3. Check residents for wetness, record results on bladder record, and give feedback on whether response was correct or incorrect.
4. Whether wet or dry, ask residents if they would like to use the toilet or urinal. If they say yes:
   - Offer assistance.
   - Record results on bladder record.
   - Give positive reinforcement by spending extra time talking with them.

If they say no:
   - Repeat the question once or twice.
   - Inform them that you will be back in 1 hour and request that they try to delay voiding until then.
   - If there has been no attempt to void in the last 2–3 hours, repeat the request to use the toilet at least twice more before leaving.
5. Offer fluids.

Targeting

1. Prompted voiding is more effective in some residents than others.
2. The best candidates are residents who show the following characteristics during the assessment period:
   - Void in the toilet, commode, or urinal (as opposed to being incontinent in a pad or garment) more than two-thirds of the time
   - Wet on ≤20% of checks
   - Show substantial reduction in incontinence frequency on 2-hour prompts
3. Residents who do not show any of these characteristics may be candidates for either:
   - Further evaluation to determine the specific type of incontinence if they attempt to toilet but remain frequently wet
   - Supportive management by padding and adult diapers, and a checking-and-changing protocol if they do not cooperate with prompting

Prompted voiding (ongoing protocol)

1. Contact the resident every 2 hours from 7 AM to 7 PM.
2. Use same procedures as for the assessment period.
3. For nighttime management, use either modified prompted voiding schedule or padding, depending on resident's sleep pattern and preferences.
4. If a resident who has been responding well has an increase in incontinence frequency despite adequate staff implementation of the protocol, the resident should be evaluated for reversible factors.

PART II

All antimuscarinic drugs have anticholinergic properties and can theoretically cause problems with memory and other central nervous system side effects. Many older incontinent patients with urgency incontinence or overactive bladder have memory loss or early dementia and are already on cholinesterase inhibitors. In these patients,

TABLE 8-16. Drug Treatment for Urinary Incontinence and Overactive Bladder

Drugs	Dosages	Mechanisms of action	Type of incontinence	Potential common adverse effects
Antimuscarinic				
Darifenacin	7.5–15 mg daily	Increase bladder capacity and diminish involuntary bladder contractions	Urge or mixed with urge predominant	Dry mouth, constipation, blurry vision, elevated intraocular pressure, cognitive impairment, delirium
Fesoterodine	4–8 mg daily		Overactive bladder with incontinence	
Oxybutynin				
Short-acting	2.5–5 mg tid			
Long-acting	5–30 mg daily			
Transdermal	3.9-mg patch changed after each 3 days			
Solifenacin	5–10 mg daily			
Tolterodine				
Short-acting	2 mg bid			
Long-acting	4 mg daily			
Trospium				
Short-acting	20 mg bid			
Long-acting	60 mg daily			
α-Adrenergic antagonists		Relax smooth muscle of urethra and prostatic capsule	Urge incontinence and related irritative symptoms associated with benign prostatic enlargement	Postural hypotension
			May be more effective in combination with an antimuscarinic drug	
Alfuzosin	10 mg qd			
Silodosin	4 mg daily			
Tamsulosin	0.4 mg qd			

α-Adrenergic agonists*

Drug	Dose	Mechanism	Indication	Side effects
Pseudoephedrine	30–60 mg tid or 60–120 mg, long acting	Stimulates contraction of urethral smooth muscle	Stress	Headache, tachycardia, elevation of blood pressure
Duloxetine	20–40 mg daily	Increases α-adrenergic tone to the urethra	Stress	Nausea
Topical estrogen[†]				
Topical cream	0.5–1.0 g/day for 2 weeks, then twice weekly	Strengthen periurethral tissues	Urge associated with severe vaginal atrophy or atrophic vaginitis	Local irritation
Vaginal estradiol ring	One ring every 3 months	Increase periurethral blood flow	Stress	
Arginine vasopressin[‡]				
DDAVP oral	0.1–0.4 mg at night	Prevents water loss from the kidney	Nocturia that is bothersome and does not respond to other treatments	Hyponatremia (serum sodium must be monitored closely at the onset of treatment)
Nasal spray	10–20 µg of nasal spray in each nostril at night			Flushing, nausea, rhinitis
Cholinergic agonist[§]				
Bethanechol	10–30 mg tid	Stimulate bladder contraction	Acute incontinence associated with incomplete bladder emptying in the absence of obstruction	Bradycardia, hypotension, bronchoconstriction, gastric acid secretion, diarrhea

*α-Adrenergic agonists are not approved by the U.S. Food and Drug Administration for this indication.
†Topical estrogen alone is not effective in relieving symptoms and should be considered an adjunctive treatment. There is also evidence that estrogen (given orally) may worsen incontinence in some women (Hendrix et al., 2005).
‡DDAVP is not approved by the U.S. Food and Drug Administration for this indication.
§Bethanechol may be helpful in selected patients after an episode of acute urinary retention; there is no evidence that it is useful on a chronic basis.

the decision to add an antimuscarinic for the bladder must be based on careful weighing of the bother of the symptoms versus the potential risks of the drugs.

The maximum effect of antimuscarinic drugs may not be achieved for up to 1 to 2 months. Therefore, patients should be educated to prevent unrealistic expectations about a quick cure and complete dryness. To maximize adherence, they should be told that many patients benefit from these drugs and some are cured, and that it may take a couple of months to achieve the desired effect. As with many other therapeutic agents, some patients respond to one drug better than others in the same class, so patients who are bothered and not responsive to one drug could be given a trial of another drug.

A new drug with a different mechanism of action (beta-3 receptor agonist) is now available (mirabegron) and appears to have similar efficacy as antimuscarinic drugs, but without the anticholinergic side effects. Mirabegron can raise blood pressure, but generally not enough to be clinically meaningful.

Among older men, symptoms of overactive bladder, including urgency incontinence, overlap with the irritative symptoms of benign prostatic hyperplasia (BPH). Men with large prostate glands (eg, estimated volume >30 g) may benefit from a 5-α reductase inhibitor. α-Adrenergic blockers (listed in Table 8-16) are effective for many older men for lower urinary tract symptoms associated with BPH but must be used carefully because of their potential to cause postural hypotension, especially among men already on cardiovascular medications. Combining an α-blocker with an antimuscarinic drug appears to be more efficacious than either alone, and the incidence of significant urinary retention with combination is very low (Kaplan et al, 2006). Phosphodiesterase inhibitors (not listed in the table) may also be effective, for these symptoms but must be used cautiously in older men with cardiovascular disease.

Carefully selected patients with bothersome nocturia and/or nocturnal incontinence may benefit from a careful trial of intranasal arginine vasopressin (DDAVP) (see Table 8-16). However, it is not approved by the U.S. Food and Drug Administration (FDA) for this indication and the incidence of hyponatremia with this agent is very high in older patients, and thus treated patients must be carefully monitored for its development. Currently, this would be an off-label use of this drug.

For stress incontinence, there are no drug treatments approved by FDA. If drug treatment is considered, it usually involves a combination of an α-agonist and estrogen. Drug treatment is appropriate for motivated patients who have mild to moderate degrees of stress incontinence, do not have a major anatomic abnormality (eg, grade 3 cystocele or ISD), and do not have any contraindications to these drugs. Pseudoephedrine is contraindicated in older patients with hypertension. Duloxetine, a selective serotonin reuptake inhibitor antidepressant, increases α-adrenergic tone to the lower urinary tract through a spinal cord mechanism. It is approved in some countries for the treatment of stress incontinence. Neither pseudoephedrine nor duloxetine is FDA approved for stress incontinence and would be used off label for this indication. Patients with stress incontinence may also respond to concomitant behavioral interventions, as described earlier.

For stress incontinence, estrogen alone is not as effective as it is in combination with an α-agonist. Estrogen is also used for the treatment of irritative voiding symptoms and urgency incontinence in women with atrophic vaginitis and urethritis. Oral estrogen is not effective, and thus, topical estrogen must be used for these symptoms; in fact, oral estrogen may actually worsen incontinence in some women (Hendrix et al, 2005). Vaginal estrogen can be prescribed five nights per week for 1 to 2 months initially and then reduced to a maintenance dose of one to three times per week. A vaginal ring that slowly releases estradiol and vaginal tablets are also available. Drug treatment for chronic "overflow" incontinence using a cholinergic agonist or an α-adrenergic antagonist is rarely efficacious. Bethanechol may be helpful when given for a brief period subcutaneously in patients with persistent bladder contractility problems after an overdistention injury, but it is seldom effective when given over the long term orally. It can cause bradycardia and bronchoconstriction. α-Adrenergic blockers may be helpful in relieving symptoms associated with outflow obstruction in some patients but are probably not efficacious for long-term treatment of overflow incontinence.

SURGERY

Surgery should be considered for older women with stress incontinence that continues to be bothersome after attempts at nonsurgical treatment and in women with a significant degree of pelvic prolapse or ISD. As with many other surgical procedures, patient selection and the experience of the surgeon are critical to success. All women being considered for surgical therapy should have a thorough evaluation, including urodynamic tests, before undergoing the procedure.

Women with mixed stress incontinence and detrusor overactivity may also benefit from surgery, especially if the clinical history and urodynamic findings suggest that stress incontinence is the predominant problem. A randomized controlled trial has demonstrated that women with a clear history of pure stress incontinence do not necessarily need urodynamic testing before surgery (Nager et al, 2012). Many modified techniques of bladder neck suspension can be done with minimal risk and are successful in achieving continence over about a 5-year period. Urinary retention can occur after surgery, but it is usually transient and can be managed by a brief period of suprapubic catheterization. Data suggest that a fascial sling is more efficacious than a Burch colposuspension, but it is also associated with more postoperative complications (Albo et al, 2007). Periurethral injection of collagen and other materials is now available and may offer patients with ISD an alternative to surgery.

Surgery may be indicated in men in whom incontinence is associated with anatomically and/or urodynamically documented outflow obstruction. Men who have experienced an episode of complete urinary retention without any clear precipitant are likely to have another episode within a short period of time and should have a prostatic resection, as should men with incontinence associated with a sufficient amount of residual urine to be causing recurrent symptomatic infections or hydronephrosis. The decision about surgery in men who do not meet these criteria must be an individual one, weighing carefully the degree to which the symptoms bother the patient, the potential benefits of surgery (obstructive symptoms often respond better than irritative symptoms), and the risks of surgery, which may be minimal with newer prostate resection techniques. A small number of older patients, especially men who have stress incontinence related to sphincter damage caused by previous transurethral surgery, may benefit from the surgical implantation of an artificial urinary sphincter.

CATHETERS AND CATHETER CARE

Catheters should be avoided in managing incontinence, unless specific indications are present. Three basic types of catheters and catheterization procedures are used for the management of urinary incontinence: external catheters, intermittent straight catheterization, and chronic indwelling catheterization.

External catheters generally consist of some type of condom connected to a drainage system. Sound design and observance of proper procedure and skin care when applying the catheter will decrease the risk of skin irritation as well as the frequency with which the catheter falls off. Patients with external catheters are at increased risk of developing symptomatic infection. External catheters should be used only to manage intractable incontinence in male patients who do not have urinary retention and who are extremely physically dependent. As with incontinence undergarments and padding, these devices should not be used as a matter of convenience because they may foster dependency.

Intermittent catheterization can help in the management of patients with incontinence associated with urinary retention. The procedure can be carried out by either the patient or a caregiver and involves straight catheterization two to four times daily, depending on catheter urine volumes and patient tolerance. In general, bladder volume should be kept to less than 400 mL. In the home setting, the catheter should be kept clean (but not necessarily sterile).

Intermittent catheterization may be useful for certain patients in acute care hospitals and nursing homes, for example, following removal of an indwelling catheter in a bladder retraining protocol (see Table 8-14). Nursing home residents, however, may be difficult to catheterize, and the anatomic abnormalities commonly found in older patients' lower urinary tracts may increase the risk of infection as a consequence of repeated straight catheterizations. In addition, using this technique in an institutional setting (which may have an abundance of organisms that are relatively resistant to many commonly used antimicrobial agents) may yield an unacceptable risk of nosocomial infections, and using sterile catheter trays for these procedures would be very expensive; thus, it may be extremely difficult to implement such a program in a typical nursing home setting.

Indwelling catheterization is still overused in acute hospital settings and increases the incidence of a number of complications, including chronic bacteriuria, bladder stones, periurethral abscesses, and even bladder cancer with long-term use. Nursing home residents, especially men, managed by chronic catheterization are at relatively high risk of developing symptomatic infections. Given these risks, it seems

TABLE 8-17. Indications for Chronic Indwelling Catheter Use

Urinary retention that
  Is causing persistent overflow incontinence, symptomatic infections, or renal dysfunction
  Cannot be corrected surgically or medically
  Cannot be managed practically with intermittent catheterization
Skin wounds, pressure ulcers, or irritations that are being contaminated by incontinent urine
Care of terminally ill or severely impaired patients for whom bed and clothing changes are uncomfortable or disruptive
Preference of patient when toileting or changing causes excessive discomfort

appropriate to recommend that the use of chronic indwelling catheters be limited to certain specific situations (Table 8-17). When indwelling catheterization is used, sound principles of catheter care should be observed to attempt to minimize complications (Table 8-18).

TABLE 8-18. Key Principles of Chronic Indwelling Catheter Care

1. Maintain sterile, closed gravity-drainage system.
2. Avoid breaking the closed system.
3. Use clean techniques in emptying and changing the drainage system; wash hands between patients in institutionalized setting.
4. Secure the catheter to the upper thigh or lower abdomen to avoid perineal contamination and urethral irritation because of movement of the catheter.
5. Avoid frequent and vigorous cleaning of the catheter entry site; washing with soapy water once per day is sufficient.
6. Do not routinely irrigate.
7. If bypassing occurs in the absence of obstruction, consider the possibility of a bladder spasm, which can be treated with a bladder relaxant.
8. If catheter obstruction occurs frequently, increase the patient's fluid intake and acidify the urine with dilute acetic acid irrigations.
9. Do not routinely use prophylactic or suppressive urinary antiseptics or antimicrobials.
10. Do not do surveillance cultures to guide management of individual patients because all chronically catheterized patients have bacteriuria (which is often polymicrobial) and the organisms change frequently.
11. Do not treat infection unless the patient develops symptoms; symptoms may be nonspecific, and other possible sources of infection should be carefully excluded before attributing symptoms to the urinary tract.
12. If a patient develops frequent symptomatic urinary tract infections, a genitourinary evaluation should be considered to rule out pathology such as stones, periurethral or prostatic abscesses, and chronic pyelonephritis.

FECAL INCONTINENCE

Fecal incontinence is less common than urinary incontinence. Its occurrence is relatively unusual in older patients who are continent with regard to urine; however, 30% to 50% of geriatric patients with frequent urinary incontinence also have episodes of fecal incontinence, especially in the nursing home population. This coexistence suggests common pathophysiological mechanisms. Evidence-based reviews are now available on this topic (Shamliyan et al, 2007; Wald, 2007).

Defecation, like urination, is a physiological process that involves smooth and striated muscles, central and peripheral innervation, coordination of reflex responses, mental awareness, and physical ability to get to a toilet. Disruption of any of these factors can lead to fecal incontinence. The most common causes of fecal incontinence are problems with constipation and laxative use, unrecognized lactose intolerance, neurological disorders, and colorectal disorders (Table 8-19). Constipation is extremely common in the geriatric population and, when chronic, can lead to fecal impaction and incontinence. The hard stool (or scybalum) of fecal impaction irritates the rectum and results in the production of mucus and fluid. This fluid leaks around the mass of impacted stool and precipitates incontinence. Constipation technically indicates less than three bowel movements per week, although many patients use the term to describe difficult passage of hard stools or a feeling of incomplete evacuation. Poor dietary and toilet habits, immobility, and chronic laxative abuse are the most common causes of constipation in geriatric patients (Table 8-20).

Appropriate management of constipation will prevent fecal impaction and resultant fecal incontinence. The first step in managing constipation is the identification of all possible contributory factors. If the constipation is a new complaint and represents a recent change in bowel habit, then colonic disease, endocrine or metabolic disorders, depression, or drug side effects should be considered (see Table 8-19).

Proper diet, including adequate fluid intake and bulk, is important in preventing constipation. Crude fiber in amounts of 4 to 6 g/day (equivalent to 3 or

---

TABLE 8-19. Causes of Fecal Incontinence

Fecal impaction
Laxative overuse or abuse
Neurological disorders
    Dementia
    Stroke
    Spinal cord disease/injury
Colorectal disorders
    Diarrheal illnesses
    Lactose intolerance
    Diabetic autonomic neuropathy
    Rectal sphincter damage

TABLE 8-20. Causes of Constipation

Diet low in bulk and fluid
Poor toilet habits
Immobility
Laxative abuse
Colorectal disorders
    Colonic tumor, stricture, volvulus
    Painful anal and rectal conditions (hemorrhoids, fissures)
Depression
Drugs
    Anticholinergic
    Narcotic
Diabetic autonomic neuropathy
Endocrine or metabolic
    Hypothyroidism
    Hypercalcemia
    Hypokalemia

4 tablespoons of bran) is generally recommended. Improving mobility, positioning of body during toileting, and the timing and setting of toileting are all important in managing constipation.

Defecation should optimally take place in a private, unrushed atmosphere and should take advantage of the gastrocolic reflex, which occurs a few minutes after eating. These factors are often overlooked, especially in nursing home settings.

A variety of drugs can be used to treat constipation (Table 8-21). These drugs are often overused; in fact, their overuse may cause an atonic colon and contribute to chronic constipation ("cathartic colon").

Laxative drugs can also contribute to fecal incontinence. Rational use of these drugs necessitates knowing the nature of the constipation and quality of the stool. For example, stool softeners will not help a patient with a large mass of already soft stool in the rectum. These patients would benefit from glycerin or irritant suppositories. The use of osmotic and irritant laxatives should be limited to no more than three or four times a week.

Fecal incontinence from neurological disorders is sometimes amenable to pelvic floor muscle training, although most severely demented patients are unable to cooperate. For patients with end-stage dementia who fail to respond to a regular toileting program and suppositories, a program of alternating constipating agents (if necessary) and laxatives on a routine schedule (such as giving laxatives or enemas three times a week) is often effective in controlling defecation.

Experience suggests that these measures should permit management of even severely demented patients. As a last resort, specially designed incontinence undergarments are sometimes helpful in managing fecal incontinence and preventing complications.

TABLE 8-21. Drugs Used to Treat Constipation

Type	Examples	Mechanism of action
Stool softeners and lubricants	Dioctyl sodium succinate Mineral oil	Soften and lubricate fecal mass
Bulk-forming agents	Bran Psyllium mucilloid	Increase fecal bulk and retain fluid in bowel lumen
Osmotic cathartics	Milk of magnesia Magnesium sulfate/citrate Lactulose Polyethylene glycol Sorbitol	Poorly absorbed and retain fluid in bowel lumen; increase net secretions of fluid in small intestine
Stimulants and irritants	Cascara Senna Bisacodyl Phenolphthalein	Alter intestinal mucosal permeability; stimulate muscle activity and fluid secretions
Enemas	Tap water Saline Sodium phosphate Oil	Induce reflex evacuations
Suppositories	Glycerin Bisacodyl	Cause mucosal irritation
Chloride ion activator	Lubiprostone	Enhances intestinal secretion; used for chronic idiopathic constipation
Opioid antagonists	Methylnaltrexone	Reduces opioid-induced constipation

Frequent changing is essential, because fecal material, especially in the presence of incontinent urine, can cause skin irritation and predispose to pressure ulcers.

Evidence Summary

Do's

- Assess for correctable underlying causes of overactive bladder and incontinence by history and targeted physical examination.
- Manage constipation.
- Utilize education and simple behavioral interventions for all incontinent patients.
- Consider drug therapy for overactive bladder and/or urge continence in women (antimuscarinic or beta-3 agonist) and men (selective α-adrenergic blocker with or without an antimuscarinic or beta-3 agonist).
- Follow symptomatic response and satisfaction with treatment after a 4- to 6-week period to determine the need to adjust the treatment plan.

Don'ts

- Send all patients for specialist consultation or urodynamics.
- Automatically prescribe medication for all older patients with symptoms of overactive bladder and incontinence.
- Prescribe oral estrogen.

Consider

- Referring selected patients for further urological, gynecological, and/or urodynamic evaluation.
- A careful trial of pharmacological therapy for older patients with overactive bladder and urge incontinence who have functional and/or cognitive impairment by carefully weighing the potential for benefit on bothersome symptoms vs the potential cognitive side effects of anticholinergic agents.

REFERENCES

Albo ME, Richter HE, Brubaker L, et al. Burch colposuspension versus fascial sling to reduce urinary stress incontinence. *N Engl J Med.* 2007;356:2143-2155.

American Medical Directors Association. *Urinary Incontinence: Clinical Practice Guideline.* Columbia, MD: AMDA; 2006.

Burgio KL, Goode PS, Johnson TM, et al. Behavioral versus drug treatment for overactive bladder in men: the Male Overactive Bladder Treatment in Veterans (MOTIVE) Trial. *J Am Geriatr Soc.* 2011;59:2209-2216.

Burgio KL, Goode PS, Locher JL, et al. Behavioral training with and without biofeedback in the treatment of urge incontinence in older women. *JAMA.* 2002;288:2293-2299.

DuBeau CE, Kraus SR, Griebling TL, et al. Effect of fesoterodine in vulnerable elderly subjects with urgency incontinence: a double-blind, placebo-controlled trial. *J Urol.* 2013. doi:10.1016/j.juro.2013.08.027.

Elbadawi A, Yalla SV, Resnick N. Structural basis of geriatric voiding dysfunction: I. methods of a prospective ultrastructural/urodynamic study and an overview of the findings. *J Urol.* 1993;150:1650-1656.

Fung CH, Spencer B, Eslami M, et al. Quality indicators for the screening and care of urinary incontinence in vulnerable elders. *J Am Geriatr Soc.* 2007;55:S443-S449.

Hendrix SL, Cochrane BB, Nygaar IE, et al. Effects of estrogen with and without progestin on urinary incontinence. *JAMA.* 2005;293:935-948.

Kaplan SA, Roehrborn CG, Rovner ES, et al. Tolterodine and tamsulosin for treatment of men with lower urinary tract symptoms and overactive bladder. *JAMA.* 2006;296:2319-2328.

Nager CW, Brubaker L, Litman HJ, et al. A randomized trial of urodynamic testing before stress-incontinence surgery. *N Engl J Med.* 2012;366:1987-1997.

Ouslander JG. Management of overactive bladder. *N Engl J Med.* 2004;350:786-799.

Ouslander JG. Quality improvement initiatives for urinary incontinence in nursing homes. *J Am Med Dir Assoc.* 2007;8:S6-S11.

Ouslander JG, Schapira M, Schnelle J, et al. Does eradicating bacteriuria affect the severity of chronic urinary incontinence among nursing home residents? *Ann Intern Med.* 1995;122:749-754.

Ouslander JG, Uman GC, Urman HN. Development and testing of an incontinence monitoring record. *J Am Geriatr Soc.* 1986;34:83-90.

Resnick NM, Yalla SV. Detrusor hyperactivity with impaired contractile function: an unrecognized but common cause of incontinence in elderly patients. *JAMA.* 1987;257:3076-3081.

Shamliyan TA, Kane RL, Wyman J, Wilt TW. Systematic review: randomized, controlled trials of nonsurgical treatments for urinary incontinence in women. *Ann Intern Med.* 2008;148:459-473.

Shamliyan T, Wyman J, Bliss DZ, et al. *Prevention of Urinary and Fecal Incontinence in Adults.* Rockville, MD: Prepared by the Minnesota Evidence-Based Practice Center for the Agency for Healthcare Research and Quality under Contract No. 290-02-0009; Evidence Report/Technology Assessment No. 161, AHRQ Publication No. 08-E003. December 2007. www.ncbi.nlm.nih.gov/books/NBK38514/.

Shamliyan T, Wyman JF, Ramakrishnan R, Sainfort F, Kane RL. Benefits and harms of pharmacologic treatment for urinary incontinence in women: a systematic review. *Ann Intern Med.* 2012;156:861-874.

Taylor JA, Kuchel GA. Detrusor underactivity: clinical features and pathogenesis of an underdiagnosed geriatric condition. *J Am Geriatr Soc.* 2006;54:1920-1932.

Wald A. Fecal incontinence in adults. *N Engl J Med.* 2007;356:1648-1655.

SUGGESTED READINGS

Boudreau DM, Onchee Y, Gray SI, et al. Concomitant use of cholinesterase inhibitors and anticholinergics: prevalence and outcomes. *J Am Geriatr Soc.* 2011;59:2069-2076.

Brown JS, Vittinghoff E, Wyman JF, et al. Urinary incontinence: does it increase risk for falls and fractures? *J Am Geriatr Soc.* 2000;48:721-725.

DuBeau CE. Therapeutic/pharmacologic approaches to urinary incontinence in older adults. *Clin Pharmacol Ther.* 2009;85:98-102.

Fink HA, Taylor BC, Tacklind JW, Rutks IR, Wilt TJ. Treatment interventions in nursing home residents with urinary incontinence: a systematic review of randomized trials. *Mayo Clin Proc.* 2008;83:1332-1343.

Fleming V, Wade WW. Overview of laxative therapies for treatment of chronic constipation in older adults. *Am J Geriatr Phamacother.* 2010;8:514-550.

Forte ML, Andrade KE, Butler M, et al. Treatments for fecal incontinence. *Comparative Effectiveness Review* No. 165, AHRQ Publication No. 15(16)-EHC037-EF; March 2016.

Gibbs CF, Johnson TM II, Ouslander JG. Office management of geriatric urinary incontinence. *Am J Med.* 2007;120:211-220.

Hägglund D. A systematic literature review of incontinence care for persons with dementia: the research evidence. *J Clin Nurs.* 2010;19:303-312.

Kay GG, Abou-Donia MB, Messer WS, et al. Antimuscarinic drugs for overactive bladder and their potential effects on cognitive function in older patients. *J Am Geriatr Soc.* 2005;53:2195-2201.

Lembo A, Camilleri M. Chronic constipation. *N Engl J Med.* 2003;349:1360-1368.

Malmstrom TK, Andresen EM, Wolinsky FD, et al. Urinary and fecal incontinence and quality of life in African Americans. *J Am Geriatr Soc.* 2010;58:1941-1945.

Markland AD, Vaughan CP, Johnson TM, et al. Incontinence. *Med Clin North Am.* 2011;95:539-554.

Ouslander JG, Schnelle JF. Incontinence in the nursing home. *Ann Intern Med.* 1995;122:438-449.

Talley KM, Wyman JF, Shamliyan TA. State of the science: conservative interventions for urinary incontinence in frail community-dwelling older adults. *Nurs Outlook.* 2011;59:215-220.

Zarowitz BJ, Ouslander JG. The application of evidence-based principles of care in older persons (issue 6): urinary incontinence. *J Am Med Dir Assoc.* 2007;8:35-45.

SELECTED WEBSITES (ACCESSED 2017)

National Association for Continence, www.nafc.org/

Simon Foundation for Continence, www.simonfoundation.org/

CHAPTER 9

Falls

Falls are a major cause of morbidity and mortality in the geriatric population. Close to one-third of those aged 65 years and older living at home suffer a fall each year. Among nursing home residents, as many as half suffer a fall each year; 10% to 25% cause serious injuries. Accidents are the fourth leading cause of death in persons older than age 65, and falls account for two-thirds of these accidental deaths. Of deaths from falls in the United States, more than 70% occur in those older than age 65. Fear of falling can adversely affect older persons' functional status and overall quality of life. An injurious fall sets off a chain of events including emergency department care, hospitalization, surgical intervention, and prolonged immobility. Repeated falls and consequent injuries can be important factors in the decision to institutionalize an older person.

Table 9-1 lists potential complications of falls. Fractures of the hip, femur, humerus, wrist, and ribs and painful soft tissue injuries are the most frequent physical complications. Many of these injuries will result in hospitalization, with the attendant risks of immobilization and iatrogenic illnesses (see Chapter 10). Fractures of the hip and lower extremities often lead to prolonged disability because of impaired mobility. A less common, but important, injury is subdural hematoma. Neurological symptoms and signs that develop days to weeks after a fall should prompt consideration of this treatable problem.

Even when the fall does not result in serious injury, substantial disability may result from fear of falling, loss of self-confidence, and restricted ambulation (either self-imposed or imposed by caregivers).

Many studies suggest that some falls can be prevented. The potential for prevention, together with the use of falling as an indicator of underlying risk for disability make understanding the causes of falls and a practical approach to the evaluation and management of gait instability and fall risk important components of geriatric care. Like many other conditions in the geriatric population, multiple factors can contribute to or cause falls, and very often more than one of these factors play an important role in an individual fall (Fig. 9-1). Some of these factors are intrinsic to the individual, such as medical and neurological conditions, sensory impairment, and age-related changes in neuromuscular function, reflexes, and gait. Others are extrinsic to the individual, such as medications, improper footwear or use of assistive devices, and environmental hazards. Falls often result from the combination of extrinsic and intrinsic factors. The multifactorial nature of falls can make evaluation and prevention of future falls challenging.

AGING AND INSTABILITY

Several age-related factors can contribute to instability and falls (Table 9-2). Most "accidental" falls are caused by one or a combination of these factors interacting with environmental hazards.

TABLE 9-1. Complications of Falls in Older Patients

Injuries
    Painful soft tissue injuries
    Fractures
        Hip
        Femur
        Humerus
        Wrist
        Ribs
Subdural hematoma
Hospitalization
    Complications of immobilization (see Chap. 10)
    Risk of iatrogenic illnesses (see Chap. 5)
Disability
    Impaired mobility because of physical injury
    Impaired mobility from fear of falling, loss of self-confidence, and restriction of ambulation
Increased risk of institutionalization
Increased risk of death

Aging changes in postural control and gait can play a major role in many falls among older persons. Increasing age is associated with diminished proprioceptive input, slower righting reflexes, diminished strength of muscles important in maintaining posture, and increased postural sway. All of these changes can contribute to falls—especially the ability to avoid a fall after encountering an environmental hazard or an unexpected trip. Changes in gait also occur with increasing age. Although these changes may not be sufficient to be labeled truly pathologic, they can increase

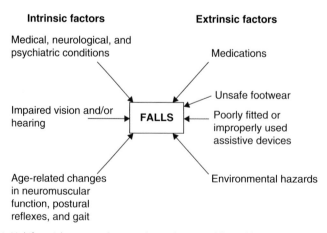

FIGURE 9-1 Multifactorial causes and potential contributors to falls in older persons.

TABLE 9-2. Age-Related Factors Contributing to Instability and Falls

Changes in postural control and blood pressure
    Decreased proprioception
    Slower righting reflexes
    Decreased muscle tone
    Increased postural sway
    Orthostatic hypotension
    Postprandial hypotension
Changes in gait
    Feet not picked up as high
    Men develop flexed posture and wide-based, short-stepped gait
    Women develop narrow-based, waddling gait
Increased prevalence of pathologic conditions predisposing to instability
    Degenerative joint disease in the neck, hips, knees, ankles, and feet
    Fractures of hip and femur
    Stroke with residual deficits
    Muscle weakness from disuse and deconditioning
    Peripheral neuropathy
    Diseases or deformities of the feet
    Impaired vision
    Impaired hearing
    Impaired cognition and judgment
    Other specific disease processes (eg, cardiovascular disease, parkinsonism—
    see Table 9-3)
Increased prevalence of conditions causing nocturia (eg, congestive heart failure,
    venous insufficiency)
Increased prevalence of dementia

susceptibility to falls. In general, older people do not pick up their feet as high, thus increasing the tendency to trip. Older men tend to develop wide-based, short-stepped gaits; older women often walk with a narrow-based, waddling gait. These gait changes have been associated with white matter changes in the brain on magnetic resonance imaging (MRI).

Orthostatic hypotension (defined as a drop in systolic blood pressure of 20 mm Hg or more when moving from a lying to a standing position) occurs in approximately 20% of older persons. This problem is especially common among people with significant comorbidity (eg, heart failure, diabetes) who are prescribed multiple antihypertensives and/or other drugs with hypotensive effects. Orthostatic hypotension may be difficult to detect because research has demonstrated that these changes can be very transient during the first few seconds after standing, or may occur as long as 3 to 5 minutes later. Although not all older individuals with orthostatic hypotension are symptomatic, this impaired physiological response could play a role in causing instability and precipitating falls. Older people can experience a postprandial fall in blood pressure as well. People with orthostatic and/or postprandial hypotension are at particular risk for near syncope and falls when treated with diuretics and antihypertensive drugs.

Several pathologic conditions that increase in prevalence with increasing age can contribute to instability and falling. Degenerative joint disease (especially of the neck, the lumbosacral spine, and the lower extremities) can cause pain, unstable joints, muscle weakness, and neurological disturbances that can contribute to falls. Healed fractures of the hip and femur can cause an abnormal and less steady gait. Residual muscle weakness or sensory deficits from a recent or remote stroke can also cause instability.

Muscle weakness as a result of disuse and deconditioning (caused by pain, bed rest during an acute illness, and/or lack of exercise) can contribute to an unsteady gait and impair the ability to right oneself after a loss of balance. Diminished sensory input, such as in diabetes and other peripheral neuropathies, visual disturbances, and impaired hearing decrease cues from the environment that normally contribute to stability and thus predispose to falls. Impaired cognitive function may result in the creation of, or wandering into, unsafe environments and may lead to falls. Podiatric problems (bunions, calluses, nail disease, joint deformities, etc) that cause pain, deformities, and alterations in gait are common, correctable causes of instability. Other specific disease processes common in older people (such as Parkinson disease and cardiovascular disorders) can cause instability and falls and are discussed later in the chapter.

CAUSES OF FALLS IN OLDER PERSONS

Table 9-3 outlines the multiple and often interacting causes of falls among older persons. They include a variety of intrinsic as well as extrinsic factors. More than half of all falls are related to medically diagnosed conditions, emphasizing the importance of a careful medical assessment for patients who fall (see below). Several studies have found a variety of risk factors for falls, including cognitive impairment, impaired lower extremity strength or function, gait and balance abnormalities, visual impairment or use of bifocals, nocturia, alcohol use, and the number and nature of medications being taken. Frequently overlooked, environmental factors can increase susceptibility to falls and other accidents. Homes of older people are often full of environmental hazards (Table 9-4). Unstable furniture, rickety stairs with inadequate railings, throw rugs and frayed carpets, steps that may not be obvious, and poor lighting should be identified on home visits. Several factors are associated with falls among older nursing home residents (Table 9-5). Awareness of these factors can help prevent morbidity and mortality in these settings.

Several factors can hinder precise identification of the specific causes for falls. These factors include lack of witnesses, inability of the older person to recall the circumstances surrounding the event, the transient nature of several causes (eg, arrhythmia, transient ischemic attack [TIA], postural hypotension), and the fact that the majority of older people who fall do not seek medical attention.

Close to half of all falls can be classified as accidental (often referred to as "mechanical"). Usually an accidental trip or a slip can be precipitated by an environmental

TABLE 9-3. Causes of Falls

Accidents (often referred to as "mechanical" falls)
   True accidents (trips, slips, etc)
   Interactions between environmental hazards and factors increasing susceptibility
   (see Table 9-2) and/or other conditions listed below
Syncope (sudden loss of consciousness)
Drop attacks (sudden leg weaknesses without loss of consciousness)
Dizziness and/or vertigo
   Vestibular disease
   Central nervous system disease
Orthostatic hypotension
   Hypovolemia or low cardiac output
   Autonomic dysfunction
   Impaired venous return
   Prolonged bed rest
   Drug-induced hypotension
   Postprandial hypotension
Drug-related causes
   Antihypertensives
   Antidepressants
   Antiparkinsonian
   Diuretics
   Sedatives
   Antipsychotics
   Hypoglycemics
   Alcohol
Specific disease processes
   Acute illness of any kind
   Cardiovascular
      Arrhythmias
      Valvular heart disease (aortic stenosis)
      Carotid sinus hypersensitivity
   Neurological causes
   Transient ischemic attack (TIA)
   Stroke (acute)
   Seizure disorder
   Parkinson disease
   Cervical or lumbar spondylosis (with spinal cord or nerve root compression)
   Cerebellar disease
   Normal-pressure hydrocephalus (gait disorder, incontinence, cognitive impairment)
   Central nervous system lesions (eg, tumor, subdural hematoma)
Urinary
   Overactive bladder
   Urge incontinence
   Nocturia

PART II

TABLE 9-4. Common Environmental Hazards

Old, unstable, and low-lying furniture
Beds and toilets of inappropriate height
Unavailability of grab bars
Uneven or poorly demarcated stairs and inadequate railing
Throw rugs, frayed carpets, cords, wires
Slippery floors and bathtubs
Inadequate lighting, glare
Cracked and uneven sidewalks
Pets that get under foot

hazard, often in conjunction with factors listed in Table 9-2. For example, tripping on the edge of a rug may be related to muscle weakness and poor elevation/dorsiflexion of the feet while walking. Thus, even if an older patient presents with what sounds like an accidental fall, assessment should include searching for factors that could make the individual more susceptible to environmental hazards. Addressing the environmental hazards begins with a careful assessment of the environment. Some older persons have developed a strong attachment to their cluttered surroundings and may need active encouragement to make the necessary changes, but many may simply take such environmental risks for granted until they are specifically identified.

Syncope, "drop attacks," and "dizziness" are commonly cited causes of falls in older persons. If there is a clear history of loss of consciousness, a cause for true syncope should be sought. Although the complete differential diagnosis of syncope is beyond the scope of this chapter, some of the more common causes of syncope in older people include vasovagal responses, carotid sinus hypersensitivity, cardiovascular disorders (eg, bradycardia, tachyarrhythmias, aortic stenosis), acute neurological events (eg, TIA, stroke, seizure), pulmonary embolus, and metabolic disturbances

TABLE 9-5. Factors Associated With Falls Among Older Nursing Home Residents

Recent admission
Dementia
Hip flexor muscle weakness
Certain activities (toileting, getting out of bed)
Psychotropic drugs causing daytime sedation
Cardiovascular medications (vasodilators, antihypertensives, diuretics)
Polypharmacy
Low staff–patient ratio
Unsupervised activities
Unsafe furniture
Slippery floors

(eg, hypoxia, hypoglycemia). A precise cause for syncope may remain unidentified in 40% to 60% of older patients.

Drop attacks, described as sudden leg weakness causing a fall without loss of consciousness, are often attributed to vertebrobasilar insufficiency and often precipitated by a change in head position. Only a small proportion of older people who fall have truly had a drop attack; the underlying pathophysiology is poorly understood, and care should be taken to rule out other causes.

Dizziness and unsteadiness are common complaints among older people who fall (as well as those who do not). A feeling of light-headedness can be associated with several different disorders but is a nonspecific symptom and should be interpreted with caution. Patients complaining of light-headedness should be carefully evaluated for postural hypotension and intravascular volume depletion.

Vertigo (a sensation of rotational movement), on the other hand, is a more specific symptom and is probably an uncommon precipitant of falls in older persons. It is most commonly associated with disorders of the inner ear, such as acute labyrinthitis, Ménière's disease, and benign positional vertigo. Vertebrobasilar ischemia and infarction and cerebellar infarction can also cause vertigo. Patients with vertigo caused by organic disorders often have nystagmus, which can be observed by having the patient quickly lie down and turning the patient's head to the side in one motion. Many older patients with symptoms of dizziness and unsteadiness are anxious, depressed, and chronically afraid of falling, and the evaluation of their symptoms is quite difficult. Some patients, especially those with symptoms suggestive of vertigo, will benefit from a thorough otological examination including auditory testing, which may help clarify the symptoms and differentiate inner ear from central nervous system (CNS) involvement.

Orthostatic hypotension is best detected by taking the blood pressure and pulse rate in supine position, after 1 minute in the sitting position, and after 1 and 3 minutes in the standing position, though transient drops in blood pressure before 1 minute do occur. A drop of more than 20 mm Hg in systolic blood pressure is generally considered to represent significant orthostatic hypotension. In many instances, this condition is asymptomatic; however, several conditions can cause orthostatic hypotension or worsen it enough to precipitate a fall. These conditions include low cardiac output from heart failure or hypovolemia, overtreatment with cardiovascular medications, autonomic dysfunction (which can result from diabetes or Parkinson disease), impaired venous return (eg, venous insufficiency), and prolonged bed rest with deconditioning of muscles and reflexes. Simply eating a full meal can precipitate a reduction in blood pressure in an older person that may be worsened when the person stands up and lead to a fall.

Drugs that should be suspected of playing a role in falls include diuretics (hypovolemia), antihypertensives and alpha blockers used for urinary symptoms (bradycardia and/or hypotension), cholinesterase inhibitors (bradycardia), antidepressants (postural hypotension), sedatives (excessive sedation), antipsychotics (sedation, muscle rigidity, postural hypotension), hypoglycemics (acute hypoglycemia), and alcohol (intoxication). Combinations of these drug types may greatly increase the risk of a fall. Many older patients are on a diuretic and one or two other antihypertensives, with consequent hypotension or postural hypotension that may precipitate a fall. Psychotropic drugs are commonly prescribed and substantially increase the risk of falls and hip fractures, especially in patients concomitantly prescribed antidepressants.

Many disease processes, especially of the cardiovascular and neurological systems, are associated with falls. Cardiac arrhythmias are common in ambulatory older persons and may be difficult to associate directly with a fall or syncope. In general, cardiac monitoring should document a temporal association between a specific arrhythmia and symptoms (or a fall) before the arrhythmia is diagnosed (and treated) as the cause of a fall.

Syncope is a symptom of aortic stenosis and is an indication to evaluate a patient suspected of having significant aortic stenosis for valve replacement. Aortic stenosis is difficult to diagnose by physical examination alone; all patients suspected of having this condition should have an echocardiogram.

Some older individuals have sensitive carotid baroreceptors and are susceptible to syncope resulting from reflex increase in vagal tone (caused by cough, straining at stool, micturition, etc), which leads to bradycardia and hypotension.

Cerebrovascular disease is often implicated as a cause or contributing factor for falls in older patients. Acute strokes (caused by thrombosis, hemorrhage, or embolus) can cause, and may initially manifest themselves in, falls. TIAs of both the anterior and posterior circulations frequently last only minutes and are often poorly described. Thus, care must be taken in making these diagnoses. Anterior circulation TIAs may cause unilateral weakness and thus precipitate a fall. Vertebrobasilar (posterior circulation) TIAs may cause vertigo, but a history of transient vertigo alone is not a sufficient basis for the diagnosis of TIA. The diagnosis of posterior circulation TIA necessitates that one or more other symptoms (visual field cuts, dysarthria, ataxia, or limb weakness, which can be bilateral) are associated with vertigo. Vertebrobasilar insufficiency, as mentioned earlier, is often cited as a cause of drop attacks; in addition, mechanical compression of the vertebral arteries by osteophytes of the cervical spine when the head is turned has also been proposed as a cause of unsteadiness and falling. Both of these conditions are poorly documented, are probably overdiagnosed, and should not be used as causes of a fall simply because nothing else can be found.

Other diseases of the brain and CNS can also cause falls. Parkinson's disease and normal-pressure hydrocephalus can cause disturbances of gait, which lead to instability and falls. Normal pressure hydrocephalus should be suspected when there is a progressive gait disorder without an obvious cause; urinary incontinence and cognitive impairment may also be present. Cerebellar disorders, intracranial tumors, and subdural hematomas can cause unsteadiness, with a tendency to fall. A slowly progressive gait disability with a tendency to fall, especially in the presence of spasticity or hyperactive reflexes in the lower extremities, should prompt consideration of cervical spondylosis and spinal cord compression. It is especially important to consider these diagnoses because treatment may improve the condition before permanent disability ensues.

Urinary tract disorders including overactive bladder, urgency incontinence, and nocturia are also associated with falling. Urinary urgency may cause a distraction, similar to the "dual-tasking" and thereby predispose to falls. Awakening at night to void, especially among people who have taken hypnotics or other psychotropic drugs, may substantially increase the risk of falls.

Despite this long list, the precise causes of many falls will remain unknown, even after a thorough evaluation. The ultimate test of the etiology for falls is its reversibility. As noted earlier in the text, we are often better at finding putative causes of geriatric conditions than in correcting them.

EVALUATING THE OLDER PATIENT WHO FALLS

Quality indicators for the identification, evaluation, and management of vulnerable older people with falls and mobility problems have been published as a component of the Assessing Care of Vulnerable Elders (ACOVE) project (Chang and Ganz, 2007). Older patients who report a fall (or recurrent falls) that is not clearly the result of an accidental trip or slip should be carefully evaluated, even if the fall has not resulted in serious physical injury. A jointly developed set of recommendations for assessing people who fall has been issued by the American Geriatrics Society, the British Geriatrics Society, and the American Academy of Orthopaedic Surgeons (Panel on Prevention of Falls in Older Persons, 2011). A thorough fall evaluation consists of a focused history, targeted physical examination, gait and balance assessment, and, in certain instances, selected laboratory studies.

The history should focus on the general medical history and medications; the patient's thoughts about what caused the fall; the circumstances surrounding it, including ingestion of a meal and/or medications; any premonitory or associated symptoms (such as palpitations caused by a transient arrhythmia or focal neurological symptoms caused by a TIA); and whether there was loss of consciousness or signs of a seizure (Table 9-6). A history of loss of consciousness after the fall (which is often difficult to document) is important and should raise the suspicion of a cardiac event (transient arrhythmia or heart block) that caused syncope or near-syncope or a seizure (especially if there has been incontinence). Falls are often unwitnessed, and older patients may not recall any details of the circumstances surrounding the event. Detailed questioning can sometimes lead to identification of environmental factors that may have played a role in the fall and to symptoms that may lead to a specific diagnosis. Many older patients will not be able to give details about an unwitnessed fall and will simply report, "I just fell down; I don't know what happened." The head, skin, extremities, and painful soft tissue areas should be assessed to detect any injury that may have resulted from a fall.

Several other aspects of the physical examination can be helpful in determining the cause(s) (Table 9-7). Because a fall can herald the onset of a variety of acute illnesses, careful attention should be given to vital signs. Fever, tachypnea, tachycardia, and hypotension should prompt a search for an acute illness (such as pneumonia or sepsis, myocardial infarction, pulmonary embolus, or gastrointestinal bleeding).

TABLE 9-6. Evaluating the Older Patient Who Falls: Key Points in the History

General medical history
History of previous falls
Medications (especially antihypertensive and psychotropic agents)
Patient's thoughts on the cause of the fall
    Was patient aware of impending fall?
    Was it totally unexpected?
    Did patient trip or slip?
Circumstances surrounding the fall
    Location and time of day
    Activity
    Situation: alone or not alone at the time of the fall
    Witnesses
    Relationship to changes in posture, turning of head, cough, urination, a meal,
      medication intake
Premonitory or associated symptoms
    Light-headedness, dizziness, vertigo
    Palpitations, chest pain, shortness of breath
    Sudden focal neurological symptoms (weakness, sensory disturbance, dysarthria,
      ataxia, confusion, aphasia)
    Symptoms of a seizure (witnessed clinic movements; incontinence of urine or stool;
      tongue biting)
Loss of consciousness
    What is remembered immediately after the fall?
    Could the patient get up, and if so, how long did it take?
    Can loss of consciousness be verified by a witness?

Postural blood pressure and pulse determinations are critical in the diagnosis and management of falls in older patients. Hypotension may be a sign of dehydration, acute blood loss (occult gastrointestinal bleeding), or a drug side effect (especially with cardiovascular medications and antidepressants). Visual acuity should be assessed for any possible uncorrected vision impairment that may have contributed to instability and falls. Use of bifocals has also been associated with falling. The cardiovascular examination should focus on the presence of arrhythmias (many of which are easily missed during a brief examination) and signs of aortic stenosis. Because both of these conditions are potentially serious and treatable, yet difficult to diagnose by physical examination, the patient should be referred for continuous monitoring and echocardiography if they are suspected. If the history suggests carotid sinus sensitivity, the carotid can be gently massaged for 5 seconds to observe whether this precipitates a profound bradycardia (50% reduction in heart rate) or a long pause (2 seconds). This must be done cautiously and should be performed only when a "crash cart" is readily available. The extremities should be examined for

TABLE 9-7. Evaluating the Older Patient Who Falls: Key Aspects of the Physical Examination

Vital signs
   Fever, hypothermia
   Respiratory rate
   Pulse and blood pressure (including orthostatic measurements)
Skin
   Turgor for hydration (over the chest; other areas unreliable)
   Pallor
   Trauma
Eyes
   Visual acuity; use of bifocals
Neck
   Range of motion (to detect possible cervical arthritis)
Cardiovascular
   Arrhythmias
   Carotid bruits
   Signs of aortic stenosis
   Carotid sinus sensitivity
Extremities
   Degenerative joint disease
   Range of motion
   Deformities
   Fractures
   Podiatric problems (calluses; bunions; ulcerations; poorly fitted, inappropriate, or worn-out shoes)
Neurological
   Mental status
   Focal signs
   Muscles (weakness, rigidity, spasticity)
   Peripheral innervation (especially position sense)
   Cerebellar (especially heel-to-shin testing)
   Resting tremor, bradykinesia, other involuntary movements
   Observation of gait and balance
     Get up and go test (Table 9-8)
Evaluation of assistive devices for hazards, such as missing tips on canes and walkers, impaired locking devices, or broken footrests and correct sizing of wheelchairs

evidence of deformities, limits to range of motion, or active inflammation that might underlie instability and cause a fall.

Special attention should be given to the feet because of deformities; painful lesions (calluses, bunions, ulcers); and poorly fitting, inappropriate, or worn-out shoes which are common and can contribute to instability and falls.

Neurological examination is also an important aspect of this assessment. Mental status should be assessed (see Chapter 6), with a careful search for focal neurological signs. Evidence of muscle weakness, rigidity, or spasticity should be noted, and signs of peripheral neuropathy (especially posterior column signs such as loss of position or vibratory sensation) should be ruled out. Abnormalities in cerebellar function (especially heel-to-shin testing and heel tapping) and signs of Parkinson disease (such as resting tremor, muscle rigidity, and bradykinesia) should be sought.

Gait and balance assessments are critical components of the examination and are probably more useful in identifying remediable problems than is the standard neuromuscular examination. Although sophisticated techniques have been developed to assess gait and balance, careful observation of a series of maneuvers is the most practical and useful assessment technique. The "get up and go" test and other practical performance-based balance and gait assessments have been developed (Table 9-8). While timing of this test has been used in research, timing in clinical practice is not essential and may distract the observer from careful assessment of gait and balance. Abnormalities on this assessment may be helpful in identifying patients who are likely to fall again and potentially remediable problems that might prevent future falls.

There is no specific laboratory workup for an older patient who falls. Laboratory studies should be ordered based on information gleaned from the history and physical examination. If the cause of the fall is obvious (such as a slip or a trip) and no suspicious symptoms or signs are detected, laboratory studies are unwarranted. If the history or physical examination (especially vital signs) suggests an acute illness, appropriate laboratory studies (eg, complete blood count, electrolytes, blood urea nitrogen, chest film, electrocardiogram) should be ordered. Because some evidence suggests that vitamin D may be helpful in fall management, evaluating patients who fall recurrently for vitamin D deficiency is appropriate. If a transient arrhythmia or heart block is suspected, ambulatory electrocardiographic monitoring should be done. Although the sensitivity and specificity of cardiac monitoring for determining the cause of falls are unknown, and many older people have asymptomatic ectopy, cardiac abnormalities detected on continuous monitoring that are clearly related to symptoms should be treated.

Because it is difficult to diagnose aortic stenosis on physical examination, echocardiography should be considered in all patients with suggestive histories and a systolic heart murmur or those who have a delay in the carotid upstroke (which may be falsely negative in older people with atherosclerosis). If the history suggests anterior circulation TIA, noninvasive vascular studies should be considered to rule out treatable vascular lesions. Computed tomography (CT) scans or MRI scans should be reserved for patients in whom there is a high suspicion of sudural hematoma or other intracranial lesion or seizure disorder. While it is a very common practice to perform these tests routinely in older patients who fall when they come to an emergency department to exclude occult injury or intracranial pathology, they are not warranted unless the history or physical exam suggests they are necessary.

TABLE 9-8. Example of a Performance-Based Assessment of Gait and Balance (Get Up and Go)

Maneuver	Normal	Adaptive	Abnormal
Sitting balance	Steady, stable	Holds onto chair to keep upright	Leans, slides down in chair
Arising from chair	Able to arise in a single movement without using arms	Uses arms (on chair or walking aid) to pull or push up and/or moves forward in chair before attempting to rise	Multiple attempts required or unable without human assistance
Immediate standing balance (first 3–5 s)	Steady without holding onto walking aid or other object for support	Steady, but uses walking aid or support grabbing objects for support	Any sign of unsteadiness (eg, other object for staggering, more than minimal trunk sway)
Standing balance	Steady, able to stand with feet together without holding onto an object for support	Steady, but cannot put feet together	
Balance with eyes closed (Romberg test)	Steady without holding onto any object with feet together	Steady with feet apart	Any sign of unsteadiness or needs to hold onto an object
Nudge on sternum (patient standing with eyes closed; examiner pushes with light, even pressure over sternum three times; reflects ability to withstand displacement)	Steady, able to withstand pressure	Needs to move feet, but able to maintain balance	Begins to fall, or examiner has to help maintain balance
Walking (usual pace with assistive device if used)	Stable, smooth gait	Use of cane, walker, holding onto furniture	Decreased step height and/or step length; unsteadiness or staggering gait

(continued)

PART II

TABLE 9-8. Example of a Performance-Based Assessment of Gait and Balance (Get Up and Go) (continued)

Maneuver	Normal	Adaptive	Abnormal
Turning balance (360°)	No grabbing or staggering; no need to hold onto any objects; steps are continuous (turn is a flowing movement)	Steps are discontinuous (patient puts one foot completely on floor before raising other foot)	Any sign of unsteadiness or holds onto an object; more than four steps to turn 360°
Neck turning (patient asked to turn head side to side and look up while standing with feet as close together as possible)	Able to turn head at least halfway side to side and able to bend head back to look at ceiling; no staggering, grabbing, or symptoms of light-headedness, unsteadiness, or pain	Decreased ability to turn side to side to extend neck, but no staggering, grabbing, or symptoms of light-headedness, unsteadiness, or pain	Any sign of unsteadiness or symptoms when turning head or extending neck
Back extension (ask patient to lean back as far as possible, without holding onto object if possible)	Good extension without holding object or staggering	Tries to extend, but range of motion is decreased or needs to hold object to attempt extension	Will not attempt, no extension seen, or staggers
Reaching up (have patient attempt to remove an object from a shelf high enough to necessitate stretching or standing on toes)	Able to take down object without needing to hold onto other object for support and without becoming unsteady	Able to get object but needs to steady self by holding onto something for support	Unable or unsteady
Bending down (patient is asked to pick up small objects, such as pen, from the floor)	Able to bend down and pick up the object and able to get up easily in single attempt without needing to pull self up with arms	Able to get object and get upright in single attempt but needs to pull self up with arms or hold onto something for support	Unable to bend down or unable to get upright after bending down or takes multiple attempts to upright self
Sitting down	Able to sit down in one smooth movement	Needs to use arms to guide self into chair or not a smooth movement	Falls into chair, misjudges distances (lands off center)

MANAGEMENT

Table 9-9 outlines the basic principles of managing older patients with instability and a history of falls. Assessment and treatment of physical injury should not be overlooked because it may be helpful in preventing recurrent falls. The American Geriatrics Society has updated its clinical practice guideline on falls (Panel on Prevention of Falls in Older Persons, 2011), and several meta-analyses have documented the effectiveness of a variety of interventions, including multicomponent programs, exercise, tai chi, and vitamin D (Bischoff-Ferrari et al, 2009; Bischoff-Ferrari et al, 2012; Cameron et al, 2012; Coussement et al, 2007; Gillespie et al, 2012; Kalyani et al, 2010; Kendrick et al, 2014; Leung et al, 2011; Robertson and Gillespie, 2013; Sherrington et al, 2011). Vitamin D in high doses such as 60,000 IU per month in a single oral dose have been associated with an increased risk of falls in older people (Bischoff-Ferrari et al, 2016). In addition, one randomized trial of exercise and Vitamin D (800 IU/day) in older women did not show a significant effect of vitamin D (Uusi-Rasi et al, 2015). Thus, the optimal role of vitamin D in fall management in older people remains uncertain.

When specific conditions are identified by history, physical examination, and laboratory studies, they should be treated in order to minimize the risk of subsequent falls, morbidity, and mortality. Table 9-10 lists examples of treatments for some of the more common conditions. This table is meant only as a general outline; most of these topics are discussed in detail in general textbooks of medicine. Because the cause of a fall in an older person is often multifactorial, multicomponent interventions are often necessary to reduce fall risk.

Physical and occupational therapy and patient education are important aspects of the management. Gait training, muscle strengthening, the use of assistive devices,

PART II

TABLE 9-9. Principles of Management for Older Patients With Complaints of Instability and/or Falls

Assess and treat physical injury
Treat underlying conditions (Table 9-10)
Prevent future falls
Provide physical and occupational therapy and education
   Gait and balance retraining (including tai chi where available)
   Muscle strengthening
   Aids to ambulation
   Properly fitted shoes
   Adaptive behaviors
Alter the environment
   Safe and proper-size furniture
   Elimination of obstacles (loose rugs, etc)
   Proper lighting
   Rails (stairs, bathroom)

TABLE 9-10. Examples of Treatment for Underlying Causes of Falls

Condition and cause	Potential treatment
Cardiovascular	
Tachyarrhythmias	Antiarrhythmics[*]
Bradyarrhythmias	Pacemaker[*]
Aortic stenosis	Valve surgery (for syncope) if indicated
Postural hypotension	
Drug-related	Elimination of drugs(s) that may contribute
Intravascular volume depletion	Rehydrate as appropriate
With venous insufficiency	Evaluate for blood loss if indicated
	Support stockings
	Leg elevation
	Adaptive behaviors
Neurologic	
Autonomic dysfunction or idiopathic	Support stockings
	Mineralocorticoids
	Midodrine
	Droxidopa
	Adaptive behaviors (eg, pausing and getting up slowly)
TIA	Aspirin and/or surgery[†]
Cervical spondylosis (with spinal cord compression)	Physical and occupational therapy
	Neck brace
	Surgery
Parkinson disease	Antiparkinsonian drugs
Visual impairment	Ophthalmological evaluation and specific treatment
Seizure disorder	Anticonvulsants
Normal-pressure hydrocephalus	Surgery (ventricular-peritoneal shunt)
Dementia	Supervised activities
	Hazard-free environment
Benign positional vertigo	Habituation exercises
	Anti-vertiginous medication
Others	
Foot disorders	Podiatric evaluation and treatment
Gait and balance disorders (miscellaneous)	Properly fitted shoes
	Physical therapy
	Exercise with balance training (including tai chi where available)
Muscle weakness, deconditioning	Lower extremity strength training

(continued)

TABLE 9-10. Examples of Treatment for Underlying Causes of Falls (*continued*)

Condition and cause	Potential treatment
Drug overuse (eg, sedatives, alcohol, other psychotropic drugs, antihypertensives)	Elimination of drug(s)
Vitamin D deficiency	Vitamin D supplementation
Recurrent falls in high-risk patients	Consider hip protectors

TIA, transient ischemic attack.
*These treatments may be indicated only if the cardiac disturbance is clearly related to symptoms.
†Risk–benefit ratio must be carefully assessed.

PART II

and adaptive behaviors (such as rising slowly, using rails or furniture for balance, and techniques of getting up after a fall) are all helpful in preventing subsequent morbidity from instability and falls.

Environmental manipulations can be critical in preventing further falls in individual patients. The environments of older individuals are often unsafe (see Table 9-4), and appropriate interventions can often be instituted to improve safety (see Table 9-10). Physical restraints (eg, vests, belts, mittens, geri-chairs) have been used in institutional settings for those individuals felt to be at high risk of falling. However, research has demonstrated no benefit or increased risk with restraints. Federal nursing home regulations and quality improvement initiatives have led to dramatically reduced use of these devices in many institutional settings; most nursing homes now aspire to be restraint free. Multifaceted interventions for fall prevention in long-term care settings have been designed and tested, but the results of these trials have been mixed (Vlayen et al, 2015).

For older patients who are at high risk for falls and hip fractures, the use of hip protectors should be considered. Clinical trials and meta-analyses have not shown definitive evidence that hip protectors reduce morbidity in a population of fallers (Honkanen et al, 2006; Kannus et al, 2000; Kiel et al, 2007; Parker et al, 2003; Sawka et al, 2007). However, in individual high-risk patients who will wear them, hip protectors may be a simple and relatively inexpensive preventive intervention to consider.

Evidence Summary

Do's

- Distinguish between falls, syncope, and seizure.
- Distinguish between "dizziness" and true vertigo.
- Assess for correctable underlying causes of falls by history and targeted physical examination.
- Pay particular attention to:
  - Uncorrected vision impairment and use of bifocals
  - Postural vital signs

- Antihypertensive medications and others that can cause hypotension
- Psychotropic medications
- Gait and balance abnormalities
- Inappropriate footwear
- Incorrect use of canes and other assistive devices
- Environmental hazards
- A simple "get up and go" test on all patients who have fallen
- Ensure safety in recurrent fallers by urgent intervention(s) to prevent injury.
- Refer patients to rehabilitation therapists (physical and occupational) whenever appropriate for detailed environmental and safety assessments, strengthening, and proper prescription and use of assistive devices.
- Consider prescribing vitamin D in doses of at least 800 IU per day, but not in very high doses (see below under Don'ts).

Don'ts

- Send all patients for extensive diagnostic studies or cardiac monitoring.
- Overtreat hypertension.
- Prescribe very high doses of vitamin D (eg, 60,000 IU per month in a single oral dose).

Consider

- Referring selected patients for tai chi if they have balance problems and classes are available.
- Recommending hip protectors in carefully selected patients who are at high risk for fracture and who are recurrently falling.

REFERENCES

Bischoff-Ferrari HA, Dawson-Hughes B, Orav EJ, et al. Monthly high-dose vitamin D treatment for the prevention of functional decline: a randomized clinical trial. *JAMA Int Med.* 2016;176:175-183.

Bischoff-Ferrari HA, Willett WC, Orav EJ, et al. A pooled analysis of vitamin D dose requirements for fracture prevention. *N Engl J Med.* 2012;367:40-49.

Bischoff-Ferrari HA, Willett WC, Wong JB, et al. Prevention of nonvertebral fractures with oral vitamin D and dose dependency: a meta-analysis of randomized controlled trials. *Arch Intern Med.* 2009;169:551-561.

Cameron ID, Gillespie LD, Robertson MC, et al. Interventions for preventing falls in older people in care facilities and hospitals. *Cochrane Database Syst Rev.* 2012;(12):CD005465. doi:10.1002/14651858.CD005465.pub3.

Chang JT, Ganz D. Quality indicators for falls and mobility problems in vulnerable elders. *J Am Geriatr Soc.* 2007;55:S327-S334.

Coussement J, De Paepe L, Schwendimann R, et al. Interventions for preventing falls in acute- and chronic-care hospitals: a systematic review and meta-analysis. *J Am Geriatr Soc.* 2007;56:29-36.

Gillespie LD, Robertson MC, Gillespie WJ, et al. Interventions for preventing falls in older people living in the community. *Cochrane Database Syst Rev.* 2012;(9):CD007146. doi:10.1002/14651858.CD007146.pub3.

Honkanen LA, Mushlin AI, Lachs M, et al. Can hip protector use cost-effectively prevent fractures in community-dwelling geriatric populations? *J Am Geriatr Soc.* 2006;54:1658-1665.

Kannus P, Parkkari J, Niemi S, et al. Prevention of hip fracture in elderly people with use of a hip protector. *N Engl J Med.* 2000;343:1506-1513.

Kalyani RR, Stein B, Valiyil R, et al. Vitamin D treatment for the prevention of falls in older adults: systematic review and meta-analysis. *J Am Geriatr Soc.* 2010;58:1299-1310.

Kendrick D, Kumar A, Carpenter H, et al. Exercise for reducing fear of falling in older people living in the community. *Cochrane Database Syst Rev.* 2014;(11):CD009848. doi:10.1002/14651858.CD009848.pub2.

Kiel DP, Magaziner J, Zimmerman S, et al. Efficacy of a hip protector to prevent hip fracture in nursing home residents: the HIP PRO randomized controlled trial. *JAMA.* 2007;298:413-422.

Leung DP, Chan CK, et al. Tai chi as an intervention to improve balance and reduce falls in older adults: a systematic and meta-analytical review. *Altern Ther Health Med.* 2011;17:40-48.

Parker MJ, Gillespie LD, Gillespie WJ. Hip protectors for preventing hip fractures in the elderly. *Cochrane Database Syst Rev.* 2003;(3):CD001255.

Panel on Prevention of Falls in Older Persons; American Geriatrics Society; British Geriatrics Society. Summary of the updated American Geriatrics Society/British Geriatrics Society clinical practice guideline for prevention of falls in older persons. *J Am Geriatr Soc.* 2011;59:148-157.

Robertson MC, Gillespie LD. Fall prevention in community-dwelling older adults. *JAMA.* 2013;1406-1407.

Sawka AM, Boulos P, Beattie K, et al. Hip protectors decrease hip fracture risk in elderly nursing home residents: a Bayesian meta-analysis. *J Clin Epidemiol.* 2007;60:336-344.

Sherrington C, Tiedemann A, Fairhall N, et al. Exercise to prevent falls in older adults: an updated meta-analysis and best practice recommendations. *N S W Public Health Bull.* 2011;22:78-83.

Uusi-Rasi K, Patil R, Karinkanta S, et al. Exercise and vitamin D in fall prevention: a randomized clinical trial. *JAMA Int Med.* 2015;175:703-711.

Vlayen E, Coussement J, Geysens G, et al. Characteristics and effectiveness of fall prevention programs in nursing homes: a systematic review and meta-analysis of randomized controlled trials. *J Am Geriatr Soc.* 2015;63:211-221.

SUGGESTED READINGS

Agency for Healthcare Research and Quality. Preventing falls in hospitals. www.ahrq.gov/professionals/systems/hospital/fallpxtoolkit/index.html. Accessed October 1, 2016.

Centers for Disease Control and Prevention. Preventing falls: a guide to implementing effective community-based fall prevention programs. www.cdc.gov/homeandrecreationalsafety/falls/community_preventfalls.html. Accessed October 1, 2016.

Taylor JA, Parmelee P, Brown H, et al. The Fall Management Program: a quality improvement initiative for nursing facilities. 2005. http://joataylor.com/resources. Accessed September 25, 2016.

Tinetti ME, Kumar C. The patient who falls. *JAMA.* 2010;303:258-266.

CHAPTER 10

Immobility

Although mobility can be achieved by using various devices, the discussion here emphasizes walking. Immobility implies a limitation in independent, purposeful physical movement of the body or of one or more lower extremities. Immobility may result from physical decline, but it can also trigger a series of subsequent diseases and problems in older individuals that produce further pain, disability, and impaired quality of life. Optimizing mobility should be the goal of all members of the healthcare team working with older adults. Small improvements in mobility can decrease the incidence and severity of complications, improve the patient's well-being, and decrease the cost and burden of caregiving. This chapter outlines the common causes and complications of immobility and reviews the principles of management for some of the more common conditions associated with immobility in the older population.

CAUSES

Immobility can be caused by a wide variety of factors. The causes of immobility can be divided into intrapersonal factors including psychological factors (eg, depression, fear of falling or getting hurt, motivation); physical changes (cardiovascular, neurological, and musculoskeletal disorders, and associated pain); interpersonal factors and the interactions older adults have with caregivers; environmental causes such as access to open, uncluttered areas for walking and policy that either facilitate or decrease opportunities to maintain mobility. Additional examples of the many factors that influence immobility are provided in Table 10-1.

The prevalence of osteoarthritis is high in older adults, although symptoms of disease may not manifest in all individuals who have radiographic changes (Allena and Golightlya, 2015). The pain and musculoskeletal changes associated with osteoarthritis can result in contractures and progressive immobility if not appropriately treated. In addition, podiatric problems associated with degenerative changes in the feet (eg, bunions and hammertoes) can likewise cause pain and contractures. These changes can result in painful ambulation and a subsequent decrease in the older individual's willingness and ability to ambulate. Patients who have had a stroke resulting in partial or complete hemiparesis/paralysis, spinal cord injury resulting in paraplegia or quadriplegia, fracture or musculoskeletal disorder limiting function, or exposure to prolonged bed rest after surgery or acute illness are at high risk for becoming immobilized. Approximately 6% of older adults in the 60- to 79-year age group experience a stroke, and this rate increases to 15% for adults aged 80 and above. About half of the individuals who suffer a stroke have residual deficits for which they require assistance, and often these deficits result in immobility. Parkinson disease (PD), another common neurological disorder found in older adults, can cause severe limitations in mobility. PD is a progressive neurological disorder that affects

TABLE 10-1 Factors That Influence Immobility

Intrapersonal factors	Interpersonal factors	Environmental factors	Policy factors

Musculoskeletal disorders
  Arthritides
  Osteoporosis
  Fractures (especially hip and femur)
  Podiatric problems
  Other (eg, Paget disease)
	Interactions with caregivers that discourage mobility and use wheelchairs for convenience	Lack of access to appropriate and safe aids for mobility	Forced immobility in hospitals and nursing homes due to regulations such as not allowing the patient to get up until seen by a therapist

Neurological disorders
  Stroke
  Parkinson disease
  Neuropathies
  Normal-pressure hydrocephalus
  Dementias
  Other (cerebellar dysfunction, neuropathies)
	Caregiving that decreases need for mobility by keeping everything easily accessible for the individual	Lack of access to areas that are open and free of clutter for safe ambulation	Falls policies that encourage sedentary responses to the fall

Cardiovascular disease
  Congestive heart failure (severe)
  Coronary artery disease (frequent angina)
  Peripheral vascular disease (frequent claudication)
	Caregiving that does not motivate or encourage mobility; walk with patients/ residents and make mobility fun	Lack of resources (eg, exercise equipment, grab bars, stair rails, rails in hallways) to help maintain mobility	Lack of policies that encourage mobility such as walk-to-dine programs or removal of wheelchairs in the dining room

Pulmonary disease Chronic obstructive lung disease (severe)			

Sensory factors
  Impairment of vision
  Decreased kinesthetic sense
  Decreased peripheral sensation			

Acute and chronic pain			
Motivation			
Fear of falling			
Nutritional status			
Mood/depression			
Medications			

approximately 1 million people in the United States, most of whom are over the age of 60. As the disease progresses, it has a major impact on the individual's function due to associated bradykinesia (slow movement) or akinesia (absence of movement), resting tremor, and muscle rigidity, as well as cognitive changes.

Severe congestive heart failure, coronary artery disease with frequent angina, peripheral vascular disease with frequent claudication, orthostatic hypotension, and severe chronic lung disease can restrict activity and mobility in many older adults because of lack of cardiovascular endurance. Peripheral vascular disease, especially in older diabetics, can cause claudication, peripheral neuropathy, and altered balance, all of which limit ambulation.

According to the National Osteoporosis Foundation (NOF), 9.9 million Americans have osteoporosis and an additional 43.1 million have low bone density. Osteoporosis and the commonly associated kyphosis results in altered balance due to an altered center of gravity and subsequent decline in mobility.

The psychological and environmental factors that influence immobility are as important as the physical changes noted. Depression, lack of motivation, apathy, fear of falling, cognitive changes and health beliefs (ie, a belief that rest and immobility are beneficial to recovery) can all influence mobility in older adults. Interpersonal factors and the physical environment can also have a major impact on mobility. Well-meaning formal and informal caregivers may provide care for older individuals rather than help the individual optimize his or her underlying function. Inappropriate use of wheelchairs, bathing, and dressing of individuals who have the underlying capability to engage in these activities results in deconditioning and immobility. Inappropriate use of mobility aids (eg, use of motorized wheelchairs and transfer devices) and lack of access to appropriate assisted devices that can optimize function and mobility (eg, canes, walkers, and appropriately placed railings), cluttered environments, uneven surfaces, and the height, shape and positioning of chairs and beds can further lead to immobility. Negotiating stairs can be a special challenge.

Drug side effects may also contribute to immobility. Sedatives and hypnotics can result in drowsiness, dizziness, delirium, and ataxia, and can impair mobility. Antipsychotic drugs (especially the typical antipsychotic agents) have prominent extrapyramidal effects and can cause muscle rigidity and diminished mobility. The treatment of hypertension can result in orthostatic hypotension or bradycardia such that the individual experiences dizziness and is unable to ambulate independently.

COMPLICATIONS OF IMMOBILITY

Immobility can lead to complications in almost every major organ system (Table 10-2). Prolonged inactivity or bed rest has adverse physical and psychological consequences. Metabolic effects include a negative nitrogen and calcium balance and impaired glucose tolerance. Older individuals can also experience diminished plasma volume and subsequent changes in drug pharmacokinetics. Immobilized older patients often become depressed, are deprived of environmental stimulation, and, in some instances, become delirious. Deconditioning can occur rapidly, especially among older individuals who have little physiological reserve.

TABLE 10-2. Complications of Immobility

Skin
    Pressure ulcers
Musculoskeletal
    A reduction in anabolic processes and an increase in catabolic processes of the
        muscle proteins
    Muscular deconditioning and atrophy
    Contractures
    Bone loss (osteoporosis)
    Myalgias and arthralgias
    Falls
Cardiovascular
    A decrease in hydrostatic pressure
    Hypovolemia
    Deconditioning
    Orthostatic hypotension
    Venous thrombosis, embolism
Pulmonary
    Decreased ventilation
    Atelectasis
    Aspiration pneumonia
Gastrointestinal
    Anorexia
    Constipation
    Fecal impaction, incontinence
Genitourinary
    Urinary infection
    Urinary retention
    Bladder calculi
    Incontinence
Metabolic
    Altered body composition (eg, decreased plasma volume)
    Negative nitrogen balance
    Impaired glucose tolerance
    Altered drug pharmacokinetics
Psychological
    Sensory deprivation
    Delirium
    Depression

Musculoskeletal complications associated with immobility include loss of muscle strength and endurance; reduced skeletal muscle fiber size, diameter, and capillarity; contractures; disuse osteoporosis; and pain. The severity of muscle atrophy is related to the duration and magnitude of activity limitation. If left unchecked, the associated muscle wasting can lead to long-term sequelae, including impaired functional capacity and permanent muscle damage and increased risk of falls. Moreover, immobility exacerbates bone turnover by resulting in a rapid and sustained increase in bone resorption and a decrease in bone formation.

The impact of immobility on skin can also be devastating. Varying degrees of immobility and decreased serum albumin significantly increase the risk for pressure ulcer development. Prolonged immobility results in cardiovascular deconditioning; the combination of deconditioned cardiovascular reflexes and diminished plasma volume can lead to postural hypotension. Postural hypotension may not only negatively influence rehabilitative efforts but also predispose to falls and serious cardiovascular events such as stroke and myocardial infarction. Likewise, deep venous thrombosis and pulmonary embolism are well-known complications of immobility. Immobility, especially bed rest, also impairs pulmonary function. Tidal volume is diminished; atelectasis may occur, which, when combined with the supine position, predisposes to developing aspiration pneumonia.

Gastrointestinal and genitourinary problems are likewise influenced by immobility. Constipation and fecal impaction may occur because of decreased mobility and inappropriate positioning to optimize defecation. Urinary retention can result from inability to void lying down and/or rectal impaction impairing the flow of urine. These conditions and their management are discussed in Chapter 8. Overall, time spent in sedentary activity exacerbates disease and impacts mortality.

ASSESSING IMMOBILE PATIENTS

Several aspects of the history and physical examination are important in assessing factors contributing to immobility among older adults (Table 10-3). Focused histories should address the intrapersonal aspect as well as the environmental issues associated with immobility. It is important to explore the underlying cause, or perceived cause, of the immobility on the part of the individual and/or the caregiver. Specific contributing factors to explore include medical conditions, treatments (eg, medications, associated treatments such as intravenous lines), pain, psychological (eg, mood and fear) state, and motivational factors. Nutrition status, particularly protein levels and evaluation of 25-hydroxy vitamin D, may be useful to consider when evaluating the older patient because these have been associated with muscle weakness, poor physical performance, balance problems, and falls. An assessment of the environment is critical and should include both the patient's physical and social environment (particularly caregiving interactions). Any and all of these factors can decrease the individual's willingness to engage in activities. A comprehensive assessment is critical and input from other members of the health-care team (eg, social work, physical therapy) can facilitate these evaluations and provide important aspects based on their expertise and focus.

In addition to the potential causes of immobility, the impact of immobility on older adults must always be considered. A comprehensive skin assessment should be done with a particular focus on bony prominences and areas of pressure against the bed, chair, splint, shoe, or any type of immobilizing device. Evaluation of lower

TABLE 10-3. Assessment of Immobile Older Patients

History
    Nature and duration of disabilities causing immobility
    Medical conditions contributing to immobility
    Pain
    Drugs that can affect mobility
    Motivation and other psychological factors
    Environment
Physical examination
    Skin
    Cardiopulmonary status
Musculoskeletal assessment
    Muscle tone and strength
    Joint range of motion
    Foot deformities and lesions
Neurological deficits
    Focal weakness
    Sensory and perceptual evaluation
Levels of mobility
    Bed mobility
    Ability to transfer (bed to chair)
    Wheelchair mobility
    Standing balance
    Gait (see Chap. 9)
    Pain with movement

extremities among those with known arterial insufficiency is critical. Cardiopulmonary status, especially intravascular volume, and postural changes in blood pressure and pulse are important to consider, particularly as these may further limit mobility. A detailed musculoskeletal examination, including evaluation of muscle tone and strength (Table 10-4), evaluation of joint range of motion, and assessment of podiatric problems that may cause pain, should be performed. Standardized and repeated assessments of overall physical capability can be helpful in gauging a patient's functional and physical ability. This exam focuses on the individual's ability to follow simple commands as well as evidence of basic underlying capability to perform activities of daily living (Resnick et al, 2013). The neurological examination should identify focal weakness as well as cognitive, sensory, and perceptual problems that can impair mobility and influence rehabilitative efforts.

Most importantly, the patient's function and mobility should be assessed and reevaluated on an ongoing basis. Assessments should include bed mobility; transfers, including toilet transfers; and ambulation and stair climbing (see Table 10-3). Pain, fear, resistance to activity, and endurance should simultaneously be considered during these evaluations. As previously noted, other members of the health-care team

TABLE 10-4. Example of How to Grade Muscle Strength in Immobile Older Patients

0 = Flaccid
1 = Trace/slight contractility but no movement
2 = Weak with movement possible when gravity is eliminated
3 = Fair movement against gravity but not against resistance
4 = Good with movement against gravity with some resistance
5 = Normal with movement against gravity and some resistance

Upper extremity:
Shoulder extension: Have the individual hold up the arm at 90°. Place your hand on the individual's upper arm between elbow and shoulder and tell the individual not to let you push down the arm.
Elbow flexion: Have the individual bend the elbow fully and attempt to straighten out the arm while telling the individual not to let you pull the arm down.
Elbow extension: While the individual still has the elbow flexed, tell him or her to try and straighten out the arm while you resist.

Lower extremity:
Hip flexion: Place your hand on the individual's anterior thigh and ask him or her to raise the leg against your resisting hand (say to individual: don't let me push your leg down).
Knee extension: Have the individual bend the leg on the bed and place one of your hands just below the individual's knee and tell the individual to try and straighten out the leg as you resist.
Ankle plantar flexion: Have the individual extend the foot against your hand.
Ankle dorsiflexion: Have the individual pull the foot up against your hand.

(eg, physical therapy, occupational therapy, and nursing) are skilled in completion of these assessments and are critical to the comprehensive evaluation of the patient.

MANAGEMENT OF IMMOBILITY

The goal in the management of any older adult is to optimize function and mobility. Medical management is central to ensuring this goal because optimal management of underlying acute and chronic disease must be addressed to ensure success. It is beyond the scope of this text to detail the management of all conditions associated with immobility in older adults, however, important general principles of the management of the most common of these conditions are reviewed. Brief sections at the end of the chapter provide an overview of key principles managing pain and the rehabilitation of geriatric patients.

ARTHRITIS

Arthritis includes a heterogeneous group of related joint disorders that have a variety of causes such as metabolic changes, joint malformation, joint trauma, and joint damage. The pathology of osteoarthritis (OA) is characterized by cartilage destruction with subsequent joint space loss, osteophyte formation, and subchondral sclerosis. OA is the most common joint disease among older adults and is the major cause of knee, hip, and back pain. OA is not, by definition, inflammatory, although hypertrophy of synovium and accumulation of joint effusions are typical. It is currently believed that the pathogenesis of OA progression revolves around a complex interplay of numerous factors: chondrocyte regulation of the extracellular matrix, genetic influences, local mechanical factors, and inflammation.

Plain film radiography has been the main diagnostic modality for assessing the severity and progression of OA. Magnetic resonance imaging (MRI) and ultrasound, however, have been noted to be more accurate and comprehensive measures of joint changes. Once diagnosed, a wide variety of modalities can be used to treat OA as well as other painful musculoskeletal conditions. Treatment can be separated into three different categories: nonpharmacological, pharmacological, and surgical. Nonpharmacological management should be the focus of interventions and include weight loss, physical therapy to strengthen related musculature, use of local ice and heat, acupuncture, and use of exercise programs to maintain strength and function.

Pharmacological management is targeted toward symptomatic relief and includes use of analgesics (discussed further later), nonsteroidal anti-inflammatory drugs (NSAIDs) and intra-articular injections with steroids and hyaluronans. In addition, topical nonsteroidals, arthroscopic irrigation, acupuncture, and nutraceuticals, which are a combination of pharmaceutical and nutritional supplements, have also been used. The most common nutraceuticals include glucosamine and chondroitin. Although there may be a placebo effect resulting in benefit to patients using glucosamine and chondroitin, there is no evidence of a significant improvement in pain. Likewise there is no evidence that vitamin D decreases pain or facilitates repair of structural damage among individuals with OA. Arthroscopic interventions have been used when there is known inflammation and when other noninvasive interventions have failed. The lack of evidence about the benefit of such procedures has not deterred the rate of arthroscopies (Adelani et al, 2016). Other surgical interventions include debridement and lavage, osteotomy, cartilage transplant, and arthroplasty. Joint replacement should be reserved for individuals with severe symptomatic disease who do not respond to more conservative interventions.

Patients referred for joint replacement should have stable medical conditions and be encouraged to lose weight and strengthen relevant muscles before the procedure. Those who have more extensive disease benefit more from the surgery than others in terms of management of pain and function and make surgery worth the risk of the commonly associated adverse events (eg, thromboembolism, infection) (Maempel et al, 2015; Tilbury et al, 2016). Optimal management often involves the use of multiple treatment modalities, and the best combination of treatments will vary from patient to patient.

Treating arthritis optimally requires a differential diagnosis because there are multiple different types of arthritic conditions and treatments may vary. For example, polymyalgia rheumatica (PMR) is a chronic inflammatory disorder of unknown cause characterized by the subacute onset of shoulder and pelvic girdle pain and early morning stiffness in men and women over the age of 50 years. Diagnosis is based on clinical assessment and laboratory evidence of inflammation. Treatment involves use of steroids, such as prednisone, although methotrexate has been used as a corticosteroid-sparing agent and may be useful for patients with frequent disease relapses and/or corticosteroid-related toxicity. Conversely, infliximab, an antibody used to treat inflammatory disorders, has not been shown to be beneficial in terms of pain management or disease progression and thus is not currently recommended for polymyalgia rheumatica. Because of the close association between polymyalgia rheumatica and temporal arteritis, any symptoms suggestive of involvement of the temporal artery—headache, jaw claudication, recent changes in vision—especially when the sedimentation rate is very high (>75 mm/h), should prompt consideration of temporal artery biopsy. Acute treatment of temporal arteritis with high-dose steroids is needed to prevent blindness. The history and physical examination can be helpful in differentiating OA from inflammatory arthritis (Table 10-5), however, other procedures are often essential.

Gout, one of the oldest recognized forms of arthritis, is characterized by intra-articular monosodium urate crystals. Gout generally presents as acute, affecting the first metatarsal phalangeal joint, mid foot, or ankle, although the knee, elbow, or wrist can also be involved. Tophi, which are subcutaneous urate deposits on extensor surfaces, can develop in later phases of the disease and are sometimes confused with rheumatoid arthritis and associated nodules. Radiographs may reveal well-defined gouty erosions in or around joints. Some patients will have elevated uric acid levels. The definitive diagnosis of gout is established by observing the presence of needle-shaped crystals in the involved joint. The goal of treatment is to terminate the acute attack and then prevent future attacks by considering underlying causes (eg, considering hypouricemic therapy). The acute phase of gout should be managed using short-term NSAIDs, colchicine, corticotropin, and corticosteroids. Treatment choices should be based on patient comorbidities (eg, renal function, gastrointestinal disease). Treatment to decrease uric acid levels should not be initiated during the acute phase because drugs such as allopurinol or probenecid may exacerbate the acute attack. Due to renal changes associated with aging, allopurinol is recommended over probenecid in older individuals. Colchicine can be used for acute management as

PART II

TABLE 10-5. Clinical Features of Osteoarthritis Versus Inflammatory Arthritis

Clinical feature	Osteoarthritis	Inflammatory arthritis
Duration of stiffness	Minutes	Hours
Pain	Usually with activity	Occurs even at rest and at night
Fatigue	Unusual	Common
Swelling	Common, but little synovial reaction	Very common, with synovial proliferation and thickening
Erythema and warmth	Unusual	Common

well as for prophylaxis. After NSAIDs, colchicine, and steroids, IL-1 inhibitors are beneficial as fourth-line therapy for acute gout attacks among individuals who do not tolerate or respond to other treatment options.

In addition to differentiating the type of rheumatological disorders the individual is experiencing whenever possible, careful physical examination can detect treatable nonarticular conditions such as tendinitis and bursitis. Bicipital tendinitis and olecranon and trochanteric bursitis are common in geriatric patients. Dramatic relief from pain and disability from these conditions can be achieved by local treatments such as the injection of steroids.

HIP FRACTURE

Worldwide, the total number of hip fractures is expected to surpass 6 million by the year 2050. This varies, however, based on country and demographic factors such as gender and ethnicity. Much of the research and focus on hip fractures has been with women. However, an increasing number of men are experiencing hip fracture and the men who fracture tend to be younger and have more comorbidities than women at the time of fracture. Men have approximately twice the risk of mortality compared to women following fracture and these risks persist for at least 2 years after the event. Although it is not clear why men tend to be a greater risk of negative outcomes postfracture, it is believed to be due to higher prevalence of underlying acute medical problems. One year after hip fracture, approximately half of affected individuals do not regain their prefracture function with regard to activities of daily living or their ability to ambulate. After 3 months, there is generally no further improvement in overall function. Individuals do, however, improve their ability to ambulate across the first 12-month recovery period. The assessment and management of falls, the major cause of hip fracture, are discussed in Chapter 9.

The degree of immobility and disability caused by a hip fracture depends on several factors including coexisting medical conditions, patient motivation and resilience, social supports, genetic factors, the nature of the fracture, and the techniques of management. Preexisting comorbid conditions such as OA, heart failure, or stroke make the recovery process all the more challenging. Patients with these underlying conditions and those with cognitive impairment are at especially high risk for poor functional recovery. However, those with cognitive impairment can benefit from rehabilitation services as much as those without impairment (Resnick et al, 2016). The location of the fracture is especially important in determining the most appropriate management plan (Figure 10-1). For displaced fractures of the femoral neck, a total hip arthroscopy may be particularly advantageous, especially for active older adults. For older adults who have multiple comorbidities, hemiarthroplasty or unipolar implants are sufficient (Rogmark and Leonardsson, 2016). Especially among frail, nonambulatory older adults, providing conservative, nonsurgical interventions that involve early transfers to sitting/wheelchair activity results in similar morbidity and mortality outcomes as when surgical repair is provided (Kawaji et al, 2016).

The current guidelines from the American College of Chest Physicians (Kearon et al, 2016) recommend that unfractionated heparin, low molecular weight heparin,

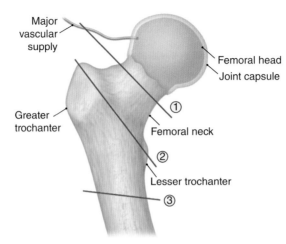

	TYPE OF FRACTURE	ANATOMY	IMPLICATIONS
①	Subcapital (intra capsular)	Disrupts blood supply to femoral head	Higher incidence of non-union and necrosis of femoral head
②	Intertrochanteric	Blood supply to femoral head intact	Lower incidence of non union and necrosis of femoral head
③	Subtrochanteric		

FIGURE 10-1 Characteristics of different types of hip fractures.

low-dose unfractionated heparin, or fondaparinux be used to prevent venous thromboembolism for patients who have had an orthopedic surgical intervention involving a hip or knee. The type of prophylaxis and length of time of treatment recommended vary by surgical intervention (Table 10-6). For periods of nonorthopedic-related bedrest due to medical conditions such as cancer or severe cardiac or lung disease, subcutaneous unfractionated heparin and the low molecular weight heparins are preferred. Aspirin is not considered a preferred option for prophylaxis as it is less effective at reducing incidence of thromboembolism than the other agents. Thus, use of aspirin should be reserved for situations in which it is the only viable option.

PARKINSON DISEASE

The first step in successful management of Parkinson disease (PD) is to recognize its presence. Pathologically, PD is associated with a progressive loss of dopamine-producing cells, especially in the substantia nigra, which sends dopamine to the corpus striatum. These structures, located in the basal ganglia, are stimulated by the neurotransmitter dopamine and are responsible for planning and controlling automatic movements of the body, such as walking, writing, or rising from a seated position. Once the level of dopamine loss has reached a threshold, individuals typically develop a triad of symptoms: bradykinesia (slow movement) or akinesia (absence

TABLE 10-6. Recommended Treatment Options for Venous Thromboembolism Prophylaxis in Immobility*

	LMWH	Fondaparinux	Apixaban	Dabigatran	Rivaroxaban	LDUH	Warfarin	UFH
Hip surgery	X	X	X	X	X	X	X	
Knee surgery	X	X	X	X	X	X	X	
Medical conditions	X							X

LMWH = low molecular weight heparin; LDUH = low-density unfractionated heparin; UFH = unfractionated heparin.

*Treatment should be for at least 10–14 days and up to 35 days.

of movement), resting tremor, and muscle rigidity. Many older patients, especially in long-term care institutions, have undiagnosed, treatable forms of parkinsonism. Some of these individuals have drug-induced parkinsonism resulting from the extrapyramidal side effects of antipsychotics (see Chapter 14). Nonmotor symptoms of PD are also common and include depression, psychosis, anxiety, sleep disturbances, dysautonomia, dementia, and others. Left untreated, parkinsonian patients eventually become immobile and can develop flexion contractures, pressure sores, malnutrition, and aspiration pneumonia.

Pharmacological treatment of PD is based on an attempt to increase the ratio of dopamine to acetylcholine in the central nervous system, specifically the nigrostriatal system. Many drugs are used in the treatment of the disease including catechol-O-methyltransferase inhibitors, dopaminergic agents, dopamine agonists, monoamine oxidase-B inhibitors, and miscellaneous treatments including amantadine (Table 10-7). Some agents are currently considered unacceptable including the anticholinergic agents, tolcapone (a catechol-O-methyltransferase inhibitor), apomorphine (a dopaminergic agent), and bromocriptine (a dopamine agonist) because the benefits of these drugs do not outweigh the potential risks. Clinical response may require dose adjustments and can take several weeks; side effects are common and often limit pharmacological treatment. Wide variations in response can also occur, including morning akinesia, peak-dose dyskinesias, and freezing episodes (sometimes referred to as the "on–off phenomenon"). Excessive dopamine can also cause sleep disturbances, delirium, and psychosis. Alternative modes of drug delivery have been considered in the treatment of PD including the use of rotigotine (Neupro), a transdermal patch. The ease of administration and maintenance of blood levels and potential for decreasing dyskinesias may have some benefit over other modes of administration.

Additional interventions for PD include the use of exercise (Duchesne et al, 2015), specifically aerobic exercise and doing the tango (Rios Romenets et al, 2015). Last, surgical options, including thalamotomy, pallidotomy, and deep brain stimulation, are gaining more attention and are a viable choice for a select group of individuals.

STROKE

To prevent the progression of immobility moving toward disability and subsequent complications, patients with completed strokes should receive prompt and intensive rehabilitative therapy. (Stroke is also discussed in Chapter 11.) In many older patients, coexisting medical conditions (eg, cardiovascular disease) limit the intensity of rehabilitation treatment that can be tolerated and thus they are not eligible for Medicare coverage in an acute inpatient or skilled nursing facility. Although all stroke patients deserve an assessment and consideration for intensive rehabilitation, the cost-effectiveness of various approaches to stroke rehabilitation is controversial, and there is no evidence to support or guide the amount of time spent in therapy sessions. The best outcomes for rehabilitation occur in formal rehabilitation settings where the focus of care is on regaining function. However, whether the rehabilitative efforts occur in the acute care hospital, special rehabilitation unit, nursing home,

TABLE 10-7. Drugs Used to Treat Parkinson Disease

Drug (brand name)	Usual dosages	Mechanism of action	Potential side effects
Catechol-O-methyltransferase inhibitor			
Dopaminergic agents			
Carbidopa, levodopa (Sinemet) (Sustained-release options and disintegrating tablet options)	40/400–200/2000 mg/day in divided doses	Increases dopamine availability and decreases peripheral dopamine metabolism	Nausea, vomiting, anorexia Dyskinesias Orthostatic hypotension Behavioral disturbances Vivid dreams and hallucinations
Tolcapone (Tasmar)	100–200 mg tid	Increases dopamine availability and decreases peripheral dopamine metabolism	Liver dysfunction
Dopamine agonists			
Bromocriptine (Parlodel)	1–1.5 mg tid or qid (initial); gradually increase to maximum of 30–40 mg in divided doses	Directly activates dopaminergic receptors	Behavioral changes Hypotension Nausea
Ropinirole	0.75–24 mg/day (patch)	Directly activates dopaminergic receptors	Dizziness, orthostasis, dyskinesias, nausea, somnolence, peripheral edema, confusion, sudden sleep onset, psychosis
Pramipexole (Mirapex)	0.5-1.5 mg tid	Dopamine agonist	Hallucinations Nausea Somnolence

Ropinirole (Requip)	3–8 mg tid	Dopamine agonist	Orthostatic hypotension Syncope Nausea Somnolence
Monoamine oxidase-B inhibitors			
Selegiline (Eldepryl) (oral and disintegrating tablets)	10 mg/day in one dose	MAO-B inhibitor	Nausea Confusion Agitation Insomnia Involuntary movements
Rasagiline (Azilect)	1 mg/day in one dose	Selective, irreversible MAO-B inhibitor	Balance difficulties Anorexia Vomiting Weight loss Depressive symptoms No dietary restrictions
Tolcapone (Tasmar)	100–200 mg tid		Liver dysfunction*
Miscellaneous			
Amantadine (Symmetrel)	100–300 mg/day†	Increases dopamine release	Delirium and hallucinations

*Top number represents carbidopa; bottom number, levodopa.
†Eliminated by kidney; dosages should be adjusted when renal function is diminished.

or at home, these efforts should involve a multidisciplinary rehabilitation team and the basic principles should remain the same (see the "Rehabilitation" section later in this chapter).

Although complete functional recovery occurs in less than half of stroke patients, immobility and its attendant complications can almost always be prevented or minimized. Treadmill training, for example, has repeatedly shown significant benefits in gait and balance among stroke survivors. There is interest in using brain–computer interfaces to facilitate rehabilitation after stroke. Innovative interventions such as motor training consisting of voluntary movements assisted by a robot device have been compared against tradition rehabilitation. There is evidence that use of the robot interventions may be helpful in augmenting, but not replacing, traditional interventions. In addition to intensive rehabilitation in the immediate poststroke period, ongoing exercise and physical activity are critical after stroke to maintain optimal function and quality of life and to prevent future strokes. The management of older patients with cerebrovascular disease is discussed further in Chapter 11.

PRESSURE ULCERS

A pressure ulcer is defined as localized damage caused to the skin and/or underlying soft tissue usually appearing over a bony prominence due to external pressure and/or sheering force. The amount of pressure necessary to occlude blood supply to the skin (and thus predispose to irreversible tissue damage) depends on the quality of the tissue and blood flow to the area. For example, in a patient with peripheral artery disease, heel pressure over a relatively short period of time may cause an ulceration to occur.

Shearing forces (such as those created when the head of a bed is elevated and the torso slides down and transmits pressure to the sacral area) contribute to the stretching and angulation of subcutaneous tissues. Friction, caused by the repeated movement of skin across surfaces such as bed sheets or clothing, increases the shearing force. This can eventually lead to thrombosis of small blood vessels, thus undermining and then destroying skin. Shearing forces and friction are worsened by loose, folded skin, which is common in older adults because of loss of subcutaneous tissue and/or dehydration. Moisture from bathing, sweat, urine, and feces compounds the damage. In light of the many risk factors and their variable influence, numerous scales have been developed to quantify a person's risk of developing pressure ulcers. The two most commonly used scales are the Braden scale (www.bradenscale.com/) and the Norton scale (www.orthotecmedical.com/pdfs/Norton.pdf). There is limited evidence to support the effectiveness of these measures in terms of identifying individuals at risk for pressure ulcers. They are noted to be low in risk, however, and use is encouraged to help identify individuals at risk so that appropriate preventive interventions can be implemented. Pressure ulcers can be classified into four stages, depending on their clinical appearance and extent (Table 10-8) and/or described as unstageable. The area of damage below the pressure ulcer can be much larger than the ulcer itself. This is caused by the manner in which pressure and shearing forces are transmitted to subcutaneous tissues. More than 90% of pressure ulcers occur in

TABLE 10-8. Clinical Characteristics of Pressure Sores

Characteristics	Diagnostic tips
Stage I Nonblanchable erythema	
Acute inflammatory response limited to epidermis	Pressure areas at stage I do not blanch when pressed
Presents as irregular area of erythema, induration, edema; may be firm or boggy	May be different with different skin pigments
Often over a bony prominence	Redness with pressure persists after 30 min; in dark skin the color may be red, blue, or a purple hue
Skin is unbroken	
Stage II Partial thickness	
Extension of acute inflammatory response through dermis to the junction of subcutaneous fat	May look like an abrasion or a blister
Appears as a blister, abrasion, or shallow ulcer with more distinct edges	It should *not* be described as a skin tear
Early fibrosis and pigment changes occur	
Stage III Full thickness skin loss	
Full-thickness skin ulcer extending through subcutaneous fat; may extend down to but not through the underlying fascia	This presents like a crater and may have undermining of the adjacent tissue
The skin may have undermining	Bone and tendon are not visible or directly palpable
Base of ulcer infected, often with necrotic, foul-smelling tissue	
Stage IV Full thickness tissue loss	
Extension of ulcer through deep fascia, so that bone, tendon, or muscle is visible at base of ulcer	Undermining is even more common and there may be sinus tracts
Osteomyelitis and septic arthritis can be present	
Unstageable/Unclassified: Full thickness skin or tissue loss with depth unknown	
Full thickness tissue loss in which the depth of the ulcer is obscured by slough or eschar in the wound bed. It is not necessary to remove the eschar if it is stable (dry, intact, and there is no surrounding erythema or fluctuance or drainage)	

PART II

the lower body—mainly in the sacral and coccygeal areas, at the ischial tuberosities, and in the greater trochanter area.

The cornerstone of management of the skin in immobile patients is prevention of pressure ulcers (Table 10-9). All preventive measures listed in Table 10-9 should be used to avoid development and/or progression of an ulcer, and intensive local skin

TABLE 10-9. Principles of Skin Care in Immobile Older Patients

Preventive
   Identify patients at risk
   Decrease pressure, friction, and skin folding
   Keep skin clean and dry
   Avoid excessive bed rest: optimize and encourage function
   Avoid oversedation
Provide adequate nutrition and hydration (30–35 kcal/kg) overall, protein (1–1.5 g/kg),
   and fluid (1 mL/kcal)
Stages I and II pressure sores
   Clean wounds with warm, normal saline or water
   Avoid pressure and moisture
   Cover open wounds with an occlusive dressing: determined based on ulcer
     condition (eg, presence of granulation, necrotic tissue), type and amount of
     drainage, surrounding tissue, and evidence of infection
   Prevent further injury and infection: use antibiotics very judiciously
   Provide intensive local skin care[*]
   Manage associated pain
Stage III pressure sores
   Debride necrotic tissue: autolytic, chemical, mechanical, sharp, or surgical options
   Cleanse and dress wound as above*
   Culture wound: treat only in cases of confirmed bacteremia, sepsis, osteomyelitis,
     and cellulitis[†]
   Manage associated pain
Stage IV pressure sores
   Take tissue biopsy for culture
   Use systemic antimicrobials as noted in stage III
   Cleanse and dress wound as above
   Have surgical consultation to consider surgical repair
   Manage associated pain

[*]Many techniques are effective (see text).
[†]Cultures and topical antimicrobials should not be used routinely (see text).

care must be instituted. Many techniques have been advocated for local skin care; none is more successful than the others. The most important factor in all these techniques is the attention that the skin gets, particularly relief from pressure. Almost any technique that involves removing pressure from the area and regularly cleansing and drying the skin will work. Alternating pressure mattresses and alternating pressure overlays are equally effective in terms of prevention and management of pressure ulcers. Likewise, addressing nutrition and hydration of the patient is critical.

Treatment of pressure ulcers includes the use of a variety of occlusive dressings depending on the stage of the wound, degree of drainage, and evidence of infection. Several nonpharmacological interventions have been used to treat pressure ulcers including positioning, use of support surfaces, nutrition, and electrotherapy.

However, none of these interventions is effective in management of the ulcer (Vélez-Díaz-Pallarés et al, 2015). Nor is there sufficient evidence to support the use of hyperbaric oxygen therapy, topical oxygen therapy, or biological dressings in the treatment of pressure ulcers. The evidence to support the use of platelet-derived growth factor is not sufficient to recommend routine use.

The management of stage III and IV pressure ulcers is more complicated. Debridement of necrotic tissue and frequent irrigation (two to three times daily), cleansing (with saline or peroxide), and dressing of the wound are essential. Eschars should be undermined and removed if they are suspected of hiding large amounts of necrotic and infected tissue. Chemical debriding agents can be helpful. The role of wound cultures and antimicrobials in the management of stage III pressure ulcers is controversial. Topical antimicrobials may be useful, especially when bacterial colony counts are high, but they are generally not recommended. Systemic antimicrobials should not be used because they do not reach sufficient concentrations in the area of the ulcer; topical therapy will be more effective unless cellulitis is present. Routine wound cultures are probably not warranted for stage III lesions because they almost always grow several different organisms and do not detect anaerobic bacteria, which are often pathogenic. Results of such cultures generally reflect colonization rather than infection. Once a lesion has progressed to stage IV, systemic antimicrobials are often necessary. Routine and anaerobic cultures of tissue or bone are most helpful in directing antimicrobial therapy. Patients with large pressure ulcers that become septic should be treated with broad-spectrum antimicrobials that will cover anaerobes, gram-negative organisms, and *Staphylococcus aureus*. In selected instances, consideration of plastic surgery for stage IV lesions is warranted.

Documentation of pressure sores is critical and should include the following components: (1) the type of ulcer, how long it has been present, and in what setting it occurred; (2) the size measured as length × width × depth in centimeters (area of the wound bed that is deepest, without a tract); (3) the color as percentage, with red indicating amount of granulation tissue, yellow indicating the amount of slough present, and black being necrotic tissue or eschar; (4) exudate as serous, serosanguinous, sanguineous, or purulent; (5) the presence or absence of odor in the wound (this should be determined after the wound is thoroughly cleaned); (6) description of the periwound tissues (eg, viable, macerated, inflamed, or hyperkeratotic); and (7) evidence of undermining (undermining is a separation of the tissues between the surface and the subcutaneous tissues).

PAIN MANAGEMENT

Pain is a major cause of immobility in older adults and immobility can cause or exacerbate painful conditions and create a vicious cycle of pain, decreased mobility, and increased pain. The American Geriatrics Society has published recommendations for the management of persistent pain in older adults, and readers are referred to this publication listed in the Web resources for more details (pain is also discussed in Chapter 3). Pain assessment and management tools are available at the Sigma Theta Tau Geriatric Pain website (www.geriatricpain.org/Pages/home.aspx).

Pain in older persons is commonly underdiagnosed and undertreated despite the availability of many assessment tools and effective therapeutic interventions. Pain is now viewed as a "fifth vital sign," and health professionals are encouraged to routinely inquire about pain. When pain is identified, it should be carefully characterized. In addition to the standard questions about location, timing, aggravating factors, and the like, a simple standardized pain scale can be helpful in rating the severity of pain. Several such scales are available, as noted earlier, with some scales being more appropriate for those with cognitive impairment who may be less able to communicate and describe their pain (www.geriatricpain.org/Pages/home.aspx). Pain during any type of activity may be diagnosed in individuals with cognitive impairment based on evidence of agitation, moaning, becoming tense or rigid during movement, grimacing, or hitting or pushing the caregiver away, among other types of behaviors.

Acute pain, such as that following an orthopedic fracture, can negatively affect the neurophysiological aspects of nociception and the overall recovery of a patient. Initially, the physiological response to acute pain is adaptive as it facilitates an immediate "fight or flight" response via the sympathetic nervous system and the neuroendocrine system. This stimulates the heart to increase blood flow to internal organs and muscles and dilates the bronchioles so that more oxygen intake is increased allowing the body to respond rapidly to the danger. Longer term, however, the impact of the sympathetic and neurochemical changes cause unpleasant symptoms and increase the risk of impaired healing and infection, hyperglycemia, lipolysis, protein catabolism, increased antidiuretic and catecholamine levels, immunosuppression, and a hypercoagulation state.

For individuals with chronic pain, such as that associated with OA, the degree to which pain interferes with activities of daily living and sleep is especially important to explore among older adults. Recurrent or persistent pain can result in complications such as a predisposition to falling because of deconditioning, fatigue, behavioral problems, depression, and impaired quality of life. It is important to discuss pain management options with older adults and to assess pain on an ongoing basis to determine if it has been resolved, if treatment is tolerable (ie, drug side effects), and if there is a need to alter the pain management regimen.

It is useful to differentiate between nociceptive pain and neuropathic pain (Table 10-10). The former includes somatic pain arising from the skin, bone, joint, muscle, or connective tissue and is often described as throbbing, visceral pain that arises from internal organs such as the large intestine or pancreas. The latter is pain from abnormal processing of sensory input by the peripheral or central nervous system. Neuropathic pain is generally described as burning, tingling, shock-like, or shooting. Differentiating pain helps guide management strategies and ensures more efficient pain relief. Pain management should consider nonpharmacological and pharmacological approaches.

Although the benefits of different types of nonpharmacological treatment for pain vary by patient population and outcomes considered, there is no evidence they cause harm and thus are worth implementing and combining with traditional

TABLE 10-10. Pain Categories and Management Options

Type of pain	Examples	Description	Treatment
Nociceptive pain: somatic	Trauma/fracture Cellulitis/inflammation	Pain associated with injury or localized inflammatory process Due to activation of small-diameter afferent nerve fibers that are sometimes called "pain" nerve fibers Fast pain nerve fibers cause sharp, stinging sensation Slow pain nerve fibers result in aching, burning type pain	Treatment of nociceptive pain requires resolution of the conditions that are activating the nociceptive fibers For example, if local inflammation is a major factor, suppression of the inflammatory reaction would be expected to resolve the pain Nonopioids, NSAIDs, opioids Nonpharmacological options (eg, ice, heat)
Nociceptive pain: visceral	Inflammation associated with peritonitis, appendicitis, cholecystitis, and ischemic-myocardial and ischemic colitis	Pain that originates from ongoing injury to the internal organs or the tissues that support them Visceral pain is also caused by obstruction of visceral tubes and lack of blood supply (ischemic) to viscera The pain is described as: Pressure-like Deep Stabbing Dull and aching Throbbing Difficult to localize Episodic Pain may be referred to adjacent or distal part of the body (eg, gallbladder pain is referred to the scapula)	Treatment of the underlying problem. Nonopioids, NSAIDs, opioids Nonpharmacological options (eg, ice, heat)

(continued)

PART II

TABLE 10-10. Pain Categories and Management Options (*continued*)

Type of pain	Examples	Description	Treatment
Neuropathic pain	Diabetic neuropathy, postherpetic neuralgia, phantom limb pain, deafferentation, and trigeminal neuralgia	Generated or sustained by the nervous system (central or peripheral) Neuropathic pain is, by definition, chronic and may escalate with time Described as shooting or burning, tingling or numbness	Neuropathic pain responds poorly to normal pain treatments, and in fact may be complicated by commonly used acute pain treatments Nonpharmacological options include such things as acupuncture and electrical nerve stimulation Pharmacological interventions include the use of topical anesthetics (eg, capsaicin cream), regional anesthetic blocks, tricyclic antidepressants, anticonvulsants, and narcotics
Psychological pain	Most patients with chronic pain have some degree of psychological disturbance There may be anxiety and/or depression Psychological distress may not only be a consequence of the pain, but may also contribute to the pain itself	Is an unpleasant feeling of a psychological, nonphysical origin	Treatment options include treating the underlying anxiety and depression Behavioral therapy such as talk therapy, relaxation training, stress management, and pain-coping skills training
Mixed pain	Postherpetic neuralgia, chronic pain postmastectomy	Acute painful conditions, often associated with acute nociceptive and acute inflammatory mechanisms This pain can transition to chronic pain states and have more neuropathic mechanisms predominating	Combination of drugs used to treat neuropathic and nonneuropathic pain may be needed Nonpharmacological interventions can be tried

pharmacological treatments. Examples of nonpharmacological approaches include cold therapy, breathing exercises and guided imagery, distraction, heat, massage, music, positioning, acupuncture, relaxation, and physical activity, particularly exercises that focus on strengthening muscles around the joint.

The mainstay of pain management is drug therapy. Table 10-11 lists drugs that can be helpful in managing pain in older adults. For persistent pain, most experts recommend initiating treatment with acetaminophen and the use of topical treatments such as capsaicin or ketamine gel or combination gels, lidocaine patches, or local intra-articular corticosteroid injections. Nonselective NSAIDs and cyclooxygenase-2 (COX-2) selective inhibitors should be avoided and considered rarely, with caution, in highly selected individuals. If pain management is not controlled with nonpharmacological interventions and acetaminophen, consideration should be given to adding an opioid when pain is impacting function and quality of life (see Table 10-11). The Centers for Disease Control and Prevention (CDC) recently released guidelines for when to start opioids for chronic pain management (Table 10-12). The side effects of opioids are well known and include respiratory depression, sedation, constipation, nausea, vomiting, and delirium. Side effects should be anticipated and a plan of care initiated as prevention. In addition there is the risk that individuals will become addicted to opioids and this can result in misuse of these medications.

Nonopioid medications to treat persistent pain include a group of treatment options referred to as adjuvant therapy and include antidepressants such as the selective serotonin reuptake inhibitors (SSRIs), tricyclic antidepressants, anticonvulsants, and topical agents. Tricyclic antidepressants were the first drugs used in this way, but due to their significant anticholinergic side effects including dry mouth, urinary retention, constipation, delirium, tachycardia, and blurred vision, they are contraindicated in older adults. SSRIs and mixed serotonin and norepinephrine reuptake inhibitors (SNRIs) are more effective in the treatment of pain, particularly neuropathic pain, and have much better side effect profiles. Anticonvulsant drugs, such as gabapentin and pregabalin, are also effective for neuropathic pain and tend to have fewer side effects than some of the older anticonvulsants. Nonsteroids and corticosteroids are effective in the management of pain, particularly when there is associated inflammation. Significant adverse effects with the use of steroids are well known and include gastrointestinal irritation, delirium, thinning of the skin, osteoporosis, fluid retention, hyperglycemia, and immunosuppression, thus treatment using steroids is generally avoided.

The benefits of muscle relaxant drugs such as cyclobenzaprine, carisoprodol, and chlorzoxazone, among others, are controversial with regard to management of pain and should be avoided because of the associated fall risk when they are used. Likewise, benzodiazepines are not likely to be effective for pain management unless used on a trial basis to treat muscle spasm. Meperidine is metabolized to normeperidine, a substance that has no analgesic properties but may impair kidney function and cause tremulousness, myoclonus, and seizures and thus should not be used. Tramadol, a drug that combines opioid-receptor binding and norepinephrine and serotonin

TABLE 10-11. Examples of Drug Groups and Associated Drugs Commonly Used to Treat Pain

Medication	Use	Benefits	Risks
Nonopioid analgesics			
Aspirin	Acute pain and inflammation such as headache	Anti-inflammatory properties Low cost	Gastrointestinal irritation Prolonged bleeding Can precipitate asthma
Salicylate salts	Chronic pain such as with osteoarthritis	Some anti-inflammatory properties Does not increase bleeding time	Gastrointestinal irritation
Acetaminophen	Acute or chronic pain such as headache or muscle aches	Does not cause stomach irritation or increase bleeding time	May cause liver irritation, particularly in individuals who drink alcohol heavily
Nonsteroidal anti-inflammatory agents (NSAIDS such as ibuprofen)	Acute or chronic pain such as headache or muscle aches	Anti-inflammatory properties Effects last longer than with aspirin	Gastrointestinal irritation Cardiovascular risks Kidney risks; liver risks
Cox-2 inhibitors	Acute or chronic pain such as headache or muscle aches	Anti-inflammatory properties Less gastrointestinal irritation than other NSAIDs	Gastrointestinal irritation Cardiovascular risks Kidney risks; liver risks
Opioid agonists			
Codeine (combined with acetaminophen)	Acute or chronic pain not relieved by other treatments	None	Some individuals may not have the enzyme to convert codeine to morphine in the liver and thus it is ineffective Tends to cause nausea/vomiting and constipation
Fentanyl	Acute or chronic pain not relieved by other treatments	Multiple methods of delivery (oral, patch, sublingual)	Risk of nausea, vomiting, constipation, abuse, and overdosage

Hydrocodone available alone or with acetaminophen	Acute or chronic pain not relieved by other treatments	Short acting Effective to suppress coughing	Risk of abuse and overdosage Risk of liver impairment
Hydromorphone	Acute or chronic pain not relieved by other treatments	None	Risk of nausea, vomiting, constipation, abuse, and overdosage
Meperidine	Acute or chronic pain not relieved by other treatments	None	Low potency, short duration of action, and unique toxicities (eg, seizures, delirium)
Morphine	Acute or chronic pain not relieved by other treatments	Available in many formulations	Risk of abuse and overdosage
Methadone	Acute or chronic pain not relieved by other treatments	Useful for intractable pain	Has a long half-life and interacts with a large number of other medications Can interfere with cardiac conduction Can cause sleep apnea High risk of overdosage
Oxycodone	Acute or chronic pain not relieved by other treatments	Often combined with agents to augment efficacy	Risk of nausea, vomiting, constipation, abuse, and overdosage
Tapentadol	Acute or chronic pain not relieved by other treatments	Dual mechanism drug with both opioid and antidepressant-like activity There is a short-acting version for acute pain and longer-acting version for chronic pain May cause less gastrointestinal side effects than other drugs	Risk of nausea, vomiting, constipation, abuse, and overdosage

(continued)

PART II

TABLE 10-11. Examples of Drug Groups and Associated Drugs Commonly Used to Treat Pain (*continued*)

Medication	Use	Benefits	Risks
Tramadol	Acute or chronic pain not relieved by other treatments	Weak opioid-like drug Less respiratory suppression	Affects neurotransmitters in the brain and can't be used with serotonin reuptake inhibitors Decreases seizure threshold Can kidney and liver damage Risk of nausea, vomiting, constipation, abuse, and overdosage
Buprenorphine	Chronic pain management	Used to relieve unpleasant withdrawal symptoms due to opioid detoxification and addiction Has a ceiling effect and dosages higher than 32 mg/day do not improve pain management	Risk of nausea, vomiting, constipation, abuse, and overdosage
Anticonvulsants			
Gabapentin	For nerve injury or neuropathic pain	Generally well tolerated	May cause some sleepiness, confusion, hyponatremia, and swelling
Pregabalin	Effective for postherpetic neuralgia, diabetic neuropathy, and fibromyalgia.	Generally well tolerated	May cause some dizziness
Carbamazepine	Trigeminal neuralgia	Generally well tolerated	Interacts with other drugs Can cause liver damage and white blood cell impairment
Valproic acid	Headache or nerve pain	Generally well tolerated	May affect platelet development

Muscle relaxants

Carisoprodol	Muscle relaxant for acute muscle pain Avoid use in chronic pain	Converted by the body into meprobamate, a barbiturate-like drug May cause physical dependence May cause kidney or liver damage
Cyclobenzaprine	Muscle relaxant for acute muscle pain	Similar to a tricyclic antidepressant May cause dizziness, drowsiness, and anticholinergic effects such as constipation, dry mouth, and confusion
Methocarbamol	Muscle relaxant for acute muscle pain	Has sedative properties so can help with nighttime sleep Drowsiness and urine discoloration (to brown, black, or green)
Baclofen	For muscle spasm	Reduces spasticity in muscles after neurological illness or injury Withdrawal should not be abrupt as it can be life-threatening Depresses the central nervous system Can cause excessive sedation

Antidepressants

Selective serotonin reuptake inhibitors (SSRIs such as sertraline)	For neuropathic pain, migraines Not effective for acute musculoskeletal pain	Work directly by increasing norepinephrine and indirectly by decreasing depression and anxiety They are nonaddictive and have a good safety profile May cause some nausea, hyponatremia, sexual problems, cognitive/personality changes among other side effects
Tricyclic antidepressants	For neuropathic pain, migraines Not effective for acute musculoskeletal pain	Anticholinergic side effects including drug mouth, urinary retention, constipation, and orthostatic hypotension

(continued)

PART II

TABLE 10-11. Examples of Drug Groups and Associated Drugs Commonly Used to Treat Pain (*continued*)

Medication	Use	Benefits	Risks
Selective serotonin and norepinephrine reuptake inhibitors	Indicated for painful diabetic peripheral neuropathy, fibromyalgia, anxiety disorder, depression, and in 2010 for chronic musculoskeletal pain including osteoarthritis and chronic low back pain	Limited side effects	Low risk given limited side effects
Topical agents			
Aspirin in chloroform or diethyl ether	Treatment for musculoskeletal pain	Limited side effects as not absorbed systemically	Skin irritation
Capsaicin	Treatment for neuropathic pain	Limited side effects as not absorbed systemically	Skin irritation
Lidocaine	Treatment of musculoskeletal pain	Limited side effects as not absorbed systemically	Skin irritation
Compounded medications that typically include lidocaine, amitriptyline, ibuprofen, gabapentin, and/ or ketoprofen	Treatment of musculoskeletal or neuropathic pain	Limited side effects as not absorbed systemically	Skin irritation

TABLE 10-12. CDC Recommendations for Determining When to Initiate or Continue Opioids for Chronic Pain

1. Nonpharmacological and nonopioid pharmacological therapies are preferred for chronic pain.
2. Consider opioid therapy only if expected benefits for both pain and function are anticipated to outweigh risks to the patient. If opioids are used, they should be combined with nonpharmacological and nonopioid pharmacological therapies, as appropriate.
3. Before starting opioid therapy for chronic pain, establish treatment goals with the patient and consider how therapy will be discontinued if benefits do not outweigh risks. Continue opioid therapy only if there is clinically meaningful improvement in pain and function that outweighs risks to patient safety.
4. Before starting and periodically during opioid therapy, discuss with the patient known risks and realistic benefits of opioid therapy and patient and clinician responsibilities for managing therapy.
5. When starting opioid therapy for chronic pain, prescribe immediate-release opioids instead of extended-release/long-acting (ER/LA) opioids.
6. When opioids are started, prescribe the lowest effective dosage.
7. Long-term opioid use often begins with treatment of acute pain. When opioids are used for acute pain, clinicians should prescribe the lowest effective dose of immediate-release opioids and should prescribe no greater quantity than needed for the expected duration of pain severe enough to require opioids. Three days or less will often be sufficient; more than 7 days will rarely be needed.
8. Evaluate benefits and harms of opioids with patients within 1 to 4 weeks of starting opioid therapy for chronic pain or of dose escalation and evaluate benefits and harms of continued therapy with patients every 3 months or more frequently.
9. Before starting and periodically during continuation of opioid therapy, evaluate risk factors for opioid-related harms and plan strategies to mitigate risk, including considering offering naloxone when factors that increase risk for opioid overdose, such as history of overdose, history of substance use disorder, higher opioid dosages (≥50 MME/day), or concurrent benzodiazepine use, are present.
10. Review the patient's history of controlled substance prescriptions using state prescription drug monitoring program (at least every 3 months) data to determine whether the patient is receiving opioid dosages or dangerous combinations that put him or her at high risk for overdose.
11. When prescribing opioids for chronic pain, do a urine drug test before starting opioid therapy and consider urine drug testing at least annually to assess for prescribed medications as well as other controlled prescription drugs and illicit drugs.
12. Avoid prescribing opioid pain medication and benzodiazepines concurrently whenever possible.
13. Offer or arrange evidence-based treatment (usually medication-assisted treatment with buprenorphine or methadone in combination with behavioral therapies) for patients with opioid use disorder.

PART II

reuptake inhibition, lowers the seizure threshold and should not be given when the individual is taking other medications with serotonergic properties.

THE ROLE OF EXERCISE TO PREVENT IMMOBILITY

Exercise is an important intervention for preventing immobility and its complications and is also discussed in Chapter 5. Participation in either nonspecific physical activity or specific aerobic or resistive exercise is associated with decreased progression of OA and can also decrease the risk of falls, both of which contribute to immobility (Chan et al, 2015; Desveaux et al, 2014; Mat et al, 2015). The specific amount of exercise needed to achieve the desired benefit varies based on individual goals and capabilities. Combining recommendations from the American College of Sports Medicine, the CDC, and the National Institutes of Health (NIH), health-care providers should recommend that older adults engage in 30 minutes of physical activity *daily*, and the activity should incorporate aerobic activity (walking, dancing, swimming, biking), resistance training, and flexibility. Exercises can be done individually or in group settings depending on the individual's preference, cognitive ability, and motivational level.

In light of the many benefits of physical activity and low risk of serious adverse events associated with low- and moderate-intensity physical activity, there is no reason to screen older adults prior to engaging in a moderate intensity exercise program (Whitfield et al, 2014). Moreover, the risks of false positives from screening and subsequent cost of additional testing are greater than the risks associated with moderate-level physical activity. Resources are readily available for older adults interested in getting more information about the type and amount of exercise to do. For example, the National Institute of Aging provides free exercise booklets that cover a basic exercise program including resistive, stretching, balance, and aerobic activities, and other materials are likewise available at no cost to individuals (www.nia.nih.gov/health/publication/go4life-dvd-everyday-exercises-national-institute-aging).

REHABILITATION

The goal of rehabilitation is to restore function and prevent further disability. Following rehabilitation, the goal of restorative or function focused care is to optimize and maintain the individual's underlying capability and level of physical function. Maintaining a philosophy of care in which function and physical activity of the individual take precedence over task completion is helpful when working with older individuals. Physiatrists and physical and/or occupational therapists can be very helpful in developing appropriate and optimal rehabilitative and maintenance goals for function and physical activity. Table 10-13 outlines some of the key principles. Careful assessment of a patient's function and underlying capability, the setting of realistic goals, prevention of secondary disabilities and complications of immobility, evaluation of the environment, and adapting of the environment to the patients' abilities (and vice versa) are all essential elements of the rehabilitation process. Moreover, ongoing motivation of the older individual as well as the caregivers is critical

TABLE 10-13. Basic Principles of Rehabilitation in Older Patients

- Optimize the treatment of underlying diseases, nutrition and hydration, and psychosocial situation.
- Optimize the physical environment with regard to encouraging function and physical activity (eg, handrails, clutter-free areas).
- Facilitate opportunities for the older individual to perform functional tasks and physical activity (eg, personal care activities, bed making, laundry, walking to meals).
- Prevent secondary disabilities and complications of immobility.
- Treat primary disabilities (eg, manage pain associated with osteoarthritis).
- Set realistic, individualized goals.
- Emphasize functional independence.
- Attend to motivation and other psychological factors of both patients and caregivers—use self-efficacy-based approaches including successful performance, role modeling, verbal encouragement, and elimination of unpleasant sensations.
- Use a team approach including all members of the health-care team, the resident/patient, and family.

to successful rehabilitation and restoration of function (Resnick et al, 2011). The expertise of an interdisciplinary team, specifically physical and occupational therapists, can be extremely valuable in assessing, treating, motivating, and monitoring patients whose mobility is impaired. Physical therapists generally attend to the relief of pain, muscle strength and endurance, joint range of motion, and gait. They use a variety of treatment modalities (Table 10-14). Occupational therapists focus on functional abilities, especially as they relate to activities of daily living. They make detailed assessments of mobility and help patients improve or adapt to their abilities to perform basic and instrumental activities of daily living. Even when mobility and function remain impaired, occupational therapists can make life easier for these patients by performing environmental assessments and recommending modifications and assistive devices that will improve the patients' ability to function independently (Table 10-15). Speech therapists are helpful in assessing and implementing rehabilitation for disorders of communication, cognition and orientation, and swallowing. Nursing and informal caregivers have the responsibility of ongoing encouragement of older adults to engage in the activities recommended by these therapists (eg, walking to the bathroom, participating in exercise classes, or completing specific strength training activities).

Rehabilitation services can be provided during an acute care hospital stay, in an inpatient rehabilitation facility (IRF), in a skilled nursing facility (SNF), an outpatient clinical setting, assisted living setting, or at home. Posthospital rehabilitation provided in an IRF, SNF, or as part of home health care may be covered by Medicare. Rehabilitation provided at an acute level of care, such as in stroke rehabilitation, is generally limited in terms of length of stay and depends on the older individual's goals and demonstration of progress toward goal achievement. IRF rehabilitation covered by Medicare requires 3 hours a day of therapy by at least two out of the three

TABLE 10-14. Physical Therapy in the Management of Immobile Older Patients

Objectives
  Relieve pain
  Evaluate, maintain, and improve joint range of motion
  Evaluate and improve strength, endurance, motor skills, and coordination
  Evaluate and improve gait and stability
  Assess the need for and teach the use of assistive devices for ambulation (wheelchairs, walkers, canes)
Treatment modalities
Exercise
  Active (isometric and isotonic)
  Passive
  Encourage sitting exercise programs
Heat
  Hot packs
  Paraffin
  Diathermy
  Ultrasound
Hydrotherapy
Ultrasound
Transcutaneous electrical nerve stimulation

therapists (physical, occupational, or speech therapy). At this level of care, the patient is seen by a physician or designated provider daily and receives 24-hour nursing rehabilitation care. Reimbursement is based on case-mix groups using the Functional Independence Measure. Rehabilitation provided in SNFs is somewhat less rigorous, although most Medicare intermediaries will require that a patient show significant rehabilitation potential and steady improvement toward some predetermined goal. At this level a physician must supervise the care, but daily visits are not required. Reimbursement is based on prospective payment according to resource utilization groups (obtained from the Minimum Data Set). Once the older individuals' goals are achieved, continued rehabilitation services can occur under Medicare Part B 3 days a week at home or in an institutional setting.

The benefit of rehabilitation services in one site, or at one level, versus another has not been well established. The outcomes vary by the condition being treated. Some of the variation may depend on the specific facility in which the care is provided and the philosophy of care that is implemented by the direct caregivers. For example, in inpatient rehabilitation settings it is critical that the time spent outside of therapy should continue to implement a rehabilitation focus of care in which older adults are encouraged to practice activities such as bathing, dressing, and ambulation in their real-world settings. If formal or informal caregivers provide care for the individual who should be doing this care himself or herself, it is unlikely that the rehabilitation

TABLE 10-15. Occupational Therapy in the Management of Immobile Older Patients

Objectives

  Restore, maintain, and improve ability to function independently

  Evaluate and improve sensory and perceptual motor function

  Evaluate and improve ability to perform activities of daily living (ADLs)

  Fabricate and fit splints for upper extremities

  Improve coping and problem-solving skills

  Improve use of leisure time

Modalities

  Assessment of mobility

    Bed mobility

    Transfers

    Wheelchair propulsion

  Assessment of other ADLs using actual or simulated environments

    Dressing

    Toileting

    Bathing and personal hygiene

    Cooking and cleaning

Visit home for environmental assessment and recommendations for adaptation

Provide task-oriented activities (eg, crafts, projects)

Recommend and teach use of assistive devices (eg, long-handled reachers, special eating and cooking utensils, sock aids)

Recommend and teach use of safety devices (eg, grab bars and railing, raised toilet seats, shower chairs)

goals will be achieved. Moreover, the individual will learn to be dependent and believe that he or she is not capable of independently performing the activity. Similarly, exemplary rehabilitation services are of little value if after completion of rehabilitation the individual is no longer encouraged to do such things as walk to the dining room. While the caregivers may be well intended and believe that "helping" and demonstrating "caring" is best shown by providing hands-on care services, this type of care only creates deconditioning and dependency, along with contractures and the other sequelae of immobility. Therefore, regardless of site of service, a rehabilitative or function-focused care approach should be implemented to maintain and optimize the function of each older individual.

Summary of Evidence

Do's

- Focus on nonpharmacological management of OA such as weight loss, physical therapy, exercise, local ice/heat treatment, and acupuncture.
- Treat the acute phase of gout with pharmacological interventions to manage symptoms including nonsteroidals, colchicines, or corticosteroids, as tolerated by the patient.

- Treat Parkinson disease with pharmacological interventions to increase the ratio of dopamine to acetylcholine in the central nervous system.
- Encourage exercise interventions in patients with stroke to improve balance and recovery.

Don'ts

- Recommend surgical interventions for OA such as debridement, lavage, ostomy, cartilage transplant, or arthroplasty.
- Start treatments to decrease uric acid levels during acute gout attacks.
- Use hyperbaric oxygen, topical oxygen, or biological dressings to treat pressure ulcers.

Consider

- Joint replacement for individuals with severe arthritis.
- Exercise as a treatment option in all older adults to optimize and maintain function.
- Innovative interventions after stroke using motor training via robotics.

REFERENCES

Adelani M, Harris A, Bowe T, et al. Arthroscopy for knee osteoarthritis has not decreased after a clinical trial. *Clin Orthop Related Res.* 2016;474:489-494.

Allena KD, Golightlya YM. Epidemiology of osteoarthritis: state of the evidence. *Curr Opin Rheumatol.* 2015;27:276–83.

Chan WC, Fai Yeung JW, Man Wong CS, et al. Efficacy of physical exercise in preventing falls in older adults with cognitive impairment: systematic review and meta-analysis. *J Am Med Dir Assoc.* 2015;16:149-154.

Desveaux L, Beauchamp M, Goldstein R, Brooks D. Community-based exercise programs as a strategy to optimize function in chronic disease: a systematic review. *Med Care.* 2014;52:216-226.

Duchesne C, Lungu O, Nadeau A, et al. Enhancing both motor and cognitive functioning in Parkinson's disease: aerobic exercise as a rehabilitative intervention. *Brain Cogn.* 2015;99:68-77.

Kawaji H, Uematsu T, Oba R, Takai S. Conservative treatment for fracture of the proximal femur with complications. *J Nippon Med Sch.* 2016;83:2-5.

Kearon C, Akl EA, Ornelas J, et al. Antithrombotic therapy for VTE disease: chest guideline and expert panel report. *Chest.* 2016;149:315-352.

Maempel JF, Riddoch F, Calleja N, Brenkel IJ. Longer hospital stay, more complications, and increased mortality but substantially improved function after knee replacement in older patients. *Acta Orthop.* 2015;86:451-456.

Mat S, Tan MP, Kamaruzzaman SB, Ng CT. Physical therapies for improving balance and reducing falls risk in osteoarthritis of the knee: a systematic review. *Age Ageing.* 2015;44:16-24.

Resnick B, Beaupre L, McGilton KS, et al. Rehabilitation interventions for older individuals with cognitive impairment post-hip fracture: a systematic review. *J Am Med Dir Assoc.* 2016;17:200-205.

Resnick B, Galik E, Boltz M. *Implementing Restorative Care Nursing in All Settings.* 2nd ed. New New York, NY: Springer Publishing; 2011.

PART II

Resnick B, Galik E, Boltz M, Wells C. Physical Capability Scale: psychometric testing. *Clin Nurs Res.* 2013;22:7-29.

Rios Romenets S, Anang J, Fereshtehnejad SM, Pelletier A, Postuma R. Tango for treatment of motor and non-motor manifestations in Parkinson's disease: a randomized control study. *Comp Ther Med.* 2015;23:175-184.

Rogmark C, Leonardsson O. Hip arthroplasty for the treatment of displaced fractures of the femoral neck in elderly patients. *Bone Joint J.* 2016;98B:291-297.

Tilbury C, Holtslag MJ, Rutger TL, et al. Outcome of total hip arthroplasty, but not of total knee arthroplasty, is related to the preoperative radiographic severity of osteoarthritis: a prospective cohort study of 573 patients. *Acta Orthop.* 2016;87:67-71.

Vélez-Díaz-Pallarés M, Lozano-Montoya I, Abraha I, et al. Nonpharmacologic interventions to heal pressure ulcers in older patients: an overview of systematic reviews (The SENATOR-ONTOP Series). *J Am Med Dir Assoc.* 2015;16:448-469.

Whitfield GP, Pettee Gabriel KK, Rahbar MH, Kohl HW III. Application of the American Heart Association/American College of Sports Medicine adult preparticipation screening checklist to a nationally representative sample of US adults aged greater than 40 years from the National Health and Nutrition Examination Survey 2001 to 2004. *Circulation.* 2014;129:1113-1120.

PART II

SUGGESTED READINGS

Boehm K, Raak C, Cramer H, Lauche R, Ostermann T. Homeopathy in the treatment of fibromyalgia—a comprehensive literature-review and meta-analysis. *Comp Ther Med.* 2014;22:731-742.

Durmus D, Alayli G, Bayrak I, Canturk F. Assessment of the effect of glucosamine sulfate and exercise on knee cartilage using magnetic resonance imaging in patients with knee osteoarthritis: a randomized controlled clinical trial. *J Back Musculoskel Rehab.* 2012;25:275-284.

Haentjens P, Magaziner J, Colón-Emeric CS, et al. Meta-analysis: excess mortality after hip fracture among older women and men. *Arch Intern Med.* 2010;152:380-390.

Hernández-Rodríguez J, Cid MC, López-Soto A, Espigol-Frigolé G, Bosch X. Treatment of polymyalgia rheumatica: a systematic review. *Arch Intern Med.* 2009;169:1839-1850.

Kim KH, Kim TH, Lee BR, et al. Acupuncture for lumbar spinal stenosis: a systematic review and meta-analysis. *Comp Ther Med.* 2013;21:535-556.

Margolis DJ, Gupta J, Hoffstad O, et al. Lack of effectiveness of hyperbaric oxygen therapy for the treatment of diabetic foot ulcer and the prevention of amputation: a cohort study. *Diabetes Care.* 2013;36:1961-1966.

Norouzi-Gheidari N, Archambault PS, Fung J. Effects of robot-assisted therapy on stroke rehabilitation in upper limbs: systematic review and meta-analysis of the literature. *J Rehab Res Dev.* 2012;49:479-495.

Panula J, Pihlajamaki H, Mattila VM, et al. Mortality and cause of death in hip fracture patients aged 65 or older: a population-based study. *BMC Musculoskel Dis.* 2011;12:105.

Tateno F, Sakakibara R, Nagao T, et al. Deep brain stimulation ameliorates postural hypotension in Parkinson's disease. *J Am Geriatr Soc.* 2015;63:2186-2189.

Tran TH, Pham JT, Shafeeq H, Manigault KR, Arya V. Role of interleukin-1 inhibitors in the management of gout. *Pharmacotherapy.* 2013;33:744-753.

SELECTED WEBSITES (ACCESSED 2017)

American Heart Association and American Stroke Association, Statistical Fact Sheet 2015 Update: Older Americans & Cardiovascular Diseases, www.heart.org/idc/groups/heart-public/@wcm/@sop/.../ucm_472923.pdf

Institute of Clinical Systems Improvement, Pressure Ulcer Treatment and Prevention Protocol, www.icsi.org/_asset/6t7kxy/PressureUlcer.pdf

National Osteoporosis Foundation, Clinician's Guide to Prevention and Treatment of Osteoporosis, 2014, www.nof.org/.../nofs-clinicians-guide-published-by-osteoporosis-international/

National Pressure Ulcer Advisory Panel, NPUAP Pressure Ulcer Stages/Categories, 2015, www.npuap.org/resources/educational-and-clinical-resources/npuap-pressure-ulcer-stages-categories/

Parkinson's Disease Foundation, Statistics on Parkinson's, www.pdf.org/en/parkinson_statistics

PAIN GUIDELINES

American Chronic Pain Association, 2016 guidelines, https://theacpa.org/uploads/documents/ACPA_Resource_Guide_2016.pdf

American Geriatrics Society, 2009 guidelines, www.americangeriatrics.org/files/documents/2009_Guideline.pdf

American Pain Society, clinical practice guidelines, http://americanpainsociety.org/education/guidelines/overview

GENERAL MANAGEMENT
STRATEGIES

CHAPTER 11

Cardiovascular Disorders

In older adults, heart disease is the leading cause of death worldwide and is the most common cause for hospitalization. Physiological changes of the cardiovascular system in aging may modify the presentation of cardiac disease.

PHYSIOLOGICAL CHANGES

In using data on physiological changes of the cardiovascular system, it is important to recognize the selection criteria of the population studied. Because the prevalence of coronary artery disease in asymptomatic individuals may be 50% in the eighth and ninth decades of life, screening to exclude occult cardiovascular disease may modify findings.

In a population screened for occult coronary artery disease, there is no change in cardiac output at rest over the third to eighth decades (Gerstenblith et al, 1987) (Table 11-1). There is a slight decrease in heart rate and a compensatory slight increase in stroke volume. This pattern is in contrast to studies in unscreened individuals, where cardiac output falls from the second to the ninth decades. Consistent with the principle of decreased responsiveness to stress in aging, during maximal exercise, other changes are manifest even in the screened population (Table 11-2). Heart rate response to exercise is decreased in older adults compared to younger individuals, reflecting a diminished β-adrenergic responsiveness in aging. Cardiac output is decreased slightly. Cardiac output is maintained by increasing cardiac volumes—increasing end-diastolic and end-systolic volumes. With this increase in workload and the work of pumping blood against less-compliant arteries and a higher blood pressure, cardiac hypertrophy occurs even in the screened elderly population.

Because myocardial reserve mechanisms are used to maintain normal function in aging, older persons are more vulnerable to developing dysfunction when disease is superimposed.

Diastolic dysfunction—retarded left ventricular filling and higher left ventricular diastolic pressure—is present both at rest and during exercise in older persons. Older persons are more dependent on atrial contraction, as opposed to ventricular relaxation, for left ventricular filling, and thus are more likely to develop heart failure if atrial fibrillation ensues. Heart failure may occur in the absence of systolic dysfunction or valvular disease.

HYPERTENSION

Hypertension is the major risk factor for stroke, heart failure, and coronary artery disease in older adults; all are important contributors to mortality and functional disability. Because hypertension is remediable and its control may reduce the incidence

TABLE 11-1. Resting Cardiac Function in Persons Aged 30 to 80 Years Old Compared With That in Persons Aged 30 Years Old

	Unscreened for occult CAD	Screened for occult CAD
Heart rate	–	–
Stroke volume	– –	+
Stroke volume index	– –	0
Cardiac output	– –	0
Cardiac index	– –	0
Peripheral vascular resistance	+ +	0
Peak systolic blood pressure	+ +	+ +
Diastolic pressure	0	0

CAD, coronary artery disease; –, slight decrease; – –, decrease; +, slight increase; + +, increase; 0, no difference.

of coronary heart disease and stroke, increased efforts at detection and treatment of high blood pressure are indicated. Investigators are learning more of the biological mechanisms leading to coronary artery disease by both reviewing the commonly known risk factors, in addition to novel genetic factors. New developments in the genetics of these illnesses may lead to different treatments to address each unique atherosclerosis pathophysiology.

Hypertension is defined as a systolic blood pressure of 140 mm Hg or greater and/or a diastolic blood pressure of 90 mm Hg or greater (per the most recent definition in 2003 by the Seventh Joint National Committee, JNC-7) (Joint National Committee, 2004). This is based on the average of two or more properly measured readings at each of two or more office visits, after an initial screening. Isolated systolic

TABLE 11-2. Performance at Maximum Exercise in Sample Screened for Coronary Artery Disease Aged 30 to 80 Years

	Compared with 30-year-olds
Heart rate	– –
End-diastolic volume	+ +
Stroke volume	+ +
Cardiac output	–
End-systolic volume	+ +
Ejection fraction	– –
Total peripheral vascular resistance	0
Systolic blood pressure	0

–, slight decrease; – –, decrease; + +, increase; 0, no difference.

hypertension is defined as a systolic pressure of 140 mm Hg or greater with a diastolic pressure of less than 90 mm Hg. With these definitions, as many as 67% of individuals older than age 60 may be hypertensive (Ostchega et al, 2007).

Despite the high prevalence of hypertension in older adults, it should not be considered a normal consequence of aging. Hypertension is the major risk factor for cardiovascular disease in older adults, and that risk increases with each decade. Both elevation of systolic blood pressure and pulse pressure are better predicators of adverse events than diastolic pressure. This is particularly relevant to older individuals, in whom isolated systolic hypertension predominates and may be present in 90% of hypertensive patients over the age of 80 (reviewed in Chobanian, 2007).

EVALUATION

The diagnosis should be made on serial blood pressures. In patients with labile hypertension, blood pressure should be averaged to make the diagnosis because these patients are at no less risk than those patients with stable hypertension. The history and physical examination should be directed toward assessing the duration, severity, treatment, and complications of the hypertension (Table 11-3). Atherosclerosis may

TABLE 11-3. Initial Evaluation of Hypertension in Older Adults

History
Duration
Severity
Treatment
Complications
Other risk factors
A directed physical examination
Blood pressure, including Osler maneuver, standing determinations, and verification of the blood pressure on the contralateral arm
Weight and body mass index
Funduscopic, vascular, and cardiorespiratory examination for end-organ damage
Palpation of the thyroid gland
Abdominal bruit and femoral bruit
Abdominal examination for enlarged kidneys, pulsatile aorta, or distended bladder
Lower extremity examination for edema and pulses
Neurological examination for focal deficits
Laboratory tests
   Urinalysis
   Electrolytes
   Estimated glomerular filtration rate
   Calcium
   Thyrotropin (TSH)
   Lipid profile
   12-lead electrocardiogram

interfere with occlusion of the brachial artery by a blood pressure cuff, leading to erroneously elevated blood pressure determinations, or "pseudohypertension." Such an effect can be determined by the Osler maneuver. The cuff pressure is raised above systolic blood pressure. If the radial artery remains palpable at this pressure, significant atherosclerosis is probably present and may account for a 10- to 15-mm Hg pressure error. Standing blood pressure and blood pressure on the contralateral side should also be determined. Initial laboratory evaluation should include urinalysis; complete blood cell count; measurements of blood electrolytes and calcium, estimated glomerular filtration rate, fasting glucose, and lipids; and 12-lead electrocardiogram (ECG). Although not all hypertension experts agree, the recent guidelines from the United Kingdom's National Institute for Health and Clinical Excellence (NICE) recommend using ambulatory blood pressure monitoring (worn for a period of 24 to 48 hours and designed to intermittently measure and record values) to confirm the diagnosis of hypertension (Krause et al, 2011).

Secondary forms of hypertension are uncommon in older adults but should be considered in treatment-resistant patients and in those with diastolic pressures greater than 115 mm Hg (Table 11-4). Pheochromocytoma is uncommon in older adults and is particularly unusual in those older than age 75. Atherosclerotic renovascular hypertension and primary hyperaldosteronism may occur more frequently in older persons. With the use of automated calcium determinations, the frequency of diagnosis of primary hyperparathyroidism is increasing, particularly in postmenopausal women. Because there is a causal link between this disorder and hypertension, the diagnosis and treatment of hyperparathyroidism may ameliorate the elevated blood pressure.

Additional considerations include obesity, obstructive sleep apnea, excessive alcohol use, and cocaine abuse. A critical review of the medications should assess for nonsteroidal anti-inflammatory agents, steroid medications, phenopropanolamine, estrogen, erythropoietin, cyclosporine, nicotine, and herbal supplements.

TREATMENT

The issue of treatment of systolic/diastolic or isolated systolic hypertension in older individuals is still being defined. The contemporary issue is not whether to treat,

---

TABLE 11-4. Secondary Hypertension in Older Persons

Renovascular disease (atherosclerotic)
Primary hyperaldosteronism
Thyroid or parathyroid disease (calcium)
Drug induced
Renal disease (decreased creatinine clearance) including renovascular disease or obstructive uropathy
Obstructive sleep apnea
Pheochromocytoma
Obesity
Alcohol excess
Cocaine use

but how aggressively to treat. Multiple large trials have demonstrated that treating hypertension in older adults decreases morbidity and mortality from coronary artery disease, heart failure, and stroke (reviewed in Joint National Committee, 2014; for NICE guidance, see Krause et al, 2011). Although there has been concern about the hazard of treating individuals with cerebrovascular disease, the evidence suggests that the presence of cerebrovascular disease is an indication for, rather than a contraindication to, hypertensive therapy.

The Eighth Joint National Committee (JNC8) recommended the following for the general population of adults aged 60 years and older. Initiate pharmacological treatment to lower blood pressure at systolic of 150 mm Hg or higher or a diastolic blood pressure of 90 mm Hg or higher and treat to a goal of a systolic blood pressure of less than 150 mm Hg and a goal diastolic blood pressure of less than 90 mm Hg. The JNC8 panel noted the corollary that if there are older patients whose treatment for high blood pressure results in lower achieved blood pressure (eg, less than 140/90 mm Hg) and this blood pressure is not associated with adverse effects on health or quality of life, the treatment does not have to be adjusted. This expert opinion was based on studies which had goals for systolic blood pressure of less than 150 mm Hg, with the average systolic blood pressure of the participants at 143 and 144 mm Hg. Many of the participants in these trials had a systolic blood pressure that was less than 140 mm Hg, which was generally well tolerated. The panel was unable to reach a consensus on the issue of the goal systolic blood pressure of less than 150 mm Hg. For those with chronic kidney disease and less than age 70 years and with a systolic blood pressure of 140 mm Hg or greater or a diastolic blood pressure of 90 mm Hg or greater, the goal systolic blood pressure is less than 140 mm Hg and diastolic blood pressure of less than 90 mm Hg. Adults of any age with diabetes mellitus whose systolic blood pressure is 140 mm Hg or greater or diastolic blood pressure is 90 or greater, should receive pharmacological treatment to achieve a goal systolic blood pressure of less than 140 mm Hg and diastolic blood pressure goal of less than 90 mm Hg.

The SPRINT trial randomized 9361 patients aged 50 years and older with a systolic blood pressure of 130 mm Hg or higher and at increased risk for cardiovascular events (but without diabetes mellitus). Additional exclusions were polycystic kidney disease, prior cerebrovascular accident, and heavy proteinuria. The intensive treatment groups had a target goal of a systolic blood pressure of less than 120 mm Hg, while the standard treatment group had a target of 140 mm Hg. Again, the patient population was aged 50 years and older. The average age of the study participants was 68 years, and about 28% were over age 75 years. Also, 48% of the study participants had an estimated glomerular filtration rate of <60 mL/min/1.73m². The study was stopped early, after a median follow-up period of over 3 years, because the intensive treatment group had lower composite outcomes than the standard treatment group. The intensive treatment group had a lower rate of fatal and nonfatal major cardiovascular events and deaths from any cause. The intensive treatment group, however, had increased rates of adverse events (The SPRINT Research Group, 2015). These adverse events were hypotension, syncope, electrolyte abnormalities, noninjurious falls, and acute kidney injury or failure. So where does that leave clinicians who are caring for older patients with this common problem? The answer is not unfamiliar for geriatricians: uncertainty. On the one hand, intensive treatment targets for individuals with hypertension lead to better outcomes for older patients. On the other hand, those who receive such intensive treatment are at higher risk of problems from such treatment. Further, SPRINT does not guide us with the goals of individuals who are aged 85 years and older. The best approach is to discuss treatment targets with each patient, use shared decision-making approaches, and monitor over time.

Some of the other treatment trials that have included individuals up to 84 years suggest that there should be no age cutoff above which high blood pressure is not treated. A study specifically directed to hypertensive patients (systolic blood pressure of 160 mm Hg or more) aged 80 years or older demonstrated a 30% reduction in the rate of fatal and nonfatal stroke, a 21% reduction in the rate of death from any cause, a 23% reduction in the rate of death from cardiovascular causes, and a 64% reduction in the rate of heart failure (Beckett et al, 2008). Relatively healthy older persons at any age should be treated unless they have severe comorbid disease that will clearly limit their life expectancy or unless the toxicity of treatment is so great that it outweighs potential benefits. The treatment goal for uncomplicated hypertension is a blood pressure of less than 150/90 mm Hg. Despite the NICE guidance, controversies on management and treatment blood pressure goals persist (Godlee, 2012). Cardiovascular outcomes may not be improved with blood pressures below 130/85 mm Hg. Systolic blood pressures below 120 mm Hg may be associated with increased all-cause mortality in those aged 85 and older (Molander et al, 2008), and higher blood pressure (an average of 158 mm/Hg) is associated with better cognitive function in those over 85 (Euser et al, 2009). Stay tuned to this area of primary care and cardiovascular care for older adults. More evidence will be available over time to help guide practice. Standard care often changes over time and nuances of treatment are important to keep in mind.

THERAPY

Guidance from the American College of Cardiology and the American Heart Association (AHA) for the treatment of hypertension in older adults has recently been published (Aronow et al, 2011). Lifestyle changes are not easily accomplished but should be attempted, including maintaining ideal body weight, limiting dietary sodium intake, eating fruits and vegetables and low-fat dairy products, reducing saturated and total fats, and engaging in aerobic exercise. Foods rich in potassium, calcium, and magnesium should be consumed. Excess sodium intake and potassium deficit have adverse effects on arterial pressure and should be reversed as part of the management of all hypertensive patients (Adrogué and Madias, 2007). Other risk factors, such as smoking, dyslipidemia, and diabetes mellitus, should also be modified. It is remarkable that only about half of people with high blood pressure have it under control.

If dietary measures fail to control blood pressure, drug therapy should be considered. Physiological and pathological changes of aging should be considered in individualizing the therapy. Changes in volumes of distribution and hepatic and renal metabolism may alter pharmacokinetics (see Chapter 14). Changes in vessel elasticity and baroreceptor sensitivity may alter responses to posture and drug-induced falls in blood pressure. The duration of most of the randomized controlled trials that have studied the pharmacological treatment of hypertension in older adults is 2 to 5 years. When one reviews the Kaplan-Meier survival curves of the outcomes of treatment trials of hypertension in older adults, the benefits of treatment begin to occur in a year or two. This may depend on the specific outcome that is measured. To get a general sense of the benefit, 1000 persons were treated for 5 years in the Syst Euro trial to prevent 29 strokes or 53 cardiovascular events. Other trials (eg, SHEP and HYVET) describe similar patterns of benefit from pharmacological treatment of hypertension in older adults. There is no clear pattern to the benefit at various ages in which treatment of hypertension is initiated.

Thiazide diuretics are usually the initial step in therapy, especially in older patients with isolated systolic hypertension. They are well tolerated, are relatively inexpensive, and can be given once a day (Table 11-5). Many older hypertensive patients can be treated with diuretics as the only medication. Low-dose thiazides—for example, 12.5 to 25 mg of chlorthalidone—are efficacious in lowering blood pressure while minimizing metabolic side effects. Many experts prefer chlorthalidone over hydrochlorothiazide as a better antihypertensive. Higher doses have a minimal additional effect on blood pressure with a more marked effect on hypokalemia. Thiazides are contraindicated in patients with gout. The provider needs to take into account multiple comorbid conditions during which a thiazide diuretic could make the patient worse (eg, urine incontinence or benign prostatic hypertrophy). Postural hypotension is uncommon, but serum potassium should be monitored. Diabetics may have increased requirements for insulin or oral hypoglycemic agents.

Although β-blockers are also recommended as initial-step therapy, several meta-analyses have called this strategy into question (reviewed in Panjrath and Messerli, 2006). These meta-analyses indicate that traditional β-blockers do have efficacy in lowering blood pressure but are not known to be effective in preventing coronary artery disease, cardiovascular mortality, or all-cause mortality in older adults. When

PART III

TABLE 11-5. Thiazide Diuretics for Antihypertensive Therapy

Advantages	Adverse effects
Well tolerated	Hypokalemia
No central nervous system side effects	Volume depletion
Relatively inexpensive	Hyponatremia
Infrequent dosing	Hyperglycemia
Good response rate	Hyperuricemia
Orthostatic hypotension uncommon	Impotence
Can be used in conjunction with other agents	
Effective in advanced age	
Effective in systolic hypertension	

compared to each other, thiazides are superior to β-blockers in older adults (MRC Working Party, 1992). In the Antihypertensive and Lipid-Lowering Treatment to Prevent Heart Attack Trial (ALLHAT), thiazides were superior to angiotensin-converting enzyme (ACE) inhibitors in reducing cardiovascular disease, stroke, and heart failure (ALLHAT Collaborative Research Group, 2002). However, another trial suggests that ACE inhibitors are superior in older subjects, particularly men, in reducing cardiovascular events and mortality, but not stroke (Wing et al, 2003). β-Blocking agents may be used as the initial drug when another indication for their use exists, such as coronary heart disease, myocardial infarction (MI), heart failure, tachyarrhythmias, or essential tremor.

If thiazides alone do not control blood pressure, a second agent is added (Table 11-6) or a thiazide is added if one of the other agents has failed. The choice should be individualized and usually selected from among β-blockers, calcium channel antagonists, ACE inhibitors, or angiotensin-receptor blockers (ARBs) (The Medical Letter, 2001). β-Blockers are indicated for treatment of angina, heart failure, previous MI, and tachyarrhythmias in association with hypertension. These agents are contraindicated in patients with cardiac conduction deficits, bradyarrhythmias, and reactive airways disease. The more water-soluble β-blockers may be well suited for the geriatric population because they enter the central nervous system less readily and thus have fewer of the central nervous system side effects such as somnolence and depression; this would be a particular advantage in older adults. However, if cardiac output is decreased, renal perfusion and glomerular filtration rate may be affected. One concern with β-blockers is the production of bradycardia with reduced cardiac output. One simple test to monitor for this side effect is the patient's response to mild exercise after each dosage increase; a failure to increase pulse by at least 10 beats per minute is an indication to reduce the dosage. If a patient is to be taken off a β-blocking agent, withdrawal should be done slowly over a period of several days to avoid rebound of original symptoms.

Calcium channel antagonists are peripheral vasodilators with the advantage of maintaining coronary blood flow. These agents appear to have increased potency with age, possibly as a result of the decreased reflex tachycardia and myocardial contractility in older adults as compared with younger individuals. Headache, sodium retention, negative inotropic effects—especially in combination with β-blockers—and conduction abnormalities may limit their use. Calcium channel antagonists are effective in reducing stroke incidence in older patients with isolated systolic hypertension (Staessen et al, 1997). However, these drugs do not significantly reduce the risk of heart failure (Blood Pressure Lowering Treatment Trialists' Collaboration, 2000). Calcium channel blocker treatment in the Syst-Eur trial was superior to placebo in slowing the decline in cognitive function of older patients with hypertension (Forette et al, 1998). No comparative data are available, however, to define whether certain classes of antihypertensive medications are superior to others in preventing cognitive decline.

ACE inhibitors are effective and well tolerated for treatment of hypertension. They are both preload and afterload reducers and thus are particularly useful in the face of congestive heart failure. They prolong survival in patients with heart failure or left

TABLE 11-6. Antihypertensive Medications

Agent*	Advantages	Disadvantages
β-Blockers	Useful in angina, previous myocardial infarction, heart failure Water-soluble agents have fewer central nervous system side effects Must be withdrawn slowly in presence of coronary artery disease	Contraindicated in cardiac conduction defects and reactive airways disease May cause bronchospasm, bradycardia, impaired peripheral circulation, fatigue, and decreased exercise tolerance
Calcium channel blockers†	Peripheral vasodilator Coronary blood flow maintained Potency increased with age or in systolic hypertension	Headaches Sodium retention Negative inotropic effect Conduction abnormality
Angiotensin-converting enzyme inhibitors	Preload and afterload reduction Use in congestive heart failure, diabetes mellitus, other nephropathy with proteinuria	Hyperkalemia Hypotension Decreased renal function Cough Angioedema
Angiotensin-receptor antagonists	Use in angiotensin-converting enzyme inhibitor–induced cough, congestive heart failure, diabetes mellitus, other nephropathy with proteinuria	Hyperkalemia Angioedema (rare)
Clonidine†	Increased renal perfusion	Somnolence, depression Dry mouth, constipation Rarely, withdrawal hypertensive crisis
α-Blockers†	Useful in benign prostatic hypertrophy	Orthostatic hypotension
Hydralazine	May be useful in systolic hypertension	Reflex tachycardia, aggravation of angina Lupus-like syndrome at high dosage
Eplerenone	Aldosterone-receptor antagonist Fewer side effects than spironolactone and avoidance of gynecomastia	Hyperkalemia Contraindicated in renal insufficiency (creatinine >2.0) and in the presence of albuminuria

*With all these agents, initiation with low dosage and careful titration may minimize side effects.
†Some of the medications within these categories are included on the 2015 Beers list of potentially inappropriate medications for older adults.

PART III

ventricular dysfunction after an MI. Long-acting agents may have an advantage in adherence. Renal function, which may deteriorate on administration of these agents, must be monitored carefully. These agents may also induce hyperkalemia and should generally not be used with a potassium-sparing diuretic. Older adults are also more vulnerable to the hypotensive effects of these drugs.

ARBs are effective in lowering blood pressure without causing cough. They and ACE inhibitors are appropriate initial therapy in patients with diabetes mellitus, renal disease, or congestive heart failure (August, 2003). ARBs are superior to β-blockers in the treatment of patients with isolated systolic hypertension and left ventricular hypertrophy (Kjeldsen et al, 2002).

Clonidine may cause somnolence and depression, but it increases renal perfusion. The clonidine transdermal patch may lessen some of these adverse effects. However, local skin reactions may occur in about 15% of users. The once-per-week application of the patch may be an asset in improving adherence. This medication is listed on the AGS Updated Beers Criteria.

The major side effect of α-blockers is orthostatic hypotension; this is especially problematic with initial doses of prazosin. Newer agents with lesser hypotensive effects are now being used to treat symptomatic benign prostatic hypertrophy. In ALLHAT, the α-blocker arm was stopped early because of a higher incidence of congestive heart failure. Consequently, α-blockers are not recommended as monotherapy for hypertension and they are also listed on the AGS Updated Beers Criteria.

Although hydralazine is usually a third-step drug, it may occasionally be used as a second-step drug in older adults because reflex tachycardia rarely occurs. If used with diuretics alone, it should be initiated in low doses, which should be increased slowly. It should not be used in the absence of a β-blocker if coronary artery disease is present.

A newer available agent is eplerenone, an aldosterone-receptor antagonist. It has a better side effect profile than spironolactone, particularly the avoidance of gynecomastia in men, but needs to be used with caution in patients with renal insufficiency and microalbuminuria, and potassium must be monitored for development of hyperkalemia.

With the newer, more effective agents, drug-resistant hypertension is unusual. In such cases, drug adherence should be monitored and sodium intake assessed. If such factors are not contributing to drug resistance, secondary causes of hypertension should be considered, especially renovascular disease and primary hyperaldosteronism.

HYPERLIPIDEMIA IN OLDER ADULTS

There are several essential points to make about the treatment of hyperlipidemia in older adults. Recent guidelines have focused on those individuals who are most likely to benefit from evidence-based statin therapy to reduce the risk of atherosclerotic cardiovascular disease (see Stone, 2013 in Suggested Readings). Recommendations for prevention are based on the foundations of a healthy lifestyle. A key aspect of the recommendations is that they are designed around fixed intensity of treatment instead of fixed target for the outcomes of the medications. The fixed target strategy would have all patients below a specific level of LDL cholesterol. The recommendations, instead, describe high-intensity statin therapy as daily dosage of statin which lowers the LDL cholesterol by ≥50%. The recommendations describe moderate-intensity therapy as a daily dosage of statin which lowers the LDL cholesterol by 30% to less than 50%. (The dosage of the statin medication, hence, may be to different endpoints for different patients.) For those between ages 65 and 74 years with known atherosclerotic cardiovascular vascular disease, the treatment guidelines recommend high-intensity statin (the same as for middle-aged adults). Moderate intensity is recommended for those over age 75 years and for those who cannot tolerate the high-intensity therapy. Decisions for those over age 75 years need to take into account the benefits and risks of treatment, as well as patient preferences. Primary prevention for those adults with an LDL cholesterol that is ≥190 mg/dL is high-intensity statin therapy. The primary prevention recommendations do not specifically comment on the care for those over age 75 years. Again, the benefits and risks of treatment should be discussed with the patient. For older patients with diabetes mellitus who are between ages 65 and 74 years, moderate statin therapy is recommended (except those whose 10-year atherosclerotic cardiovascular risk is estimated to be ≥7.5% and hence would benefit from high-intensity statin). Patients should have their 10-year risk of atherosclerotic cardiovascular disease recalculated about every 4 to 6 years. The risk assessment tools, by the way, are designed to take into account patients between ages 40 and 79 years. The U.S. Preventive Services Task Force Recommendation Statement on statin use for primary prevention of cardiovascular disease described no specific choice of one statin over another (U.S. Preventive Services Task Force, 2016).

The use of statins for the primary prevention of cardiovascular disease in older patients remains a dilemma. Most of all the treatment trials of statin therapy in which older adults are enrolled have no information on cognitive or functional endpoints. There is an absence of clear evidence of the use of statins for primary prevention in adults older than age 75 years and uncertainty of the risks of therapy. Clinicians should discuss the potential benefits and risks with their patients in an approach of shared decision making (Gurwitz et al, 2016).

STROKE AND TRANSIENT ISCHEMIC ATTACKS

Although the incidence of stroke has declined dramatically, it is still a major medical problem affecting approximately 50,000 individuals in the United States every year. It is the third leading cause of death and is also a major cause of morbidity, long-term disability, and hospital admissions. Stroke is clearly a disease of older adults; approximately 75% of strokes occur in those older than age 65. The incidence of stroke rises steeply with age, being 10 times greater in the 75- to 84-year-old age group than in the 55- to 64-year-old age group.

Table 11-7 lists the types and outcomes of stroke. In cerebral infarct, thrombosis, usually arteriosclerotic, is the most common cause, with embolization from an ulcerated plaque or myocardial thrombosis being less frequent causes. Table 11-8 lists outcomes for survivors.

TABLE 11-7. Stroke

Cause	Relative frequency, %	Mortality rate, %
Subarachnoid hemorrhage	10	50
Intracerebral hemorrhage	15	80
Cerebral infarction (thrombosis and embolism)	75	40

Table 11-9 lists the modifiable risk factors for ischemic stroke. Hypertension is the major risk factor. Systolic hypertension is associated with a three- to fivefold increased risk for stroke. Hypertension accelerates the formation of atheromatous plaques and damages the integrity of vessel walls, predisposing to thrombotic occlusion and cerebral infarction. Hypertension also promotes growth of microaneurysms in segments of small intracranial arteries. Those lesions are sites of intracranial hemorrhage and lacunar infarcts.

Whether diabetes mellitus is a modifiable risk factor remains an unresolved issue. Tight glycemic control trials in type 2 diabetes have not shown improved outcomes for stroke.

Patients with a history of transient ischemic attacks (TIAs) are at substantial risk for subsequent stroke, particularly within the first few days. Completed stroke as a sequel of TIA is reported to occur in 12% to 60% or more of untreated TIA patients. In retrospective studies of patients with completed stroke, previous TIA is reported to have occurred in 50% to 75% of patients.

The keystone to the diagnosis of stroke is a clear history of sudden, acute neurological deficit.

The American Heart Association uses the five "suddens" in its public education campaign: sudden weakness, sudden speech difficulty, sudden visual loss, sudden dizziness, and/or sudden severe headaches. When the history is not clear, especially if the deficit could have had a gradual onset, consideration should be given to a mass lesion (eg, brain tumor or subdural hematoma). Brain scanning with computed tomography or magnetic resonance imaging is required to distinguish cerebral infarction from intracerebral hemorrhage. Initial laboratory testing should include a glucose level, complete blood count, troponin, and prothrombin time and partial

TABLE 11-8. Outcome for Survivors of Stroke

Outcome	Percentage
No dysfunction	10
Mild dysfunction	40
Significant dysfunction	40
Institutional care	10

TABLE 11-9. Modifiable Risk Factors for Ischemic Stroke

Alcohol consumption (>5 drinks/day)
Asymptomatic carotid stenosis (>50%)
Atrial fibrillation
Elevated total cholesterol level
Hypertension
Obesity
Physical inactivity
Smoking

thromboplastin time, especially if thrombolysis is considered. Except for the glucose level, the blood testing should not delay the initial decision for initiation of intravenous fibrinolytic therapy (as noted below). Electroencephalography is helpful only occasionally in the differential diagnosis. An ECG should be performed routinely in cases of TIA or stroke because it may relate the episode to MI or cardiac arrhythmia. Invasive techniques are usually unnecessary in stroke patients.

In older adults, symptoms acceptable as evidence of cerebral ischemia are often misinterpreted. Table 11-10 lists the presenting symptoms for TIA in the carotid and vertebral–basilar systems.

TREATMENT

The U.S. Food and Drug Administration has approved, and committees of the AHA and the American Academy of Neurology have published guidelines endorsing, the use of tissue plasminogen activator (tPA) within 3 hours of onset of ischemic stroke. The earlier that the treatment is started, the better the result. The AHA and the European Stroke Organization have recently updated their guidelines to extend the treatment window to 4.5 hours (Wechsler, 2011). Thrombolytic therapy increases the risk for early death and intracranial hemorrhage but decreases the combined endpoint of death or dependency at 3 to 6 months. The use of intravenous tPA among warfarin-treated patients (international normalized ratio [INR] ≤1.7) was not associated with increased symptomatic intracranial hemorrhage risk compared with non-warfarin-treated patients (Xian et al, 2012). In two large randomized trials, the use of aspirin initiated within 48 hours after onset of stroke and continued for 2 weeks or until discharge reduced rates of death or dependency at discharge or at 6 months. A meta-analysis found no evidence that anticoagulants in the acute phase of stroke improve functional outcomes (therapies of acute stroke reviewed in van der Worp and van Gijn, 2007).

Supportive care remains a cornerstone of initial treatment for those who do and do not receive fibrinolytic treatment. Thoughtfully evaluate the underlying cause of each abnormal finding while carefully managing blood pressure (by lowering by 15% among those with markedly elevated blood pressure), correcting hypoxia, correcting hypoglycemia, administering antipyretic medication, assessing the underlying

TABLE 11-10. Transient Ischemic Attack: Presenting Symptoms

Symptom	Carotid	Vertebrobasilar
Paresis	+++	++
Paresthesia	+++	+++
Binocular vision	0	+++
Vertigo	0	+++
Diplopia	0	++
Ataxia	0	++
Dizziness	0	++
Monocular vision	++	0
Headache	+	+
Dysphasia	+	0
Dysarthria	+	+
Nausea and vomiting	0	+
Loss of consciousness	0	0
Visual hallucinations	0	0
Tinnitus	0	0
Mental change	0	0
Drop attacks	0	0
Drowsiness	0	0
Light-headedness	0	0
Hyperacusis	0	0
Weakness (generalized)	0	0
Convulsion	0	0

+++, most frequent; 0, least frequent.

cause of infection of those with fever, and managing hypovolemia. Provide care on comprehensive specialized stroke units with early rehabilitation and appropriate stroke care order sets. Provide deep venous thrombosis prophylaxis for those who are immobilized. Assess swallowing prior to starting eating or drinking or the administration of oral medications. Those with suspected pneumonia or urinary tract infection should be treated with appropriate antibiotics. Those with less severe deficits should be mobilized with assistance early in their course of recovery. Placement of an indwelling urinary catheter is not recommended as it is associated with an increased risk of associated urinary tract infection. In summary, there are multiple details to address in the overall care of the patient with an acute stroke.

For primary prevention of stroke, adequate blood pressure reduction, smoking cessation, treatment of hyperlipidemia, glucose control in patients with diabetes, use of antithrombotic therapy in patients with atrial fibrillation, and antiplatelet therapy in patients with MI are effective and supported by evidence from several randomized trials (Straus et al, 2002). These same strategies are effective in secondary prevention of stroke, as is carotid endarterectomy in patients with severe carotid artery stenosis.

Lowering blood pressure in hypertensive individuals is effective in the secondary prevention of hemorrhagic and ischemic stroke. There are multiple nuances to lowering blood pressure in the context of an acute ischemic stroke in a patient who is otherwise eligible for tPA. Bring systolic blood pressure down to less than 185 mm Hg and diastolic blood pressure to less than 110 mm Hg prior to administering tPA. Avoid giving tPA to those with severely uncontrolled blood pressure who have not been controlled, and maintain blood pressure of 180/105 during the first 24 hours of therapy for those who have been treated with tPA. For those who have not received fibrinolytic treatment, the key theme for managing blood pressure in the first 24 hours to avoid hypoperfusion to the area of the brain which is still in jeopardy (see the American Heart Association/American Stroke Association Guidelines by Jauch et al, 2013 for important specifics). The long-term benefits of antihypertensive treatment extend to patients older than 80 years (Gueyffier et al, 1999). Thiazide diuretics, ACE inhibitors, and long-acting calcium channel blockers, as treatment for hypertension, reduce the incidence of stroke. β-Blockers are less efficacious. In patients with a recent ischemic stroke, systolic blood pressures in the range of 120 of 140 mm Hg were associated with a lower risk of recurrent stroke than blood pressures below or above this range (Ovbiagele et al, 2011). Selection of a specific class of drugs is discussed earlier in this chapter.

Patients with atrial fibrillation have a mortality rate double that of age- and sex-matched controls without atrial fibrillation. The risk of stroke with nonrheumatic atrial fibrillation is approximately 5% a year. Adjusted-dose warfarin and aspirin reduce stroke in patients with atrial fibrillation, and warfarin is substantially more efficacious than aspirin (Hart et al, 2007). Major extracranial hemorrhage is minimally increased in warfarin-treated patients. Excess bleeding risk with warfarin in older patients can be similar to the low rates achieved in the randomized trials (Caro et al, 1999; Fang et al, 2006). Therapy with clopidogrel plus aspirin is not an alternative to warfarin because it is less effective and significantly increases the risk of bleeding (ACTIVE Writing Group, 2006). Strokes that occur in patients receiving warfarin or aspirin are not more severe than those occurring in placebo-treated patients. Stroke risks and benefits of antithrombotic therapy are similar for patients with paroxysmal or chronic atrial fibrillation (Hart et al, 2000). Direct thrombin inhibitors and factor Xa inhibitors are discussed later in the "Arrhythmias" section.

The risk of ischemic stroke is increased after an MI, particularly in the first month. Aspirin reduces the risk of nonfatal stroke in patients who have experienced an MI (Antiplatelet Trialists' Collaboration, 2002). Aspirin decreases the risk of stroke in patients with previous TIA or stroke. Oral administration of aspirin is recommended within 24 to 48 hours of the stroke onset at a dosage of 325 mg for most patients. Clopidogrel is modestly more effective than aspirin in decreasing risk of the combined endpoint of stroke, MI, or vascular death (Straus et al, 2002). The overall usefulness of clopidogrel in the context of acute stroke has not been well established, per the stroke guidelines.

Carotid endarterectomy decreases the risk of stroke or death in patients with symptomatic carotid disease and severe carotid artery stenosis (70%–99%). In patients with symptomatic moderate carotid artery stenosis (50%–69%), benefits were more marginal. Carotid stenting is less invasive than endarterectomy, but in a study of patients with symptomatic carotid stenosis of 60% or more, the rates of death and stroke at 1 and 6 months were lower with endarterectomy than with stenting (Mas et al, 2006). Patients with lesser degrees of stenosis (<50%) may be harmed by surgery. For people with asymptomatic carotid disease, the optimal therapy is unclear. However, identifying carotid artery stenosis in asymptomatic individuals can involve expensive and invasive diagnostic procedures. The costs of screening large numbers of asymptomatic people outweigh the benefits to the number of individuals screening would identify.

STROKE REHABILITATION

Table 11-11 presents factors in the prognosis for rehabilitation of elderly stroke patients. Although the benefit of stroke rehabilitation is controversial, it should be initiated early in the course if it is to be of benefit. Stroke patients may fare better in acute rehabilitation facilities than in skilled nursing facilities (Beeuwkes Buntin et al, 2010; Kane, 2011). Generally, most neurological return occurs during the first month after the stroke. By the end of the third month, little, if any, further return can be expected. Not all dysfunctions result in the same level of disability. Motor loss is often the least disabling. Perceptual and/or sensory loss, aphasia, loss of balance, hemicorporal neglect, hemianopsia, and/or cognitive damage may cause more severe and often untreatable disabilities.

In the immediate rehabilitation stage, treatment is directed toward avoiding complications such as pressure sores, contractures, phlebitis, pulmonary embolism, aspiration pneumonia, and fecal impaction.

In the next stage of rehabilitation, treatment is directed toward reeducating muscles (affected areas) and enhancing remaining capabilities (unaffected areas) (reviewed in Dobkin, 2005). Table 11-12 describes measures to be taken during this phase. In patients 3 to 9 months within a first stroke, constraint-induced movement therapy produced significant and clinically relevant improvements in arm motor function (Wolf et al, 2006).

When the patient stops making progress after intensive therapy, the goal of rehabilitation shifts to finding ways for the patient to cope with the dysfunction. At this stage, the patient is assessed for the need for braces and assistive devices for both

---

TABLE 11-11. Factors in Prognosis for Rehabilitation

Availability and implementation of sound program
Mentation
Motivation
Prognosis for neurological return
Vigor

TABLE 11-12. Stroke Rehabilitation

Acute phase
   Change of patient's position at least every 2 h
   Positioning of patient's joints to prevent contractures
   Positioning of patient to prevent aspiration pneumonia
   Range-of-motion exercises
Later phase
   Activities of daily living training
   Ambulation training
   Functional activities for affected side
   Muscle reeducation exercises
   Perceptual training
   Training in transfer technique

ambulation and performance of activities of daily living. With a sound program of rehabilitation, most older patients who survive a stroke can return to the community.

CORONARY ARTERY DISEASE

The frequency of both coronary artery disease and MI increases with age. Older patients have more severe disease than younger patients, and the mortality rate is higher after an acute MI.

Hypertension is the major risk factor for coronary artery disease in older adults. Hypercholesterolemia and cigarette smoking become less important risk factors in this age group, although they are still significant. Risk factor reduction should include the preventive strategies to manage the ABCS: Aspirin when appropriate, Blood pressure control, Cholesterol management, and Smoking cessation (Lloyd-Jones et al, 2016). A recently released risk factor calculator (www.cvriskcalculator.com) helps clinicians and their Medicare patients better estimate the long-term benefit and risks from cardiovascular preventive therapies. Future treatments for coronary artery disease may focus on the underlying mechanism of disease to prevent plaque disruption and thrombosis, beyond the traditional focus of reducing stenosis (reviewed in Libby, 2013 in Suggested Readings).

Angina pectoris has a similar presentation in both older adults and in younger patients, with familiar pain characteristics and radiation. Pharmacologically, acute episodes of angina pectoris can be treated with sublingual nitroglycerin, which should be taken in the sitting position to avoid severe orthostatic hypotension. Primary therapy for chronic stable angina is aspirin and β-blockers. Both are underused in older persons, especially after acute MI. Secondary therapy includes long-acting nitrates and calcium channel blockers, but their use may be limited by orthostatic hypotension in older patients.

Younger patients with chronic symptomatic coronary artery disease benefit from revascularization. Procedure-related mortality increases with age both after coronary

PART III

artery bypass graft (Alexander et al, 2000) and after percutaneous coronary intervention (Batchelor et al, 2000). In those without significant comorbidity, mortality approaches that seen in younger patients. One-year outcomes in older patients with chronic angina are similar with regard to symptoms, quality of life, and death or nonfatal infarction with invasive versus optimized medical strategies (Pfisterer et al, 2003). Older patients with angina refractory to standard drug therapy have a choice between an early invasive strategy that carries a certain early intervention risk and an optimized medical strategy that carries a chance of late hospitalization and revascularization. After 1 year, quality-of-life outcomes and survival will be similar.

Older patients with an acute MI often present with symptoms other than chest pain (Table 11-13). Treatment of the older patient with acute MI is similar to that of the younger patient. The key themes to remember in the immediate treatment are aspirin, P2Y12 inhibitor medication (eg, clopidogrel or ticagrelor), and anticoagulation. Details and explanations are nicely described in pocket card guidelines available at http://eguidelinecentral.com. Initial β-blocker should be given in the first 24 hours, except for those with contraindications. Particular attention should be paid to the pharmacotherapy in older patients. The dosages of the medications for acute coronary syndrome and acute MI should be adjusted by weight and/or creatinine clearance to reduce adverse drug events. Management decisions for older patients should be patient centered and take into account the patient's goals and preferences. Further, the decisions need to take into account the patient's comorbidities, functional and cognitive status, and life expectancy.

The current treatment for non-ST elevation acute coronary syndrome with refractory angina is to perform an urgent/immediate diagnostic angiography with the intent to perform revascularization, if appropriate, based on the coronary anatomy for those with refractory angina or hemodynamic or electrical instability (without serious comorbidities to such procedures) (reviewed in Shahian et al, 2012). Likewise, the treatment for patients with ST elevation myocardial infarction is primary percutaneous coronary intervention (PCI), when it can be done within 2 hours of the onset of symptoms. If PCI is unavailable in rural communities, thrombolytics should be administered to eligible patients with ST elevation myocardial infarction with symptom onset within 12 hours. The patient should subsequently be transferred to a PCI capable center. Additional details regarding treatment are available on the Guideline Central home page (http://eguideline.guidelinecentral.com).

TABLE 11-13. Presenting Symptoms of Myocardial Infarction

Chest pain
Confusion
Dyspnea
Rapid deterioration of health
Syncope
Worsening congestive heart failure

No specific trials in older patients have assessed percutaneous coronary intervention versus thrombolysis for treatment of acute MI. However, subgroup analyses indicate better outcomes with percutaneous coronary intervention (reviewed in Ting et al, 2006). Coronary artery surgery can be performed with excellent symptomatic results in older patients but with increased morbidity and mortality. The strongest indication for surgery is angina pectoris refractory to medical management. In patients with left main coronary artery disease, surgery significantly improves survival over medical therapy. Patients with three-vessel disease may also have improved survival. In older adults, however, improved survival must be considered in light of the patient's projected life expectancy and the higher operative risk.

Long-term administration of β-blockers to patients after MI improves survival. Pooled analysis of intravascular ultrasound studies demonstrates that β-blockers can slow progression of coronary atherosclerosis (Sipahi et al, 2007). Despite these data, physicians are reluctant to administer β-blockers to many patients, such as older patients (Krumholz et al, 1998) and those with chronic pulmonary disease, left ventricular dysfunction, or non-Q-wave MI. However, all of these subgroups benefit from β-blocker therapy after MI (Gottlieb et al, 1998). Given the higher mortality rates in these subgroups, the absolute reduction in mortality was similar to or greater than that among patients with no specific risk factors. Other secondary prevention interventions should include aspirin, clopidogrel (for those treated with invasive therapy), ACE inhibitors (for those where specific indications exist, or angiotensin receptor blockers, for those who are intolerant of ACE inhibitors), and aldosterone blockers (where specific indications exist). Patients should be educated about blood pressure management, cholesterol management, and smoking cessation. Cardiac rehabilitation programs decrease total and cardiac mortality rates. Recent programs of the Department of Health and Human Services have been designed to promote the use of cardiac rehabilitation services. Observational studies support that doses of aspirin greater than 75 to 81 mg do not enhance efficacy, whereas larger doses are associated with an increased incidence of bleeding events (reviewed in Campbell et al, 2007). Intensive low-density lipoprotein cholesterol-lowering therapy has been shown to be beneficial in high-risk older patients with established cardiovascular disease (Wenger et al, 2007). Current data do not support adding ezetimibe to statin therapy to lower cholesterol in prevention of vascular disease (Kastelein et al, 2008).

VALVULAR HEART DISEASE

CALCIFIC AORTIC STENOSIS

Pathologically, degenerative calcification of the aortic and mitral valves is common among older adults; it is found at autopsy in approximately one-third of individuals older than age 75. For many years, degenerative aortic stenosis was thought to be caused by the passive accumulation of calcium on the surface of the aortic valve leaflet. However, the etiology of aortic valve disease has a similar pathophysiology to that of vascular atherosclerosis (Rajamannan et al, 2007). Aortic valve sclerosis is common in elderly persons (29% in the Cardiovascular Health Study) and is

PART III

associated with an increase in the risk of death from cardiovascular causes and the risk of MI, even in the absence of hemodynamically significant obstruction of left ventricular outflow (Otto et al, 1999). The frequency of aortic stenosis increases with age, appearing at autopsy in approximately 4% to 6% of those older than age 65. Isolated aortic stenosis is more common among men than women except in those older than age 80, where women predominate. Aortic insufficiency may coexist with calcific aortic stenosis, although regurgitation is usually mild and a regurgitant murmur is usually not heard.

The usual clinical presentation of aortic stenosis in older adults consists of fatigue, syncope, angina pectoris, and congestive heart failure. Some patients with aortic stenosis may be identified by incidental findings on an echocardiogram. Because systolic murmurs are a frequent finding in older adults, differentiation of mitral regurgitation, aortic sclerosis, or aortic stenosis by auscultation is a challenge. The location of the murmur is usually along the lower left sternal border and apex and often does not radiate to the axilla or carotids. It is characteristically a crescendo–decrescendo late systolic murmur ending before the second heart sound. Table 11-14 describes aspects that may help differentiate mitral regurgitation from aortic murmurs.

Differentiating aortic stenosis from aortic sclerosis can be difficult in older adults. The typical murmur and pulse of aortic stenosis may be modified in older adults. Systemic hypertension may shorten the systolic murmur of stenosis, giving it the characteristic of an aortic sclerosis murmur. Loss of vascular elasticity may modify the pulse pressure, so that the typical pulse contour of aortic stenosis is absent. Therefore, the physical examination alone is not reliable in diagnosing aortic stenosis in older adults. The addition of Doppler flow studies to echocardiography has improved the diagnostic accuracy of noninvasive procedures for aortic stenosis. The initial method for the assessment of an older adult with aortic stenosis is transthoracic echocardiogram. There are important stages of aortic stenosis from asymptomatic to symptomatic severe (based on clinical presentation, the valve hemodynamics, and the hemodynamic

TABLE 11-14. Differentiation of Systolic Murmurs				
	Postpercutaneous coronary angioplasty*	Amyl nitrate	Valsalva	Squatting
Aortic sclerosis	↑†	↑	↓	↑
Aortic stenosis	↑	↑↓	↓	↑
Idiopathic Hypertrophic Subaortic stenosis	↑	↑↑	↑↑	↓↓
Mitral regurgitation	—	↓	↓	—

*Best following a premature ventricular contraction.
†Effect of maneuver on intensity of murmur.

consequences). An evaluation of the surgical or the interventional risk should consider the patient's comorbidities, frailty, and procedural specific impediments. Cardiac catheterization for hemodynamic assessment is recommended for symptomatic patients when noninvasive tests are inconclusive or during important decision making.

Surgical mortality for valve replacement is higher in older individuals, but results have improved. Patients with severe aortic stenosis should be evaluated by a multidisciplinary heart valve team when an intervention is considered. Surgical aortic valve replacement is recommended for those who meet the indications for aortic valve replacement with low or intermediate surgical risk. Risk assessment is performed by taking into account the patient's Society of Thoracic Surgeons (STS) score, frailty, major organ system dysfunction (which is not to be improved postoperatively), or procedure-specific impediments. Excellent early and late outcomes of aortic valve replacement in people aged 80 and older have been described (Filsoufi et al, 2008). Significant coexistent coronary artery disease should be treated with bypass surgery at the time of valve replacement. In general, a biological prosthetic valve is preferred. Transcatheter aortic valve replacement has been shown to reduce death and hospitalization, with a decrease in symptoms, as an alternative to surgery in high-risk patients (Kodali et al, 2012; Makkar et al, 2012). The TAVR (transcatheter aortic valve replacement) procedure is recommended for those who meet indication for aortic valve replacement and who have a high surgical risk for aortic valve replacement (Nishimura et al, 2014).

CALCIFIED MITRAL ANNULUS

Mitral ring calcification is a disease of older adults and is most frequently found in patients older than age 70. It is reported in 9% of autopsies in individuals older than age 50 and has a striking increase with advancing age, particularly in women, in whom it rises from 3.2% in women younger than age 70 to 44% in women older than age 90.

This lesion often results in mitral insufficiency or conduction abnormalities and rarely in stenosis. It is an important contributing factor to congestive heart failure in older adults and is a site for endocarditis. As many as two-thirds of patients with mitral annulus calcification present with an apical systolic murmur of mitral regurgitation.

Echocardiography is the best technique for diagnosing mitral annulus calcification. Regurgitation is usually mild to moderate, and surgery is usually indicated only if endocarditis is superimposed. There is a higher incidence of cerebral embolism in this disorder, and thus anticoagulation with warfarin (Coumadin) may be indicated. Transesophageal Echocardiogram is better able to visualize the degree of severity of the mitral valve lesions.

MITRAL VALVE PROLAPSE

Mucoid degeneration affects mainly the mitral valve. This process allows stretching of the mitral valve leaflet under normal intracardiac pressure, with subsequent prolapse into the left atrium during systole.

Although the classic murmur is late systolic, the murmur can occur anytime in systole. Mucoid degeneration of the mitral valve has been described in approximately 1% of autopsies on patients older than age 65. It is associated with mitral insufficiency; left atrial dilatation and regurgitant murmurs are common. Mitral insufficiency caused by this disorder is usually well tolerated and rarely requires surgery. Some patients with this syndrome have abnormal ECGs and chest pain suggestive of coronary artery disease; sudden death has been reported. (Evaluation and treatment are reviewed in Foster, 2010).

Death directly from valve disease is usually related to rupture of the chordae tendineae. Although mucoid degeneration also predisposes to infective endocarditis, prophylaxis for subacute bacterial endocarditis is no longer recommended by the AHA (Wilson et al, 2007). Newer interventional cardiology procedures are available at referral centers to repair primary mitral regurgitation using a simple clip (or two) of the regurgitant valves.

IDIOPATHIC HYPERTROPHIC SUBAORTIC STENOSIS

In older adults, idiopathic hypertrophic subaortic stenosis (IHSS) may be misdiagnosed as aortic valve stenosis or mitral regurgitation. Presenting symptoms are similar to those of aortic stenosis or coronary artery disease. The presence of a bisferious arterial pulse in the presence of a systolic ejection murmur and in the absence of an aortic regurgitation murmur should suggest IHSS. The IHSS murmur usually does not radiate to the carotids. Squatting, which increases left ventricular filling, usually decreases the murmur of IHSS. Factors that decrease left ventricular volume (Valsalva maneuver, standing) increase the intensity of the murmur.

Documentation of IHSS is accomplished by echocardiography, usually transthoracic followed by transesophageal.

Therapy usually relies on β-adrenergic antagonists. Symptoms may be worsened by cardiac glycosides, which increase myocardial contractility, and diuretics, which create volume depletion. Atrial fibrillation is poorly tolerated and may require cardioversion in the rapidly deteriorating patient. Interventional cardiology procedures are available at referral centers to address this condition. During the procedure the operator injects ethanol into the hypertrophic area of the intraventricular septum. This leads to a controlled infarction of this muscle with improvement in the hemodynamics. In patients refractory to medical therapy, surgery should be considered after cardiac catheterization to assess severity of outflow obstruction and state of coronary artery flow.

ARRHYTHMIAS

Although the prevalence of arrhythmias increases with age, most older patients without clinical heart disease are in normal sinus rhythm.

Atrial fibrillation occurs in 5% to 10% of asymptomatic ambulatory older adults and more frequently in hospitalized patients. It is usually associated with underlying heart disease; the causes are the same as in younger individuals. Important extracardiac causes to consider include hypertension, obesity, hyperthyroidism, alcohol consumption/drugs, and sleep apnea. The most common symptom of those with atrial fibrillation is palpitations. Some patients are completely asymptomatic, while others present with fatigue, dyspnea, chest pain, hypotension, syncope, confusion, dizziness, or heart failure. Pulse pressure has been demonstrated to be an important risk factor for incident atrial fibrillation (Mitchell et al, 2007). Long-term treatment of hypertension with ACE inhibitors, ARBs, or β-blockers reduces the risk for atrial fibrillation (Schaer et al, 2010).

The initial assessment of the patient with suspected or proven atrial fibrillation involves characterizing the pattern of the arrhythmia (paroxysmal, persistent, long-standing persistent, or permanent), determining its cause, defining associated cardiac and extracardiac disease, and assessing thromboembolic risk. Patients with recent-onset atrial fibrillation and hemodynamic instability or angina should undergo urgent cardioversion (Falk, 2001). If the patient's condition is stable, heart rate should be controlled with intravenous diltiazem, or a β-blocker. If atrial fibrillation persists and onset is ≤48 hours, cardioversion may be attempted after initiation of heparin therapy. If onset is >48 hours, treatment should include 3 weeks of anticoagulation prior to cardioversion, unless a transesophageal echocardiogram reveals no atrial thrombus at presentation. Anticoagulation for persistent and intermittent atrial fibrillation was discussed earlier in the section on treatment of stroke and TIAs. In patients with atrial fibrillation, the choice of antithrombotic therapy should be individualized based on shared decision making after a discussion of the risks of stroke and bleeding, and the patient's values and preferences. The choice of antithrombotic therapy should be based on the risk of thromboembolism, irrespective of whether the pattern is paroxysmal, persistent, or permanent. For those with nonvalvular atrial fibrillation, the CHA_2DS_2-VASc score should be used to assess the risk of stroke (January et al, 2014). Those with a nonvalvular atrial fibrillation with a prior stroke, TIA, or a CHA_2DS_2-VASc score of 2 or more should receive oral anticoagulation with either warfarin (with an INR 2.0 to 3.0) or one of the newer agents (dabigatran, rivaroxaban, or apixaban). The newer agents are preferred if the INR is difficult to maintain. There are specifications for the dosage adjustment of the newer anticoagulant medications for varying degrees of renal impairment and these medications are not recommended for patients with end-stage chronic kidney disease who are or who are not on dialysis. Aspirin or no therapy is recommended when the patient has a CHA_2DS_2-VASc score of 1. Reassess the need for and the choice of the antithrombotic therapy at regular intervals to review the stroke and bleeding risks. Additional details regarding the management of atrial fibrillation are reviewed in recent guidelines (January et al, 2014). For long-term rate control, verapamil, diltiazem, and β-blockers should be the initial drugs of choice. β-Adrenergic blockers are especially effective in the presence of thyrotoxicosis and increased sympathetic tone. Digoxin should be considered only in patients with congestive heart failure secondary to impaired systolic ventricular function. In some patients, combinations of these drugs may be needed to control ventricular response. The maintenance dose of digoxin is usually lower in older adults because of decreased muscular

TABLE 11-15. Manifestations of Sick Sinus Syndrome

Angina pectoris
Congestive heart failure
Dizziness
Insomnia
Memory loss
Palpitations
Syncope

mass and decreased renal clearance. In patients with recurrence of persistent atrial fibrillation after electrical cardioversion and in patients with heart failure, rate control is not inferior to rhythm control (repeated cardioversion or antiarrhythmics) for prevention of death and morbidity from cardiovascular causes (Marshall et al, 2004; Roy et al, 2008; Van Gelder et al, 2002). Sinus rhythm can be maintained long term by means of circumferential pulmonary vein ablation with a significant decrease in both the severity of symptoms and the left atrial diameter (indications and outcomes reviewed in Wazni et al, 2011).

The incidence of premature ventricular contractions increases with age and occurs in approximately 10% of ECGs and in 30% to 40% of Holter monitorings. The decision to treat with antiarrhythmic therapy is difficult except in the immediate post-MI period, when it is recommended. Criteria for therapy in older patients are the same as for therapy in younger patients. The half-life of antiarrhythmic drugs is prolonged in elderly people. Therapy should be initiated at lower doses, and blood levels should be monitored (see Chapter 14).

The sick sinus syndrome is particularly common among older patients. Diagnosis is made by Holter monitor. Table 11-15 lists the symptoms of sick sinus syndrome, which are usually related to decreased organ perfusion. There is no satisfactory medical therapy. Symptomatic patients may require pacemakers, which do not seem to decrease mortality in this syndrome but can alleviate symptoms. A pacemaker may be indicated in patients with cardiac side effects from drugs used to control tachycardias in the bradycardia–tachycardia syndrome.

HEART FAILURE

Although congestive heart failure is prevalent in older adults, it is often overdiagnosed. Pedal and pretibial edema is not sufficient to warrant the diagnosis. Venous stasis may produce a similar picture. Care is needed to establish the presence of other signs of congestive heart failure (eg, cardiac enlargement, S_3 heart sound, basilar crackles, jugular venous distention, enlarged liver). Determination of ejection fraction by echocardiography assists in the diagnosis. NICE recommendations for the diagnosis of heart failure were updated in 2010, with echocardiography as the initial diagnostic test in individuals with a previous MI and measurement of serum natriuretic peptide in those without a previous MI (Mant et al, 2011). Assessment by a specialist should be considered. The NICE treatment recommendations are also reviewed in Mant et al, 2011.

More than 75% of cases of overt heart failure in older patients are associated with hypertension or coronary heart disease. Diastolic dysfunction, not systolic dysfunction, is the primary cause of heart failure in older patients and is associated with marked increases in all-cause mortality (Bursi et al, 2006; Redfield et al, 2003). Diuretics should be used to treat pulmonary congestion or peripheral edema, and β-blockers should be used to control heart rate. Few large randomized controlled trials studying the drug treatment of diastolic heart failure have been designed, and trials studying digoxin and ARBs have shown minimal benefit (Shah and Gheorghiade, 2008). Comorbidities common in patients with diastolic heart failure, including hypertension, coronary artery disease, atrial fibrillation, and diabetes mellitus, should be treated.

The mainstays of therapy for congestive heart failure as a result of systolic dysfunction in older patients, as in younger patients, are diuretics for fluid overload, ACE inhibitors or ARBs, β-blockers, and aldosterone blockers (reviewed in McMurray, 2010). Tolerance of medications may be lower and side effects of medications require closer and more frequent monitoring in older patients. To improve function and survival, all patients with chronic symptomatic congestive heart failure that is associated with reduced systolic ejection or left ventricular remodeling should be treated with ACE inhibitors. β-Blockers also improve symptoms and survival (McAlister et al, 2009). Low doses of spironolactone decrease mortality in severe heart failure (The Medical Letter, 1999), and eplerenone, a mineralocorticoid inhibitor with fewer side effects than spironolactone, has been shown to be of benefit in patients with mild symptoms (Zannad et al, 2011). Hydralazine in combination with nitrate medications is recommended as a second line treatment for those who cannot tolerate ACE inhibitors or ARBs. Digoxin is recommended for worsening or severe heart failure due to left ventricular systolic dysfunction despite first and second line treatment for heart failure. Aspirin should be prescribed for those with heart failure and atherosclerotic arterial disease. Statin use in adults with heart failure should be confined to those with coronary heart disease.

If symptoms persist despite medical therapy, referral to a specialist should be done. Cardiac resynchronization therapy with or without a defibrillator should be considered (Mant et al, 2011; Sun and Joglar, 2011).

Although low serum concentrations of digoxin (0.5–0.9 ng/mL) have been shown to reduce mortality and hospitalization in older heart failure patients, the use of digitalis preparations must be approached with caution (Ahmed, 2007). Once begun on digoxin, patients tend to remain on it long after the indications have ceased. Subtle signs of toxicity may be missed, as the drug accumulates in the presence of decreased renal function. Because of decreases in lean body mass and glomerular filtration rate, lower doses of digoxin are generally required in older patients. Initial maintenance doses should be lower, and blood levels should be monitored to avoid toxic levels. Because the therapeutic window is narrowed in older adults, patients who have been on digoxin therapy for long periods of time after an acute episode of cardiac decompensation not related to arrhythmias should be considered for discontinuation of digoxin. Weight should be monitored closely so that digoxin can be

---

TABLE 11-16. Calculation of the Ankle–Brachial Index

Formula
  Ankle–brachial index = highest right (left) ankle pressure (mm Hg)/highest arm
    pressure (mm Hg)
Interpretation of Calculated Index
  Above 0.90—normal
  0.71–0.90—mild obstruction
  0.41–0.70—moderate obstruction
  0.00-0.40—severe obstruction

Data from White C: Intermittent claudication, *N Engl J Med*. 2007 Mar 22;356(12):1241-1250.

reinstated before congestive symptoms occur. With such evaluation and monitoring, some older patients on chronic digoxin therapy for other than antiarrhythmic treatment may not require digoxin therapy.

PERIPHERAL VASCULAR DISEASE

The prevalence of peripheral vascular disease (PVD) increases with age. Cigarette smoking and diabetes mellitus are the strongest risk factors. The risk of limb loss for patients without diabetes is low. Cardiovascular disease is the major cause of death (reviewed in White, 2007, from which this section was modified). Typical intermittent claudication is present in 20% of patients, and many patients present with atypical symptoms of leg fatigue, difficulty in walking, and atypical leg pain. (Also see Chapter 10 for a discussion of PVD and its effects on mobility.)

The examination should focus on pulses, hair loss, skin color, and trophic skin changes of the lower legs and feet. The initial screening test is calculation of the ankle–brachial index (Table 11-16). A result of 0.9 or less is adequate to make the diagnosis of peripheral arterial disease. In uncertain diagnosis, further imaging with duplex ultrasound, computed tomographic angiography (CTA), or magnetic resonance angiography (MRA) may be useful. The gold standard is invasive digital subtraction angiography if an endovascular intervention is planned.

Evidence Summary

Do's

- Treat hypertension in older adults, including those over age 80 and those who have had a stroke.
- Monitor standing blood pressure in patients on antihypertensive therapy.
- Use the CHA_2DS_2-VASc score to assess thromboembolic risk for patients with nonvalvular atrial fibrillation.
- Administer β-blockers to patients after an acute MI.
- Perform echocardiogram as part of the assessment of a patient with heart failure.
- Measure serum natriuretic peptide in patients with clinical features suggestive of heart failure.

Don'ts
• Use short-acting calcium channel antagonists for long-term therapy of hypertension.
• Withhold anticoagulation for atrial fibrillation because of fall risk.

Consider
• Limiting initial therapy with β-blockers in older patients with hypertension to those with compelling indications, such as coronary heart disease, MI, heart failure, or certain arrhythmias.
• Thiazide diuretics or angiotensin-converting enzyme inhibitors as first-line therapy of hypertension.
• Percutaneous coronary intervention over thrombolysis for treatment of acute MI.
• Aortic valve replacement for aortic stenosis, including in patients over age 80.

Treatment includes risk factor modification (quitting smoking, lowering lipids, controlling hypertension, and managing diabetes), an exercise program, and antiplatelet therapy. Antiplatelet therapy is initiated with low-dose aspirin. Clopidogrel may be considered as an alternative. Cilostazol (100 mg twice a day) has been shown to improve walking distance, whereas pentoxifylline appears to be no better than placebo. If warranted for symptomatic relief, revascularization (endovascular or surgical) may be considered when the risk–benefit ratio is favorable.

REFERENCES

ACTIVE Writing Group on behalf of the ACTIVE Investigators. Clopidogrel plus aspirin versus oral anticoagulation for atrial fibrillation in the Atrial Fibrillation Clopidogrel Trial with Irbesartan for Prevention of Vascular Events (ACTIVE W): a randomised controlled trial. *Lancet.* 2006;367:1903-1912.

Adrogué HJ, Madias NE. Sodium and potassium in the pathogenesis of hypertension. *N Engl J Med.* 2007;356:1966-1978.

Ahmed A. Digoxin and reduction in mortality and hospitalization in geriatric heart failure: importance of low doses and low serum concentrations. *J Gerontol A Biol Sci Med Sci.* 2007;62A:323-329.

Alexander KP, Anstrom KJ, Muhlbaier LH, et al. Outcomes of cardiac surgery in patients > or = 80 years: results from the National Cardiovascular Network. *J Am Coll Cardiol.* 2000;1:731-738.

ALLHAT Collaborative Research Group. Major outcomes in high-risk hypertensive patients randomized to angiotensin-converting enzyme inhibitor or calcium channel blocker vs diuretic. The Antihypertensive and Lipid-Lowering Treatment to Prevent Heart Attack Trial (ALLHAT). *JAMA.* 2002;288:2981-2997.

Antiplatelet Trialists' Collaboration. Collaborative meta-analysis of randomized trials of antiplatelet therapy for prevention of death, myocardial infarction and stroke in high risk patients. *BMJ.* 2002;324:71-86.

Aronow WS, Fleg JL, Pepine CJ, et al. ACCF/AHA 2011 expert consensus document on hypertension in the elderly: a report of the American College of Cardiology Task Force on Clinical Expert Consensus documents in collaboration with the American Academy of Neurology, American Geriatrics Society, American Society for Preventive Cardiology, American Society of Hypertension, American Society of Nephrology, Association of Black Cardiologists, and European Society of Hypertension. *J Am Coll Cardiol.* 2011;57:2037-2114.

August P. Initial treatment of hypertension. *N Engl J Med.* 2003;348:610-617.

Batchelor WB, Anstrom KJ, Muhlbaier LH, et al. Contemporary outcome trends in the elderly undergoing percutaneous coronary interventions: results in 7,472 octogenarians. National Cardiovascular Network Collaboration. *J Am Coll Cardiol.* 2000;36:723-730.

Beckett NS, Peters R, Fletcher AE, et al. Treatment of hypertension in patients 80 years of age or older. *N Engl J Med.* 2008;358:1887-1898.

Beeuwkes Buntin M, Hoverman Colla C, Deb P, et al. Medicare spending and outcomes after postacute care for stroke and hip fracture. *Med Care.* 2010;48(9):776-784.

Blood Pressure Lowering Treatment Trialists' Collaboration. Effects of ACE inhibitors, calcium antagonists, and other blood pressure-lowering drugs: results of prospectively designed overviews of randomized trials. *Lancet.* 2000;356:1955-1964.

Bursi F, Weston SA, Redfield MM, et al. Systolic and diastolic heart failure in the community. *JAMA.* 2006;296:2209-2216.

Campbell CL, Smyth S, Montalescot G, et al. Aspirin dose for the prevention of cardiovascular disease. *JAMA.* 2007;297:2018-2024.

Caro JJ, Flegel KM, Orejuela ME, et al. Anticoagulant prophylaxis against stroke in atrial fibrillation: effectiveness in actual practice. *Can Med Assoc J.* 1999;161:493-497.

Chobanian AV. Isolated systolic hypertension in the elderly. *N Engl J Med.* 2007;357:789-796.

Dobkin BH. Rehabilitation after stroke. *N Engl J Med.* 2005;352:1677-1684.

Euser SM, van Bemmel T, Schram MT, et al. The effect of age on the association between blood pressure and cognitive function later in life. *J Am Geriatr Soc.* 2009;57:1232-1237.

Falk RH. Atrial fibrillation. *N Engl J Med.* 2001;344:1067-1078.

Fang MC, Go AS, Hylek EM, et al. Age and the risk of warfarin-associated hemorrhage: the anticoagulation and risk factors in atrial fibrillation study. *J Am Geriatr Soc.* 2006;54:1231-1236.

Filsoufi F, Rahmanian PB, Castillo JG, et al. Excellent early and late outcomes of aortic valve replacement in people aged 80 and older. *J Am Geriatr Soc.* 2008;56:255-261.

Forette F, Seux ML, Staessen JA, et al. Prevention of dementia in randomized double-blind placebo-controlled Systolic Hypertension in Europe (Syst-Eur) Trial. *Lancet.* 1998;352:1347-1351.

Foster E. Mitral regurgitation due to mitral-valve prolapse. *N Engl J Med.* 2010;363:156-165.

Gerstenblith G, Renlund DG, Lakatta EG. Cardiovascular response to exercise in younger and older men. *Fed Proc.* 1987;46:1834-1839.

Godlee F. Controversies over hypertension guidelines. *BMJ.* 2012;344:e653.

Gottlieb SS, McCarter RJ, Vogel RA. Effects of beta-blockade on mortality among high-risk and low-risk patients after myocardial infarction. *N Engl J Med.* 1998;339:489-497.

Gueyffier F, Bulpitt C, Borssel JP, et al. Antihypertensive drugs in very old people: a subgroup meta-analysis of randomized controlled trials. *Lancet.* 1999;353:793-796.

Gurwitz JH, Go AS, Fortmann SP. Statins for primary prevention in older adults—uncertainty and the need for more evidence. *JAMA.* 2016;316(19):1971-1972.

Hart RG, Pearce LA, Aguilar MI, et al. Met-analysis: antithrombotic therapy to prevent stroke in patients who have nonvalvular atrial fibrillation. *Ann Intern Med.* 2007;146:857-867.

Hart RG, Pearce LA, Rothbart RM, et al. Stroke with intermittent atrial fibrillation: incidence and predictors during ASA therapy. *J Am Coll Cardiol.* 2000;35:183-187.

January CT, Wann LS, Alpert JS et al. 2014 AHA/ACC/HRS guideline for the management of patients with atrial fibrillation: a report for the American College of Cardiology/American Heart Association Task Force on Practice Guidelines and the Heart Rhythm Society. *J Am Coll Cardiol.* 2014. doi:10.1016/j.jacc.2014.03.022.

Jauch EC, Saver JL, Adams HP, et al. Guidelines for the early management of patients with acute ischemic stroke: a guideline for healthcare professionals from the American Heart Association/American Stroke Association. *Stroke.* 2013;44:870-947.

Joint National Committee. *The Seventh Report of the Joint National Committee on Prevention, Detection, Evaluation, and Treatment of High Blood Pressure.* Bethesda, MD: National Institutes of Health; 2004.

Joint National Committee. 2014 evidence-based guideline for the management of high blood pressure in adults. Report from the Panel Members Appointed to the Eighth Joint National Committee (JNC8). *JAMA.* 2014;311(5):507-520.

Kane RL. Finding the right level of post-hospital care: "We didn't realize there was any other option for him." *JAMA.* 2011;305(3):284-293.

Kastelein JJP, Akdim F, Stroes ESG, et al. Simvastatin with or without ezetimibe in familial hypercholesterolemia. *N Engl J Med.* 2008;358:1431-1443.

Kjeldsen SE, Dahlof B, Devereux RB, et al. Effects of losartan on cardiovascular morbidity and mortality in patients with isolated systolic hypertension and left ventricular hypertrophy. A Losartan Intervention for End Point Reduction (LIFE) substudy. *JAMA.* 2002;288:1491-1498.

Kodali SK, Williams MR, Smith CR, et al. Two-year outcomes after transcatheter or surgical aortic-valve replacement. *N Engl J Med.* 2012;366:1685-1695.

Krause T, Lovibond K, Caulfield M, et al. Management of hypertension: summary of NICE guidance. *BMJ.* 2011;343:1-6.

Krumholz HM, Radford MJ, Wang Y, et al. National use and effectiveness of β-blockers for the treatment of elderly patients after acute myocardial infarction. *JAMA.* 1998;280:623-629.

Lloyd-Jones DM, Huffman MD, Karmali KN, et. al. Estimating longitudinal risks and benefits from cardiovascular preventive therapies among Medicare patients: the Million Hearts Longitudinal ASCVD risk assessment tool: a special report from the American Heart Association and the American College of Cardiology. *Circulation.* 2016;134.

Makkar RR, Fontana GP, Jilaihawi H, et al. Transcather aortic-valve replacement for inoperable severe aortic stenosis. *N Engl J Med.* 2012;366:1696-1704.

Mant J, Al-Mohammad A, Swain S, et al. Management of chronic heart failure in adults: synopsis of the National Institute for Health and Clinical Excellence Guideline. *Ann Intern Med.* 2011;155:252-259.

Marshall DA, Levy AR, Vidaillet H, et al. Cost-effectiveness of rhythm versus rate control in atrial fibrillation. *Ann Intern Med.* 2004;141:653-661.

Mas J-L, Chatellier G, Beyssen B, et al. Endarterectomy versus stenting in patients with symptomatic severe carotid stenosis. *N Engl J Med.* 2006;355:1660-1671.

McAlister FA, Wiebe N, Ezekowitz JA, et al. Meta-analysis: beta-blocker dose, heart rate reduction, and death in patients with heart failure. *Ann Inten Med.* 2009;150:784-794.

McMurray JJV. Systolic heart failure. *N Engl J Med.* 2010;362:228-238.

Mitchell GF, Vasan RS, Keyes MJ, et al. Pulse pressure and risk of new-onset atrial fibrillation. *JAMA.* 2007;297:709-715.

Molander L, Lovheim H, Norman T, et al. Lower systolic blood pressure is associated with greater mortality in people aged 85 and older. *J Am Geriatr Soc.* 2008;56:1853-1859.

MRC Working Party. Medical Research Council trial of treatment of hypertension in older adults: principal results. *BMJ.* 1992;304:405-412.

Nishimura RA, Otto CM, Sorajja P, et al. 2014 AHA/ACC guideline for management of patients with valvular heart disease—a report of the American College of Cardiology/American Heart Association Task Force on practice guidelines. *J Am Coll Cardiol.* 2014;63(22):e57-e185.

Ostchega Y, Dillon CF, Hughes JP, et al. Trends in hypertension prevalence, awareness, treatment, and control in older U.S. adults: data from the National Health and Nutrition Examination Survey 1988 to 2004. *J Am Geriatr Soc.* 2007;55:1056-1065.

Otto CM, Lind BK, Kitzman DW, et al. Association of aortic-valve sclerosis with cardiovascular mortality and morbidity in the elderly. *N Engl J Med.* 1999;341:142-147.

Ovbiagele B, Diener H-C, Yusuf S, et al. Level of systolic blood pressure within normal range and risk of recurrent stroke. *JAMA.* 2011;306:2137-2144.

Panjrath GS, Messerli FH. Beta-blockers for primary prevention in hypertension: era bygone? *Prog Cardiovasc Dis.* 2006;49:76-87.

Pfisterer M, Buser P, Osswald S, et al. Outcome of elderly patients with chronic symptomatic coronary artery disease with an invasive vs optimized medical treatment strategy: one-year results of the randomized TIME trial. *JAMA.* 2003;289:1117-1123.

Rajamannan NM, Bonow RO, Rahimtoola SH. Calcific aortic stenosis: an update. *Nat Clin Pract Cardiovasc Med.* 2007;4:254-262.

Redfield MM, Jacobsen SJ, Burnett JC, et al. Burden of systolic and diastolic ventricular dysfunction in the community: appreciating the scope of the heart failure epidemic. *JAMA.* 2003;289:194-202.

Roy D, Taljic M, Nattel S, et al. Rhythm control versus rate control for atrial fibrillation and heart failure. *N Engl J Med.* 2008;358:2667-2677.

Schaer BA, Schneider C, Jick SS, et al. Risk for incident atrial fibrillation in patients who receive antihypertensive drugs. *Ann Intern Med.* 2010;152:78-84.

Shah SJ, Gheorghiade M. Heart failure with preserved ejection fraction. *JAMA.* 2008;300:431-433.

Shahian DM, Meyer GS, Yeh RW, et. al. Percutaneous coronary interventions without on-site cardiac surgical backup. *N Engl J Med.* 2012;366:1814-1823.

Sipahi I, Tuzcu M, Wolski KE, et al. Beta-blockers and progression of coronary atherosclerosis: polled analysis of 4 intravascular ultrasonography trials. *Ann Intern Med.* 2007;147:10-18.

Staessen JA, Fagard R, Thijs L, et al. Morbidity and mortality in the placebo-controlled European trial on isolated systolic hypertension in the elderly. *Lancet.* 1997;350:757-764.

Straus SE, Majumdar SR, McAlister FA. New evidence for stroke prevention: scientific review. *JAMA.* 2002;288:1388-1395.

Sun S, Joglar JA. Cardiac resynchronization therapy: prospect for long-lasting heart failure remission. *J Investig Med.* 2011;59:887-892.

The Medical Letter. Spironolactone for heart failure. *Med Lett Drugs Ther.* 1999;41:81-84.

The Medical Letter. Drugs for hypertension. *Med Lett Drugs Ther.* 2001;43:17-22.

The SPRINT Research Group. A randomized trial of intensive versus standard blood-pressure control. *N Engl J Med.* 2015;373:2103-2116.

Ting HH, Yang E, Rihal CS. Narrative review: reperfusion strategies for ST-segment elevation myocardial infarction. *Ann Intern Med.* 2006;145:610-617.

U.S. Preventive Services Task Force. Statin use for the primary prevention of cardiovascular disease in adults—U.S. Preventive Services Task Force recommendation statement. *JAMA.* 2016;316(19):1997-2007.

van der Worp HB, van Gijn J. Acute ischemic stroke. *N Engl J Med.* 2007;357:572-579.

Van Gelder IC, Hagens VE, Bosker HA, et al. A comparison of rate control and rhythm control in patients with recurrent persistent atrial fibrillation. *N Engl J Med.* 2002;347:1834-1840.

Wazni O, Wilkoff B, Saliba W. Catheter ablation for atrial fibrillation. *N Engl J Med.* 2011;365:2296-2304.

Wechsler LR. Intravenous thrombolytic therapy for acute ischemic stroke. *N Engl J Med.* 2011;364:2138-2146.

PART III

Wenger NK, Lewis SJ, Herrington DM, et al. Outcomes of using high- or low-dose atorvastatin in patients 65 years of age or older with stable coronary disease. *Ann Intern Med.* 2007;147:1-9.

White C. Intermittent claudication. *N Engl J Med.* 2007;356:1241-1250.

Wilson W, Taubert KA, Gewitz M, et al. Presentation of infective endocarditis. *Circulation.* 2007;116:1736-1754.

Wing LMH, Reid CM, Ryan P, et al. A comparison of outcomes with angiotensin-converting-enzyme inhibitors and diuretics for hypertension in the elderly. *N Engl J Med.* 2003;348:583-592.

Wolf SL, Winstein CJ, Miller JP, et al. Effect of constraint-induced movement therapy on upper extremity function 3 to 9 months after stroke. *JAMA.* 2006;296:2095-2104.

Xian Y, Liang L, Smith EE et al. Risks of intracranial hemorrhage among patients with acute stroke receiving warfarin and treated with intravenous tissue plasminogen activator. *JAMA.* 2012;307:2600-2608.

Zannad F, McMurray JJV, Krum H, et al. Eplerenone in patients with systolic heart failure and mild symptoms. *N Engl J Med.* 2011;364:11-21.

SUGGESTED READINGS

Amsterdam EA, Wenger NK, Brindis RG, et. al. 2014 AHA/ACC Guidelines for the management of patients with non-ST-elevation acute coronary syndromes: a report of the American College of Cardiology/American Heart Association Task Force on Practice Guidelines. *J Am Coll Cardiol.* 2014;64(24):e139-e228.

Carabello BA. Aortic stenosis. *N Engl J Med.* 2002;346:677-682.

Chen MA. Heart failure with preserved ejection fraction in older adults. *Am J Med.* 2009;122:713-723.

Haider AW, Larson MG, Franklin SS, et al. Systolic blood pressure, diastolic blood pressure, and pulse pressure as predictors of risk for congestive heart failure in the Framingham heart study. *Ann Intern Med.* 2003;138:10-16.

Kane GC, Karon BL, Mahoney DW, et al. Progression of left ventricular diastolic dysfunction and risk of heart failure. *JAMA.* 2011;306:856-863.

Kitzman DW, Little WC, Brubaker PH, et al. Pathophysiological characterization of isolated diastolic heart failure in comparison to systolic heart failure. *JAMA.* 2002;288:2144-2150.

Kostis JB, Cabrera J, Cheng JQ, et al. Association between chlorthalidone treatment of systolic hypertension and long-term survival. *JAMA.* 2011;306:2588-2593.

Libby P. Mechanisms of acute coronary syndromes and their implications for therapy. *N Engl J Med.* 2013;368:2004-2013.

Mitka M. New guidance covers ways to prevent and treat hypertension in elderly patients. *JAMA.* 2011;305:2394-2398.

Stone NJ, Robinson J, Lichtenstein AH, et al. 2013 ACC/AHA guideline on the treatment of blood cholesterol to reduce atherosclerotic cardiovascular risk in adults: a report of the American College of Cardiology/American Heart Association Task Force on Practice Guidelines. *Circulation.* 2013. doi:10.1161/01.cir.0000437738.63853.7a/-/DC1.

Van Gelder IC, Groenveld HF, Crijns HJGM. Lenient versus strict rate control in patients with atrial fibrillation. *N Engl J Med.* 2010;362:1363-1373.

Wilber DJ, Pappone C, Neuzel P, et al. Comparison of antiarrhythmic drug therapy and radiofrequency catheter ablation in patients with paroxysmal atrial fibrillation. *JAMA.* 2010;303:333-340.

PART III

CHAPTER 12

Decreased Vitality

DECREASED VITALITY IN THE CONTEXT OF FRAILTY

Older adults frequently report decreased vitality, which has a host of underlying causes. This chapter outlines metabolic factors that may lead to decreased energy in the older adults: endocrine disease, anemia, poor nutrition, and infection. Lack of exercise is discussed in Chapter 5. Although the topic of frailty is outlined in Chapter 1, this chapter will provide some essential clinical points to assist primary care providers at the bedside.

- **When to consider the diagnosis of frailty**
  Older individuals should be considered for frailty at times of vulnerability or of an anticipated threat. Examples of such threat would be at the time of an injury or trauma. Likewise, the assessment should be made at the time of surgery or of elective surgery. Further, the assessment should be performed early in a hospital course or at the time of consideration for the start of chemotherapy. Finally, the assessment should be considered in the setting of weight loss, of falls, or in the setting of multiorgan system dysregulation. In short, one should consider the diagnosis of frailty during the time of an assessment of a vulnerable older patient.
- **How to make the diagnosis of frailty**
  The criteria for frailty has been defined by the frailty phenotype and the Canadian Study of Health and Aging Clinical Frailty Scale. Each of these tools is described in Chapter 1.
- **How to use frailty to help guide decision making**
  The frailty screening tools should lead to a more thorough assessment of the whole patient. Frailty frames the context of important decisions for older patients, but it is also the starting point for further evaluation of why the person has become frail. This evaluation should review the medical causes (including multiple comorbid illnesses, as well as many of the conditions described later in this chapter), their medications, the patient's behavioral health needs, their social needs, and the meaning of the current situation to the individual. This biopsychosocial approach is the starting point for the assessment of a frail older patient.
  Frailty should not preclude access to health care, but instead should guide the development of the most appropriate care plan to match with the patient's needs. This plan should take into account the patient's goals and preferences.

PART III

- **How to help a frail older patient**

  Several key points need to be made regarding the clinical management of frail older patients. First, look for the underlying medical problems that could be culminating in frailty. Second, carefully take into account unaddressed social and behavioral health needs of the individual. A social worker as part of your team can help fill in the details here. Next, review the medications for potential adverse drug events, including medications that have been prescribed for many years. In short, critically review the indications for these meds and whether the medication could be contributing to the patient's current state. A clinical pharmacist as a part of an interdisciplinary team could help guide this assessment. Then, think about the overall prognosis of the patient. Consider using an online tool for this, such as www.eprognosis.org. Next, make sure that the patient has had the opportunity to express what is most important to him or her. This patient input frames the discussion of his or her goals and preferences. From there, define if the patient has an advance directive. If not, make sure to engage the patient in this process. Consider your role in communicating about the patient's frailty with other providers who are consulting in the patient's care. This will likewise help in their shared decision making with the patient. Make sure to initiate nutritional support and an appropriate physical therapy assessment into the interdisciplinary care of the individual. Finally, provide appropriate monitoring of the patient's care plan over time.

- **Defining the trajectory of frailty**

  Individuals who are frail often respond poorly to a perturbation in their health or environment. Some may move to a state of adult failure to thrive, which may be a predeath state of decline over a period of weeks to months. Others may move quickly to multisystem failure and death. Still others may be able to withstand the threat and plateau out at a new functional state. Primary care providers should review the trajectory of older patients as they assess patients who have become frail. To do this one might graph the weight of an individual over time. Likewise, one could review (and graph) the functional status of the patient 1, 3, and 6 months prior. A busy practice may make it difficult to take a moment to review the overall trajectory of the patient over time, but it is a worthwhile investment. Alternatively, one might simply ask the patient or family caregiver for his or her perspective of the vulnerability trajectory over the prior several months. This may give a better understanding of the course of the patient's condition.

  While decline to functional dependency may flow from frailty, it is not inevitable. A holistic approach to the individual and defining "what is fixable" serves as the framework to guide clinicians in their care of vulnerable older patients. Some of the main themes in helping frail individuals over time are best addressed in supporting their psychosocial needs. Some of the additional considerations in the assessment of a frail patient are also noted in the topics of this chapter.

ENDOCRINE DISEASE

CARBOHYDRATE METABOLISM

Over 11 million older adults in the United States have diabetes mellitus, making up approximately 26% of all older adults. Approximately a third of these individuals are undiagnosed. Each year in America there are about 400,000 new cases of diabetes diagnosed among persons aged 65 years and older. In short, diabetes mellitus affects the lives of millions of older adults in our country.

Approximately 50% of older people have glucose intolerance with normal fasting blood sugar levels. Although poor diet, obesity, and lack of exercise may account for some of these findings, aging itself is associated with deteriorating glucose tolerance. This is primarily attributable to a change in peripheral glucose utilization, although beta-cell dysfunction and decreased insulin secretion are also contributing factors. Glucose intolerance alone is not sufficient to diagnose diabetes mellitus. However, such individuals are at increased risk of developing diabetes mellitus. Prediabetes is identified as impaired fasting glucose (fasting plasma glucose level of 100–125 mg/dL), as impaired glucose tolerance (plasma glucose level of 140–199 mg/dL 2 hours after 75 g of glucose), or as a glycosylated hemoglobin of 5.7% to 6.4% (reviewed in Inzucchi, 2012 and in the "Professional" section of the American Diabetes Association website at www.diabetes.org). Lifestyle modification, including weight loss and exercise, prevents or forestalls the development of type 2 diabetes in individuals with glucose intolerance (Diabetes Prevention Program Research Group, 2002; reviewed in Gillies et al, 2007).

The U.S. Preventive Services Task Force (USPSTF) recommended that adults aged 40 to 70 years old who are overweight or obese should receive a blood glucose screen as part of their cardiovascular risk assessment (Selph et al, 2015). The USPSTF noted that clinicians should provide, or refer patients with abnormal blood glucose for, intensive behavioral counseling to promote a healthful diet and physical activity. The recommendation further noted that screening for diabetes did not improve the mortality rate after 10 years of follow-up in two trials, but was found to decrease mortality rates in a lifestyle intervention study with 23 years of follow-up. Treating adults with impaired fasting glucose and impaired glucose tolerance tests was associated with delayed progression to diabetes.

Both the USPSTF and the American Diabetes Association (ADA) recommend intensive behavioral counseling, a healthful diet, and physical activity for patients at risk for diabetes (Selph et al, 2015).

The high number of older adults with diabetes is in part related to the aging of our population and, as well, related to the increasing rates of adults who are overweight and obese. The incidence of diabetes increases continuously with advancing age until age 65 and then levels off. Many older Americans develop diabetes after age 65 (incident diabetes), while others have had diabetes as middle-aged adults and continue with this condition as they age. Those who experienced the onset of diabetes as middle-aged adults are more likely to develop retinopathy as they age, compared to those who develop diabetes at an advanced age, but there is no difference (middle-age onset vs advanced-age onset) in the likelihood of developing cardiovascular disease or peripheral neuropathy. The study on which this epidemiologic description is based is a cross-sectional survey of diabetes complications among a large population of individuals who had developed diabetes in their middle age and in late life. Hence developing diabetes late in life puts that individual at risk for developing end-organ damage. Clearly this illness leads to important complications that have an impact on the morbidity and mortality of millions of people in their advancing age. However, as noted below, treatment should be prescribed in the context of the whole patient. Putting a frail 85-year-old on a strict regimen may make her life less worth living. The single best reference on this topic is a consensus report prepared by the American Diabetes Association titled *Diabetes in Older Adults* (Kirkman et al, 2012).

The diagnosis of diabetes should be made based on a fasting plasma glucose level of ≥126 mg/dL or a glycosylated hemoglobin of ≥6.5% and confirmed by either test. The American Diabetes Association further notes that the diagnosis of diabetes can also be made with a 2-hour plasma glucose ≥200mg/dL during a 75-g oral glucose challenge test. In absence of unequivocal hyperglycemia, results should be confirmed by repeat testing. If the patient has discordant test results, the value that is abnormal should be repeated. If the value on the repeated test is abnormal, then the patient should be considered to have diabetes. Further discussion of the 2017 classification and diagnosis of diabetes is available at www.diabetes.org. Initial evaluation in patients with type 2 diabetes should include glycosylated hemoglobin level, fasting lipid profile, basic metabolic panel, a spot urine albumin-to-serum creatinine ratio, and thyroid function tests for older women. The presenting symptoms of diabetes mellitus do not change with advancing age, except that many older patients with diabetes may have comorbid conditions. The symptoms of polydipsia and polyuria are just as likely in older patients as in middle-aged individuals. The additional symptoms may include weight loss, fatigue, lethargy, falls in the prior year, and concurrent infections. It is imperative to define the older individual's ability to perform basic and instrumental activities of daily living. The clinician should likewise ask about other important medical conditions, such as kidney disease, hypertension, cardiovascular or peripheral vascular diseases, or hyperlipidemia. The key physical examination findings of diabetes in an older adult would include an assessment of blood pressure, of body mass index, and of any change in weight. The bedside examination would further focus on a cognitive screen such as the Mini-Cog, a depression screen with the PHQ-2 tool, a funduscopic examination, a hearing screen, a gait and balance examination with the Timed Up and Go test, a cardiovascular examination, and a foot examination.

Providers caring for older adults with diabetes must take into account the heterogeneity of individuals when setting and prioritizing treatment goals. Some older adults with diabetes have little comorbidity and are quite active. Others may have multiple diabetes-related comorbid illnesses, frailty, functional limitations, and/or cognitive impairment. The approach to treatment for the older patient must take into account the individual's unique health needs and goals. The therapeutic goal for relatively healthy, nonfrail older diabetic patients is the same as that for younger patients: normal fasting plasma glucose without hypoglycemia. The American Diabetes Association (www.diabetes.org website in the Professional Resources online) recommends that the treatment goals for older adults with diabetes who are highly functional and cognitively intact with a significant life expectancy should be the same as goals developed for younger adults. Generally, the approach to older patients should take into account the patient's medical condition, functional status, and mental and social needs. Further, some of the glycemic goals should be relaxed while understanding that hyperglycemia leading to symptoms or risks of acute complications should be avoided. The risk of diabetic ketoacidosis is generally smaller than in middle-aged and in younger adults.

Hypoglycemia may in fact pose greater risk for some than hyperglycemia. This is a good example of narrowing the therapeutic window described in Chapter 4. Older adults are at particular risk of hypoglycemia because of insulin deficiency necessitating insulin therapy and renal insufficiency. Further, older adults may have unrecognized cognitive deficits resulting in difficulty in some of the executive function required to manage the complex self-care activities of diabetes management. Among older diabetic patients, the presence of multiple comorbid illnesses or functional impairments is a more important predictor of limited life expectancy and diminishing expected benefits of intensive glucose control than is age alone (Huang et al, 2008). Although glycemic control may provide benefit in many older individuals, the greater risk of hypoglycemia in older adults must be considered when managing diabetes mellitus in this population (Ligthelm et al, 2012). Large randomized trials in patients with type 2 diabetes suggest that tight glycemic control burdens patients with complex treatment programs, hypoglycemia, weight gain, and costs and offers uncertain benefit in return (Montori and Fernandez-Balsells, 2009). There is also an association between tight glycemic control (HbA1c <7%) and a greater risk of hip fracture (Puar et al, 2012). In community-dwelling, nursing home–eligible individuals with diabetes mellitus, HbA1c of 8.0% to 8.9% is associated with better functional outcomes at 2 years than HbA1c of 7.0% to 7.9% (Yau et al, 2012). The American Geriatrics Society now recommends a HbA1c target of 8.5% to 9% for older patients with diabetes who have very complex health problems (those who require long term care or who have end-stage chronic illnesses or moderate to severe cognitive impairment or two or more functional dependencies). Quality-of-life considerations need to be taken into account in this situation.

Because most patients with adult-onset diabetes are obese, weight reduction should be attempted, although only approximately 10% will maintain a prolonged weight loss. Dietary fats should be reduced. Aerobic exercise can both delay the onset of type 2 diabetes mellitus and improve insulin resistance in individuals with established disease (Boulé et al, 2001). A combination of aerobic and resistance training is effective in lowering HbA1c levels in patients with type 2 diabetes mellitus (Church et al, 2010). Diet plus exercise is more effective than diet alone.

Several groups of oral hypoglycemic agents and noninsulin, injectable medications for diabetes, each with a different mechanism of action, are now available.

Metformin is the first-line agent in the treatment of older adults with type 2 diabetes mellitus. Comparative effectiveness and safety of medications for type 2 diabetes and clinical practice guidelines have been published (Bennett et al, 2011; Inzucchi et al, 2015; Qaseem et al, 2012). Table 12-1 outlines the mechanisms of action of these medications, the particular nuances for prescribing in older adults, and general cost considerations. The cost of medication needs to be factored into the overall care plan, especially considering that these medications will be needed over a long period of time. Specific contraindications are outlined, as well as strategies to monitor for possible side effects. A key point to keep in mind is high risk of drug–drug interactions. The clinician is encouraged to use computer software tools to assess for such interactions, prior to prescribing and during routine care.

Some older patients cannot achieve glycemic control in spite of optimal antihyperglycemic medications. Insulin treatment may be initiated in these individuals while adjusting the patient's baseline regime. Be aware of the complexity of the medication regimes for the patients and consider working with a diabetic educator who can assist with guiding the patient's medications, lifestyle counseling, and nutrition. The benefits and risks of tight control should be discussed with the patient in a mode of shared decision making.

The treatment of diabetes mellitus has become considerably more complex in the context of the development of multiple newer medications. The core of all treatment remains healthy eating, weight control, increased physical activity, and diabetes education. Monotherapy with metformin is initiated at the time of diagnosis or soon thereafter, unless there are contraindications. If hemoglobin A1c targets are not attained after about 3 months of monotherapy, dual therapy is initiated with one of six treatment options including a sulfonylurea, a thiazolidinedione, a DPP-4 inhibitor, an SGLT2 inhibitor, a GLP-1 receptor agonist, or basal insulin. The choice of which agent should be added to metformin is based on the patient's comorbid diseases, the hypoglycemic risks, possible side effects of the medications (including weight gain), and costs of the medications. If the patient's hemoglobin A1c targets are still not achieved after 3 months of dual therapy, a three-drug combination is advised. Likewise, a combination injectable therapy is considered for those who still do not achieve target of treatment.

Glucose control is a cornerstone of treatment for older individuals with diabetes mellitus. Reducing hyperglycemia reduces the onset and progression of microvascular complications. The benefit of tight glucose control on cardiovascular complications is less certain. A modest benefit is likely to be present, but emerges only after years of improved control. Overly aggressive control of glucose in some older patients with more advanced disease may not provide significant benefit and may in fact pose risks. The overall approach should take into account the benefits of glucose control and risks of adverse effects of the medications (primarily hypoglycemia) as well as the patient's age and health status. Modulation of the intensiveness of blood glucose lowering depends on the patient and disease features (reviewed in Inzucchi et al, 2015).

The control of the older person's glucose is in the context of that person's overall cardiovascular risk reduction. Diabetics are at increased risk of macrovascular disease.

TABLE 12-1. Common Noninsulin Medications for Diabetes Mellitus in Older Adults

Class/medication examples	Mechanism of action	Key principles when prescribing to older adults*	Additional notes
Biguanides: Metformin	Inhibit hepatic glucose production	Obtain estimated GFR prior to prescribing. Initial and subsequent dosing should be conservative—avoid maximum dosage. Monitor renal function carefully and avoid if estimated GFR between 30 and 45 ml/minute/1.73 meter² (See additional notes.) May benefit cardiovascular outcomes. Discontinue prior to iodinated contrast imaging in patients with estimated GFR between 30–60 mL/min/1.73 m², a liver disease, alcoholism, heart failure, or if intra-arterial iodinated contrast. Reassess in 48 hours after stable renal function. Several drug–drug interactions notable. $	FDA black box warning: lactic acidosis. Contraindicated in: 1. Acute and chronic metabolic acidosis. 2. Estimated GFR less than 30 mL/min/1.73 m² 3. Hypoxia. 4. Dehydration. Hepatic impairment is a risk factor for the development of lactic acidosis with this medication. Nausea, vomiting, diarrhea are common side effects.
Second-generation sulfonylureas: Glipizide Glimepiride	Increase beta-cell insulin secretion	Watch for hypoglycemia and weight gain. Conservative initial and subsequent dosage recommended. Several drug–drug interactions notable. $	Glyburide is a Beers medication and should not be used in older adults, hence is not included as an example Rx. Contraindicated in patients with hypersensitivity to the medication; sulfonamide derivatives. Contraindicated to use this medication concurrently with other sulfonamide-containing medication classes.

(continued)

PART III

TABLE 12-1. Common Noninsulin Medications for Diabetes Mellitus in Older Adults *(continued)*

Class/medication examples	Mechanism of action	Key principles when prescribing to older adults*	Additional notes
Meglitinides: Repaglinide Nateglinide	Increase insulin secretion	Decreased postprandial glucose. Watch for hypoglycemia and weight gain. Frequent dosing schedule (prior to meals). Increased hypoglycemic risk in debility, elderly, malnourished. Several drug–drug interactions notable. $$	Contraindicated in patients with hypersensitivity to the medication. Headache.
Thiazolidinediones: Pioglitazone Rosiglitazone	Increase insulin sensitivity	Assess liver function tests prior to starting Rx and during treatment. Edema, heart failure. Increased weight. Bone fractures in women. Increased LDL possible with rosiglitazone; increased HDL both meds. Increased MI for rosiglitazone, hence this med is highly restricted. Macular edema. Several drug–drug interactions notable. $	FDA black box warning: Can cause or worsen heart failure in some patients. Contraindicated in patients with New York Heart Association Class 3 or 4 heart failure. Contraindicated in patients with hypersensitivity to the medication. Concerns about increased risk of bladder cancer from pioglitazone.
Alpha-glucosidase inhibitors: Acarbose Miglitol	Slow intestinal carbohydrate absorption	No hypoglycemia. Flatulence and diarrhea may result in intolerance in older adults. Decreased postprandial glucose. Several drug–drug interactions notable. $$	Contraindicated in context of numerous gastrointestinal disorders; diabetic ketoacidosis, and hypersensitivity to the medication.

Drug	Mechanism	Effects	Notes
DPP-4 inhibitors: Sitagliptin Saxagliptin Linagliptin Alogliptin	Increase insulin secretion Decrease glucagon secretion	No hypoglycemia. Take into account renal function when dosing. Angioedema/urticaria and other important dermatologic side effects. Possible pancreatitis, pancreatic neoplasia. More heart failure hospitalizations. Several drug–drug interactions notable. $$$	Prescribe cautiously if at all in those with preexisting heart failure. Particular caution noted in patients with a history of pancreatitis. Severe arthralgia has been reported.
Bile acid sequestrants: Colesevelam	Decrease hepatic glucose production Increase incretin levels	No hypoglycemia. Complex lipid changes. Constipation. Several drug–drug interactions notable. $$$	Contraindicated in patients with (1) history of bowel obstruction, (2) serum triglyceride level of more than 500 nh/dL, (3) history of hypertriglyceridemia associated pancreatitis.
Dopamine-2 agonists: Bromocriptine	Modulate hypothalamic regulation of metabolism Increase insulin sensitivity	No hypoglycemia. Possible decrease in cardiovascular events. Dizziness/syncope/headache. Several drug–drug interactions notable. $$$	Contraindicated in patients with any sensitivity to bromocriptine, ergot alkaloids. Nausea and fatigue. Rhinitis.
SGLT2 inhibitors: Canagliflozin Dapagliflozin Empagliflozin	Block renal glucose reabsorption, increasing glucose in urine	No hypoglycemia. Decreased weight. Decreased blood pressure. Increased serum potassium possible. Several drug–drug interactions notable. $$$	FDA alert: Increased risk of renal injury for canagliflozin and dapagliflozin. Multiple additional safety alerts in years 2015 and 2016. Increased genitourinary infections. Polyuria. Volume depletion with implications. Increased LDL.

(continued)

PART III

TABLE 12-1. Common Noninsulin Medications for Diabetes Mellitus in Older Adults (*continued*)

Class/medication examples	Mechanism of action	Key principles when prescribing to older adults*	Additional notes
GLP-1 receptor agonists: Exenatide Liraglutide Albiglutide Dulaglutide	Increase insulin secretion Decrease glucagon secretion Slow gastric emptying Increase satiety	No hypoglycemia. Decreased weight. Decrease in some cardiovascular risk factors. Headache. Not recommended in patients with severe renal impairment. Several drug–drug interactions notable. $$$	FDA black box warning: C-cell thyroid tumors and avoid in patients with personal or family history of medullary thyroid carcinoma. Possible pancreatitis, pancreatic neoplasia. Nausea/vomiting/diarrhea. Tachycardia. Requires injection.
Amylin mimetics: Pramlintide	Decrease pancreatic glucagon secretion Delay gastric emptying Increase satiety	Decreased postmeal glucose. Decreased weight. Lower the individual's insulin dosage requirement. May cause headache. Several drug–drug interactions notable. $$$	FDA black box warning: Co-administration with insulin may lead to severe and persistent hypoglycemia. Nausea/vomiting. Must reduce insulin dose simultaneously to avoid hypoglycemia. Injectable at separate site. Do *not* mix with insulin. Frequent dosing required.

*Cost: low, $; moderate, $$; high, $$$.

Other atherosclerotic risk factors such as smoking, dyslipidemia, and hypertension should be addressed. Therapy of these risk factors may be of greater benefit than tight glucose control in older diabetics. Blood pressure control reduces both micro- and macrovascular complications in type 2 diabetes (United Kingdom Prospective Diabetes Study Group, 1998). There is no evidence from randomized trials to support a strategy of lowering systolic blood pressure below 135 to 140 mm Hg in persons with type 2 diabetes mellitus (Cushman et al, 2010). A meta-analysis of cholesterol-lowering and blood pressure–lowering trials demonstrated large, significant effects on reducing macrovascular disease in type 2 diabetes (Huang et al, 2001). However, this meta-analysis analyzed studies with predominantly middle-aged partcipants, although one study had middle-aged and older patients up to age 73. Angiotensin-converting enzyme (ACE) inhibitors and angiotensin-receptor blockers (ARBs) attenuate progression of nephropathy in both type 1 and type 2 diabetic patients with hypertension and in normotensives with microalbuminuria. They also attenuate decline in renal function in normotensive, normoalbuminuric type 2 diabetic patients (reviewed in Strippoli et al, 2006). The antihypertensive regimen of diabetics should include an ACE inhibitor or ARB, and such therapy should be initiated in normotensive albuminuric patients. Intensified multifactorial intervention with tight glucose regulation and the use of renin–angiotensin system blockers, aspirin, and lipid-lowering agents has been shown to reduce the risk of nonfatal cardiovascular disease and the rates of death from cardiovascular causes and death from any cause (Gaede et al, 2008).

Table 12-2 describes multiple issues that need to be considered in the care of older individuals with diabetes mellitus. Common comorbidities and geriatric syndromes are noted along with the context of the care for the older adult. Essential points are outlined to help guide the approach to help the patient. The approach to care of older persons with diabetes in the long-term care setting requires a few additional comments. Treatment should be individualized. Diabetes education the staff of the skilled nursing facility is fundamental. Additional points are outlined in the table.

Older adults with diabetes are a heterogeneous population. They may differ in their duration of diabetes mellitus, their rate of microvascular complications, their macrovascular complications, their comorbid illnesses, their geriatrics syndromes, their functional abilities, and their prognosis. The management of older individuals with diabetes mellitus should emphasize gaining skills and confidence to live healthier lives. The focus of chronic disease self-management includes healthy eating, being active, adhering to medications, learning coping skills, and monitoring blood glucose. The most common strategies for delivering these behaviors to populations have been through Chronic Disease Self-Management Programs and Diabetes Self-Management Programs. This evidence-based program results in a variety of improvements in health outcomes. In a 6-month randomized controlled trial of Chronic Disease Self- Management, the participants who received the intervention had improvements in exercise, cognitive symptom management, communication with physicians, self-reported health, health distress, fatigue, disability, and social/role activity limitations. In a 2-year follow-up study, the participants continued with

TABLE 12-2. Common Clinical Conditions to Consider in the Care of Older Individuals With Diabetes Mellitus

Condition	Special considerations for older adults	Essential points
Multiple comorbid conditions	The presence of multiple comorbid illnesses or functional impairment is a more important predictor of limited life expectancy and diminishing expected benefits of intensive glucose control, than age alone.	Older adults who have no or minor microvascular complications of diabetes, are free of concurrent illnesses, and have an estimated life expectancy of 10–15 years should have hemoglobin A1c target of <7%, if it can be safely achieved.
Functional impairment	Aging and diabetes are both associated with functional impairment. Multiple comorbid conditions each can cause debility.	Assess functional status regularly, as it is a key determinant in the framework for defining diabetes treatment goals. Physical activity interventions improve function in older persons with and without diabetes.
Cognitive impairment	Alzheimer disease and multi-infarct dementia occur twice as often in older persons with diabetes than in age-matched nondiabetic persons. Diabetes self-management requires executive function skills.	Cognitive impairment increases the risk of developing hypoglycemia for older persons with diabetes. Also, a history of severe hypoglycemia increases the risk of dementia. Periodically screen for cognitive impairment using standard tools, particularly in those with impairment in instrumental activities of daily living and decline in basic self-cares. Neuropsychological evaluation should be considered for those in whom dementia is suspected.
Injurious falls and fractures	Women with diabetes have a higher risk of hip and proximal humeral fractures. Avoiding high or low glucose may decrease the risk of falls.	Assess falls risk and perform functional assessment periodically in older adults with diabetes.

Polypharmacy	Older adults with diabetes take medications that are prescribed to control comorbidities and to reduce the risk of diabetes complications. Costs of many diabetes meds are high.	Focus attention on medication reconciliation, ongoing review of the indications for each Rx, medication adherence, and barriers. Medication management requires executive function.
Depression	Diabetes in older adults is associated with a high prevalence of depression, which if untreated can lead to poor self-care, poor lifestyle choices, higher dementia rates, and higher mortality.	Screen for and treat depression in this high-priority population.
Vision and or hearing impairment	Vision impairment occurs in about 20% of older adults with diabetes. Hearing impairment occurs at twice the usual rate.	Screen for glaucoma every 12 months for older adults with diabetes (covered by Medicare Part B). Control glucose and blood pressure to decrease risk of diabetic retinopathy. Screen at time of diagnosis.
Urine incontinence	Higher rates of urinary incontinence, especially among older women who have diabetes.	Assess urinary incontinence and treat as in older patients with no diabetes. Uncontrolled hyperglycemia can increase urine amount and frequency.
Persistent pain	Higher rates of pain, often from peripheral neuropathy, are associated with multiple adverse outcomes, including higher health-care costs.	Assess pain at each visit in older patients with diabetes. Implement strategies to ameliorate pain and promote functional independence.
Cardiovascular risk factors	Treat with consideration of the timeframe of benefit and the individual patient. Blood pressure control and lipid management goals can be relaxed in context of palliative care.	Treatment of hypertension is indicated in the context of almost all patients. Lipid-lowering meds and aspirin are reasonable if life expectancy is more than a year or two.

(continued)

PART III

TABLE 12-2. Common Clinical Conditions to Consider in the Care of Older Individuals With Diabetes Mellitus (*continued*)

Condition	Special considerations for older adults	Essential points
Skilled nursing home care	Diabetes prevalence: 22% Caucasian and 36% non-Caucasian residents. Compared to matched residents with no diabetes, more falls, cognitive decline, cardiovascular disease, depression, and functional dependencies.	Establish glycemic goals and make careful choices of glucose-lowering agents. Therapeutic should be reviewed to avoid unintended weight loss. Provide staff education on diabetes care.
End-of-life care	Higher rates of premature death.	Primary goals: comfort, symptom management, quality of life, dignity.
Lipid control	High rates of hyperlipidemia in older adults.	Lifestyle modification is recommended with highest level of evidence. Lipid management should be done in the context of the timeframe of benefit.
Chronic kidney disease	High rates of chronic kidney disease with advancing age in older individuals with diabetes. Renal insufficiency increases risk of hypoglycemia in older adults.	Screen with serum creatinine and check urine microalbumin levels. Maintain optimal blood glucose control if it can be done safely. Note the important contraindications to some diabetes medications with worsening renal function.
Obesity	The prevalence of obesity is high in older adults with diabetes Older adults with sarcopenic obesity are at risk of functional decline similar to that seen in frailty.	Lifestyle modification and weight loss are key strategies to improve outcomes.

their gains in self-efficacy and decreased their health distress and their emergency department visits, as well as their outpatient visits.

The goals for glycemic control are less well established for hospitalized than for ambulatory patients. However, data suggest that maintaining blood glucose at 80 to 110 mg/dL in critically ill patients reduces mortality and that hyperglycemia adversely affects wound healing and increases the risk for infection (reviewed in Inzucchi, 2006). Although sliding scale insulin regimens are frequently used in hospitalized patients with diabetes, it is the opinion of the authors that they should not be used. The University of Washington has developed an algorithm to replace sliding scale insulin orders (Fig. 12-1).

Older adults have an increased incidence of hyperosmolar hyperglycemic state (HHS). The overall incidence is one case per 1000 person years. The most common age of patients with this condition is between 60 and 70 years. Those at risk for this condition include nursing home populations, those who have comorbidities that could limit hydration, debility, and dementia. Characteristic symptoms and signs help the physician distinguish this syndrome from diabetic ketoacidotic (DKA) coma. Whereas DKA frequently develops over hours, HHS typically develops over days to weeks. Focal or generalized seizures are common in HHS and unusual in uncomplicated DKA. The fluid deficit is greater in HHS, thus leading to a higher serum sodium and more marked rise in blood urea nitrogen. Therapy in HHS must therefore address the volume and hyperosmolar state of the patient. Because these patients may be quite sensitive to insulin, lowering of glucose should be done cautiously. Volume replacement should be initiated with normal saline. This therapy alone may reduce blood glucose levels, as renal perfusion is enhanced and glucose is lost in the urine. If, after 1 hour of volume repletion, blood glucose levels are not reduced, a bolus of 20 U of regular insulin should be administered intravenously. If glucose levels do not respond, an insulin drip may be started. Such an approach should allow repletion of volume without lowering serum osmolarity too rapidly.

THYROID

The changes with aging in the hypothalamic-pituitary-thyroid axis have been reviewed (Habra and Sarlis, 2005). Although thyroid function is generally normal in aging, clinicians should be aware of the norms for thyroid function tests for this age group (Table 12-3). Primary care providers should keep thyroid disease in their differential diagnosis when evaluating older patients with a wide spectrum of clinical complaints. The majority of data indicate that thyroxine (T_4) levels are normal. Triiodothyronine (T_3) levels may be lower in healthy older people when compared to younger individuals, but are still in the normal range. It has been suggested that the lower T_3 levels reported in several studies are caused by undiagnosed illness and the low T_3 syndrome described later. Thyroid-stimulating hormone (TSH) levels are also normal, whereas the TSH response to thyroid-releasing hormone (TRH) is decreased in males and normal in females. Thus, the TRH test is less valuable in older males. Metabolic clearance of thyroid hormones is decreased in aging. With intact feedback loops, normal thyroid function is maintained despite this change. However, with

PART III

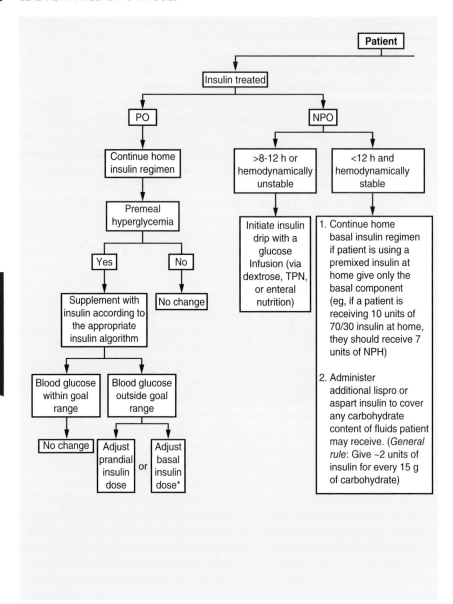

FIGURE 12-1 Flow diagram for treatment of hospitalized (nonintensive care unit) patients with type 2 diabetes mellitus. CHF, congestive heart failure; NPH, neutral protamine Hagedorn (insulin); NPO, nothing by mouth; PO, by mouth; TPN, total parenteral nutrition. (*Reproduced with permission from Ku S. Algorithms replace sliding scale insulin orders.* Drug Ther Topics. *2002;31:49-53.*)

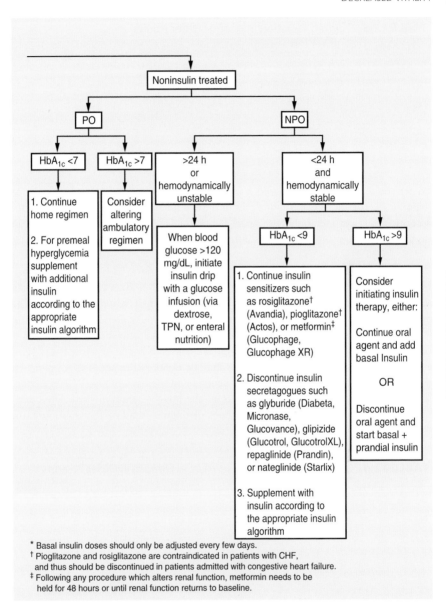

* Basal insulin doses should only be adjusted every few days.
† Pioglitazone and rosiglitazone are contraindicated in patients with CHF,
  and thus should be discontinued in patients admitted with congestive heart failure.
‡ Following any procedure which alters renal function, metformin needs to be
  held for 48 hours or until renal function returns to baseline.

FIGURE 12-1 (*Continued*)

TABLE 12-3. Thyroid Function in Normal Older Adults

Normal	Decreased
T_4	TSH response to TRH in males
Free T_4	Thyroid hormone production rate
T_3	Metabolic clearance rate of thyroid hormone
TSH	

TSH, thyroid-stimulating hormone; TRH, thyroid-releasing hormone.

exogenous replacement of thyroid hormone, such regulatory mechanisms are not maintained; thyroid replacement doses in older adults should be lower to take into account the lower metabolic clearance. Laboratory evaluation tests most useful in thyroid disease are summarized in Table 12-4.

Hypothyroidism

Hypothyroidism is primarily a disease of those aged 50 to 70 years. Goiter is rarely seen with hypothyroidism in older adults except when it is iodide induced. The prevalence of undiagnosed hypothyroidism in healthy older people has varied from 0.5% to 2% in multiple studies; consequently, a general screening program is not cost-effective. The diagnosis of hypothyroidism is usually made by a low free T_4 and an elevated TSH. Because total T_4 levels may be depressed in seriously ill patients, diagnosis of hypothyroidism should not be made on the basis of low T_4 levels alone. Table 12-5 lists laboratory characteristics of the low T_4 syndrome associated with nonthyroidal illness. Not all free T_4 methods distinguish the low T_4 syndrome from

TABLE 12-4. Laboratory Evaluation of Thyroid Disease in Older Persons

	Hypothyroidism	Hyperthyroidism
T_4	E	E
TSH	E	E
Free T_4	E	E
T_3	O	D
Radioactive iodine uptake	O	D
TRH test	D (females)	D (females)
	O (males)	O (males)
Reverse T_3	D	D
TSH stimulation	D	O
T_3 suppression	O	O

TSH, thyroid-stimulating hormone; TRH, thyroid-releasing hormone; E, test for initial evaluation; O, not helpful in diagnosis or not indicated; D, helpful in confirming diagnosis or in differentiation of difficult cases.

TABLE 12-5. Thyroid Function Tests in Nonthyroidal Illness

	Low T_4 syndrome	Low T_3 syndrome
T_4	Decreased	Normal
Free T_4	Normal or increased	Normal
T_3	Decreased	Decreased
Reverse T_3	Normal or increased	Normal or increased
Thyroid-stimulating hormone	Normal	Normal

hypothyroidism; physicians should be aware of the type of determination and interpretation used in their laboratory. Because the T_3 level may be in the normal range in hypothyroidism, this is not a helpful test. The low T_3 level associated with a host of acute and chronic nonthyroidal illnesses also contributes to the poor specificity of this test in hypothyroidism. Approximately 75% of circulating T_3 is derived from peripheral conversion from T_4. The enzymes that convert T_4 to T_3 or reverse T_3 are under metabolic control. During illness, more T_4 is converted to reverse T_3, leading to the characteristic laboratory findings of the low T_3 syndrome.

The radioactive iodine uptake is also not helpful because normal values are so low that they overlap with hypothyroidism. The TRH stimulation test can be used in females, but decreased responsiveness to TRH in older males does not allow this test to distinguish normal from pathologic states. In males, a TSH stimulation test may help confirm the presence of hypothyroidism.

Hypothyroidism may be accompanied by other laboratory abnormalities. Creatine phosphokinase (CPK) levels may be elevated. A normocytic, normochromic anemia, which responds to thyroid hormone replacement, may be present. There is an increased incidence of pernicious anemia in hypothyroidism, but the microcytic anemia of iron deficiency remains the most common anemia associated with hypothyroidism.

The symptoms and signs of hypothyroidism may be overlooked when such complaints as fatigue, memory loss, and decreased hearing are ascribed to aging without further investigation. Although TSH is recommended in the evaluation of older patients with cognitive impairment, the frequency of hypothyroidism as a cause of cognitive impairment is very uncommon. The prevalence of hypothyroidism among older adults who are ill, however, is sufficient to support screening for hypothyroidism in this population, comprising individuals who have already presented themselves for care.

Therapy for hypothyroidism should be started at 0.025 to 0.05 mg of sodium levothyroxine (Synthroid) per day and increased by the same dose at 1- to 3-week intervals. The decreased metabolic clearance rate of thyroid hormone in aging may lead to a lower maintenance dose of T_4. The physician should monitor heart rate response and symptoms of angina and, in the laboratory, the TSH level. When indicated for symptomatic cardiovascular disease, a β-blocker may be added to the

T$_4$ regimen. Recent clinical guidelines on treatment of hypothyroidism emphasize a few important points (reviewed in Jonklaas et al, 2014). The absorption of levothyroxine may be decreased in older adults and may also be decreased by concomitant medication use (eg, calcium carbonate and ferrous sulfate). Further, the clinician is advised to watch for adverse effects of thyroid hormone including atrial fibrillation and osteoporotic fractures.

Subclinical Hypothyroidism

Subclinical hypothyroidism is characterized by increased serum TSH concentrations with normal free T$_4$ and free T$_3$ levels. It occurs in 3% of men and 8% of women in the general population. The prevalence in women over 60 years of age increases to 15% to 18%. These patients may be identified when they present with a general complaint and blood tests reveal the pattern noted previously. The presentation is nonspecific, and symptoms are usually subtle. In a prospective follow-up study, based on the initial TSH level (4 to 6, >6 to 12, or >12 mIU/L), the incidence of overt hypothyroidism after 10 years was 0%, 42.8%, and 76.9%, respectively (Huber et al, 2002). The incidence of overt disease was increased in those with positive microsomal antibodies. Subclinical hypothyroidism is associated with an increased risk of coronary heart disease (CHD) events and CHD mortality in those with higher TSH levels, particularly in those with a TSH concentration of 10 mIU/L or greater (Rodondi et al, 2010), and is associated with left ventricular diastolic dysfunction that is improved with T$_4$ therapy (Biondi et al, 1999). Others have not found an association of subclinical hypothyroidism with cardiovascular disorders or mortality (Cappola et al, 2006). The decision to treat patients remains controversial (Fatourechi, 2007). Contributing to this controversy is the question of the age-specific distribution of TSH (Surks and Hollowell, 2007). This is further complicated by data showing reduced mortality risk in untreated mild hypothyroid subjects over the age of 85 years (Mariotti and Cambuli, 2007). A Cochrane Database Review described 12 randomized controlled trials of levothyroxine replacement versus placebo for patients with subclinical hypothyroidism. The authors concluded that replacement did not result in improved survival or decreased cardiovascular morbidity. Health-related quality of life and symptoms were no different between the two groups. Some evidence indicates that levothyroxine benefits lipid profiles and left ventricular function. In summary, the clinician is guided to use clinical judgment and to define the patient's preference in making decisions regarding this condition.

Myxedema Coma

Most patients with myxedema coma are older than age 60 (Table 12-6). In approximately 50% of the cases, the coma is induced in the hospital by treating hypothyroid patients with hypnotics. A neck scar, from previous thyroid surgery, is a clue to the cause of coma. Because patients with this disorder die of respiratory failure, hypercapnia requires prompt attention. These patients should be treated in an intensive care setting, with intubation and respiratory assistance instituted at the first sign of respiratory failure. The cerebrospinal fluid protein level is often more than 100 mg/dL

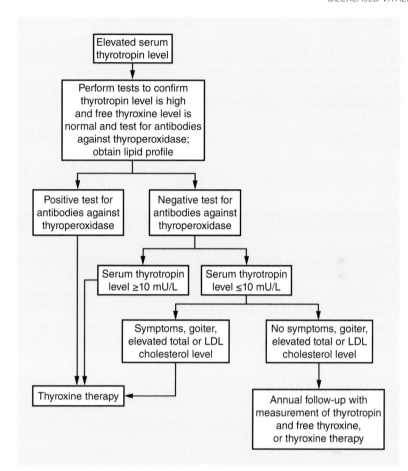

FIGURE 12-2 An algorithm for the management of subclinical hypothyroidism. LDL, low-density lipoprotein. (*Reproduced with permission from Cooper DS. Subclinical hypothyroidism,* N Engl J Med. *2001 Jul 26;345(4):260-265.*)

TABLE 12-6. Myxedema Coma

Usually older than age 60 years
50% induced by hypnotics
Neck scar
Hypothermia
Delayed relaxation of tendon reflex
Respiratory failure and apnea

and should not in itself be used as an indicator of other central nervous system pathology. Therapy includes an initial dose of T_4 intravenously (reviewed in Jonklaas et al, 2014). Although studies have not been done to demonstrate the efficacy of glucocorticoids in this syndrome, it is generally recommended that these patients receive doses appropriate for the stressed state and preceding the administration of levothyroxine. Patients with concomitant adrenal insufficiency will require continued steroid therapy.

Hyperthyroidism

The prevalence of hyperthyroidism in older adults is 1% to 2%. Older women have this illness twice as often as older men. The most common clinical features in older adults are tachycardia, weight loss, and fatigue. Ophthalmopathy is infrequent. Approximately one-third have no goiter. Toxic multinodular goiter is more frequent in older persons than in the young. Severe nonthyroidal disease may disguise thyrotoxicosis (apathetic hyperthyroidism). Congestive heart failure (CHF), stroke, and infection are common disorders associated with masked hyperthyroidism. There should be a high threshold of suspicion for hyperthyroidism in older adults. Unexplained heart failure or tachyarrhythmia, recent onset of a psychiatric disorder, or profound myopathy should raise questions about masked hyperthyroidism. The triad of weight loss, anorexia, and constipation, which may raise the possibility of neoplastic disease, occurs in 15% of older thyrotoxic patients. Diagnosis is made by T_4, T_3, and/or radioactive iodine uptake (see Table 12-4). The ultrasensitive TSH assays can differentiate hyperthyroidism from normal. In the absence of acute nonthyroidal disease, this test alone may confirm the clinical diagnosis of hyperthyroidism. In the presence of acute illness, concomitant determination of TSH and free T_4 may be more appropriate. A T_3 suppression test should not be done in older adults because of the risk of angina or myocardial infarction.

Therapy is usually by radioactive iodine ablation. Often patients are first treated with antithyroid medications to control hyperthyroidism and deplete the thyroid gland of hormone prior to the radioactive iodine treatment (reviewed in Cooper, 2005). Surgery is reserved for patients with thyroid glands that are causing local obstructive symptoms.

Severe thyrotoxicosis is treated with antithyroid drugs (preferably propylthiouracil because it blocks peripheral conversion of T_4 to T_3) to inhibit new hormone synthesis, iodides to block thyroid hormone secretion, and β-blockers to decrease the peripheral manifestations of thyroid hormone action. In older adults with underlying cardiac disease, β-blocker therapy may be a problem; thus the cardiovascular response must be closely monitored. In patients allergic to antithyroid medications or where β-blockers are contraindicated, calcium ipodate (Oragrafin), 3 g every 3 days, can be used because it inhibits peripheral conversion of T_4 to T_3. Dexamethasone 2 mg every 6 hours inhibits peripheral conversion of T_4 to T_3 and may be added to any of the above regimens.

For the management guidelines of hyperthyroidism and other causes of thyrotoxicosis from the American Thyroid Association, see Ross et al, 2016.

Subclinical Hyperthyroidism

Subclinical hyperthyroidism is defined as a combination of serum TSH of less than 0.45 mIU/L and normal serum free T_4 and T_3. This clinical condition is noted when a clinician orders thyroid function tests in the context of case finding. Subclinical hyperthyroidism is associated with a 24% increase in mortality, a 29% increase in CHD mortality, and 69% incident atrial fibrillation in 9 years (Collet et al, 2012), and older subclinical hyperthyroid individuals are significantly more likely to have cognitive dysfunction than those who are euthyroid (hazard ratio, 2.26) (Ceresini et al, 2009). If the TSH level is less than 0.1 mIU/L, treatment is generally recommended with iodine-131 ablation. In patients with a TSH level of 1.0 to 4.5 mIU/L and atrial fibrillation, cardiovascular disease, or low bone density, or those with multinodular goiter, treatment is also recommended. If treatment is deferred, TSH and free T_4 and T_3 should be measured in 6 months.

HYPERPARATHYROIDISM

One-third of patients with hyperparathyroidism are older than age 60. Symptoms are the same in older adults as in those who are younger, but may be overlooked. Bone demineralization, weakness, and joint complaints may be ascribed to aging when they may actually indicate parathyroid disease. This condition has been recognized more in the setting of patients who receive a serum calcium level as a part of their evaluation during standard blood testing on hospitalization or emergency department visits. The clinical profile of individuals presenting with this disease has shifted in Western countries from the hypercalcemic symptoms to no specific symptoms (Marcocci and Cetani, 2011). A National Institutes of Health workshop has developed guidelines for surgery in patients with asymptomatic primary hyperthyroidism (Bilezikian et al, 2002, and reviewed in Marcocci and Cetani, 2011). Surgery is recommended if one of the following is present: serum calcium concentration greater than 1.0 mg/dL above upper limit of normal; 24-hour urinary calcium greater than 400 mg; creatinine clearance reduced by 30%; bone mineral density T-score lower than –2.5 at any site; and age less than 50 years. In those older than 50, surgery can be delayed with monitoring for these criteria.

Table 12-7 contrasts some of the basic patterns of the common laboratory tests in hyperparathyroidism with those of other metabolic bone diseases that are common in older adults.

VASOPRESSIN SECRETION

Basal vasopressin levels are unaltered in normal older individuals. Infusion of hypertonic saline, however, leads to a greater increase in plasma vasopressin in older compared with younger persons. In contrast to the response to the hyperosmolar challenge, volume changes related to the assumption of upright posture are associated with less of a vasopressin response in older subjects as compared with the young. Both of these findings might be explained by impaired baroreceptor input to the supraoptic nucleus. These findings may influence volume status and water homeostasis. Volume expansion decreases osmoreceptor sensitivity. Hypertonic saline infusion

TABLE 12-7. Laboratory Findings in Metabolic Bone Disease

Disease	Ca	P	Alk	PTH
Hyperparathyroidism	High	Low/normal	High/normal	High
Osteomalacia	Low/normal	Low	High/normal	High
Hyperthyroidism	High	High	High/normal	Low
Osteoporosis	Normal	Normal	Normal	Normal/high
Paget disease	Normal/high	Normal/high	High	Normal

Ca, calcium; P, phosphorus; Alk, alkaline phosphatase; PTH, parathyroid hormone.

results in volume expansion and thus decreases osmoreceptor sensitivity. If baroreceptor input is impaired in older adults, volume expansion would lead to a lesser dampening effect, and thus, the vasopressin response to hyperosmolar stimuli would be increased.

Hyponatremia is a serious and often overlooked problem of the older patient (reviewed in Ellison and Berl, 2007; Sterns, 2015). This syndrome is often associated with one of three general causes: (1) decreased renal blood flow with a decreased ability to excrete a water load, (2) diuretic administration leading to water intoxication (this condition is rapidly corrected by discontinuing diuretics), or (3) excess vasopressin secretion. Although a host of pulmonary disorders (eg, pneumonia, tuberculosis, tumor) and central nervous system disorders (eg, stroke, meningitis, subdural hematoma) are associated with the syndrome of inappropriate secretion of antidiuretic hormone (SIADH) in any age group, older adults seem more prone to develop this complication. Certain drugs, such as chlorpropamide and barbiturates, may cause this syndrome more frequently in older individuals.

In addition to treatment directed at correcting the underlying cause, water restriction and hypertonic saline are indicated when the patient is symptomatic or the sodium level is below 120 mEq/L. Demethylchlortetracycline therapy may be needed in resistant patients with SIADH. This agent induces a partial nephrogenic diabetes insipidus and thus corrects the hyponatremia. Serum creatinine and blood urea nitrogen should be closely monitored.

ANABOLIC HORMONES

Aging is associated with a decline in anabolic hormones (Lamberts et al, 1997). The declining activity of the growth hormone insulin-like growth factor-1 (IGF-1) axis with advancing age may contribute to the decrease in lean body mass and the increase in mass of adipose tissue that occur with aging. Increased lean body mass and decreased fat mass have been demonstrated to occur in men and women with growth hormone treatment. Men had marginal improvement of muscle strength and maximum oxygen consumption (VO_{2max}), but women had no significant change. Adverse effects were frequent, including glucose intolerance and diabetes (Blackman et al, 2002; Liu et al, 2007).

Normal male aging is accompanied by a decline in testicular function, including a fall in serum levels of total testosterone and bioavailable testosterone. Only some men become hypogonadal. Androgens have many important physiological actions, including effects on muscle, bone, and bone marrow. However, little is known about the effects of the age-related decline in testicular function on androgen target organs. Studies of testosterone supplementation in older males demonstrate significant increases in lean body mass and significant decreases in biochemical parameters of bone resorption with testosterone treatment. Testosterone supplementation in older men with low-normal testosterone concentration did not affect functional status or cognition (Emmelot-Vonk et al, 2008). However, there was a significant increase in hematocrit and a sustained stimulation of prostate-specific antigen (Gruenewald and Matsumoto, 2003). Based on these results, growth hormone administration and testosterone supplementation cannot be recommended at this time for older men with normal or low-normal levels of these anabolic hormones. Although clinical trial data are limited, current practice guidelines recommend testosterone replacement therapy in symptomatic men with low testosterone levels to improve bone mineral density; muscle mass, strength, and physical performance; sexual function; and quality of life (Kazi et al, 2007; Kenny et al, 2010; Page et al, 2005; Snyder et al 2016). There is no effect on the 6-minute walking ability and no impact on vitality. Further it is noted that some studies of testosterone effects screened very large populations of men to enroll patients. Clinicians should bear in mind the limitations of research testosterone replacement therapy outcomes when prescribing to older men with multiple comorbid conditions. The clinical practice guideline also highlights numerous conditions that preclude the use of testosterone: breast cancer or prostate cancer, a prostate nodule or a prostate-specific antigen level greater than 4 ng/mL, or greater than 3 ng/mL in men at high risk of prostate cancer such as African Americans or men with first-degree relatives with prostate cancer, a hematocrit that is greater than 50%, untreated severe obstructive sleep apnea, severe lower urinary tract symptoms, or poorly controlled heart failure (see the Suggested Readings). Overall, the disadvantages of testosterone replacement outweigh the advantages.

ANEMIA

Anemia is common in older adults, but should not be attributed simply to old age. Anemia is defined as a hemoglobin <7.5 mmol/dL in women and <8.1 mmol/dL in men. Increased weakness, fatigue, and a mild anemia should not be dismissed as a manifestation of aging. In healthy older individuals, there is generally no change in normal levels of hemoglobin from younger adult values. A low hemoglobin concentration at old age signifies disease and is associated with increased mortality, disability, and hospitalization (Dong et al, 2008; Izaks et al, 1999; Longo, 2005; Maraldi et al, 2006; Penninx et al, 2006), although the actual mechanism has not been elucidated. Higher red cell distribution width (RDW) is also a predictor of mortality in community-dwelling older adults with and without age-associated diseases (Patel et al, 2010). The biological mechanisms underlying this association are unknown.

PART III

Signs and symptoms of anemia may be subtle. Table 12-8 lists some of these manifestations. Anemia should be considered in these circumstances. If anemia is present, a directed and thoughtful diagnostic evaluation is indicated to define the cause. The appearance of the peripheral blood smear along with the history and physical examination should direct the diagnostic evaluation as described below. However, despite intensive evaluation, unexplained anemia predominates in older adults (Artz and Thirman, 2011). Unexplained anemia is characterized by a hypoproliferative mild-to-moderate anemia with suppressed serum erythropoietin.

IRON DEFICIENCY

Iron deficiency is the most common anemia with a known etiology in older adults. Laboratory findings include hypochromia, microcytosis, low reticulocyte count, decreased serum iron, increased total iron-binding capacity (TIBC), low transferrin saturation, and absent bone marrow iron stores. A low serum iron and elevated TIBC indicate iron deficiency even in the absence of changes in red cell morphology. Because transferrin is reduced in many diseases, the TIBC may be normal or low in older patients with iron deficiency. However, a transferrin saturation of less than 10% would suggest iron deficiency even in the presence of a low TIBC. A low serum ferritin level is valuable in confirming the diagnosis because serum ferritin levels are below 12 mg/L in iron-deficiency anemia. Because inflammatory disease can elevate ferritin levels and liver disease can influence ferritin levels in either direction, the diagnosis of iron deficiency based on a ferritin level must be made with knowledge of the clinical situation.

Once iron deficiency is identified, it should be treated, and the cause of the anemia must be identified and corrected. Poor dietary intake of iron may contribute to iron deficiency in older adults. A dietary evaluation is important, both for foods that contain iron and for substances such as tea, which inhibit iron absorption. However, even in the presence of poor nutrition, evaluation for a bleeding lesion must be completed.

The stool should be examined for occult blood. Evaluation for a gastrointestinal lesion should be carried out in a patient with unexplained iron deficiency, even if the stool is negative for occult blood. Although gastrointestinal bleeding may be caused by medications (especially certain analgesics, steroids, and alcohol), a gastrointestinal lesion must be excluded. Diverticulosis is a common cause of bleeding. Vascular

TABLE 12-8. Signs and Symptoms of Anemia

Weakness	Ischemic chest pain
Postural hypotension	Congestive heart failure
Syncope	Exertional dyspnea
Falls	Pallor
Confusion	Tachycardia
Worsened dementia	

ectasia of the cecum and ascending colon is increasingly a recognized cause of bleeding in older adults.

Replacement of iron should usually be by daily oral administration. The hemoglobin should improve in 10 days and be normal in approximately 6 weeks. Normal bone marrow iron stores should occur in an additional 4 months. If the anemia does not improve, one should consider nonadherence, continued bleeding, or an incorrect diagnosis. In nonadherent patients, or when oral iron is not tolerated, parenteral iron replacement is indicated. Tolerance should be monitored with a test dose, and the patient should be closely observed for an acute reaction. Severe reactions occur less frequently with ferric gluconate, but a test dose should be used as well. Parenteral iron should not be used routinely, but it is an important therapeutic modality in the appropriate clinical situation. A review of iron-deficiency anemia is listed in the Suggested Readings (Camaschella, 2015).

CHRONIC DISEASE

The anemia of chronic disease (ACD) may display many similarities with iron-deficiency anemia (reviewed in Keel and Abkowitz, 2009; Weiss and Goodnough, 2005). In older adults, this anemia is frequently associated with chronic inflammatory diseases or neoplasia. There is a defect in bone marrow red cell production and a shortening of erythrocyte life span. The finding of hypochromia, low reticulocyte count, and low serum iron may lead to confusion with iron deficiency. When a high TIBC does not confirm the presence of iron deficiency, a ferritin level can differentiate the two anemias. It is low in iron deficiency and high-normal or elevated in ACD. Treatment is addressed to the underlying chronic illness because there is no specific therapy for this type of anemia.

SIDEROBLASTIC ANEMIA

Sideroblastic anemia should be considered in an older patient with hypochromic anemia who does not have iron deficiency or a chronic disease. Serum iron and transferrin saturation are increased. Hence, synthesis is defective, leading to increased iron stores and the diagnostic finding of ringed sideroblasts in the marrow.

In older adults, sideroblastic anemia is commonly of the acquired type. The idiopathic group is usually refractory; only a few patients have a partial response to pyridoxine, but all should have a trial of pyridoxine. Although the prognosis is fairly good, approximately 10% of patients develop acute myeloblastic leukemia. Secondary sideroblastic anemia may be associated with underlying diseases such as malignancies and chronic inflammatory diseases. Certain drugs and toxins can induce sideroblastic anemia (eg, ethanol, lead, isoniazid, chloramphenicol). The drug-induced syndromes are corrected by administering pyridoxine. Table 12-9 lists the tests that will assist in the differential diagnosis of hypochromic anemias.

VITAMIN B$_{12}$ AND FOLATE DEFICIENCY

Both vitamin B$_{12}$ and folate deficiency may occur on a nutritional basis, although folate deficiency is more common (reviewed by Stabler, 2013 in Suggested Readings).

TABLE 12-9. Differential Tests in Hypochromic Anemia

Item	Iron deficiency	Chronic disease	Sideroblastic anemia
Serum iron	Low	Low	High
Total iron-binding capacity	Usually increased*	Low	Normal
Transferrin saturation	Low	Low	High
Ferritin	Low	High	Normal
Bone marrow iron	Absent	Adequate	Increased ringed sideroblasts

*May be normal or even low in older adults.

Older people who live alone or who are alcoholics are most likely to have poor nutrition. Poor dietary intake of fresh fruits and vegetables may lead to folate deficiency; lack of meat, poultry, fish, eggs, and dairy products may lead to vitamin B_{12} deficiency. Vitamin B_{12} deficiency also occurs with the loss of intrinsic factor (pernicious anemia) and in gastrointestinal disorders associated with malabsorption of vitamin B_{12}.

The laboratory findings are similar in the two deficiencies and include macrocytosis, hyperchromasia, hypersegmented neutrophils, and megaloblasts in the marrow. Leukopenia and thrombocytopenia may be present, and serum lactic dehydrogenase and bilirubin may be increased. The two are differentiated by measuring serum vitamin B_{12} and folate levels.

Treatment is with vitamin B_{12} (at an oral replacement dosage of 1000 to 2000 mcg/day) or folic acid, as appropriate. However, because folate will correct the hematological disorder but not the neurological abnormalities of vitamin B_{12} deficiency, a correct diagnosis is essential before treatment.

ERYTHROPOIETIN

A longitudinal analysis of erythropoietin (Epo) levels in the Baltimore Longitudinal Study on Aging revealed a significant rise in Epo levels with age (Ershler et al, 2005). Subjects who developed anemia but did not have hypertension or diabetes had the greatest rise in Epo slope over time, whereas those with hypertension or diabetes had the lowest slope. In very advanced age or in those with compromised renal function, an inadequate compensatory mechanism leads to anemia.

Epo effectively corrects the anemia in patients with chronic kidney disease (CKD) who do not yet require dialysis and may improve anemia-induced symptoms and cardiovascular function and perhaps decrease mortality (Jones et al, 2004). An adequate response to Epo requires the maintenance of sufficient iron stores. Iron status should be evaluated and iron supplements given when there is evidence of iron deficiency. The benefits of reduced blood transfusion and anemia-related symptoms should be weighed against the risk of Epo (eg, stroke, vascular access loss, and hypertension) as reviewed in the Suggested Readings. The FDA recommendation indicates that patients with CKD, who are not on dialysis, should have a hemoglobin (Hgb) count of 10 g/dL prior to starting treatment. However, better outcomes have been demonstrated with Hgb values above 11 g/dL (hematocrit of 33%). There is also evidence for little benefit and potential risk for maintaining Hgb levels ≥13 g/dL (hematocrit 39%). In patients with heart failure or ischemic heart disease who are receiving hemodialysis, the administration of Epo to raise the hematocrit above 42% is not recommended. These patients have an increased risk of nonfatal acute myocardial infarction (Besarab et al, 1998). The recommended target is Hgb levels between 11 and 12 g/dL. Future recommendations may be lower because of the boxed warning to adjust Epo dose to maintain the Hgb level necessary to avoid the need for blood transfusion.

The FDA has issued a black box safety alert indicating that treating the anemia of cancer with Epo in patients who are not receiving chemotherapy offers no benefit and may cause serious harm (Steensma, 2008). As in CKD, the FDA recommendation is to gradually increase the Hgb concentration to the lowest level sufficient to avoid blood transfusions in patients who are receiving chemotherapy.

The preferred therapy for anemia of chronic disease (ACD) is correction of the underlying disorder, rather than transfusion or Epo therapy. Studies in humans of therapy with Epo in ACD have been limited. Although one of the hallmarks of ACD is reduced bone marrow response to endogenous or exogenous Epo, some patients may respond. Epo has been helpful in ACD in patients with rheumatoid arthritis or acquired immunodeficiency syndrome (AIDS) who have low Epo levels (<500 mU/mL).

With the present FDA recommendations and cautions, Epo therapy in older adults should be reserved for those who meet the criteria for therapy described earlier.

NUTRITION

A discussion of nutrition and aging is limited by the lack of adequate studies, defined methods, and standards. Although it is generally accepted that intake moderately above recommended allowances is optimal, animal studies demonstrate increased longevity with lower caloric levels than recommended. In establishing nutritional requirements in humans, we must contend with the multiple factors that confine interpretation of available data, for example, genetic factors, social environment, economic status, selection of food, and weak methods of assessing nutritional status.

Several national surveys have assessed nutrition in older adults. Taken as a whole, these surveys do not indicate poor nutritional status or marked deficiency among older individuals in the United States, and suggest that intake relates more to health and poverty than to age.

VITAMINS, PROTEIN, AND CALCIUM

Table 12-10 summarizes nutritional requirements in older adults and demonstrates that there is no general increase in vitamin requirements with age. Studies on vitamin metabolism and requirements reveal no correlation between age and the requirement

PART III

TABLE 12-10. Nutritional Requirements in Older Persons

Vitamins	Unchanged in older persons
Protein	0.5 to >1.0 g/kg/day
Amino acids	Unchanged to increased
Calcium	850–1020 mg/day
Calories	Declines by 12.4 cal/day/year (maturity to senescence)

for vitamins A, B_1, B_2, or C. Vitamin B_6 and vitamin B_{12} requirements also do not increase with age. However, because folate and vitamin B_{12} deficiencies are associated with an increased incidence of coronary artery disease and predict cognitive decline (Morris et al, 2012), vitamin D deficiency is associated with osteoporosis, and vitamins A, C, and E have antioxidant effects, and because most people do not consume an optimal amount of all vitamins alone, some authors recommend that all adults take vitamin supplements (Fletcher and Fairfield, 2002).

Studies on protein requirements are not in agreement. Based on nitrogen balance studies, estimates of protein requirement varied from 0.5 to more than 1.0 g/kg daily. In an analysis of the Women's Health Initiative, higher protein consumption, as a fraction of energy, is associated with a strong, independent, dose-responsive lower risk of incident frailty in older women (Beasley et al, 2010). Data on amino acid requirements are also conflicting; some data show increased requirements with age, and other data show no change.

For calcium, the recommended daily allowance for women and men over 70 years of age is 1200 mg (from the Food and Nutrition Board of the Institute of Medicine of the National Academies 2010). This includes the amount taken in by one's diet and by supplement. Data on the correlation of dietary calcium intake and osteoporosis are conflicting. However, calcium and vitamin D supplementation do improve postmenopausal osteoporosis. It may be necessary to use calcium and vitamin D supplements to ensure adequate intake.

NUTRITIONAL DEFICIENCY AND PHYSIOLOGICAL IMPAIRMENTS

There is little evidence to correlate age-associated nutritional deficiency with clinical findings. There was no significant correlation between vitamin A levels and dark adaptation, epithelial cells excreted, or percentage of keratinization. Despite their proposed antioxidant effects, neither vitamin E nor vitamin C supplementation reduced the risk of major cardiovascular events (Sesso et al, 2008). Older people with limited sun exposure may be at risk of vitamin D deficiency. Older individuals in nursing homes require at least 800 IU of vitamin D per day, double the usual recommended daily requirement to maintain normal vitamin D levels. Total 25-hydroxy vitamin D [25(OH)D] levels should be measured. However, the recommended therapeutic target serum level varies. The International Osteoporosis Foundation recommends a target of 30 ng/mL, whereas an Institute of Medicine report suggests a level of 20 ng/mL (Rosen, 2011). The threshold concentration of 25(OH)D associated with increased risk for relevant clinical disease events is likely near 20 ng/mL (De Boer et al, 2012). Until recently, vitamin D was considered only as one of the calciotropic hormones. Recent data have demonstrated that vitamin D has an important role in cell differentiation, function, and survival (Montero-Odasso and Duque, 2005). Muscle and bone are significantly affected by the presence or absence of vitamin D. In bone, vitamin D stimulates bone turnover while protecting osteoblasts from apoptosis, whereas in muscle it maintains the function of type II fibers, preserving strength and preventing falls. Both osteoporosis and sarcopenia have been linked to the development of frailty in older adults. In the Cardiovascular Health Study, vitamin D deficiency was associated with poorer physical performance, lower muscle strength, and prevalent mobility and activities of daily living disability (Houston et al, 2011). In noninstitutionalized older adults, serum 25(OH) D levels had an independent, inverse association with cardiovascular disease and all-cause mortality (Ginde et al, 2009). Vitamin D functions as an endocrine inhibitor of the renin-angiotensin system, the likely link to cardiovascular disease (Li, 2011). Vitamin D deficiency is associated with increased autoimmunity and an increased susceptibility to infection (Aranow, 2011).

Although data on the effect of vitamin D supplementation have been conflicting, a recent meta-analysis demonstrated a benefit of vitamin D in preventing falls (Jackson et al, 2007). Recent studies of older women who had a prior fall and low baseline levels of 25(OH)D show that high dose of monthly vitamin D were associated with an increased risk of falls when compared to a low-dose comparison group (Bischoff-Ferrari et al, 2016). The USPSTF has concluded that vitamin D supplementation can reduce fracture risk and that the effects on cancer risk are uncertain (Chung et al, 2011). The recommended dose for supplementation has varied from 800 to 2000 IU daily (Bischoff-Ferrari et al, 2012; Heany, 2012; Holick, 2011; Muir and Montero-Odasso, 2011). Studies on the effects of vitamin D supplementation have generally used fixed doses and not measured baseline 25(OH)D levels. The dose may be too low for those with marked deficiency, and those with high levels would not benefit. The Endocrine Society has recommended 800 IU per day for adults aged 70 and older. They further describe that 1500 to 2000 IU daily may be required to raise the blood levels of 25(OH)D above 30 ng/mL. (For the Endocrine Society practice guideline on evaluation, treatment, and prevention of vitamin D deficiency, see Holick et al, 2011.) The National Osteoporosis Foundation recommends that adults aged 50 and older take 800 to 1000 IU per day (for details see www.cme/nof.org/). Data are conflicting on correlation of dietary calcium intake and osteoporosis. Problems in assessing this correlation include reduced calcium intake in older adults, altered calcium and phosphorus ratio, decreased protein intake, and acid–base balance.

REVERSAL OF DEFICIENCY BY SUPPLEMENTATION

There is no impairment of vitamin or protein absorption in older adults; low vitamin levels in older adults can be reversed by administration of oral supplementation. Because these deficiencies can be corrected by dietary supplementation, they are most likely related to decreased intake.

CALORIC NEEDS

A study of 250 individuals aged 23 to 99 demonstrated an age-associated decline in total caloric intake at the rate of 12.4 cal/day for a year. A yearly decline in basal metabolic rate accounted for 5.23 cal/day, while 7.6 cal/day related to reduction in other requirements, including physical exercise (McGandy et al, 1966).

DIETARY RESTRICTION AND FOOD ADDITIVES

In rats, mice, *Drosophila,* and other lower organisms, caloric restriction delays maturation and increases life span. The mechanism, however, is not understood, but studies suggest that it may be related to decreased levels of IGF-1. Animals fed isocaloric diets but decreased protein have an increased life span. Based on the free radical theory of aging, it has been proposed that reducing agents would prolong life. Although the data are conflicting, some studies support this hypothesis. In certain animal models, caloric restriction decreases the incidence and delays the onset of disease, including chronic glomerulonephritis, muscular dystrophy, and carcinogenesis. In humans, however, body weight below ideal is not associated with increased life span, and in primates, caloric restriction is not associated with increased life span (see the section "Hallmarks of Aging" in Chapter 1).

Although the influence of dietary fiber on colonic carcinoma and diverticular disease is controversial, the use of dietary fiber to maintain bowel regularity has significant support, especially in older adults, where constipation may present a difficult clinical problem. When dietary intake of fiber is low, bran can be used as a supplement, particularly in cereals and breads or as bran powder. Intake of bran can be adjusted to maintain normal bowel movements. Adequate fluid intake should also be ensured.

Although the food industry is slowly responding, most canned foods still contain large amounts of added sodium and sugar. Because some of these are less expensive than fresh or frozen foods, older adults with limited incomes may use such prepared foods exclusively. When refined carbohydrates or sodium need to be restricted, these patients should be educated about the use of canned products.

OBESITY

The prevalence of obesity among older persons is growing. Although increased mortality rate from all causes extends into the seventh decade, controversy exists about the potential harms of obesity in older adults and the relation between obesity in old age and total or disease-specific mortality (Zamboni et al, 2005; see also Chapter 5). Most population-based studies that have described the relationship between weight categories and survival of older adults have identified a "J-shaped" relationship between body mass index (BMI) and all-cause mortality. A meta-analysis indicated that a BMI in the overweight range (BMI 25–29.9 kg/m^2) is not associated with a significantly increased risk of mortality in older adults, whereas a BMI in the moderately obese range (BMI >30 kg/m^2) is associated with only a modest (10%) increase in mortality risk (Janssen and Mark, 2007). Other reports have described serious mortality implications of higher grades of obesity (Flegal et al, 2013). Central fat and relative loss of fat-free mass are relatively more important than BMI in determining the health risk associated with obesity in older ages. However, obesity causes serious medical complications, impairs quality of life, can exacerbate the age-related decline in physical function, and can lead to frailty (Schroeder, 2007; Villareal et al, 2005). The prevalence of many of the medical complications associated with obesity—for example, hypertension, diabetes, cardiovascular disease, and osteoarthritis—increases with age. All components of the metabolic syndrome are prevalent in older populations. High BMI is associated with an increased risk of knee osteoarthritis in older persons. Obesity is associated with pulmonary function abnormalities, obesity-hypoventilation syndrome, and obstructive sleep apnea (Memtsoudis et al, 2013). An increase in urinary incontinence is associated with increased BMI. Obesity is associated with an increased risk of several types of cancer including breast, colon, pancreas, renal, bladder, and prostate. Self-reported functional capacity, particularly mobility, is markedly diminished in overweight and obese compared with lean older adults. Older persons who are obese (BMI >30 kg/m^2) have a greater rate of nursing home admissions than those who are not obese. Obesity impairs quality of life in older persons. Beneficial effects of obesity include an increased bone mineral density and decreased osteoporosis and hip fracture in older men and women.

Weight-loss therapy improves physical function, quality of life, and the medical complications associated with obesity in older persons (Villareal et al, 2005). Weight-loss therapy that minimizes muscle and bone losses is recommended for older persons who are obese and who have functional impairments or metabolic complications that can benefit from weight loss. The primary approach is to achieve lifestyle change. Modest goals are key components of a weight management program for older adults. A modest reduction in energy intake (500–700 kcal/day) is recommended. Regular physical activity is particularly important in obese older persons to improve physical function and help preserve muscle and bone mass. The available data are insufficient to determine the efficacy and safety of pharmacotherapy for obesity in older persons. Bariatric surgery is the most effective weight-loss therapy for obesity. Perioperative morbidity and mortality are greater but relative weight loss and improvement in obesity-related medical complications are lower in older than in younger patients. Bariatric surgery should be reserved for a select group of older subjects who have disabling obesity that can be ameliorated with weight loss and who meet the criteria for surgery.

INFECTIONS

Although it is proposed that alterations in host defense mechanisms predispose older adults to certain infections, there is little evidence to support this hypothesis. It may well be that environmental factors, physiological changes other than in the immune system, and specific diseases are the major elements in the increased frequency of certain infections in older adults (Table 12-11).

Because older persons more often have acute and chronic illnesses necessitating hospitalization and have longer hospital stays, they are at greater risk for nosocomial

TABLE 12-11. Factors Predisposing to Infection in Older Adults

More frequent and longer hospital stays
   Nosocomial infections
      Gram-negative bacilli
      Staphylococcus aureus
Physiological changes
   Lung
   Bladder
   Skin
   Glucose homeostasis
Chronic disease
   Malignancy
      Multiple myeloma and leukemia
      Immunosuppression from therapy
Diabetes mellitus
   Urinary tract infection
   Soft tissue infections
   Osteomyelitis
Prostatic hypertrophy
   Urinary tract infection
Host defenses
   Phagocytosis unaltered
   Complement unaltered
   Cellular and humoral immunity diminished

infections. A recent review of infections in older adults describes this and other vulnerabilities (Yoshikawa and Norman, 2016 in Suggested Readings). Such hospitalizations put older patients at greater risk for gram-negative and *Staphylococcus aureus* infections. Further, some of the techniques in which the health professionals insert and maintain indwelling urinary catheters contribute to the risk of catheter-associated urinary tract infection. The failure to use alternative strategies for urine collection and the lack of professional competencies in the avoidance of catheter-related urinary tract infections increases the risks of infection (Saint, 2016). Physiological alterations (see Chapter 1)—in the lungs, bladder function, and the skin—and glucose homeostasis may also predispose older adults to infections.

The incidence of malignancies is increased in older adults. Many of these neoplastic disorders, especially those of the hematological system, are associated with a higher frequency of infection. Immunosuppression during therapy is also a predisposing factor. The prevalence of diabetes mellitus is higher in older adults, thus predisposing them to more frequent urinary tract, soft tissue, and bone infections. Prostatic hypertrophy with obstruction predisposes the older male to urinary tract infections.

Phagocytic function appears to be unaltered in aging, as is the complement system. Cell-mediated immunity and, to a lesser extent, humoral immunity are diminished in aging. The role that these changes play in predisposing older individuals to infection has not been well defined. To learn more about the mechanism of lower respiratory infection see the review noted in Suggested Readings (Mizgerd, 2008).

Many infections occur more frequently in older adults and are often associated with a higher morbidity and mortality. Atypical presentation of infection in some older patients may delay diagnosis and treatment. Underreporting of symptoms, impaired communication, coexisting diseases, and altered physiological responses to infection may contribute to altered presentations.

As an example, failure of patients to seek medical evaluation is one factor in the higher morbidity and mortality of appendicitis in older adults. Difficulties in communication may also alter presentation. Infections not directly involving the central nervous system may precipitate delirium in older adults, particularly in individuals with preexisting dementia. The mechanism by which this occurs has not been completely defined (Fick et al, 2002). Acute unexplained functional deterioration should also alert the physician to a potential acute infectious process.

Existing chronic disease may mask an acute infection. Septic arthritis usually occurs in a previously abnormal joint. It may be difficult to distinguish clinically between exacerbation of the underlying arthritis and acute infection. Therefore, the physician should not be hesitant to examine synovial fluid in elderly patients with acute exacerbation of joint disease.

Febrile response may be blunted or absent in some older individuals with bacterial infections. This may obscure diagnosis and delay therapy. A poor febrile response may also be a negative prognostic factor. Conversely, a febrile response is more likely to indicate a bacterial rather than viral illness in older patients, particularly in the very old. The absence of leukocytosis in older patients should also not exclude consideration of a bacterial infection.

Antibiotic therapy in older adults, as in the young, is based on the site of the infection and directed to the specific organism isolated. A review of antibiotic therapy for community-acquired pneumonia is included in Suggested Readings (Lee et al, 2016; Musher and Thorner, 2014). Likewise, a review of urinary tract infection in older women and urinary tract infection in older men is included in Suggested Readings (Mody and Juthani-Mehta, 2015; Schaefer and Nicolle, 2016).

The spectrum of pathogens causing common infections in older adults is often different than that in younger adults (Table 12-12). The frequency of gram-negative bacilli increases in each category. Pneumonia is the most frequent cause of death caused by infection in older patients. *Streptococcus pneumoniae*, human rhinovirus, and influenza are the most common causes of pneumonia in the older people (Jain et al, 2015), but gram-negative bacilli increase in prevalence, particularly in the nursing home setting. Pneumonia in nursing homes or long-term care facilities is considered as health-care–associated pneumonia with a broader spectrum of pathogens than community-acquired pneumonia. These patients have worse outcomes and require a broader spectrum of antibiotics (Venditti et al, 2009). Annual immunization against influenza is recommended for all persons 65 years of age and older (Grohskopf et al, 2016). A recommendation on seasonal influenza is updated in the late summer of each year by the Advisory Committee on Immunization Practices.

TABLE 12-12. Pathogens of Common Infections in Older Adults

Infection	Common pathogens in adults	Common pathogens in older adults
Pneumonia	*Streptococcus pneumoniae* Anaerobic bacteria	*Streptococcus pneumoniae* Anaerobic bacteria *Haemophilus influenzae* gram-negative bacilli
Urinary tract	*Escherichia coli*	*Escherichia coli* *Proteus* sp. *Klebsiella* sp. *Enterobacter* sp. *Enterococcus*
Meningitis	*Streptococcus pneumoniae* *Neisseria meningitidis*	*Streptococcus pneumoniae* *Listeria monocytogenes* gram-negative bacilli
Septic arthritis	*Neisseria gonorrhoeae* *Staphylococcus aureus*	*Staphylococcus aureus* gram-negative bacilli

Efforts are made each year to get the right strains of influenza to increase the chance that the vaccine will be effective. Both 23-valent pneumococcal polysaccharide and the 13-valent pneumococcal polysaccharide should be routinely administered in a series to all adults aged 65 years and older (Tomczyk et al, 2014). PCV13 is given first, followed by PPSV23 6 to 12 months later. Repeated dosage of PPSV23 should be given in approximately 5 years.

Nearly 50% of infective endocarditis cases occur in older adults. The underlying cardiac lesion is often caused by atherosclerotic and degenerative valve diseases, as well as by prosthetic valves. Bacterial meningitis is an infection primarily of early childhood and late adulthood. Mortality in the older individuals ranges from 50% to 70%. *S pneumoniae* is the most frequent pathogen, but older patients may be infected with *Listeria monocytogenes* or gram-negative bacilli.

Residents in long-term care facilities (LTCFs) are at great risk for infection. Older age and comorbidities complicate recognition of infection (eg, typically defined fever is absent in more than one-half of LTCF residents with serious infections). The Infectious Diseases Society of America provided guidelines for evaluation of fever and infection in LTCF residents (High et al, 2009). The Centers for Disease Control and Prevention (CDC) has also provided a resource on antibiotic stewardship for nursing homes (www.cdc.gov/longtermcare/index.html). Further, a book on infections in long-term care is noted in Suggested Readings (Yoshikawa and Ouslander, 2006). Infection should be suspected in LTCF residents with decline in functional status, increasing confusion, incontinence, falling, deteriorating mobility, reduced food intake, or failure to cooperate with staff. Fever is defined as a single oral temperature of >100°F (37.8°C), repeated oral temperature of >99°F (37.2°C), or an increase in temperature of >2°F (–16.7°C). A complete blood count (CBC) should be performed if an infection is suspected. An elevated white blood cell (WBC) count of 14,000 cells/mm^3 or a left shift >6% warrants a careful assessment for bacterial infection. Urinalysis and urine cultures should not be performed for asymptomatic residents. In residents with long-term indwelling urethral catheters, evaluation is indicated for fever, shaking chills, hypotension, or delirium. In older adult nursing home residents, blood cultures have a low yield and rarely influence therapy. If pneumonia is clinically suspected, pulse oximetry should be performed for residents with a respiratory rate of >25. Chest radiograph should be performed if hypoxemia is documented or suspected. At the onset of a suspected respiratory viral infection outbreak, nasopharyngeal wash or swab should be obtained for virus isolation and rapid diagnostic testing for influenza A virus and other common viruses. If a resident exhibits symptoms of colitis (eg, severe fever, abdominal cramps, and/or diarrhea, with or without blood and/or WBCs in the stool), initial evaluation for *Clostridium difficile* should be performed.

The incidence of tuberculosis is on the rise again. Older persons of both sexes among all racial and ethnic groups are especially at risk for tuberculosis. This cohort has lived through a period of higher incidence of tuberculosis, has probably not been treated with isonicotinic acid hydrazide (INH) prophylaxis, and may have predisposing factors such as physiological changes, malnutrition, and underlying disease that may lead to reactivation. Older patients are also at increased risk for primary infection. This is particularly the case for older patients in LTCFs.

Tuberculosis screening programs should be implemented in LTCFs because of this increased risk and because of the potential to prevent active disease among patients whose skin test converts to a strongly positive reaction (see Chapter 16). The American Thoracic Society now recommends preventive therapy for certain types of patients regardless of age, including insulin-dependent diabetic patients, those on steroids and other immunosuppressive treatment, patients with end-stage renal disease, and patients who have lost a large amount of weight rapidly (see Nahid, 2016 in Suggested Readings). A useful rule in geriatric care is to suspect tuberculosis when a patient is inexplicably failing.

Several studies suggest that bacteriuria is associated with increased mortality in older persons. However, other studies do not confirm this finding. Most of these nonconforming studies did not differentiate between the effect of bacteriuria and age and/or concomitant disease on mortality. When adjusted for age, fatal diseases associated with bacteriuria account for the increase in mortality among older patients with bacteriuria.

Several previous studies in older hospitalized or institutionalized patients have not revealed antimicrobial therapy for bacteriuria to be effective because of the high rate of recurring infection. One study in older ambulatory nonhospitalized women with asymptomatic bacteriuria demonstrated that short-course antimicrobial therapy is effective in eliminating bacteriuria in most of the women for at least a 6-month period. Survival was not an outcome measure.

Bacteriuria in older persons is common and usually asymptomatic. At present, in the absence of obstructive uropathy, no evidence exists to support the routine use

PART III

of antimicrobial therapy for asymptomatic bacteriuria in older persons. Among bacteriuric patients with urinary incontinence and no other symptoms of urinary tract infection, the bacteriuria should be eradicated as part of the initial assessment of the incontinence (see Chapter 8).

The incidence of herpes zoster (HZ) increases with aging. In a prospective vaccine trial, the incidence of herpes was 11.8 cases per 1000 persons per year in those more than 60 years of age, whereas the incidence rate in all ages is 1.2 to 3.4 per 1000 persons per year (reviewed in Schmader, 2007). Increasing age is also the strongest risk factor for developing postherpetic neuralgia (PHN). Acyclovir, famciclovir, and valacyclovir reduce acute pain and the duration of chronic pain if started within 72 hours of rash onset. Analgesics for relief of acute pain are important. Those with moderate to severe pain may require opioids. The addition of corticosteroids or gabapentin may be considered if pain persists. Corticosteroids have not been shown to reduce the incidence of PHN in older patients. Topical lidocaine patch, gabapentin, and pregabalin are FDA approved for treatment of PHN, but nortriptyline and opioids have also been shown to be of benefit. In some cases, combination therapy may be necessary. A live, attenuated varicella-zoster vaccine has been developed and shown to be safe and to reduce the incidence of HZ (hazard ratio, 0.45), including ophthalmic HZ (hazard ratio, 0.37), and hospitalizations for HZ (hazard ratio, 0.35) (Simberkoff et al, 2010; Tseng et al, 2011).

Vaccination recommendations also include tetanus vaccination with Td every 10 years. This should be replaced at least once with Tdap to cover pertussis immunization, since the immune response to pertussis has been shown to wane.

DISORDERS OF TEMPERATURE REGULATION

Temperature dysregulation in older individuals demonstrates the narrowing of homeostatic mechanisms that occurs with advancing age. Older adults may have a mean oral body temperature lower than 98.6°F (37°C), and older nursing home residents may have lower body temperature and fail to demonstrate a diurnal rise (Gomolin et al, 2005). Older persons are less able to adjust to extremes of environmental temperatures. Hypo- and hyperthermic states are predominantly disorders of older adults. Despite underreporting of these disorders, there is evidence that morbidity and mortality increase during particularly hot or cold periods, especially among ill older adults. Much of this illness is caused by an increased incidence of cardiovascular disorders (myocardial infarction and stroke) or infectious diseases (pneumonia) during these periods.

Hypothermia is a common finding among older adults during the winter, when homes are heated at less than 70°F (21°C).

PATHOPHYSIOLOGY

Impaired temperature perception, diminished sweating in hyperthermia, and abnormal vasoconstrictor response in hypothermia are major pathophysiological mechanisms in these disorders.

HYPOTHERMIA

Hypothermia is defined as a core temperature (rectal, esophageal, tympanic) below 95°F (35°C). Essential to the diagnosis is early recognition with a low-recording thermometer.

Table 12-13 illustrates the clinical spectrum of hypothermia. Because early signs are nonspecific and subtle, a high index of suspicion must exist to allow an early diagnosis. A history of known or potential exposure is helpful, but older patients can become hypothermic at modest temperatures. Frequently, the most difficult differential diagnosis in more severe hypothermia is hypothyroidism. A previous history of thyroid disease, a neck scar from previous thyroid surgery, and a delay in the relaxation phase of the deep tendon reflexes may assist in diagnosing hypothyroidism. Patients may sometimes be mistaken for dead. Case reports reveal patients who have survived after being discovered without respiration and pulse.

The most significant early complications are arrhythmias and cardiorespiratory arrests. Later complications involve the pulmonary, gastrointestinal, and renal systems. Electrocardiogram (ECG) abnormalities are frequent. The most specific ECG finding is the J wave (Osborn wave) following the QRS complex. This abnormality disappears as temperature returns to normal.

General supportive therapy for severe hypothermia consists of intensive care management of complicated multisystem dysfunctions. Every attempt should be made to assess and treat any contributing medical disorder (eg, infection, hypothyroidism, hypoglycemia). Hypothermia in older patients should promptly be treated as sepsis unless proven otherwise. While patients should have continuous ECG monitoring, central lines should be avoided if possible because of myocardial irritability.

PART III

TABLE 12-13. Clinical Presentation of Hypothermia		
Early signs (89.6°–95°F [32°–35°C])	Late signs (82.4°–86°F [28°–30°C])	Later signs (<82.4°F [28°C])
Fatigue	Cold skin	Very cold skin
Weakness	Hypopnea	Rigidity
Slowness of gait	Cyanosis	Apnea
Apathy	Bradycardia	No pulse—ventricular fibrillation
Slurred speech	Atrial and ventricular arrhythmias	Areflexia
Confusion		
Shivering (±)	Hypotension	Unresponsiveness
Cool skin	Semicoma and coma	Fixed pupils
Sensation of cold (±)	Muscular rigidity	
	Generalized edema	
	Slowed reflexes	
	Poorly reactive pupils	
	Polyuria or oliguria	

Because there is delayed metabolism, most drugs have little effect on a severely hypo-thermic patient, but they may cause problems once the patient is rewarmed. It is preferable to stabilize the patient and immediately undertake specific rewarming techniques. Serious arrhythmias, acidosis, and fluid and electrolyte disorders will usually respond to therapy only after rewarming has been accomplished.

Passive rewarming is generally adequate for those with mild hypothermia (>89.6°F [>32°C]). Active external rewarming has been associated with increased morbidity and mortality because cold blood may suddenly be shunted to the core, further decreasing core temperature; peripheral vasodilatation can precipitate hypovolemic shock by decreasing circulatory blood volume. For more severe hypothermia (<89.6°F [<32°C]), core rewarming is necessary. Several techniques for core rewarming have been used, but positive results have been reported only from small, uncontrolled studies. Peritoneal dialysis and inhalation rewarming may be the most practical tech-niques in the majority of institutions.

Mortality is usually greater than 50% for severe hypothermia. It increases with age and is particularly related to underlying disease.

HYPERTHERMIA

Heat stroke is defined as a failure to maintain body temperature and is characterized by a core temperature of >105°F (>40.6°C), severe central nervous system dysfunc-tion (psychosis, delirium, coma), and anhidrosis (hot, dry skin). The two groups primarily affected are older adults who are chronically ill and the young undergoing strenuous exercise. Mortality is as high as 80% once this syndrome is manifest.

There are multiple predisposing factors for heat stroke in older adults, but most often there is a prolonged heat wave (reviewed in O'Malley, 2007). The diagno-sis requires a high level of suspicion. In view of the poor survival, efforts must be directed toward prevention. Older patients should be cautioned about the dangers of hot weather. For those at particularly high risk, temporary relocation to more protected environments should be considered.

Early manifestations of heat exhaustion are nonspecific (Table 12-14). Later, severe central nervous system dysfunction and anhidrosis develop.

TABLE 12-14. Clinical Presentation of Hyperthermia

Early signs	Later signs
Dizziness	Central nervous system dysfunction
Weakness	Psychosis
Sensation of warmth	Delirium
Anorexia	Coma
Nausea	Anhidrosis
Vomiting	Hot, dry skin
Headache	
Dyspnea	

TABLE 12-15. Complications of Heat Stroke

Myocardial damage
  Congestive heart failure
  Arrhythmias
Renal failure (20%–25%)
Cerebral edema
  Seizures
  Diffuse and focal findings
Hepatocellular necrosis
  Jaundice
  Liver failure
Rhabdomyolysis
  Myoglobinuria
Bleeding diathesis
  Disseminated intravascular coagulation
Electrolyte disturbances
Acid–base disturbances
  Metabolic acidosis
  Respiratory alkalosis
Infection
  Aspiration pneumonia
  Sepsis
Dehydration and shock

Table 12-15 lists some of the more serious complications resulting from heat damage to organ systems. Once the full syndrome has developed for any length of time, the prognosis is very poor. While management at this stage requires intense multisystem care, the key is rapid specific therapy consisting of cooling to 102°F (38.9°C) within the first hour. Ice packs and ice-water immersion are superior to convection cooling with alcohol sponge baths or electric fans.

Prevention appears to be the most appropriate approach to manage temperature dysregulation in older adults. Educating older adults to their susceptibility to hypo- and hyperthermia in extremes of environmental temperature, education about appropriate behavior in such conditions, and close monitoring of the most vulnerable older adults should help reduce the morbidity and mortality from these disorders.

Evidence Summary

Do's

- Screen overweight or obese patients between ages 40 and 70 years for diabetes.
- Recognize that lifestyle modification, including weight loss and exercise, are cornerstone strategies to help forestall type 2 diabetes mellitus in those with glucose intolerance.
- Treat other atherosclerotic risk factors (smoking, dyslipidemia, hypertension) in diabetic patients.

- Assess for hypothyroidism in older adults who present with fatigue, memory loss, and decreased hearing.
- Screen older adults for vitamin D deficiency.
- Assess for primary hyperparathyroidism in patients with fracture and low bone mineral density.

Don'ts

- Use metformin in patients with renal insufficiency or heart failure.
- Use thiazolidinediones in patients with heart failure.
- Recommend testosterone supplementation in older men with low-normal testosterone concentrations.

Consider

- Life expectancy and quality of life in setting goals for glucose control.

REFERENCES

American Diabetes Association. Older adults. Sec 11. In: Standards of Medical Care in Diabetes—2017. *Diabetes Care.* 2017;40(Suppl 1):S99-S104.

Aranow C. Vitamin D and the immune system. *J Investig Med.* 2011;59:881-886.

Artz AS, Thirman MJ. Unexplained anemia predominates despite an intensive evaluation in a racially diverse cohort of older adults from a referral anemia clinic. *J Gerontol A Biol Sci Med Sci.* 2011;66A:925-932.

Beasley JM, LaCroix AZ, Neuhouser ML, et al. Protein intake and incident frailty in the Women's Health Initiative Observational Study. *J Am Geriatr Soc.* 2010;58:1063-1071.

Besarab A, Bolton K, Browne JK et al. The effects of normal as compared to low hematocrit values in patients with cardiac disease who are receiving hemodialysis and epoetin. *N Engl J Med.* 1998;339:584-590.

Bennett WL, Maruther NM, Singh S, et al. Comparative effectiveness and safety of medications for type 2 diabetes: an update including new drugs and drug combinations. *Ann Intern Med.* 2011;154:602-613.

Bergström I, Landgren BM, Freyschuss B. Primary hyperparathyroidism is common in postmenopausal women with forearm fracture and low bone mineral density. *Acta Obstet Gynecol Scand.* 2007;861:61-64.

Bilezikian JP, Potts JT, Fuleihan GE-H, et al. Summary statement from a workshop on asymptomatic primary hyperparathyroidism. *J Clin Endocrinol Metab.* 2002;87:5353-5361.

Biondi B, Fazio S, Palmieri EA, et al. Left ventricular diastolic dysfunction in patients with subclinical hypothyroidism. *J Clin Endocrinol Metab.* 1999;84:2064-2067.

Bischoff-Ferrari HA, Dawson-Hughes B, Orav J, et al. Monthly high dose vitamin D treatment for the prevention of functional decline: a randomized clinical trial. *JAMA Intern Med.* 2016. doi:10.1001/jamainternmed.2015.7148.

Bischoff-Ferrari HA, Willett WC, Orav EJ, et al. A pooled analysis of vitamin D dose requirements for fracture prevention. *N Engl J Med.* 2012;367:40-49.

Blackman MR, Sorkin JD, Munzer T, et al. Growth hormone and sex steroid administration in healthy aged women and men: a randomized controlled trial. *JAMA.* 2002;288:2282-2292.

Boulé NG, Haddad E, Kenny GP, et al. Effects of exercise on glycemic control and body mass in type 2 diabetes mellitus: a meta-analysis of controlled clinical trials. *JAMA.* 2001;286:1218-1227.

Cappola AR, Fried LP, Arnold, AM, et al. Thyroid status, cardiovascular risk, and mortality in older adults. *JAMA*. 2006;295:1033-1041.

Ceresini G, Lauretani F, Maggio M, et al. Thyroid function abnormalities and cognitive impairment in elderly people: results of the Invecchiare in Chianti Study. *J Am Geriatr Soc*. 2009;57:89-93.

Chung M, Lee J, Terasawa T, et al. Vitamin D with or without calcium supplementation for prevention of cancer and fractures: an updated meta-analysis for the U.S. Preventive Services Task Force. *Ann Intern Med*. 2011;155:827-838.

Church TS, Blair SN, Cocreham S, et al. Effects of aerobic and resistance training on hemoglobin A1c levels in patients with type 2 diabetes: a randomized controlled trial. *JAMA*. 2010;304:2253-2262.

Collet TH, Gussekloo J, Bauer DC, et al. Subclinical hyperthyroidism and the risk of coronary heart disease and mortality. *Arch Intern Med*. 2012;172:799-809.

Cooper DS. Antithyroid drugs. *N Engl J Med*. 2005;352:905-917.

Cooper DS. Subclinical hypothyroidism. *N Engl J Med*. 2001;345:260-265.

Cushman WC, Evans GW, Byington RP, et al. Effects of intensive blood-pressure control in type 2 diabetes mellitus. *N Engl J Med*. 2010;362:1575-1585.

De Boer IH, Levin G, Robinson-Cohen C, et al. Serum 25-hydroxyvitamin D concentration and risk for major clinical disease events in a community-based population of older adults. *Ann Intern Med*. 2012;156:627-634.

Diabetes Prevention Program Research Group. Reduction in the incidence of type 2 diabetes with lifestyle intervention or metformin. *N Engl J Med*. 2002;346:393-403.

Dong XQ, Mendes de Leon C, Artz A, et al. A population-based study of hemoglobin, race, and mortality in elderly persons. *J Gerontol Med Sci*. 2008;63A:873-878.

Ellison DH, Berl T. The syndrome of inappropriate antidiuresis. *N Engl J Med*. 2007;356:2064-2072.

Emmelot-Vonk MH, Verhaar HJ, Nakhai Pour HR, et al. Effect of testosterone supplementation on functional mobility, cognition, and other parameters in older men: a randomized controlled trail. *JAMA*. 2008;2:39-52.

Ershler WB, Sheng S, McKelvey J, et al. Serum erythropoietin and aging: a longitudinal analysis. *J Am Geriatr Soc*. 2005;53:1360-1365.

Fatourechi V. Upper limit of normal serum thyroid-stimulating hormone: a moving and now and aging target? *Endo J*. 2007;92:4560-4562.

Fick DM, Agostini JV, Inouye SK. Delirium superimposed on dementia. *J Am Geriatr Soc*. 2002;50:1723-1732.

Flegal KM, Kit BK, Orpana H et al. Association of all-cause mortality with overweight and obesity using standard body mass index categories: a systematic review and meta-analysis. *JAMA*. 2013;309(1):71-82.

Fletcher RH, Fairfield KM. Vitamins for chronic disease prevention: clinical applications. *JAMA*. 2002;287:3127-3129.

Gaede P, Lund-Anderson H, Parving H-H, et al. Effect of a multifactorial intervention on mortality in type 2 diabetes. *N Engl J Med*. 2008;358:580-591.

Gillies CL, Abrams KR, Lambert PC, et al. Review: lifestyle or pharmacologic interventions prevent or delay type 2 diabetes in impaired glucose tolerance. *BMJ*. 2007;334:299-307.

Ginde AA, Scragg R, Schwartz RS, et al. Prospective study of serum 25-hydoxyvitamin D level, cardiovascular disease mortality, and all-cause mortality in older U.S. adults. *J Am Geriatr Soc*. 2009;57:1595-1603.

PART III

Gomolin IH, Aung MM, Wolf-Klein G, et al. Older is colder: temperature range and variation in older people. *J Am Geriatr Soc.* 2005;53:2170-2172.

Grohskopf L, Sokolow LZ, Broder KR et al. Prevention and control of seasonal influenza with vaccines: recommendations of the Advisory Committee on Immunizations Practices, 2016-2017 influenza season. *MMWR.* 2016;65(5):1-54.

Gruenewald DA, Matsumoto AM. Testosterone supplementation therapy for older men: potential benefits and risks. *J Am Geriatr Soc.* 2003;51:101-115.

Habra M, Sarlis NJ. Thyroid and aging. *Rev Endocr Metab Disord.* 2005;6:145-154.

Heany RP. Vitamin D: baseline status and effective dose. *N Engl J Med.* 2012;367:77-78.

High KP, Bradley SF, Gravenstein S, et al. Clinical practice guideline for the evaluation of fever and infection in older adult residents of long-term care facilities: 2008 update by the Infectious Disease Society of America. *J Am Geriatr Soc.* 2009;57:375-394.

Holick MF. Vitamin D: a D-lightful solution for health. *J Investig Med.* 2011;59:872-880.

Holick MF, Brinkley NC, Bischoff-Ferrari HA, et al. Evaluation, treatment, and prevention of vitamin D deficiency: an Endocrine Society clinical practice guideline. 2011;96:1911-1930.

Holman RR, Farmer AJ, Davies MJ, et al. Three-year efficacy of complex insulin regimens in type 2 diabetes. *N Engl J Med.* 2009;361:1736-1747.

Houston DK, Tooze JA, Davis CC, et al. Serum 25-hydroxyvitamin D and physical function in older adults: the Cardiovascular Health Study All Stars. *J Am Geriatr Soc.* 2011;59:1793-1801.

Huang ES, Meigs JB, Singer DE. The effect of interventions to prevent cardiovascular disease in patients with type 2 diabetes mellitus. *Am J Med.* 2001;111:633-642.

Huang ES, Zhang Q, Gandra N, et al. The effect of comorbid illness and functional status on the expected benefits of intensive glucose control in older patients with type 2 diabetes: a decision analysis. *Ann Intern Med.* 2008;149:11-19.

Huber G, Staub J-J, Meier C, et al. Prospective study of the spontaneous course of subclinical hypothyroidism: prognostic value of thyrotropin, thyroid reserve, and thyroid antibodies. *J Clin Endocrinol Metab.* 2002;87:3221-3226.

Inzucchi SE. Diagnosis of diabetes. *N Engl J Med.* 2012;367:542-550.

Inzucchi SE. Management of hyperglycemia in the hospital setting. *N Engl J Med.* 2006;355:1903-1911.

Inzucchi SE, Bergenstal RM, Buse JB et al. Management of hyperglycemia in type 2 diabetes, 2015: a patient-centered approach. Update to a position statement of the American Diabetes Association and the European Association for the Study of Diabetes. *Diabetes Care.* 2015;38:140-149.

Izaks GJ, Westendorp RG, Knook DL. The definition of anemia in older persons. *JAMA.* 1999;281:1714-1717.

Jackson C, Gaugris S, Sen SS, et al. The effect of cholecalciferol (vitamin D_3) on the risk of fall and fracture: a meta-analysis. *QJM.* 2007;100:185-192.

Jain S, Self WH, Wunderink S, et al. Community-acquired pneumonia requiring hospitalization among U.S. adults. *N Engl J Med.* 2015;373:415-427.

Janssen I, Mark AE. Elevated body mass index and mortality risk in the elderly. *Obesity Rev.* 2007;8:41-59.

Jones M, Ibels L, Schenkel B, et al. Impact of epoetin alfa on clinical end points in patients with chronic renal failure: a meta-analysis. *Kidney Int.* 2004;65:757-767.

Jonklaas J, Bianco AC, Baurer AJ, et al. Guidelines for the treatment of hypothyroidism: prepared by the American Thyroid Association task force on thyroid hormone replacement. *Thyroid.* 2014;24(12):1670-1751.

Kazi M, Geraci SA, Koch CA. Considerations for the diagnosis and treatment of testosterone deficiency in elderly men. *Am J Med.* 2007;120:835-840.

Keel SB, Abkowitz JL. The microcytic red cell and the anemia of inflammation. *N Engl J Med.* 2009;361:1904-1906.

Kenny AM, Kleppinger A, Annis K, et al. Effects of transdermal testosterone on bone and muscle in older men with low bioavailable testosterone levels low bone mass, and physical frailty. *J Am Geriatr Soc.* 2010;58:1134-1143.

Kirkman MS, Jones Briscoe V, Clark N, et al. Diabetes in older adults. *Diabetes Care.* 2012;35:2650-2664.

Ku S. Algorithms replace sliding scale insulin orders. *Drug Ther Topics.* 2002;31:49-53.

Lamberts SWJ, van den Beld AW, van der Lely A-J. The endocrinology of aging. *Science.* 1997;278:419-424.

Li YC. Molecular mechanism of vitamin D in the cardiovascular system. *J Investig Med.* 2011;59:868-871.

Ligthelm RJ, Kaiser M, Vora J, et al. Insulin use in elderly adults: risk of hypoglycemia and strategies for care. *J Am Geriatr Soc.* 2012; 60:1564-1570.

Lorig KR, Sobel DS, Stewart AL, et al. Evidence suggesting that a chronic disease self-management can improve health status while reducing hospitalization: a randomized trial. *Med Care.* 1999;37(1): 5-14.

Lorig KR, Ritter P, Stewart AL, et al. Chronic disease self-management program: 2-year health stats and health care utilization outcomes. *Med Care.* 2001;39(11):1217-1223.

Liu H, Bravata DM, Olkin I, et al. Systematic review: the safety and efficacy of growth hormone in the healthy elderly. *Ann Intern Med.* 2007;146:104-115.

Longo DL. Closing in on a killer: anemia in elderly people. *J Gerontol Biol Sci Med Sci.* 2005;60A:727-728.

Maraldi C, Ble A, Zuliani G, et al. Association between anemia and physical disability in older patients: role of comorbidity. *Aging Clin Exp Res.* 2006;8:485-492.

Marcocci C, Cetani F. Primary hyperthyroidism. *N Engl J Med.* 2011;365:2389-2397.

Mariotti S, Cambuli VM. Cardiovascular risk in elderly hypothyroid patients. *Thyroid.* 2007;17:1067-1073.

McGandy RB, Barrows CH Jr, Spanias A, et al. Nutrient intakes and energy expenditures in men of different ages. *J Gerontol.* 1966;21:581-587.

Memtsoudis SG, Besculides MC, Mazumdar M. A rude awakening: the perioperative sleep apnea epidemic. *N Engl J Med.* 2013;368:2352-2353.

Miller M. Hyponatremia and arginine vasopressin dysregulation: mechanisms, clinical consequences, and management. *J Am Geriatr Soc.* 2006;54:345-353.

Montero-Odasso M, Duque G. Vitamin D in the aging musculoskeletal system: an authentic strength preserving hormone. *Mol Aspects Med.* 2005;26:203-219.

Montori VM, Fernandez-Balsells M. Glycemic control in type 2 diabetes: time for an evidenced-based about face? *Ann Intern Med.* 2009;150:803-808.

Morris MS, Selhub J, Jacques PF. Vitamin B-12 and folate status in relation to decline in scores on the Mini-Mental State Examination in the Framingham Heart Study. *J Am Geriatr Soc.* 2012;60:1457-1464.

Muir SW, Montero-Odasso M. Effect of vitamin D supplementation on muscle strength, gait, and balance in older adults: a systematic review and meta-analysis. *J Am Geriatr Soc.* 2011;59:2291-2300.

O'Malley PG. Commentary on heat waves and heat-related illness. *JAMA.* 2007;298: 917-919.

PART III

Page ST, Amory JK, Bowman FD, et al. Exogenous testosterone (T) alone or with finasteride increases physical performance, grip strength, and lean body mass in older men with low serum T. *J Clin Endocrinol Metab.* 2005;90:1502-1510.

Patel KV, Semba RD, Ferrucci L, et al. Red cell distribution width and mortality in older adults: a meta-analysis. *J Gerontol A Biol Sci Med Sci.* 2010;65A:258-265.

Penninx BWJH, Pahor M, Woodman RC, et al. Anemia in old age is associated with increased mortality and hospitalization. *J Gerontol Biol Sci Med Sci.* 2006;61A:474-479.

Puar TH, Khoo JJ, Cho LW, et al. Association between glycemic control and hip fracture. *J Am Geriatr Soc.* 2012;60:1493-1497.

Qaseem A, Humphrey LL, Sweet DE, et al. Oral pharmacologic treatment of type 2 diabetes mellitus: a clinical practice guideline from the American College of Physicians. *Ann Intern Med.* 2012;156:218-231.

Rodondi N, den Elzen WPJ, Bauer DC, et al. Subclinical hypothyroidism and the risk of coronary heart disease and mortality. *JAMA.* 2010;304:1365-1374.

Rosen CJ. Vitamin D insufficiency. *N Engl J Med.* 2011;364:248-254.

Ross DS, Burch HB, Cooper DS, et al. 2016 American Thyroid Association guidelines for diagnosis and management of hyperthyroidism and othe causes of thyrotoxicosis. *Thyroid.* 2016;26(10):1343-1421.

Saint S, Green MT, Krein SL et. al. A program to prevent catheter-associated urinary tract infection in acute care. *N Engl J Med.* 2016;374:2111-2119.

Schmader K. Herpes zoster and postherpetic neuralgia in older adults. *Clin Geriatr Med.* 2007;23:615-632.

Schroeder SA. We can do better: improving the health of the American people. *N Engl J Med.* 2007;357:1221-1228.

Selph S, Dana T, Blazina I, et al. Screening for type 2 diabetes mellitus: a systematic review for the U.S. Preventive Services Task Force. *Ann Intern Med.* 2015;162:765-776.

Sesso HD, Buring JE, Christen WG, et al. Vitamins E and C in the prevention of cardiovascular disease in men: the Physician's Health Study II randomized controlled trial. *JAMA.* 2008;300:2123-2133.

Simberkoff MS, Arbeit RD, Johson GR, et al. Safety of herpes zoster vaccine in the Shingles Prevention Study: a randomized trial. *Ann Intern Med.* 2010;152:545-554.

Snyder PJ, Bhasin GR, Cunningham AM, et al. Effects of testosterone in older men. *N Engl J Med.* 2016;374:611-624.

Steensma DP. Is anemia of cancer different from chemotherapy induced anemia? *J Clin Oncol.* 2008;26:1022-1024.

Sterns RH. Disorders of plasma sodium: causes, consequences, and correction. *N Engl J Med.* 2015;372(1):55-65.

Strippoli GF, Craig MC, Schena FP, et al. Review: ACE inhibitors delay onset of microalbuminuria in diabetes without nephropathy and reduce mortality in diabetic nephropathy. *J Am Soc Nephrol.* 2006;17:S153-S155.

Surks MI, Hollowell JG. Age-specific distribution of serum thyrotropin and antithyroid antibodies in the US population: implications for the prevalence of subclinical hypothyroidism. *J Clin Endocrinol Metab.* 2007;92:4575-4582.

Tomczyk S, Bennett NM, Gierke R, et al. Use of 13-valent pneumococcal conjugate vaccine and 23-valent pneumococcal polysaccharide among adults aged >=65 years: recommendations of the Advisory Committee on Immunization Practices (ACIP). *MMWR.* 2014;63(37):822-825.

Tseng HF, Smith N, Harpaz R, et al. Herpes zoster vaccine in older adults and the risk of subsequent herpes zoster disease. *JAMA*. 2011;305:160-166.

United Kingdom Prospective Diabetes Study (UKPDS) Group. Effect of intensive blood-glucose control with metformin on complications in overweight patients with type 2 diabetes: UKPDS 34. *Lancet*. 1998b;352:854-865.

United Kingdom Prospective Diabetes Study (UKPDS) Group. Tight blood pressure control and risk of macrovascular and microvascular complications in type 2 diabetes: UKPDS 38. *BMJ*. 1998c;317:703-712.

Venditti M, Falcone M, Carrao S, et al. Outcomes of patients hospitalized with community-acquired, health care-associated, and hospital-acquired pneumonia. *Ann Intern Med*. 2009;150:19-26.

Villar H, Saconato H, Valente O, et al. Thyroid hormone replacement for subclinical hypothyroidism. *Cochrane Database Syst Rev*. 2007;(3):CD003419.

Villareal DT, Apovian CM, Kushner RF, et al. Obesity in older adults: technical review and position statement of the American Society for Nutrition and NAASO, the Obesity Society. *Am J Clin Nutr*. 2005;82:923-934.

Weiss G, Goodnough LT. Anemia of chronic disease. *N Engl J Med*. 2005;352:1011-1023.

Yau CK, Eng C, Cenzer IS, et al. Glycosylated hemoglobin and functional decline in community-dwelling nursing home-eligible elderly adults with diabetes mellitus. *J Am Geriatr Soc*. 2012;60:1215-1221.

Zamboni M, Mazzali G, Zoico E, et al. Health consequences of obesity in the elderly: a review of four unresolved questions. *Int J Obesity*. 2005;29:1011-1029.

SUGGESTED READINGS

Bartlett JG. Antibiotic-associated diarrhea. *N Engl J Med*. 2002;346:334-339.

Bentley DW, Bradley S, High K, et al. Practice guideline for evaluation of fever and infection in long-term care facilities. *J Am Geriatr Soc*. 2001;49:210-222.

Bouchama A, Knochel JP. Heat stroke. *N Engl J Med*. 2002;346:1978-1988.

Brady MA, Perron WJ. Electrocardiographic manifestations of hypothermia. *Am J Emerg Med*. 2002;20:314-326.

Camaschella C. Iron-deficiency anemia. *N Engl J Med*. 2015;372:1832-1843.

Chandalia M, Garg A, Lutjohann D, et al. Beneficial effects of high dietary fiber intake in patients with type 2 diabetes mellitus. *N Engl J Med*. 2000;342:1392-1398.

Davis PJ, Davis FB. Hyperthyroidism in patients over the age of 60 years. *Medicine (Baltimore)*. 1974;53:161-181.

Elia M, Ritz P, Stubbs RJ. Total energy expenditure in the elderly. *Eur J Clin Nutr*. 2000;54:S92-S103.

Endocrine Society Clinical Practice Guideline. Testostrone therapy in adult men with androgen deficiency syndromes. *J Clin Endocrinol Metab*. 2010;95(6) 2536-2559.

Federman DD. Hyperthyroidism in the geriatric population. *Hosp Pract*. 1991;26:61-76.

Finucane TE. "Tight control" in geriatrics: the emperor wears a thong. *J Am Geriatr Soc*. 2012;60:1571-1575.

Gambert SR. Effect of age on thyroid hormone physiology and function. *J Am Geriatr Soc*. 1985;33:360-365.

Gress TW, Nieto J, Shahar E, et al. Hypertension and antihypertensive therapy as risk factors for type 2 diabetes mellitus. *N Engl J Med*. 2000;342:905-912.

PART III

Hak AE, Pols HAP, Visser TJ, et al. Subclinical hypothyroidism is an independent risk factor for atherosclerosis and myocardial infarction in elderly women: the Rotterdam study. *Ann Intern Med.* 2000;132:270-278.

Ismail-Beigi F, Moghissi E, Tiktin M, et al. Individualizing glycemic targets in type 2 diabetes mellitus: implications of recent clinical trials. *Ann Intern Med.* 2011;154:554-559.

KDIGO Clinical Practice Guideline for Anemia in Chronic Disease. *Kidney Int Suppl.* 2012;2:331-335.

Lipschitz DA. An overview of anemia in older patients. *Older Patient.* 1988;2:5-11.

Mateen FJ, Mills EJ. Aging and HIV-related cognitive loss. *JAMA.* 2012:308:349-350.

Mizgerd JD. Acute lower respiratory tract infection. *N Engl J Med.* 2008;358:716-727.

Mody L, Manisha-Mehta M. *JAMA.* 2015;311(8):844-854.

Mylonakis E, Calderwood SB. Infective endocarditis in adults. *N Engl J Med.* 2001;345:1318-1330.

Nahid P, Dorman SE, Alipanah N, et al. Official American Thoracic Society/Centers for Disease Control and Prevention/Infectious Diseases Society of America Clinical Practice Guidelines: Treatment of Drug-Susceptible Tuberculosis. *Clin Infect Dis.* 2016;63(7): e147-e195.

Oxman MN, Levin MJ, Johnson GR, et al. A vaccine to prevent herpes zoster postherpetic neuralgia in older adults. *N Engl J Med.* 2005;352:2271-2284.

Schaefer AJ, Nicolle LE. Urinary tract infections in older men. *N Engl J Med.* 2016;374:562-571.

Stabler SP. Vitamin B12 deficiency. *N Engl J Med.* 2013;368:149-160.

Stead WW, To T, Harrison RW, et al. Benefit-risk considerations in preventive treatment for tuberculosis in elderly persons. *Ann Intern Med.* 1987;107:843-845.

The ORIGIN Trial Investigators. Basal insulin and cardiovascular and other outcomes in dysglycemia. *N Engl J Med.* 2012;367:319-328.

Thomas FB, Mazzaferi EL, Skillman TB. Apathetic thyrotoxicosis: a distinctive clinical and laboratory entity. *Ann Intern Med.* 1970;72:679-685.

Trivalle C, Doucet J, Chassagne P, et al. Differences in the signs and symptoms of hyperthyroidism in older and younger patients. *J Am Geriatr Soc.* 1996;44:50-53.

Tuomilehto J, Lindstrom J, Eriksson JG, et al. Prevention of type 2 diabetes mellitus by changes in lifestyle among subjects with impaired glucose tolerance. *N Engl J Med.* 2001;344:1343-1350.

United Kingdom Prospective Diabetes Study Group. Efficacy of atenolol and captopril in reducing risk of macrovascular and microvascular complications in type 2 diabetes: UKPDS 39. *BMJ.* 1998;371:713-719.

United Kingdom Prospective Diabetes Study Group. Intensive blood-glucose control with sulphonylureas or insulin compared with conventional treatment and risk of complications in patients with type 2 diabetes (UKPDS 33). *Lancet.* 1998a;352:837-852.

Yoshikawa TT, Norman D. Infectious diseases in geriatric medicine. *Clin Geriatr Med.* 2016;32:415-634.

Yoshikawa TT, Ouslander JG. *Infection Management for Geriatrics in Long-Term Care Facilities.* 2nd ed. Boca Raton, FL: CRC Press; 2006.

CHAPTER 13

Sensory Impairment

Because as many as 75% of older adults have significant visual or auditory dysfunction not reported to their physicians, adequate screening for these problems is important. These disorders may limit functional activity and lead to social isolation and depression. Correction of remediable conditions may improve ability to perform daily activities. The key clinical points include:

1. The prevalence of vision problems increases with age and many of the common causes are treatable disorders.
2. There are multiple rehabilitation strategies to maximize the functional independence of an individual with low vision.
3. The prevalence of hearing impairment increases progressively with age and some types of hearing loss can be corrected.
4. The combination of vision and hearing impairment may predispose to falls and the development of functional dependence.

PHYSIOLOGICAL AND FUNCTIONAL CHANGES

The visual system undergoes many changes with age (Table 13-1). Decreases in visual acuity in old age may be caused by morphological changes in the choroid, pigment epithelium, and retina, or by decreased function of the rods, cones, and other neural elements. Older patients frequently have difficulties turning their eyes upward or sustaining convergence. Intraocular pressure slowly increases with age.

The refractive error may become either more hyperopic (where vision is better for distant objects than for near objects) or more myopic (where it is difficult to see objects that are far away). In younger persons, hyperopia may be overcome by the accommodative power of the ciliary muscle on the young lens. However, with age, this latent hyperopia becomes manifest because of loss of accommodative reserve.

Other older patients may show an increase in myopia with age, caused by changes within the lens. The crystalline lens increases in size with age as old lens fibers accumulate in the lens nucleus. The nucleus becomes more compact and harder (nuclear sclerosis), increasing the refractive power of the lens and worsening the myopia.

Another definitive refractive change of aging is the development of presbyopia from nuclear sclerosis of the lens and atrophy of the ciliary muscle. As a result, the closest distance at which one can see clearly slowly recedes with age. The result is the inability to focus sharply for near vision. At approximately age 45, the near point of accommodation is so far that comfortable reading and near work become cumbersome and difficult. Corrective lenses are then needed to enable the patient to move that point closer to the eyes.

TABLE 13-1. Physiological and Functional Changes of the Eye With Advancing Age

Functional change	Physiological change	Implications
Visual acuity	Morphological change in choroid, pigment epithelium, or retina Decreased function of rods, cones, or other neural elements	Patient education materials, signage, prescription medication instructions may need to be presented with increased font
Extraocular motion	Difficulty in gazing upward and maintaining convergence	
Intraocular pressure	Increased pressure	
Refractive power	Increased hyperopia and myopia Presbyopia Increased lens size Nuclear sclerosis (lens) Ciliary muscle atrophy	Increased risk of glare.
Tear secretion	Decreased tearing Decreased lacrimal gland function Decreased goblet cell secretion	Increase risk of dry eyes, conjunctivitis.
Corneal function	Loss of endothelial integrity Posterior surface pigmentation	Difficulty adjusting to sudden change in lighting.

Diminished tear secretion in many older patients, especially postmenopausal women, may lead to dryness of the eyes, which can cause irritation and discomfort. This condition may endanger the intactness of the corneal surface. The treatment consists mainly in substitution therapy, with artificial tears instilled at frequent intervals.

The corneal endothelium often undergoes degenerative changes with aging. Because these cells seldom proliferate during adult life, the cell population is decreased. This may leave an irregular surface on the anterior chamber side, where pigments may accumulate. This type of endothelial dystrophy is frequently seen in older patients, and dense pigment accumulation may slightly decrease visual acuity. In some patients, the endothelial dystrophy may spontaneously progress and lead to corneal edema. Such cases require corneal transplants.

VISUAL IMPAIRMENT AND BLINDNESS

The prevalence of visual problems and blindness increases with age. In 2014, the rate of any trouble seeing, even with glasses or contacts, was 11.5% in Americans aged 65 to 74 years and 16.5% among those aged 75 and older. The most common causes of eye diseases (not counting refractive error) listed in order from most prevalent to least prevalent are cataracts, diabetic retinopathy, open-angle glaucoma, and late-age-related macular degeneration (Klein and Klein, 2013). Screening for visual

TABLE 13-2. Ophthalmological Screening Covered by Medicare Fee-for-Service

Visual acuity in the Welcome to Medicare Visit	Ability to read newspaper-sized print
Medicare provides coverage for annual glaucoma screening for high-risk groups:	A direct ophthalmoscopy examination
• Individuals with diabetes mellitus	A dilated eye exam with pressure measurement.
• Family history of glaucoma	
• African Americans aged 50 and older	
• Hispanic Americans aged 65 and older	

impairment is a required aspect of the Welcome to Medicare Visit. Screening for glaucoma is recommended for individuals at high risk (Table 13-2). Medicare does not pay for eyeglasses except for an initial pair after cataract surgery. Some Medicare Advantage programs may cover eyeglasses for their members.

Senile Cataract

Opacification of the crystalline lens is a frequent complication of aging. The Centers for Disease Control and Prevention (CDC) notes that the prevalence rates of cataracts increase with each decade of life starting around age 40. By age 80, 70% of whites have a cataract compared to about 53% of blacks and 61% of Hispanic Americans. The development of age-related cataract is a painless, progressive, but variable, process. Cataract formation is typically bilateral and often asymmetrical. Patients usually complain of problems with night driving, reading road signs, and difficulty with fine print.

The cause of age-related cataracts is unknown, but the opacifications in the lens are associated with the breakdown of the g-crystalline proteins. Epidemiological data and basic research suggest that ultraviolet light may be a contributing factor in cataract development. The pathological process may occur in either the cortex or the nucleus of the lens. Cortical cataracts have various stages of development. Early in the process, opacities are in the periphery and do not decrease visual acuity. At the mature stage, opacifications are more widespread and involve the pupillary area, leading to a slow decrease in visual acuity. In the mature stage, the entire lens becomes opaque. The nuclear cataract does not have these stages of development, but is a slowly progressing central opacity, which frequently shows a yellowish discoloration, therefore preventing certain colors from reaching the retina.

Cataracts of mild degree may be managed by periodic examination and changing eyeglasses to match the changing refractive error over an extended period. Ultraviolet lenses may decrease the sensitivity to glare. When a cataract progresses to the point where it interferes with activities, cataract surgery is generally indicated. The surgeon may use several methods to remove it, and the decision regarding the best method for each patient should be made by the ophthalmologist.

PART III

In intracapsular cataract extractions, the entire cataract and surrounding capsule are removed in a single piece. This removes the entire opacity. In extracapsular cataract extractions, the cataractous lens material and a portion of the capsule are removed. The posterior capsule is left in place to hold an intraocular lens implant.

The intraocular lens is surgically placed inside the iris and is expected to remain permanently in place. This lens corrects the focus of the eyes and permits central and peripheral vision; object size is increased by only 1%. It is appropriate for patients with cataracts in one or both eyes and is particularly useful for patients unable to wear a contact lens. The monofocal intraocular lens can be chosen to provide good near or far vision and glasses prescribed to compensate for the other type of vision (Table 13-3). Some intraocular lenses have different focusing powers within the same lens. These are called multifocal and accommodative lenses. They can reduce patients' dependence on glasses by giving clear vision for more than one set distance.

Contact lenses correct the focus of the eye, permit both central and peripheral vision, and increase apparent object size by 6%. However, handling contact lenses is difficult for some individuals, and most lenses must be removed and inserted daily. Extended-wear contact lenses are available, and approximately 50% to 70% of older patients are able to wear them after surgery. Contacts are useful in patients who have had cataract surgery in one or both eyes. The lenses correct for distant vision, but eyeglasses are required for reading. Bifocal lenses are available and may add to the quality of life of the individual.

Visual impairment is a known risk factor for falls and fractures, while patients who have had cataract surgery have a lower risk for hip fracture (Tseng et al, 2012).

Glaucoma

The glaucomas are a group of eye disorders characterized by increased intraocular pressure, progressive excavation of the optic nerve head with damage to the nerve fibers, and a specific loss in the visual field. Visual field testing should be performed. Initial changes lead to peripheral vision loss, with loss of central vision as the disease progresses. Most cases of primary glaucoma occur in older patients. Data from the CDC show that the prevalence of glaucoma increases with advancing age. Black Americans aged 40 years and older are at the greatest risk of developing glaucoma compared to people of other races. By age 80, about 8% of black Americans have glaucoma compared to about 5% of all others. Black Americans risk rises to nearly 12% after age 80 compared to 8% of whites and 10% of Hispanic Americans.

TABLE 13-3. Restoring Vision After Cataract Surgery—Intraocular Lenses

Correct central and peripheral vision
Increase image size by 1%.
Can be used after surgery on one or both eyes
Are useful for older adults unable to wear contact lenses
Require bifocal eyeglasses
Introduce added surgical and postsurgical complications

Angle-closure glaucoma is an acute and relatively infrequent type of glaucoma, characterized by a sudden painful attack of increased intraocular pressure accompanied by a marked loss in vision (see Table 13-4). Angle closure glaucoma is a surgical disease. The immediate treatment consists of normalizing the intraocular pressure by the application of miotic eye drops or other medication (such as acetazolamide or osmotic agents). The definitive treatment, however, is surgical excision of a peripheral piece of iris or, more frequently now, by laser iridectomy, ensuring free flow of aqueous humor. Because the disease is usually bilateral, some physicians propose prophylactic iridectomy on the second eye.

Chronic open-angle glaucoma is the more frequent variety of primary glaucoma. (See Kwon et al, 2009, for a review.) It is the third leading cause of blindness in the United States and the leading cause of blindness among black Americans (see www.cdc.gov/visionhealth/data/index.html for a description of the epidemiology). The irido-corneal angle is open, but aqueous outflow is diminished. The neuroretinal rim of the optic nerve becomes progressively thinner, leading to optic-nerve cupping. Its cause is the loss of retinal ganglion cell axons. Primary open-angle glaucoma is characterized by an insidious onset, slow progression, and the appearance of typical defects of the visual fields (see Table 13-4). Early in the disease, intraocular pressure is only moderately elevated, and optic nerve head excavation progresses slowly and sometimes asymmetrically. While central visual acuity may remain normal for a long time, the defects in the peripheral visual field are characteristic and gradually progressive. Initially, there is a paracentral scotoma, which may coalesce. A nasal step of the visual field is another important sign, although there are multiple possible visual field findings based on the stage of the disease. This nasal step refers to a deficit along the horizontal line of the affected eye. The patient may be entirely unaware of their visual field defects until very late into their course. Finally, the entire field will constrict and eventually involve the visual centers (Broadway, 2012).

The treatment for chronic open-angle glaucoma is usually medical, with miotics of various kinds used first (Boland et al, 2013). Medical treatment decreases the intraocular pressure and protects against visual field loss. Prostaglandins are currently the most effective topical medications for decreasing intraocular pressure. However, these medications are more likely to cause conjunctival hyperemia. Important systemic adverse effects of some of the classes of glaucoma medications warrant coordination of care between the opthamologist and the primary care provider. This is particularly important for the miotic eye drops (see Table 13-5). Surgery or laser therapy is indicated only if disease progresses on maximal medical therapy (Boland et al, 2013). Glaucoma eye medications should be reconciled and resumed as soon as older patients are hospitalized and transitioned to postacute settings of care.

Age-Related Macular Degeneration

The macular area of the retina lying at the posterior pole of the globe is the site of highest visual acuity. This area depends entirely on choriocapillaris for nutrition. Any disturbance in the vessel wall of the choroidal capillaries, in the permeability or thickness of the Bruch membrane, or in the retinal pigment epithelium may interfere with

TABLE 13-4. Signs and Symptoms Associated With Common Visual Problems in Older Adults

Signs and symptoms	Cataract	Open-angle glaucoma	Angle-closure glaucoma	Macular degeneration	Temporal arteritis	Diabetic retinopathy	Conjunctivitis	Foreign body	Subconjunctival hemorrhage
Pain			X		X		X	X	
Red eye			X				X	X	X
Fixed pupil			X						
Retinal vessel changes					X	X			
Retinal exudates				X		X			
Optic disk changes		X							
Sudden visual loss			X		X				
Loss of peripheral vision		X							
Glare intolerance	X								
Elevated intraocular pressure		X	X						
Loss of visual acuity	X			X		X			

TABLE 13-5. Potential Adverse Effects of Ophthalmic Solutions

Drug	Organ system	Responses
β-Blockers (eg, timolol)	Cardiovascular	Bradycardia, hypotension, syncope, palpitation, congestive heart failure
	Respiratory	Bronchospasm
	Neurological	Mental confusion, depression, fatigue, light-headedness, hallucinations, memory impairment, sexual dysfunction
	Miscellaneous	Hyperkalemia
Adrenergics (eg, epinephrine, phenylephrine)	Cardiovascular	Extrasystoles, palpitation, hypertension, myocardial infarction
	Miscellaneous	Trembling, paleness, sweating
Cholinergic/ anticholinesterases (eg, pilocarpine, echothiophate)	Respiratory	Bronchospasm
	Gastrointestinal	Salivation, nausea, vomiting, diarrhea, abdominal pain, tenesmus
	Miscellaneous	Lacrimation, sweating
Anticholinergics (eg, atropine)	Neurological	Ataxia, nystagmus, restlessness, mental confusion, hallucination, violent and aggressive behavior
	Miscellaneous	Insomnia, photophobia, urinary retention

PART III

the exchange of nutrients and oxygen from the choroidal blood to the central retina. Such disturbances occur frequently in older patients. Age-related degeneration of the macula is one of the most frequent causes of visual loss in older adults and is the commonest cause of legal blindness (20/200 or worse) (see Chakravarthy et al, 2010, for a review). White Americans have the highest risk of developing age-related macular degeneration. This disease affects more than 14% of white Americans aged 80 and older. By comparison, this illness is very uncommon among older blacks, Hispanics, and individuals of other races. In addition to older age, risk factors include family history of the disorder, cigarette smoking, low dietary intake or plasma concentrations of antioxidant vitamins and zinc, and white race for "wet" lesions (Fine et al, 2000). Age-related macular degeneration (AMD) is a common disease caused by the interplay of genetic predisposition and exposure to modifiable risk factors. Two susceptibility genes have been identified (*CFH* and *LOC387715*). Carrying the susceptibility alleles of either increases the risk between three- and eight-fold, whereas having two copies of the susceptibility alleles in both genes increases the risk 50-fold (Schaumberg et al, 2007). The combined effect of these polymorphisms carries an attributable risk of 60% (Haines and Pericak-Vance, 2007). Cigarette smoking and obesity multiply the risks associated with these variants. High lifetime exposure to sunlight is also a risk factor.

Ophthalmoscopic findings vary and do not always parallel loss of vision. In the geographic atrophy form of degeneration, there are areas of depigmentation alternating with zones of hyperpigmentation caused mainly by changes in the retinal pigment epithelium. In another form, the degeneration involves the Bruch membrane, leading to the pigmentation of well-circumscribed, roundish yellow areas. As lesions coalesce and involve the central macula, there is progressive worsening of vision to legal blindness (see de Jong, 2006).

The second type of degeneration features an acute exudative pathology as a consequence of neurovascularization. Here an elevated focus in the macular area at first contains serous fluid but later contains blood derived from blood vessels sprouting from the choroid to the subretinal space. The blood may become organized and form a plaque. Geographic atrophy AMD may produce a slow deterioration of central vision. Neurovascular AMD can cause a rapid distortion and loss of central vision.

In all these cases, central visual acuity will be markedly affected (see Table 13-4). Reading, driving, and recognizing faces become difficult. The atrophic type has no proven treatment or prevention. Verteporfin photodynamic (PTD) therapy has been shown to be beneficial in the treatment of advanced wet-type AMD (reviewed in Bourla and Young, 2006). PTD therapy combines the intravenous infusion of the light-sensitive dye verteporfin with low-intensity laser targeted to the neovascular tissue, causing occlusion of the abnormal choroidal vessels. However, recent therapy has been directed to vascular endothelial growth factor (VEGF) antagonism (reviewed in Chakravarthy et al, 2010). VEGF may play a critical role in the pathogenesis of neovascularization. Several VEGF antagonists, both systemic and intraocular injections, are available, but ranibizumab given monthly by intravitreal injection is the first drug demonstrated to not only slow progression but to improve vision in patients with neovascular AMD. Total blindness does not occur, as patients retain peripheral vision and therefore are able to perform activities that do not necessitate acute central vision. In the United Kingdom guidance by the National Institute for Health and Clinical Excellence has resulted in ranibizumab being adopted as the treatment of choice. However, the high cost of ranibizumab, along with the much cheaper and positive clinical experience with bevacizumab (Martin et al, 2011), has resulted in the majority of patients in the United States and other countries being treated with the latter drug. Medicare Part B pays for 80% of the costs of either of these medications and the patient pays the 20% copay. Visual rehabilitation is an important part of therapy for AMD. Patients may benefit from reading glasses or magnification devices. Clinical depression may occur as a consequence of reductions in quality of life and should be treated.

Diabetic Retinopathy

In the geriatric population, a significant amount of visual loss is attributed to diabetic retinopathy (see www.cdc.gov/visionhealth/data/index.html). The CDC again notes that the prevalence of this disease increases with advancing age, particularly among Hispanic Americans aged 50 years and older. Among adults aged 75 and older, 19% of Hispanic Americans had the disease, compared to 7% of blacks and

TABLE 13-6. Aids to Maximize Visual Function

Magnifying device
Lighting intensifiers without glare
Tinted glasses to reduce glare
Night light to assist in adaptation
Large-print newspapers, books, and magazines
Increased font size in electronic devices
Increased font size for prescription medication bottle instructions (ask pharmacist)

whites. In adult-onset diabetes with background changes, the visual loss is usually related to vascular changes in and around the macula leading to central visual loss. Leakage of serous fluid from vessels surrounding the macula leads to macular edema and deterioration of visual acuity. This may respond to laser photocoagulation.

Hemorrhages within the macula may lead to more permanent visual loss. A loss of retinal capillaries may lead to macular ischemia and poor prognosis of visual recovery. Intensive blood glucose control and tight blood pressure control reduce the risk of microvascular disease, including retinopathy in type 2 diabetes (see Chapter 12). Panretinal and focal retinal laser photocoagulation reduces the risk of visual loss in patients with severe diabetic retinopathy and macular edema, respectively (reviewed in Mohamed et al, 2007). There is currently insufficient evidence for routine use of other treatments, such as VEGF antagonists.

GENERAL FACTORS

Table 13-4 summarizes the general patterns of signs and symptoms associated with common visual problems of older adults. In addition to the specific treatment discussed earlier, some simple techniques, such as use of a magnifying device, large-print reading material, lighting intensifiers, and reduction of glare, can help maximize visual function (Table 13-6). Community resources to help the individual adapt to low vision can be accessed through the Veterans Affairs or the area agency on aging throughout the United States.

Clinicians should also be aware of the significant systemic absorption of ophthalmic medications (Anand and Eschmann, 1988). The particular concern is for β-blocker eye drops. These agents may lead to other organ system dysfunction and interact with other medications (Table 13-5). The patient's other medical problems and medications should be assessed, and the minimum dose to achieve the desired effect should be used. Patients should also be monitored for systemic toxicity.

HEARING

This section covers information related to hearing problems in older adults: a review of the auditory system, tests used to screen for and evaluate hearing, effects of aging on hearing performance, specific pathological disorders affecting the auditory system, and how treatment is likely (or not) to help.

PART III

Hearing problems are common in older adults, especially in a highly industrialized society where noise and age interact to cause hearing loss. The prevalence of hearing problems increases with increasing age in the United States. The majority of adults who had trouble hearing described their problem as a mild healing loss. Less than 2% of adults who indicated that they had any trouble hearing were deaf. In short, the degree of hearing troubles and the implications can vary within a given older population. In the 2005–2006 cycle of the National Health and Nutrition Examination Survey, hearing loss was present in 63% of those surveyed aged 70 and older. (See Pacala and Yueh, 2012, for a review of epidemiology, evaluation, and management of hearing loss in older adults.) The prevalence of hearing loss is higher in lower-income adults, those with lower education levels, and those who had an occupational exposure to noise. Exposure to recreational sound (eg, rock concerts, and ear plugs from iPhones) may change the hearing problems of our society over time. The health implications of hearing loss for older adults include and increased risk of cognitive impairment, falls, and depression, as well as a decline in the individual's quality of life. Screening is endorsed by most professional organizations, including the U.S. Preventive Services Task Force. Screening tests that reliably detect hearing loss are the whisper test administered in a standard fashion (2 feet from the patient), use of an audioscope, a handheld combination otoscope and audiometer, and a self-administered questionnaire, the Hearing Handicap Inventory for the Elderly–Screening (reviewed in Bogardus et al, 2003; Yueh et al, 2003). Hearing loss screening is a required element of the initial Welcome to Medicare Visit as well as the annual Medicare Wellness Visit. All patients with hearing loss should be referred to an audiologist for audiometric testing. This step is particularly relevant for those who have a hearing loss affecting the quality of their communication and especially those who were provided with or could afford to purchase a hearing aid (if such is required). Cerumen accumulation is common in older adults and can lead to significant hearing loss. Hearing loss in older adults is usually of the sensorineural type, caused by damage of the hearing organ, the peripheral nervous system, and/or the central nervous system. Individuals with hearing loss require hearing aids, aural rehabilitation, and understanding as the major avenues of remediation. Different approaches to the treatment plan are required for individuals with varying problems of magnification versus discrimination.

THE AUDITORY SYSTEM

On a functional basis, the auditory system can be divided into three major parts: peripheral, brain stem, and cortical areas. Each part of the hearing system has unique functions, which combine to allow hearing and understanding of speech. Table 13-7 lists auditory functional problems that are important to the primary care provider.

The main functions of the peripheral auditory system are to change sound into a series of electrical impulses and to transmit those to the brain stem. The major brain stem function is binaural interaction. Binaural interaction allows localization of sound and extraction of a signal from a noisy environment. The cortex brings sound to consciousness and allows interpretation of speech and initiation of appropriate reactions to sound signals.

TABLE 13-7. Functional Components of the Auditory System

A. Transmission of signals in the periphery
  1. Molecular motion (ear canal)
  2. Mechanical vibration (eardrum and ossicles)
  3. Hydromechanical motion (inner ear)
  4. Electrical impulse (eighth nerve)
B. Binaural interaction in the brainstem
  1. Localization and lateralization of sound
  2. Extraction of signals from environmental noise
C. Speech processing in the cortex
  1. Conscious sensation of hearing
  2. Interpretation of speech
  3. Initiation of response to sound

ASSESSMENT

Although the U.S. Preventive Services Task Force currently does not recommend screening of older adults for hearing loss, careful history may reveal symptomatic individuals who otherwise deny a deficit. Assessment of hearing function can be divided into three kinds of hearing tests: standard, binaural, and difficult speech. The standard tests are useful for evaluating the peripheral system, binaural tests for evaluating the brain stem, and difficult speech tests for evaluating cortical problems (Table 13-8). Table 13-9 outlines the clinical assessment of an older patient who presents with acute or subacute hearing loss. Standard tests are performed by presenting pure tones or single words at varying intensity. An audiometer (AudioScope, Welch-Allyn, Inc.) that will deliver pure tones is available for office screening of hearing deficits.

Tympanic membrane movement is assessed with a probe. Loudness comparison assesses the individual's ability to balance intensity of sound coming from both ears;

TABLE 13-8. Assessment of Hearing

A. Standard test measures
  1. Sensitivity for tones and speech
  2. Speech discrimination/understanding
  3. Movement of tympanic membrane
B. Binaural tests
  1. Loudness comparison
  2. Lateralization
  3. Masking of level differences
C. Difficult speech tests
  1. Monotonic degraded tasks
  2. Dichotic tasks
D. Welcome to Medicare Visit/Annual Wellness Visit screening for hearing impairment

Hearing testing is covered by Medicare if ordered by a physician, for the purpose of diagnosing a hearing or balance disorder.

TABLE 13.9. Initial Evaluation of an Older Patient With Acute or Subacute Hearing Loss

A. History
1. Recent infection or sinus problem
2. Trauma or falls
3. Exposure to loud noises
4. Associated symptoms: balance troubles, pain, drainage or bleeding from the ear, tinnitus, neurological symptoms, history of cerumen impaction, history of diabetes mellitus

B. Review of medication list
1. Antibiotics: erythromycin, azithromycin, aminoglycosides
2. Cisplatin
3. Herbal medications

C. Physical examination
1. Otoscopic examination
2. Hearing screen
3. Examination of the cranial nerves
4. Gait and balance assessment

---

lateralization tests the individual's ability to fuse sounds from both ears; and masking level differences assess the ability to pick out specific sounds from a background of noise. Monotonic degraded tasks present difficult sounds such as noise background, filtered sound, and time-compressed speech; dichotic tasks simultaneously present sense and nonsense speech, which the individual is asked to repeat.

AGING CHANGES

Many changes in the peripheral and central auditory system during aging have effects on the hearing mechanism (Table 13-10). These changes lead to diminished performance by older subjects, including the loss of sensitivity and distortion of signals that succeed in passing to higher levels, difficulty in localizing signals and in taking advantage of two-ear listening, difficulty understanding speech under unfavorable listening conditions, and problems with language, especially when aging is compounded by stroke.

Three major factors enhance the progression of hearing loss with advancing age: previous middle-ear disease, vascular disease, and exposure to noise. These factors alone, however, do not account for the hearing loss of old age, called *presbycusis*. Although clinically and pathologically complex, this is a distinct progressive sensorineural hearing loss associated with aging. The deterioration is not limited to the peripheral sensory receptor and includes brain stem and cortical functions. Presbycusis affects 60% of individuals older than age 65 in the United States. However, only a fraction of these have a functional deficit necessitating aural rehabilitation. The health implications of hearing loss in older adults are outlined in Table 13-11.

TABLE 13-10. Effects of Aging on the Hearing Mechanism and Hearing Performance in Older Adults

Effects of aging on the hearing mechanism
- Atrophy and disappearance of cells in the inner ear
- Angiosclerosis in the inner ear
- Calcification of membranes in the inner ear
- Bioelectric and biomechanical imbalances in the inner ear
- Degeneration and loss of ganglion cells and their fibers in the eighth cranial nerve
- Eighth nerve canal closure, with destruction of nerve fibers
- Atrophy and cell loss at all auditory centers in the brainstem
- Reduction of cells in auditory areas of the cortex

Hearing performance in older adults
  A. Peripheral pathology
      1. Hearing loss for pure tones
      2. Hearing loss for speech
      3. Problems understanding speech
  B. Brainstem pathology
      1. Problems localizing sounds
      2. Problems in binaural listening
  C. Cortical pathology
      1. Problems with difficult speech
      2. Language problems

SENSITIVITY

Beginning with the third decade of life, there is deterioration in the hearing threshold. At first, sensitivity at the high frequencies declines gradually. This age-associated loss has been confirmed in populations not exposed to high levels of noise. This gradual

TABLE 13-11. Health Implications of Hearing Loss in Older Adults

  A. Increased risk for
      1. Depression, anxiety, and poor self-esteem
      2. Cognitive impairment
      3. Delirium
      4. Falls
      5. Difficulties in managing instrumental activities of daily living: shopping, driving, money management, telephone calls, transportation
  B. Impact on quality of life
      1. Loneliness and difficulty in sustaining social networks and relationships
      2. Isolation and loss of social connections
      3. Frustration of family members
      4. Poor communication during routine interactions
  C. Misunderstanding of health explanations and patient instructions

impairment is sensorineural and can be tested by pure-tone audiometry, which reveals useful information about the physiological condition of hearing but does not disclose some important aspects of deterioration.

SPEECH

Although there is a close relationship between pure-tone loss and the ability to hear speech, the audiogram does not precisely measure hearing for speech. To assess this auditory function, speech audiometry can be performed by presenting the undistorted test words above threshold intensities in the absence of background noise.

Older people with hearing impairment may have difficulty understanding speech under less-favorable conditions, as with background noise, under poor acoustic conditions, or when speech is rapid. This difficulty may be caused in part by the longer time required by higher auditory centers to identify the message. Such hearing loss may necessitate testing of desired signals with the presentation of a competing signal. This will more accurately reflect hearing of speech in social circumstances.

Speech occurring in rooms that cause long reverberations is also much less intelligible to older individuals. Auditory temporal discrimination and auditory reaction time and frequency discrimination also decline with age. Because consonant sounds are of higher frequency and shorter duration, the loss of high-frequency hearing in older adults may affect these sounds, which encode much of speech information. Lipreading may compensate to some extent for this effect on understanding speech, but other factors of processing information still remain.

LOUDNESS

A common auditory problem of older individuals is abnormal loudness perception. This can occur as hypersensitivity to sounds of high intensity and appears as increased "loudness recruitment," in which gradually increasing loudness, such as amplified sound, is unpleasantly harsh and difficult to tolerate. In older adults with hearing impairment, this abnormality is manifest when a speaker is asked to speak louder or the output of a hearing aid is increased. It may result from a sensorineural loss attributable to changes in the hair cells of the inner ear.

LOCALIZATION

Sound localization contributes to effectiveness of signal detection and helps with discrimination. Loss of directional hearing results in greater hearing difficulty in a noisy environment. Localization is disturbed in older adults with hearing loss and may be partly caused by the aging brain's deranged processing of interaural intensity differences and time delays. A strongly asymmetrical hearing loss also disturbs localization.

TINNITUS

Tinnitus, an internal noise generated within the hearing system, occurs in many types of hearing disorders at all ages, but is much more frequent in older adults. Tinnitus, however, is not necessarily associated with hearing loss and may occur in older adults without hearing impairment. Estimates of prevalence of tinnitus in the United States are about 10%, with the majority of persons with tinnitus being 40 to 80 years of age (Peifer et al, 1999). Treatment is generally unsatisfactory.

OTHER HEARING DISORDERS

One of the most easily treatable but too easily overlooked causes of hearing loss is cerumen that occludes the external auditory canal (Table 13-12). Cerumen usually affects low-frequency sounds and complicates existing hearing impairments.

Hearing loss in the geriatric patient may be caused by scarring of the tympanic membrane. In tympanosclerosis, there is calcification of the tympanic membrane that results in stiffening of the drumhead.

Otosclerosis may cause fixation of the ossicular chain and lead to a conduction hearing loss. The bony capsule may also be affected, leading to sensorineural loss. Paget disease may also lead to both kinds of hearing loss and should be evaluated radiologically and by an alkaline phosphatase determination.

Ototoxic medication is an acquired cause of hearing loss producing cochlear damage. The aminoglycoside antibiotics require special caution. At high doses, ethacrynic acid and furosemide may be ototoxic.

High doses of aspirin may cause a reversible hearing impairment. Unfortunately, except for aspirin, removal of the offending drug usually does not reverse the sensorineural loss.

Sound trauma is an environmental factor with neurosensory consequences. Superimposed on the changes of aging, sound trauma can have a severe impact on a patient's communicative ability.

Vascular or mass lesions may affect hearing at one of several levels, including the middle and inner ear, auditory nerve, brain stem, and cortex.

AURAL REHABILITATION

Every individual who has communication difficulties caused by a permanent hearing loss should have an ear, nose, and throat evaluation to rule out remediable disease and then an audiological evaluation to assess the roles of amplification and aural rehabilitation. Table 13-13 lists the factors that should be considered during the evaluation for a hearing aid. In those with severe impairment, in addition to a hearing aid, aural rehabilitation with speech reading may be necessary. Table 13-14 outlines the advantages and disadvantages of various types of hearing aids while Table 13-15 notes important features of over-the-counter wearable hearing assistive devices. A few points should be noted when guiding an older patient who may benefit from a hearing aid. A consultation with a trusted audiologist is worthwhile because the causes of hearing loss can be quite important to the overall health of the individual. Also, the audiologist can counsel the patient with information about the size of the device, the costs, and the daily use of the device. The over-the-counter wearable devices may be cheaper, but the professional evaluation and management of an audiologist is likely best in the long run.

PART III

TABLE 13-12. Medical Conditions That Present With Hearing Loss in Older Adults

Signs and symptoms	Cerumen impaction	Ménière disease	Sudden sensorineural hearing loss	Otosclerosis	Cholesteatoma	Acoustic neuroma
Hearing impairment	Unilateral or bilateral	Fluctuating	Unilateral	Generally unilateral	Generally unilateral	Unilateral
Vertigo		x	Possible		x	x
Tinnitus		x				
Fullness and pressure sensation in the ear	x	x				
Ear pain					x	
Ear drainage					x	
Other features						Facial weakness; difficulty swallowing

TABLE 13-13. Factors to Consider in Evaluation of an Older Adult for a Hearing Aid

Exclude contraindicating medical or other correctable problem.

Greatest satisfaction is achieved with aid if loss is 55–80 dB; there is only partial help if loss is >80 dB.

Less satisfaction is achieved when poor discrimination is present.

Aid is specifically designed for face-to-face conversation; patient's expectations should be realistic.

Aid may need to be combined with lip reading.

Loudness perception abnormalities may make the aid unacceptable.

More severe hearing loss requires aid worn on the body rather than behind-the-ear device.

Assess for monaural or binaural aids.

Assess for patient's ability to handle aid independently.

Assess patient's motivation, expectations, and attitude in using an aid.

Patients may initially be resistant to using a hearing aid. Patient and family counseling may overcome this resistance and improve use of and satisfaction with a hearing aid. The newer models of devices and newer features may be explained to individuals to help them better understand how the devices can fit with their unique situation. Realistic expectations should be explained to the patient. Hearing aids are most useful in one-on-one conversations and are less effective in noisy, group settings. They are also less useful in improving understanding of less-familiar accents and languages, for example, a British accent in a movie or television production. Such understanding can be improved by use of the closed caption feature on television. Facing the speaker and lipreading also improves understanding. Improvements and modifications in design and construction of hearing aids, now digital, have enabled a greater proportion of the hearing-impaired population to profit from amplification. The old adage that hearing aids will not help people with sensorineural loss is simply not true. The aid can be adjusted to a specific frequency rather than all frequencies, thus decreasing loudness problems, improving discrimination, and making the aid more acceptable. Binaural aids improve sound localization and discrimination. Finally, Table 13-16 highlights important strategies health professionals should use in communicating with older patients who have serious hearing impairments.

The hearing aid that is worn on the body (as opposed to behind-the-ear or in-the-ear) provides the greatest amplification but is necessary only for patients with the most severe hearing loss. The controls are large and therefore more easily managed by some elderly persons. However, many older people prefer behind-the-ear or in-the-ear devices. The in-the-ear devices are small and cosmetically more acceptable, but more difficult to manipulate. Some older people with visual or dexterity problems may find the batteries troublesome to manage. Currently, not all state Medicaid programs cover hearing aids, Veterans Affairs insurance covers only those with service-connected hearing loss, and Medicare does not cover hearing aids.

PART III

TABLE 13-14. Some Advantages and Disadvantages of Various Styles of Hearing Aids

Style	Degree of hearing loss	Advantages	Comfort and fit	Comments
Completely in the canal	Mild to moderate	Almost invisible Less occlusion of pinna Easier to use with headphones More cosmetically appealing than larger aids	+	User's dexterity may be a problem Small size may limit features May cost more than canal or in-the-ear aids
Canal	Mild to moderate	Telecoil available in some models May be able to use with headphones	++	Shorter battery life User's dexterity may be a problem Small size may limit available features
In the ear	Mild to severe	Ease of handling Comfortable fit Options: telecoil, directional microphone More power than completely-in-the-canal aids or canal aids	++	More conspicuous than completely-in-the-canal or canal aids May be difficult to use with headphones
Behind the ear	Mild to profound	Greatest power Options: telecoil, directional microphone, direct audio input Earmold can be exchanged separately	+	More conspicuous May be more difficult to insert than the in-the-ear aids Difficult to use with headphones
Body aid	Severe to profound	Greatest separation of microphone from receiver reduces feedback	+	Most conspicuous Picks up noise from rubbing on clothing
Bone conduction	Mild to severe	Bypasses middle ear Used if ear canal is unable to tolerate aid or earmold		Microphone is on chest or on waist, but speech is directed at ear level

+ comfortable; ++ more comfortable

TABLE 13-15. Essential Points That a Health Professional Should Know About Over-the-Counter Wearable Hearing Devices

A. Background information
  1. A new assistive technology that is intended for mild to moderate hearing loss.
  2. In the United States, the Food and Drug Administration has determined that these devices cannot be marketed for the intended purpose of addressing hearing loss.
  3. May be subject to regulatory requirements and laws for hearing aids.
  4. Costs of OTC devices range from $50 to $500 per product, compared to the average consumer price of a midlevel hearing aids of $1,000 to $6,000 per pair (description for hearing aid includes bundle of devices and professional services in year 2017).
  5. The costs of OTC devices and the costs of hearing aids are not covered by Medicare.
B. Who might use such an OTC wearable hearing device?
  1. Consumers with mild to moderate hearing impairment.
  2. Those who wish to avoid the testing and treatment required for a standard hearing aid.
  3. Those who wish an affordable hearing device.
  4. Those whose attitudes and beliefs about hearing loss may make them avoid hearing aids.
C. How an OTC wearable hearing device differs from a hearing aid
  1. No need to see a physician for a medical exam or sign a waiver of this exam as required for a hearing aid.
  2. No need to see an audiologist.
  3. Less expensive and hence may improve access to treatment of hearing loss.
  4. May include a built-in self-assessment of hearing.
  5. Not as sophisticated as hearing aid in filtering out the background noise.
  6. No professional instruction of the patient on how to fit, use, and maintain.
  7. May match with the individual's needs, preference, and budget.

PART III

This constitutes a major out-of-pocket expense. Pocket talkers are less expensive and may be used by those who cannot afford hearing aids.

Hearing aids may improve the quality of life of older individuals who receive them; however, the studies that have assessed the benefit of hearing aids note several limitations. Most studies evaluated the benefit of hearing aid use in the context of free access to hearing aids. Since the costs of a hearing aid are not covered by Medicare, the costs and benefits should be taken into account by clinicians.

Surgical treatment of sensorineural hearing loss is safe and effective in older adults with severe hearing loss not corrected by hearing aids. Middle ear implant devices and cochlear implants are emerging options for such individuals. Table 13-17 outlines important aspects that health professionals should understand about cochlear implants.

TABLE 13-16. Strategies to Improve a Health Professional's Communication With an Older Patient Who Has a Hearing Impairment

- Decrease the level of background noise and complexity of the environment by moving to a quiet room.
- Define if the patient has a hearing aid and if it is functioning.
- Offer to use a voice amplifier for the visit.
- Examine the patient's ears to define if there is a remedial solution (eg, cerumen impaction).
- Speak slower instead of louder.
- Use "teach back" as a technique to affirm if the patient heard and understood important aspects of the instructions.
- Make the topic of the conversation clear at the start of the conversation.
- Consider engaging an audiologist, a speech-language pathologist, or an occupational therapist to assist in the assessment and in developing a treatment plan.
- Consider a hearing aid app for the individual's smartphone (eg, Petralex hearing aid in year 2017).
- Consider the need for an alternative communication pathway (eg, communication board) for those individuals with a severe impairment.

TABLE 13-17. Essential Points That a Health Professional Should Know About Cochlear Implants

A. Background information
   1. A cochlear implant is an internal device that is implanted during a surgical procedure
   2. An external device transmits radio frequencies to the internal components via a magnetic link across the skin.
   3. The device electronically stimulates the auditory nerves in the cochlea, allowing the individual with hearing loss to perceive sound.
   4. Medicare covers surgical placement, programming, and follow-up after cochlear implantation as a prosthetic device.
B. What are the indications for a cochlear implant?
   1. Patient has moderately severe bilateral sensorineural hearing loss.
   2. Individual is still struggling to hear despite appropriate fitting hearing aids.
   3. Unilateral cochlear implant improves hearing and quality of life.
   4. Bilateral cochlear implant improves sound localization.
C. How a cochlear implant differs from a hearing aid
   1. The reported incidence of infectious complications after placement of cochlear implant is up to 4%, whereas there is no such risk for a hearing aid.
   2. Surgical wound complications are the most common infections for older adults, although the rate of such infections has decreased with newer surgical techniques.

TASTE

Aging is associated with a significant loss of lingual papillae and an associated diminution of ability to taste. Salivary secretion also diminishes, thus decreasing solubilization of flavoring agents. Upper dentures may cover secondary taste sites and decrease taste acuity.

Olfactory bulbs also show significant atrophy with old age. In a population-based, cross-sectional study of adults aged 53 to 97, the prevalence of impaired olfaction by olfaction testing was 24.5% and increased with age to 62.5% of 80- to 97-year-olds (Murphy et al, 2002). Taste and olfactory changes together may account for the lessened interest in food shown by older adults. Olfactory impairment is associated with amnestic mild cognitive impairment and the progression of amnestic mild cognitive impairment to Alzheimer disease (Roberts et al, 2016).

POLYNEUROPATHY

Patients with polyneuropathy have impairments in balance and an increased risk for falls and falls causing injury (Richardson, 2002). (See Chapter 9 on falls.) Epidemiological data on polyneuropathy are relatively limited. In a study from Italy of subjects aged 55 and older, the prevalence of polyneuropathy was 11%. Diabetes mellitus was the most common risk factor (44% of patients with polyneuropathy). The next most common risk factors were alcoholism, nonalcoholic liver disease, and malignancy (Beghi and Monticelli, 1998). In a natural history study of type 2 diabetes mellitus, 42% of the diabetic population had nerve conduction abnormalities consistent with polyneuropathy after 10 years (Partanen et al, 1995). The prevalence of diabetes mellitus in older persons is increasing, and therefore, the prevalence of polyneuropathy is likely to increase as well. Poor vitamin B_{12} levels (deficient B_{12} status and low serum B_{12}) are associated with worse sensory and motor peripheral nerve function in older adults (Leishear et al, 2012).

In chronic polyneuropathies, such as diabetes mellitus, symptoms usually begin in the lower extremities, and sensory symptoms usually precede motor symptoms. In demyelinating polyneuropathies, such as Guillain-Barré syndrome, weakness rather than sensory loss is more typical. The physical examination should focus on the sensory examination, including pin prick, light touch, vibration, cold, and proprioception, and on muscle strength testing and appearance of muscle wasting. Likewise, a gait and balance assessment and a foot examination would complete the physical examination. Extensive diagnostic testing is usually not necessary in a patient with mild symptoms and a known underlying diagnosis such as diabetes mellitus or alcohol abuse. In patients with no clear etiology, electrodiagnostic testing should be the initial diagnostic study (Dyck et al, 1996). Rutkove (2012) has described an algorithm for a diagnostic approach to polyneuropathy. Laboratory tests, which might include a complete blood count, erythrocyte sedimentation rate, thyroid-stimulating hormone, serum and urine protein electrophoresis, blood glucose, glycohemoglobin, vitamin B_{12} level, antinuclear antibody, rheumatoid factor, heavy metals, and HIV, should be directed by the electrodiagnostic testing results.

PART III

Treatment should address the underlying disease process and alleviation of symptoms. Avoidance of toxins, such as alcohol or drugs, is the most important step. In patients with diabetes, tight control may help maintain nerve function (see Chapter 12). In painful neuropathies, tricyclic antidepressants are effective, as is gabapentin. Duloxetine also be considered for treatment of diabetic peripheral neuropathy. In patients with weakness, physical therapy evaluation is important, and use of ankle–foot orthosis, splints, and walking-assistance devices can improve function. Proper foot and nail care is important in reducing risk for foot ulcers.

Evidence Summary

Do's

- Screen for visual and auditory dysfunction in older adults.
- Refer all patients with age-related macular degeneration (AMD) for visual rehabilitation.
- Optimize blood glucose control and tight blood pressure control to reduce retinopathy in type 2 diabetes.
- Evaluate for treatable causes of hearing loss such as cerumen impaction and chronic otitis media.
- Refer patients with definite hearing loss to an audiologist.

Consider

- Cataract surgery when cataract progresses to interfering with activities.
- Glaucoma when defects in the peripheral visual field are present.
- AMD when central visual acuity is affected.

REFERENCES

Anand KB, Eschmann E. Systemic effects of ophthalmic medication in the elderly. *NY State J Med.* 1988;88:134-136.

Beghi E, Monticelli ML. Chronic symmetric symptomatic polyneuropathy in the elderly: a field screening investigation of risk factors for polyneuropathy in two Italian communities. *J Clin Epidemiol.* 1998;51:697-702.

Bogardus ST, Yueh B, Shekelle PG. Screening and management of adult hearing loss in primary care: clinical applications. *JAMA.* 2003;289:1986-1990.

Boland MV, Ervin AM, Friedman DS, et al. Comparitive effectiveness of treatments for open-angel glaucoma: a systematic review for the U.S. Preventive Services Task Force. *Ann Intern Med.* 2013;158:271-279.

Bourla DH, Young TA. Age-related macular degeneration: a practical approach to a challenging disease. *J Am Geriatr Soc.* 2006;54:1130-1135.

Broadway DC. Visual field testing for glaucoma—a practical guide. *Community Eye Health.* 2012;25(79-80):66-70.

Chakravarthy U, Evans J, Rosenfeld PJ. Age related macular degeneration. *BMJ.* 2010;340:526-530.

de Jong, PTVM. Age-related macular degeneration. *N Engl J Med.* 2006;355:1474-1485.

Dyck PJ, Dyck PJB, Grant IA, et al. Ten steps in characterizing and diagnosing patients with peripheral neuropathy. *Neurology.* 1996;47:10-17.

Fine SL, Berger JW, Maguire MG, et al. Age-related macular degeneration. *N Engl J Med.* 2000;342:483-492.

Haines JL, Pericak-Vance MA. Rapid dissection of the genetic risk of age-related macular degeneration. *JAMA.* 2007;297:401-402.

Klein BE, Klein R. Projected prevalences of eye-related diseases. *Invest Opthalmol Vis Sci.* 2013;54(14). doi:10,1167/iovs.13-12782.

Kwon YH, Fingert JH, Kuehn MH, et al. Primary open-angle glaucoma. *N Engl J Med.* 2009;360:1113-1124.

Leishear K, Boudreau RM, Studenski SA, et al. Relationship between vitamin B12 and sensory and motor peripheral nerve function in older adults. *J Am Geriatr Soc.* 2012;60:1057-1063.

Martin DF, Maguire MG, Ying G, et al. Ranibizumab and bevacizumab for neovascular age-related macular degeneration. *N Engl J Med.* 2011;364:1897-1908.

Mohamed Q, Gillies MC, Wong TY. Management of diabetic retinopathy: a systematic review. *JAMA.* 2007;298:902-916.

Murphy C, Schubert CR, Cruickshanks KJ, et al. Prevalence of olfactory impairment in older adults. *JAMA.* 2002;288:2307-2312.

Pacala JT, Yueh B. Hearing deficits in the older patient: "I didn't notice anything." *JAMA.* 2012;307:1185-1194.

Partanen J, Niskonen L, Lehtinen J, et al. Natural history of peripheral neuropathy in patients with non-insulin dependent diabetes mellitus. *N Engl J Med.* 1995;89:89-94.

Peifer KJ, Rosen GP, Rubin AM. Tinnitus: etiology and management. *Clin Geriatr Med.* 1999;15:193-204.

Richardson JK. Factors associated with falls in older patients with diffuse polyneuropathy. *J Am Geriatr Soc.* 2002;50:1767-1773.

Roberts RO, Christianson TJH, Kremers WK, et al. Association between olfaction dysfunction and amnestic mild cognitive impairment and Alzheimer disease dementia. *JAMA Neurol.* 2016;73(1):93-101.

Rutkove SB. Overview of polyneuropathy. *UpToDate 2015.* www.uptodate.com. Last updated December 1, 2015.

Schaumberg DA, Hankinson SE, Guo Q, et al. A prospective study of 2 major age-related macular degeneration susceptibility alleles and interactions with modifiable risk factors. *Arch Ophthalmol.* 2007;125:55-62.

Tseng VL, Yu F, Lum F, Coleman AL. Risk of fractures following cataract surgery in Medicare beneficiaries. *JAMA.* 2012;308:493-501.

Yueh B, Shapiro N, MacLean CH, et al. Screening and management of adult hearing loss in primary care: scientific review. *JAMA.* 2003;289:1976-1985.

SUGGESTED READINGS

Folk JC, Stone EM. Ranibizumab therapy for neovascular age-related macular degeneration. *N Engl J Med.* 2010;363:1648-1655.

Friedland DR, Runge-Samuelson C, Baig H, et al. Case-control analysis of cochlear implant performance in elderly patients. *Arch Otolaryngol Head Neck Surg.* 2010;136:432-438.

Jager RD, Mieler WF, Miller JW. Age-related macular degeneration. *N Engl J Med.* 2008;358:2606-2617.

Lin FR. Hearing loss in older adults—who's listening? *JAMA*. 2012;307:1147-1148.

Zahng X, Saaddine JB, Chou C-F, et al. Prevalence of diabetic retinopathy in the United States, 2005-2008. *JAMA*. 2010:304:649-656

SELECTED WEBSITES (ACCESSED 2017)

American Academy of Audiology, www.audiology.org

American Academy of Ophthalmology, www.aao.org/

American Glaucoma Society, www.glaucomaweb.org/

American Macular Degeneration Foundation, www.macular.org

Healthy Hearing, www.healthyhearing.com

Hearingaidhelp.com, www.hearingaidhelp.com/

Glaucoma Research Foundation, Learn about Glaucoma, www.glaucoma.org/

Lighthouse for the Blind and Visually Impaired, www.lighthouse-sf.org/

Macular Degeneration Foundation, www.eyesight.org/

Macular Degeneration Partnership, www.amd.org

National Academy of Sciences, Engineering and Medicine. Hearing Health Care for Adults: Priorities for Improving Access and Affordability. Blazer DG, Domnitz S, Liverman CT eds. Committee on Accessible and Affordable Hearing Health Care for Adults; Board on Health Sciences Policy; Health and Medicine Division. http//www.nap.edu/23446

National Eye Institute, Facts about Age-Related Macular Degeneration, https://nei.nih.gov/health/maculardegen/armd_facts

University of Texas Science Center, School of Medicine, Hearing Handicap Inventory for the Elderly Screening, http://teachhealthk-12.uthscsa.edu/activity/activity-8e-measuring-hearing-handicap-elders

U.S. National Library of Medicine, Clinical Advisory: NIDCD/VA Clinical Trial Finding Can Benefit Millions with Hearing Loss, www.nlm.nih.gov/databases/alerts/hearing.html

CHAPTER 14

Drug Therapy

Many geriatric patients are "walking chemistry sets" because they are prescribed multiple drugs in complex dosage schedules. Polypharmacy is common in older people because of the presence of multiple chronic medical conditions, the proven efficacy of an increasing number of drugs for these conditions, and practice guidelines that recommend their use. Polypharmacy has been defined variably in the literature with the threshold varying between 5 and 10 routine medications. This may be the result of older people seeing multiple prescribing clinicians who do not communicate with each other and a lack of a comprehensive medication list either electronically or in hard copy.

The nature of drug therapy in managing chronic disease has changed greatly. Many conditions can be better controlled, but at a cost. In many instances, however, complex drug regimens are unnecessary; they are costly and predispose to nonadherence and adverse drug reactions. Many older patients are prescribed multiple drugs, take over-the-counter drugs, and are then prescribed additional drugs to treat the side effects of medications they are already taking. This scenario can result in an upward spiral in the number of drugs being taken resulting in polypharmacy.

Several important pharmacological and nonpharmacological considerations influence the safety and effectiveness of drug therapy in the geriatric population. This chapter focuses on these considerations and gives practical suggestions for prescribing drugs for older patients. Drug therapy for specific geriatric conditions is discussed in several other chapters throughout this text.

NONPHARMACOLOGICAL FACTORS INFLUENCING DRUG THERAPY

Discussions of geriatric pharmacology frequently center on age-related changes in drug pharmacokinetics and pharmacodynamics. Detailed reviews of these areas are provided in the Suggested Readings section at the end of the chapter. Although these changes are often of clinical importance, nonpharmacological factors can play an even greater role in the safety and effectiveness of drug therapy in the geriatric population. Several steps make drug therapy safe and effective (Fig. 14-1). Many factors can interfere with these steps in the geriatric population; most of them come into play before pharmacological considerations arise.

Effective drug therapy requires accurate diagnoses. Many older patients underreport symptoms; patient complaints may be vague and multiple. Symptoms of physical diseases frequently overlap with symptoms of psychological illness. To add to this complexity, many diseases present with atypical symptoms. Consequently, making the correct diagnoses and prescribing the appropriate drugs are often difficult tasks in the geriatric population.

PART III

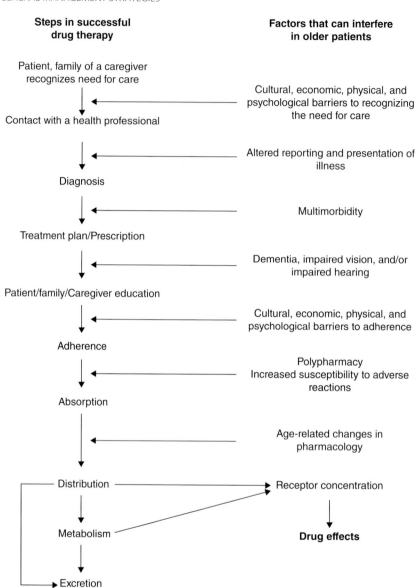

Steps in successful drug therapy

Patient, family of a caregiver recognizes need for care

Contact with a health professional

Diagnosis

Treatment plan/Prescription

Patient/family/Caregiver education

Adherence

Absorption

Distribution

Metabolism

Excretion

Factors that can interfere in older patients

Cultural, economic, physical, and psychological barriers to recognizing the need for care

Altered reporting and presentation of illness

Multimorbidity

Dementia, impaired vision, and/or impaired hearing

Cultural, economic, physical, and psychological barriers to adherence

Polypharmacy
Increased susceptibility to adverse reactions

Age-related changes in pharmacology

Receptor concentration

Drug effects

FIGURE 14-1 Factors that can interfere with successful drug therapy.

Healthcare professionals tend to treat symptoms with drugs rather than to evaluate the symptoms thoroughly. Because older patients often have multiple problems and complaints and consult several health-care professionals, they can readily end up with prescriptions for several drugs. Moreover, older patients or their family members sometimes exert pressure on health-care professionals to prescribe medication, thus adding to the tendency for polypharmacy. This pressure is intensified by direct-to-consumer advertising of drugs.

Older patients typically see many different clinicians, each of whom may prescribe medications. Frequently, neither the patients nor the health-care providers have a clear picture of the total drug regimen. New patients undergoing initial geriatric assessment should be asked to empty their medicine cabinets and to bring all bottles to their first appointments. Simple medication records, such as the one recommended by the U.S. Food and Drug Administration and shown in Figure 14-2, carried by the patient and maintained as an integral part of the overall medical record, may help eliminate some of the polypharmacy and nonadherence common in the geriatric population. Such records should be updated at each patient visit. Drug regimens should be simplified whenever possible, and patients should be instructed to discard old medications. Incorporation of medication lists into electronic medical records with medication reconciliation at each visit can be very helpful in maintaining an accurate medication list, reducing polypharmacy and improving adherence. Each time a new drug is added, a good principle is to consider if one can be discontinued.

Adherence plays a central role in the success of drug therapy in all age groups (see Fig. 14-1). In addition to the tendency for polypharmacy and complex dosage schedules, older patients face other potential barriers to adherence. The chronic nature of illness in the geriatric population can play a role in nonadherence. The symptomatic consequences of these illnesses are often delayed (as opposed to the more dramatic effects of acute illnesses), and thus adherence may be poor because the patient is not experiencing symptoms resulting from the illness. Diminished hearing, impaired vision, poor literacy, and poor short-term memory can interfere with patient education and adherence. Individuals with mild cognitive impairment may be at particular risk for nonadherence to medication regimens (Campbell et al, 2012). Problems with transportation can make getting to a pharmacy difficult. Outpatient prescriptions are now covered by Medicare to some extent, but many older persons still have to pay for some of the costs of their drugs from a limited income. Even if the older person gets to the pharmacy, can afford the prescription, understands the instructions, and remembers when to take it, the use of childproof bottles and tamper-resistant packaging may hinder adherence in those with arthritic or weak hands.

Several strategies can improve adherence in the geriatric population (Table 14-1). As few drugs as possible should be prescribed, and the dosage schedule should be as simple as possible. All drugs should be given on the same dosage schedules whenever possible, and the administration should correspond to a daily routine in order to enhance the consistency of taking the drugs and adherence. For many drugs, once-daily dosing is available and should be prescribed when clinically appropriate. Relatives or other caregivers should be instructed in the drug regimen, and they, as well as others (eg, home health aides and pharmacists), should be enlisted to help the older patient comply. Specially designed pill dispensers and frequent human reminders can be useful. Geriatric patients and their health-care providers should keep an updated record of the drug regimen (see Fig. 14-2) and discuss missed doses and overall

Be an Active Member of Your Health Care Team

My Medicine Record

DEPARTMENT OF HEALTH AND HUMAN SERVICES
Food and Drug Administration

FDA

Name (Last, First, Middle Initial): _____   Birth Date (mm/dd/yyyy): _____

	What I'm Using Rx – Brand & generic name; OTC – Name & active ingredients	What It Looks Like Color, shape, size, markings, etc.	How Much	How to Use / When to Use	Start / Stop Dates	Why I'm Using / Notes	Who Told Me to Use / How to Contact
	— Enter ALL prescription (Rx) medicine (include samples), over-the-counter (OTC) medicine, and dietary supplements —						
Ex:	XXXX/xxxxxxxxxx	20 mg pill; small, white, round	40 mg; use two 20 mg pills	Take orally, 2 times a day, at 8:00 am & 8:00 pm	1-15-11	Lowers blood pressure; check blood pressure once a week; blood test on 4-15-11	Dr. X (800) 555-1212
1							
2							
3							
4							
5							
6							
7							
8							

www.fda.gov/Drugs/ResourcesForYou/ucm079489.htm

(888) INFO-FDA
www.fda.gov/usemedicinesafely

These are my medicines as of
(Enter date as mm/dd/yyyy): _____

FORM FDA 3664 (3/11)   Page 1 of 4   PSC Publishing Services (301) 443-6740   EF

Be an Active Member of Your Health Care Team

My Medicine Record

DEPARTMENT OF HEALTH AND HUMAN SERVICES
Food and Drug Administration

FDA

My Personal Contacts

My Name (Last, First, Middle Initial) | Birth Date (mm/dd/yyyy)

Contact Information

Emergency Contact

Name | Relationship

Contact Information

Primary Care Physician

Name

Contact Information

Pharmacy / Drugstore

Name

Contact Information

Allergic Reaction or Other Problem I've Had With...
any medicine, dietary supplement, food, skin cleaner, medical tape
Describe in space below.

My Medical Conditions and Operations
Describe in space below.

Questions I Should Ask About Medicines or Dietary Supplements

❖ **Fill in the record for any new medicine, prescription (Rx) or over-the-counter (OTC), or dietary supplement, or ask my doctor or pharmacist to help me fill it in. Make sure I can read what is written on the record.**

❖ **When I review the record, or a change is made, ask:**
   • Can I use a generic form?
   • When should I start to feel differently? When should I report back to the doctor?
   • Will this take the place of anything else I am using?
   • Are there any special directions for using this?

   • Should I avoid any other medicines, dietary supplements, or treatments while using this?
   • Should I avoid any drinks, foods, other substances, or activities while using this?
   • What are the possible side effects from this? Is there anything I should watch for? What do I do if I get a side effect?
   • Will I need any tests (blood tests, x-rays, other) to make sure it is working as it should? When? How will I get the results?
   • What should I do if I miss a dose? What do I do if I use too much?
   • Where and how can I get more written information about this?

FORM FDA 3664 (3/11)   Page 2 of 4   www.fda.gov/Drugs/ResourcesForYou/ucm079489.htm   (888) INFO-FDA   www.fda.gov/usemedicinesafely

FIGURE 14-2 Example of a basic medication record recommended by the U.S. Food and Drug Administration.

Be an Active Member of Your Health Care Team

My Medicine Record

 DEPARTMENT OF HEALTH AND HUMAN SERVICES
Food and Drug Administration

How to Use My Medicine Record

- **Use this record** with the **"Be An Active Member of Your Health Care Team"** pamphlet, found at:
  www.fda.gov/Drugs/ResourcesForYou/UCM079529#pamphlet

- **Save "My Medicine Record"** on your personal computer (PC). Type information into the fields with your keyboard. You can also print the record and enter the information with a pencil.

- **Enter ALL prescription medicines you use**, including any medicine samples you are given.

- **Enter ALL over-the-counter medicines and dietary supplements** (including vitamins, minerals, and herbals) you use, whether you use them all the time or only some of the time.

- **Print and share the record** with your doctors, pharmacists, or other health professionals at ALL your visits.

- **Keep a printed copy** with you all the time. It is a good idea to give a copy to a friend or loved one.

Review this record and update it on your PC or by hand when you:

- Stop or start a medicine or dietary supplement

- Make a change in anything you use

- Visit your doctor, pharmacist, or other health professional

What I'm Using

- **Prescription (Rx) medicine** – enter the brand and generic name of the medicine, including any samples you are given

- **Over-the-Counter (OTC) medicine** – enter the name and active ingredient(s), including OTCs you use for allergies, stomach ache, heartburn, nausea; OTC pain relievers you use for minor aches and pains, headache, fever; OTC cold medicines,

laxatives, sleeping pills, and others prescribed by your doctor, such as aspirin

- Dietary supplements, including vitamins, minerals, and herbals

What it Looks Like

- Form (pill, tablet, capsule, liquid, injection, suppository, cream, lotion, eye or ear drops, etc.)

- Shape, color, size, and scoring (any lines on the medicine) or other markings

How Much

- Dose that you are directed to use either by the doctor or pharmacist or by the directions on the label

- If you are to use a dose which is different than the dose the medicine comes in, note the number you use (for example, you are supposed to use 40 mg, and it comes in 20 mg pills, put "40 mg; use two 20 mg pills" or "2 pills")

How to Use / When to Use

- **How to use** – such as "swallow with water; do not chew" or "take by mouth with food" or "two times a day")

- **When to use** – the time, or time of day, you use it (such as "10:00 pm" or "at bedtime")

Start / Stop Dates

- Date you started using it. If you are only supposed to use it for a period of time, put the date you should stop using it

- If it is something you use sometimes, such as an OTC you use only when you have a headache, put "when needed"

Be an Active Member of Your Health Care Team

My Medicine Record

 DEPARTMENT OF HEALTH AND HUMAN SERVICES
Food and Drug Administration FDA

How to Use My Medicine Record

Why I'm Using / Notes

- The reason why you are using it, such as "high blood pressure".

- Any special directions on how to use the medicine, such as whether to take it with or without food

- Any tests that are needed to find out it is working as it should, and dates you need the tests

- How and where to keep or store it, if not at room temperature

Who Told Me to Use / How to Contact

- Name and contact information of the doctor, nurse, or pharmacist (or other) who prescribed or told you to use it

My Personal Contacts

- Contact information for you, someone you want contacted in an emergency, your doctor, pharmacy, or pharmacist. Under "Contact Information," enter phone number or e-mail address. An extra space is there for an extra contact person, if needed.

Allergic Reaction or Other Problem I've Had With...

- Any medicine, dietary supplement, food, skin cleaner, medical tape with which you have had a problem

- Also enter anything that could have an effect on your use, such as pregnancy, breast feeding, trouble swallowing tablets, or trouble remembering to use. Include problems with ingredients, such as colors, flavors, starches, or sugars.

My Medical Conditions and Operations

- Any diseases, illnesses, or medical conditions, such as asthma, diabetes, heart disease, high blood pressure, kidney disease, or cancer

- Any conditions or problems you often treat with prescription or over-the-counter medicine or dietary supplements, such as acid stomach or allergies

- Operations you've had

Questions I Should Ask About Medicines or Dietary Supplements

- Fill in the record for any new medicine or dietary supplement, or ask your doctor or pharmacist to help you fill it in. Make sure you can read what is written. If you can't read it, others may have trouble reading it, too. Use these questions when you review the record with your health professionals or when a change is made in something you use.

FIGURE 14-2 *(Continued)*

TABLE 14-1. Strategies to Improve Adherence With Drug Therapy in the Geriatric Population

1. Make drug regimens and instructions as simple as possible.
   a. Use the same dosage schedule for all drugs whenever feasible (eg, once or twice per day).
   b. Time the doses in conjunction with a daily routine.
2. Instruct relatives and caregivers on the drug regimen.
3. Enlist others (eg, home health aides, pharmacists) to help ensure compliance.
4. Make sure the older patient can get to a pharmacist (or vice versa), can afford the prescriptions, and can open the container.
5. Use aids (such as special pillboxes and drug calendars) whenever appropriate.
6. Perform careful medication adjudication and patient/family education at the time of every hospital discharge.
7. Keep updated medication records (see Fig. 14-2) and review them at each visit.
8. Review knowledge of and compliance with drug regimens regularly.

adherence with their primary care clinician. For older patients who are hospitalized, medication reconciliation, consolidation, and education should be performed at the time of discharge, because posthospital medication discrepancies are common in the older population and can have serious consequences (Coleman et al, 2005). Patients and families need to be carefully instructed on which medications have been discontinued and where dosages have been changed. Medication misuse can result in avoidable emergency room visits. A handful of medications (anticoagulants, antimicrobials, cardiovascular drugs, hypoglycemics, and psychotropics) account for a substantial portion of these visits (Budnitz et al, 2011). Medications should be brought to appointments, and patients and families should show all medications to their physicians, particularly on initial visits to new primary care physicians or at a consultation with a specialist. Health-care professionals should regularly inquire about other medications being taken (prescribed by other physicians or purchased over the counter) and review their patients' knowledge of and adherence to the drug regimen.

ADVERSE DRUG REACTIONS AND INTERACTIONS

Primum non nocere ("first, do no harm"), a watchword phrase in the practice of medicine, is nowhere more applicable than when drugs are being prescribed for the geriatric population. Concerns are frequently heard about inappropriate prescribing of medications with serious side effects in older people. Numerous studies over the last three decades have described the frequency of "inappropriate" drug therapy in a variety of settings. For example, a study of over 200,000 inpatient surgical admissions in patients aged 65 and older found that one-quarter had received a potentially inappropriate medication (Finlayson et al, 2011). The American Geriatrics Society has recently completed a comprehensive review and updated the Beers Criteria, which detail potentially inappropriate medications for older adults as well as drug–drug and drug–disease interactions that should be avoided. Readers are referred to this resource for information on specific drugs to assist in preventing adverse drug reactions and interactions (American Geriatrics Society Beers Criteria Update Expert Panel, 2015). There is also a valuable guide for use of these criteria (Steinman et al, 2015).

Adverse drug reactions are the most common form of iatrogenic illness (see Chapter 5). The incidence of adverse drug reactions in hospitalized patients increases from approximately 10% in those between 40 and 50 years of age to 25% in those older than age 80 (Lazarou et al, 1998). They account for between 3% and 10% of hospital admissions of older patients each year and result in several billion dollars in yearly health-care expenditures. Many drugs can produce distressing, and sometimes disabling or life-threatening, adverse reactions (Table 14-2). Psychotropic drugs, all drugs with substantial anticholinergic activity, hypoglycemic agents, anticoagulants, and cardiovascular agents are common causes of serious adverse reactions in the geriatric population. In part, this is because of the narrow therapeutic-to-toxic ratio of many of these drugs and the sensitivity of the aging brain to anticholinergic drugs. In some instances, age-related changes in pharmacology, such as diminished renal excretion and prolonged duration of action, predispose to adverse reactions. Some side effects can have a therapeutic benefit and may be key factors in drug selection (see below).

Because symptoms can be nonspecific or may mimic other illnesses, adverse drug reactions may be ignored or unrecognized. Patients and family members should be educated to recognize and report common and potentially serious adverse reactions, especially after new medications are prescribed. In some instances, another drug is prescribed to treat these symptoms, thus contributing to polypharmacy and increasing the likelihood of an adverse drug interaction. The problem of polypharmacy is exacerbated by visits to multiple physicians, who may prescribe still more drugs, and the use of multiple pharmacies. Medication records kept by the patient (see Fig. 14-2) and the patient's primary care clinician and the increasing use of electronic medical records should help prevent unnecessary polypharmacy when many physicians are involved.

Several drugs commonly prescribed for the geriatric population can interact with adverse consequences (American Geriatrics Society Beers Criteria Update Expert Panel, 2015; Hines and Murphy, 2011). Table 14-3 lists some of the more common potential adverse drug–drug interactions. The more common types are drug displacement from protein-binding sites by other highly protein-bound drugs, induction or suppression of the metabolism of other drugs, and additive effects of different drugs on blood pressure and mental function (mood, level of consciousness, etc). Interactions among drugs metabolized by the cytochrome P450 system in the liver are especially common (see Wilkinson, 2005, for a review). Because many older patients are treated with warfarin for atrial fibrillation or venous thrombosis, clinicians must be aware of the many potential drug–drug and drug–nutrient interactions with this medication (Holbrook et al, 2005).

PART III

TABLE 14-2. Examples of Common and Potentially Serious Adverse Drug Reactions in the Geriatric Population

Drug	Common adverse reactions
Analgesics (see Chap. 10)	
Anti-inflammatory agents, aspirin	Gastric irritation and ulcers
	Chronic blood loss
Narcotics	Constipation
Antimicrobials	
Aminoglycosides	Renal failure
	Hearing loss
Other antimicrobials	Diarrhea
Antiparkinsonian drugs (see Chap. 10)	
Dopaminergic agents	Nausea
	Delirium
	Hallucinations
	Postural hypotension
Anticholinergics	Dry mouth
	Constipation
	Urinary retention
	Delirium
Cardiovascular drugs (see Chap. 11)	
Angiotensin-converting enzyme (ACE) inhibitors	Cough
	Impaired renal function
Antiarrhythmics	Pulmonary toxicity, bradycardia, hypotension (amiodarone)
Anticoagulants	Bleeding complications
Antihypertensives	Hypotension, postural hypotension, falls, near syncope
Calcium channel blockers	Decreased myocardial contractility
	Edema
	Constipation
Diuretics	Dehydration
	Hyponatremia
	Hypokalemia
	Incontinence
Digoxin	Arrhythmias
	Nausea
	Anorexia
Nitrates	Hypotension
Statins	Myopathy
	Hepatotoxicity

(continued)

TABLE 14-2. Examples of Common and Potentially Serious Adverse Drug Reactions in the Geriatric Population (*continued*)

Drug	Common adverse reactions
Hypoglycemic agents	
Insulin	Hypoglycemia
Oral agents	Edema (glitazones)
	Diarrhea (metformin)
Lower urinary tract drugs (see Chap. 8)	
Antimuscarinics	Dry mouth, eyes
Oral agents	Constipation
	Esophageal reflux
α-Blockers	Postural hypotension
Psychotropic drugs (see Tables 14-8 and 14-9)	
Antidepressants	(See Chap. 7)
Antipsychotics	Death
	Sedation
	Hypotension
	Extrapyramidal movement disorders
	Glucose intolerance
	Weight gain
Cholinesterase inhibitors	Falls
	Syncope
	Nausea
	Diarrhea
Lithium	Weakness
	Tremor
	Nausea
	Delirium
Sedative and hypnotic agents	Excessive sedation
	Delirium
	Gait disturbances and falls
Others	
Alendronate, risedronate	Esophageal ulceration
Aminophylline, theophylline	Gastric irritation
	Tachyarrhythmias
Carbamazepine	Anemia
	Hyponatremia
	Neutropenia

Source: For a complete list, see American Geriatrics Society Beers Criteria Update Expert Panel, 2015.

PART III

TABLE 14-3. Examples of Potentially Clinically Important Drug–Drug Interactions

Interaction	Examples	Potential effects
Interference with drug absorption	Antacids interacting with digoxin, isoniazid, antipsychotics, enteral tube feedings, and liquid phenytoin, iron, and ciprofloxacin	Diminished drug effectiveness
Displacement from binding proteins	Warfarin, oral hypoglycemics, and other highly protein-bound drugs	Enhanced effects and increased risk of toxicity
Altered distribution	Digoxin and quinidine	Increased risk of toxicity
Altered metabolism	Antifungals, erythromycin, clarithromycin SSRIs, with antihistamines, calcium channel blockers, and others[*]	Decreased metabolism, increased levels of toxicity
Altered excretion	Lithium and diuretics	Increased risk of toxicity and electrolyte imbalance
Pharmacological antagonism	Antimuscarinic drugs (for the bladder) and cholinesterase inhibitors	Decreased effectiveness
Pharmacological synergism	α-Blockers (for lower urinary tract symptoms in men) and antihypertensives	Increased risk of hypotension

SSRI, selective serotonin reuptake inhibitor.
*See Wilkinson, 2005.
Source: For a complete list, see American Geriatrics Society Beers Criteria Update Expert Panel, 2015.

In addition to the potential to interact with other drugs, several drugs can interact adversely with underlying medical conditions in the geriatric population, creating "drug–patient" interactions (American Geriatrics Society Beers Criteria Update Expert Panel, 2015; see Table 14-4 for examples). A good example of this problem is the increased risk of hospitalization for congestive heart failure (CHF) among older patients taking diuretics who are told to take a nonsteroidal anti-inflammatory drug (Heerdink et al, 1998).

Health-care professionals should have a thorough knowledge of the more common drug side effects, adverse reactions to drugs, and potential drug interactions in the geriatric population. Multiple applications are available to clinicians for use on their computers, tablets, and cell phones that can assist in making information readily available to avoid adverse drug reactions and interactions. Careful questioning about side effects should be an important part of reviewing the drug regimen at each visit. Many institutions use computers to detect potential adverse drug interactions and to prevent their occurrence. Special attention should be given to the potential

TABLE 14-4. Examples of Potentially Clinically Important Drug–Patient Interactions

Drug	Patient factors	Clinical implications
Diuretics	Diabetes	Decreased glucose tolerance
	Poor nutritional status	Increased risk of dehydration and electrolyte imbalance
	Urinary frequency, urgency	Incontinence may result
Angiotensin-converting enzyme (ACE) inhibitors	Renovascular disease (severe)	Worsening renal function
β-Blockers	Stress incontinence	Precipitate incontinence (cough)
	Diabetes	Sympathetic response to hypoglycemia may be masked
	Chronic obstructive lung disease	Increased bronchospasm
	Congestive heart failure (CHF)	Decreased myocardial contractility
	Peripheral vascular disease	Increased claudication
Narcotic analgesics	Chronic constipation	Worsening symptoms, fecal impaction
Antimuscarinics, tricyclic antidepressants, antihistamines, and other drugs with anticholinergic effects	Constipation, glaucoma, prostatic hyperplasia, reflux esophagitis	Worsening of symptoms
Antipsychotics	Parkinsonism	Worsening of immobility
Psychotropics	Dementia	Further impairment of cognitive function
Nonsteroidal anti-inflammatory drugs	CHF, on diuretics	Increased risk of exacerbation of CHF

PART III

for any newly prescribed drug to interact with drugs already being taken or with underlying medical or psychological conditions. Many drugs can be stopped safely as demonstrated by use of the Beers Criteria, STOPP criteria (Screening Tool of Older Persons' Potentially Inappropriate Prescriptions) (Brown et al, 2016; O'Conner et al, 2016), and other strategies such as the Good Palliative-Geriatric Practice algorithm (Garfinkel and Mangin, 2010). Consultant pharmacists with specialized expertise in geriatrics can be extremely helpful in recommending deprescribing strategies, including drug holidays and "N of 1 trials" to determine if the patient is benefiting or having adverse effects from specific medications.

AGING AND PHARMACOLOGY

Several age-related biological and physiological changes are relevant to pharmacology (Table 14-5). Except for changes in renal function, however, the effects of these age-related changes on dosages of specific drugs for individual patients are variable and difficult to predict. In general, an understanding of the physiological status of each patient (accounting for factors such as state of hydration, nutrition, and cardiac output) and how that status affects the pharmacology of a particular drug is more important to clinical efficacy than are age-related changes. Drug delivery systems, such as oral sustained-release preparations and skin patches, may be useful in designing strategies to account for the effect of aging changes on pharmacodynamics and to make many drugs safer in the geriatric population. Given these caveats, the effects of aging on each pharmacodynamic process are briefly discussed in the following sections.

ABSORPTION

Several age-related changes can affect drug absorption (see Table 14-5). Most studies, however, have failed to document any clinically meaningful alterations in drug absorption with increasing age. Absorption, therefore, appears to be the pharmacological parameter least affected by increasing age.

DISTRIBUTION

In contrast to absorption, clinically meaningful changes in drug distribution can occur with increasing age. Serum albumin, the major drug-binding protein, tends to decline, especially in hospitalized patients. Although the decline is small, it can substantially increase the amount of free drug available for action. This effect is of

TABLE 14-5. Age-Related Changes Relevant to Drug Pharmacology

Pharmacological parameter	Age-related changes
Absorption	Decreases in absorptive surface splanchnic blood flow Increased gastric pH Altered gastrointestinal motility
Distribution	Decreases in total body water, lean body mass, serum albumin Increased fat Altered protein binding
Metabolism	Decreases in liver blood flow, enzyme activity, enzyme inducibility
Excretion	Decreases in renal blood flow, glomerular filtration rate, tubular secretory function
Tissue/receptor sensitivity	Alterations in receptor number, receptor affinity, second-messenger function, and cellular and nuclear responses

particular relevance for highly protein-bound drugs, especially when they are used simultaneously and compete for protein-binding sites (see Table 14-3).

Age-related changes in body composition can prominently affect pharmacology by altering the volume of distribution (Vd). The elimination half-life of a drug varies with the ratio of Vd to drug clearance. Thus, even if the rate of clearance of a drug is unchanged with age, changes in Vd can affect a drug's half-life and duration of action.

Because total body water and lean body mass decline with increasing age, drugs that distribute in these body compartments—such as many antimicrobial agents, digoxin, lithium, and alcohol—may have a lower Vd and can therefore achieve higher concentrations from given amounts of drugs. On the other hand, drugs that distribute in body fat, such as many of the psychotropic agents, have a large Vd in geriatric patients. The larger Vd will thus cause prolongation of the half-life unless the clearance increases proportionately, which is unlikely to happen with increasing age.

METABOLISM

The effects of aging on drug metabolism are complex and difficult to predict. They depend on the precise pathway of drug metabolism in the liver and on several other factors, such as gender and amount of smoking (Wilkinson, 2005). The pharmacokinetics and elimination of drugs commonly used in older adults are now readily available on the Internet and several applications.

Even when liver function is obviously impaired, as by intrinsic liver disease or right-sided CHF, the effects of aging on the metabolism of specific drugs cannot be precisely predicted. It is *not* safe to assume, however, that geriatric patients with normal liver function tests can metabolize drugs as efficiently as can younger individuals.

The cytochrome P450 system in the liver has been extensively studied. More than 30 isoenzymes have been identified and classified into families and subfamilies. Genetic mutations in some of these enzymes, while relatively uncommon, can impair metabolism of specific drugs. Although aging may affect this system, the effects of commonly used drugs are probably more important (Wilkinson, 2005).

EXCRETION

The tendency for renal function to decline with increasing age can affect the pharmacokinetics of several drugs (and their active metabolites) that are eliminated predominantly by the kidney. These drugs are cleared from the body more slowly, their half-lives (and duration of action) are prolonged, and there is a tendency to accumulate to higher (and potentially toxic) drug concentrations in the steady state.

Several considerations are important in determining the effects of age on renal function and drug elimination:

1. There is wide interindividual variation in the rate of decline of renal function with increasing age. Thus, although renal function is said to decline by 50% between the ages of 20 and 90 years, this is an *average* decline. A 90-year-old individual may not have a creatinine clearance of only 50% of normal. Applying average declines to individual elderly patients can result in over- or underdosing.

2. Muscle mass declines with age; therefore, daily endogenous creatinine production declines. Because of this decline in creatinine production, serum creatinine may be normal at a time when renal function is substantially reduced. Serum creatinine, therefore, does not reflect renal function as accurately in elderly people as it does in younger persons.

3. A number of factors can affect renal clearance of drugs and are often at least as important as age-related changes. State of hydration, cardiac output, and intrinsic renal disease should be considered in addition to age-related changes in renal function.

Several formulas and nomograms have been used to estimate renal function in relation to age. Table 14-6 shows one of the most widely used and accepted formulas. Other commonly used equations for creatinine clearance or glomerular filtration rate are the Modification of Diet in Renal Disease (MDRD) equation, which is used by many clinical laboratories to estimate glomerular filtration rate, and the CKD-EPI equation. These formulae may be useful in *initial estimations* for the purpose of drug dosing in the geriatric population. However, they may over- or underestimate creatinine clearance in individual patients. Clinical factors (such as state of hydration and cardiac output), which vary over time, should be considered in determining drug dosages. Overestimation of creatinine clearance could potentially lead to serious adverse drug reactions, for example, with direct oral anticoagulants (Schwartz, 2016).

When drugs with narrow therapeutic-to-toxic ratios are being used, actual measurements of creatinine clearance and drug blood levels (when available) should be used.

TISSUE AND RECEPTOR SENSITIVITY

A proportion of the drug or its active metabolite will eventually reach its site of action. Age-related changes at this point—that is, responsiveness to given drug concentrations (without regard to pharmacokinetic changes)—are termed *pharmacodynamic changes*. Older persons are often said to be more sensitive to the effects of drugs. For some drugs, this appears to be true. For others, however, sensitivity to drug effects may decrease rather than increase with age. For example, older persons may be more sensitive to the sedative effects of given blood levels of benzodiazepines but less sensitive to the effects of drugs mediated by α-adrenergic receptors. There

---

TABLE 14-6. Renal Function in Relation to Age*

Cockcroft–Gault Equation

$$\text{Creatinine clearance} = \frac{(140 - \text{age}) \times \text{body weight (kg)}}{72 \times \text{serum creatinine level}} (\times\, 0.85 \text{ for women})$$

*Several other factors can influence creatinine clearance (see text).
Data from Cockcroft DW, Gault MH. Predictions of creatinine clearance from serum creatinine, *Nephron.* 1976;16(1):31-41.

are several possible explanations for these changes (see Table 14-5). The effects of age-related pharmacodynamic changes on dosages of specific drugs for individual geriatric patients remain largely unknown.

GERIATRIC PRESCRIBING

GENERAL PRINCIPLES

Several considerations make the development of specific recommendations for geriatric drug prescribing very difficult. These include the following:

1. Multiple interacting factors influence age-related changes in drug pharmacology.
2. There is wide interindividual variation in the rate of age-related changes in physiological parameters that affect drug pharmacology. Thus, precise predictions for individual older persons are difficult to make.
3. The clinical status of each patient (including such factors as state of nutrition and hydration, cardiac output, and intrinsic renal and liver disease) must be considered in addition to the effects of aging.
4. As more research studies with newer drugs are carried out in well-defined groups of older subjects, more specific recommendations will be possible.

Adherence to several general principles can make drug therapy in the geriatric population safer and more effective (Table 14-7).

TABLE 14-7. General Recommendations for Geriatric Prescribing

1. Evaluate geriatric patients thoroughly to identify all conditions that could (a) benefit from drug treatment, (b) be adversely affected by drug treatment, and (c) influence the efficacy of drug treatment.
2. Manage medical conditions without drugs as often as possible.
3. Know the pharmacology of the drug(s) being prescribed.
4. Consider how the clinical status of each patient could influence the pharmacology of the drug(s).
5. Avoid potentially serious adverse drug–drug interactions.
6. For drugs or their active metabolites eliminated predominantly by the kidney, use a formula to approximate age-related changes in renal function and adjust dosages accordingly.
7. If there is a question about drug dosage, start with smaller doses and increase gradually.
8. Drug blood concentrations can be helpful in monitoring several potentially toxic drugs used frequently in the geriatric population.
9. Help ensure adherence by paying attention to impaired intellectual function, diminished hearing, and poor vision when instructing patients and labeling prescriptions (and by using other techniques listed in Table 14-1).
10. Monitor older patients frequently for adherence, drug effectiveness, and adverse effects, and adjust drug therapy accordingly.

PART III

GERIATRIC PSYCHOPHARMACOLOGY

Psychotropic drugs can be broadly categorized as antidepressants (discussed in detail in Chapter 7), antipsychotics (Table 14-8), and sedative–hypnotics (Table 14-9). These drugs are probably the most misused class of drugs in the geriatric population and cause a high incidence of adverse reactions. Several studies show that more than half of nursing home residents are prescribed at least one psychotropic drug and that these prescriptions are changed frequently. Other studies suggest that psychotropic drugs are commonly prescribed inappropriately in the nursing home setting. Federal rules and emphasize avoiding the use of frequent "as needed" dosing for nonspecific symptoms (eg, agitation, wandering) and the inappropriate use of these drugs as chemical restraints. The appropriate use of antipsychotics for psychosis and several behavioral symptoms associated with dementia must, however, be distinguished from their use as "chemical restraints."

Several considerations can be helpful in preventing the misuse of psychotropic drugs in the geriatric population:

1. There are strong pressures to prescribe medications related to multimorbidity, clinical practice guidelines, and patient/family pressure. The benefit–harm ratio needs to be considered for each prescription.
2. Psychological symptoms (depression, anxiety, agitation, insomnia, paranoia, disruptive behavior) are often caused or exacerbated by medical conditions in geriatric patients. A thorough medical evaluation should therefore be done before symptoms are attributed to psychiatric conditions alone and psychotropic drugs are prescribed.

TABLE 14-8. Examples of Antipsychotic Drugs*

Drug	Usual geriatric daily dose range (mg)	Potential for Side Effects		
		Relative sedation	Hypotension	Extrapyramidal effects[†]
Aripiprazole	2.5–20[‡]	Moderate	Moderate	Moderate
Haloperidol (Haldol)	0.25–5	Low	Low	Very high
Olanzapine (Zyprexa)	2.5–10	Low	Low	Low
Quetiapine (Seroquel)	12.5–150	Moderate	Moderate	Low
Risperidone (Risperdal)	0.25	Low	Low	Low
Ziprasidone (Geodon)	20–40	Low	Moderate	Low

*Other agents are also available. All of the second-generation antipsychotics have been associated with increased mortality, and their efficacy in treating behavioral symptoms associated with dementia has been questioned (see text).
[†]Rigidity, bradykinesia, tremor, akathisia.
[‡]Geriatric dosage ranges are not well studied.

TABLE 14-9. Examples of Sedative–Hypnotics Approved for Insomnia by the U.S. Food and Drug Administration*

	Dose (mg)	Duration of action	Half-life (h)[†]
Benzodiazepines[‡]			
Lorazepam (Ativan)	0.5–2.5	Short	10–20
Temazepam (Restoril)	7.5–30	Intermediate	8–15
Benzodiazepine receptor agonists			
Eszopiclone (Lunesta)	1–3	Intermediate	5–7
Zaleplon (Sonata)	5–20	Ultra short	1
Zolpidem (Ambien)	5–10	Short	3
Zolpidem extended release (Ambien CR)	6.5 or 12.5	Short	3[§]
Melatonin receptor agonist			
Ramelteon	8	Short	2–5

*Other drugs are also approved.
[†]Half-life includes active metabolites.
[‡]Long-acting benzodiazepines should be avoided in geriatric patients.
[§]Duration of action is larger because of extended-release preparation.

3. Reports of psychiatric symptoms, such as agitation, are often presented to physicians by family caregivers and nursing home personnel who are inexperienced in the description, interpretation, and differential diagnosis of these symptoms. "Agitation" or "disruptive behavior" may, in fact, have been a reasonable response to an inappropriate interaction or situation created by the caregiver. Psychotropic drugs should therefore be prescribed only after the physician has clarified what the symptoms are and what correctable factors might have precipitated them.

4. Psychological symptoms and signs, like physical symptoms and signs, can be nonspecific in the older patient. Therefore, appropriate drug treatment often depends on an accurate psychiatric diagnosis. Psychiatrists and psychologists experienced with geriatric patients should be consulted, when available, to identify and help target psychotropic drug treatment to the major psychiatric problem(s).

5. Many nonpharmacological treatment modalities can either replace or be used in conjunction with psychotropic drugs in managing psychological symptoms. Behavioral modification, environmental manipulation, supportive psychotherapy, group therapy, recreational activities, and other related techniques can be useful in eliminating or diminishing the need for drug treatment (see Chapter 6).

6. Within each broad category of psychotropic drug there are considerable differences among individual agents in effects, side effects, and potential interactions with other drugs and medical conditions. Rational prescription of these drugs necessitates careful consideration of the characteristics of each drug in relation to the individual patient.

7. Because geriatric patients are, in general, more sensitive to the effects and side effects of psychotropic drugs, initial doses should be lower, increases should be gradual, and monitoring should be frequent.

8. Careful, ongoing assessment of the response of target symptoms and behaviors to psychotropic drugs is essential. In addition to reports from patients themselves, objective observations by trained and experienced professionals should be continuously evaluated in order to adjust psychotropic drug therapy.

Nonpharmacological approaches should be used before psychotropic drugs are prescribed, unless the patient is clearly psychotic and/or an immediate danger to himself or herself or others. A variety of nonpharmacological measures can be effective in older adults with agitation or excessive anxiety. Behavioral and other nonpharmacological therapeutic approaches are discussed in some of the Suggested Readings at the end of this chapter (see also Chapter 6). These measures, however, have not been shown to be highly effective, and are often unavailable, impractical, inappropriate, or unsuccessful (Brasure et al, 2016). Patients with severe impairment of cognitive function can be especially difficult to manage with nonpharmacological measures alone, particularly when their physical and/or verbal agitation is interfering with their care (or the care of others around them). Thus, drug treatment of physical and/or verbal agitation is necessary in some patients.

All psychotropic drugs must be used judiciously in geriatric patients because of their potential side effects. The most common and potentially disabling side effects of psychotropic drugs fall into four general categories: changes in cognitive status (eg, sedation, delirium, dementia) and extrapyramidal, anticholinergic, and cardiovascular effects. Psychotropic drugs can contribute to cognitive impairment and are associated with hip fractures in the geriatric population. Extrapyramidal side effects are most common with several older antipsychotic drugs but may occur with newer atypical antipsychotics (see Table 14-8). These effects, which include pseudoparkinsonism (rigidity, bradykinesia, tremor), akathisia (restlessness), and involuntary dystonic movements (such as tardive dyskinesia), can be severe and may cause substantial disability. Rigidity and bradykinesia can lead to immobility and related complications. Akathisia can make the patient appear more anxious and agitated and can lead to the inappropriate prescription of more medication. Tardive dyskinesia can cause permanent disability as a consequence of continuous orolingual movements and difficulty with eating.

The use of antipsychotics to treat the neuropsychiatric symptoms of dementia is highly controversial (Maher et al, 2011; Schneider et al, 2006; Sink et al, 2005). All of the second-generation antipsychotics have been associated with an increase in mortality as well as weight gain. Atypical antipsychotics now have black box warnings from the U.S. Food and Drug Administration because of the increased risk of death associated with their use. The U.S. Centers for Medicare & Medicaid Services has a campaign to improve the appropriateness and reduce the use of these drugs in nursing homes. For severely demented patients who develop physical or verbal agitation without an obvious underlying cause, empiric treatment with acetaminophen has shown some efficacy (Husebo et al, 2011).

Insomnia, like agitation, can be the manifestation of depression or physical illness. It is a very common complaint in geriatric patients, and causes of sleep disorders such as sleep apnea, nocturia, and periodic leg movements should be sought. Nonpharmacological measures (such as increasing activity during the day, diminishing nighttime noise, and ensuring cooler nighttime temperatures) are sometimes helpful. Cognitive behavioral therapy can also be useful in older patients without cognitive impairment. Several alternatives are available for drug treatment of insomnia (see Table 14-9). The long-term effects of chronic hypnotic use in the geriatric population are unknown, but rebound insomnia can become a problem in patients who use hypnotics (especially benzodiazepine hypnotics and melatonin) regularly and then discontinue them. Whatever the indication, it is extremely important that, after a hypnotic drug is prescribed, the patient be closely monitored for the effects of the drug on the target symptoms and side effects and that the drug regimen be adjusted accordingly.

Evidence Summary

Do's

- Simplify drug regimens as much as possible.
- "Start low and go slow," but increase doses to maximum if appropriate based on response.
- Carefully assess for drug effectiveness and side effects.
- Help ensure adherence by education, attention to out-of-pocket costs, and availability of caregivers' support for patients with cognitive impairment.
- Utilize the expertise and education available through pharmacists.
- Keep careful medication records and review them at each visit.

Don'ts

- Automatically prescribe all drugs that may be indicated in younger patients for older patients with multiple comorbidities.
- Use two drugs when one may be effective.
- Make drug regimens unnecessarily complicated.
- Use multiple psychotropic drugs, except in very limited circumstances.
- Prescribe antipsychotics for behavioral symptoms associated with dementia unless underlying treatable conditions have been excluded and nonpharmacological interventions have failed or unless the patient is an immediate danger to himself or herself or others.

Consider

- Drug–drug and drug–disease interactions when prescribing for older patients.
- Using specially designed pillboxes or technological approaches (eg, devices that help monitor adherence) for selected patients.

REFERENCES

American Geriatrics Society Beers Criteria Update Expert Panel. American Geriatrics Society 2015 updated Beers Criteria for potentially inappropriate medication use in older adults. *J Am Geriatr Soc.* 2015;63:2227-2246.

PART III

Brasure M, Jutkowitz E, Fuchs E, et al. Nonpharmacologic interventions for agitation and aggression in dementia. *Comparative Effectiveness Review* No. 177. (Prepared by the Minnesota Evidence-Based Practice Center under Contract No. 290-2012-00016-I.) AHRQ Publication No. 16-EHC019-EF. Rockville, MD: Agency for Healthcare Research and Quality; February 2016. www.effectivehealthcare.ahrq.gov/reports/final.cfm.

Brown JD, Hutchinson LC, Li C, et al. Predictive validity of the Beers and Screening Tool of Older Persons' Prescriptions (STOPP) criteria to detect adverse drug events, hospitalizaions, and emergency department visits in the United States. *J Am Geriatr Soc.* 2016;64:22-30.

Budnitz DS, Lovegrove MC, Shehbab N, Richards CL. Emergency hospitalizations for adverse drug events in older Americans. *N Engl J Med.* 2011;365:2002-2012.

Campbell NL, Boustani, MA, Skopeljia EN, et al. Medication adherence in older adults with cognitive impairment: an evidence-based systematic review. *Am J Geriatr Pharmacother.* 2012;10:165-177.

Cockcroft DW, Gault MH. Predictions of creatinine clearance from serum creatinine. *Nephron.* 1976;16:31-41.

Coleman EA, Smith JD, Raha D, et al. Posthospital medication discrepancies. *Arch Intern Med.* 2005;165:1842-1847.

Finlayson E, Maselli J, Steinman MA, et al. Inappropriate medication use in older adults undergoing surgery: a national study. *J Am Geriatr Soc.* 2011;59:2139-2144.

Garfinkel D, Mangin D. Feasibility study of a systematic approach for discontinuation of multiple medications in older adults. *Arch Intern Med.* 2010;170:1648-1654.

Heerdink ER, Leufkens HG, Herings RMC, et al. NSAIDs associated with increased risk of congestive heart failure in elderly patients taking diuretics. *Arch Intern Med.* 1998;158:1108-1112.

Hines LE, Murphy JE. Potentially harmful drug–drug interactions in the elderly: a review. *Am J Geriatr Pharmacother.* 2011;9:364-377.

Holbrook AM, Pereira JA, Labiris R, et al. Systematic overview of warfarin and its drug and food interactions. *Arch Intern Med.* 2005;165:1095-1106.

Husebo BS, Ballard C, Sandvik R, Nilsen OB, Aarsland D. Efficacy or treating pain to reduce behavioural disturbances in residents of nursing homes with dementia: cluster randomized trial. *BMJ.* 2011;343:d4065.

Lazarou J, Pomeranz BH, Corey PN. Incidence of adverse drug reactions in hospitalized patients: a meta-analysis of prospective studies. *JAMA.* 1998; 279:1200-1205.

Maher M, Maglione M, Bagley S, et al. Efficacy and comparative effectiveness of atypical antipsychotic medications for off-label uses in adults. *JAMA.* 2011;306:1359-1369.

O'Conner MN, O'Sullivan DO, Gallegher PF, et al. Prevention of hospital acquired adverse drug reactions using Screening Tool of Older Persons' Prescriptions and Screening Tool to Alert to Right Treatment Criteria: a cluster randomized controlled trial. *J Am Geriatr Soc.* 2016;64:1558-1566.

Schneider LS, Tariot PN, Dagerman KS, et al. Effectiveness of atypical antipsychotic drugs in patients with Alzheimer's disease. *N Engl J Med.* 2006;355:1525-1538.

Schwartz, J. Potential effet of substituting estimated glomerlar filtration rate for estimated creatinine clearance for dosing of direct oral anticoagulants. *J Am Geriatr Soc.* 2016;64:1996-2002.

Sink KM, Holden KF, Yaffe K. Pharmacological treatment of neuropsychiatric symptoms of dementia: a review of the evidence. *JAMA.* 2005;293:596-608.

Steinman MA, Beizer JL, DuBeau CE, et al. How to use the American Geriatrics Society 2015 Beers Criteria—a guide for patients, clinicians, health systems, and payors. *J Am Geriatr Soc.* 2015;63:e1-e7.

Wilkinson GR. Drug metabolism and variability among patients in drug response. *N Engl J Med.* 2005;352:2211-2221.

SUGGESTED READINGS

Bowie MW, Slattum PW. Pharmacodynamics in older adults: a review. *Am J Geriatr Pharmacother.* 2007;5:263-303.

Selma TP, Beizer JL, Higbee MD. *Geriatric Dosage Handbook.* 21st ed. Hudson, OH: Lexi-Comp; 2015.

Steinman MA, Hanlon JT. Managing medications in complex elders. *JAMA.* 2010;304:1592-1601.

CHAPTER 15

High-Value Health Services

One metaphor for geriatrics is a set of chopsticks—one labeled "chronic disease care" and the other "gerontology." Both need to work in coordination in order to achieve good geriatric care. The latter refers largely to the contents of this book: the syndromes associated with aging, the atypical presentations of disease, and diseases closely linked to aging. Chronic disease management (addressed in Chapter 4) is complicated by the difficulties of managing multiple, simultaneous, interactive problems. Health care for older persons consists largely of addressing the problems associated with multiple chronic illnesses.

Indeed, multimorbidity is the key challenge in geriatric care. Effective responses to the situation should emphasize close monitoring and rapid intervention when there are early signs of change. The goal of chronic disease management is catastrophe prevention. However, medical care continues to be practiced as though it consisted of a series of discrete encounters. What is needed is a systematic approach to chronic care that encourages clinicians to recognize the overall course expected for each patient and to manage treatment within those parameters. The fee-for-service payment system encourages routinely scheduled doctor visits, when good care would utilize frequent monitoring observations at a distance. Chapter 4 traces a number of strategies designed to improve the management of chronic disease. Geriatricians have long recognized that care in one sector affects care in other areas. For example, nursing home residents use fewer hospital resources than older persons receiving home and community-based care, even though they are likely frailer.

Several initiatives are under way that may help address this interdependence. The Patient Protection and Affordable Care Act specifically addressed attention to transitions for patients discharged from hospitals. Payments for hospital readmissions are denied in some situations, and penalties for excessive rates of 30-day readmissions are being levied. The accountable care organization concept calls for better integration of hospital care, primary care, postacute care, and nursing home care. It may extend to recognizing the need for better social integration as well. The health-care home effort to incent practices for more comprehensive care represents a step in this direction.

A prerequisite for effectively coordinating medical and social care is shared goals. Care for frail older persons has been impeded by an artificial dichotomy between medical and social interventions. This separation has been enhanced by funding policies, such as the auspices of Medicare and Medicaid, but it also reflects the philosophies of the dominant professions. Until the differences in goals are reconciled, there is little hope for integrated care. Medical practice has been driven by what may be termed a therapeutic model. The basic expectation from medical care is that it will make a difference, whereas the goals of a social model are directed more at compensation and coping with extant limitations. But both can converge in a common commitment to maximizing people's quality of life.

PART III

With frail older patients the difference is typically not reflected in an improvement in the patient's status. Indeed, for many chronically ill patients, decline is inevitable, but good care should at least delay the rate of that decline. Because many patients do get worse over time, it may be difficult for clinicians to see the effects of their care. The invisibility of this benefit makes it particularly hard to create a strong case for investing in such care.

Appreciating the benefits of good care in the context of slowing decline in function (or quality of life) over time requires a comparison between what happens and what would have occurred in the absence of that care. In effect, the yield from good care is the difference between what is observed and what is reasonable to expect; but without the expected value, the benefit may be hard to appreciate.

The inability to document these benefits of good care has many implications. It is hard to drum up public support for making substantial investments in an activity that is associated with decline. To be seen as something worth investing in, there must be evidence of benefit. Likewise, those who work in the field can become frustrated and even angry if they fail to see any results from their hard labor.

Figure 15-1 (which also appears in Chapter 4) provides a theoretical model of how a comparator is needed to demonstrate the effects of good chronic care (either medical or social or both). Both trajectories show decline, but the slope associated with better care is less acute. The area between them represents the effects of good care. Unfortunately, that benefit is invisible unless specific steps are taken to demonstrate the difference between the observed and expected course. Appreciating the need to make this benefit visible is essential to make the political and social case for a greater investment in chronic disease and long-term care (LTC). Without such evidence, people simply see decline and view this area as not worth investing in.

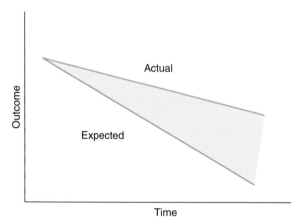

FIGURE 15-1 Measuring the effects of good chronic care. Both trajectories show decline, but the slope of expected care is steeper. The yellow area between the lines represents the effects of good care.

The alternative model, usually associated with social services, is compensatory care. Under the alternative model, usually associated with social services, a person is assessed to determine deficits, and a plan of care is developed to address the identified deficits. Good care is defined as providing services that meet the profile of dependencies and thereby allow the client to enjoy as normal a lifestyle as possible without incurring any adverse consequences.

These two approaches seem at odds, but they are compatible. Although there is some risk of encouraging dependency with excessive support, providing needed services should enhance functioning or at least slow its decline. Care for the frail older patient requires a synthesis of medical and social attention. One thing is certain: If the medical and social systems are to work together harmoniously, they must share a common set of goals. The first step in collaboration is to identify the common ground to ensure both elements are working in the same direction. Both approaches (and their synthesis) can be captured in the comparative model of change described previously. Indeed, until some proof of effectiveness is widely demonstrated it will be hard to garner public or professional support for the needed investments in care.

A third option draws on both these elements. The general lack of enthusiasm for chronic care stands in stark contrast to support for hospice care. The latter offers two advantages: (1) It represents a way to avoid futile care and hence save money and reduce suffering. (2) Its goals are attainable. It seeks to make the end of life as positive an experience as possible, ironically by removing many of the restrictions traditional care has imposed. We might well ask why we have better rules for the dying than for the living. Hospice care implies an explicit decision to forgo aggressive treatment. Palliative care represents an effort to make such care more compatible with traditional medical care, emphasizing comfort but not precluding more aggressive actions. (Hospice care is discussed in Chapter 18.)

The medical care system has generally not facilitated the interaction with social care. Managed care could provide a framework for achieving this coordination, but the track record so far does not suggest that the incentives are yet in place to produce this effect. A few notable programs have been able to merge funding and services for this frail population. Probably the best example of creative integration is seen in the Program of All-Inclusive Care for the Elderly (PACE), which uses pooled capitated funding from Medicare and Medicaid to provide integrated health and social services to older persons who are deemed to be eligible for nursing home care but who are still living in the community (Kane, Bershadsky, and Bershadsky, 2006; Wieland, 2006). The PACE programs have increased, but they are limited because they target a very specific group (persons receiving both Medicare and Medicaid who are eligible for nursing home care but live in the community) and they are expensive. They also require enrollees to change doctors to those employed by PACE. PACE services include the following:

• Primary Care (including doctor and nursing services)	• Adult Day Care
• Hospital Care	• Recreational Therapy

PART III

- Medical Specialty Services
- Prescription Drugs
- Nursing Home Care
- Emergency Services
- Home Care
- Physical and Occupational Therapy
- Transportation

- Dentistry
- Meals
- Nutritional Counseling
- Social Services
- Social Work Counseling
- Laboratory/X-ray Services

States and the federal government are making a heavy investment in managed care to serve the so-called dually eligible (for Medicare and Medicaid) in a hope that integration will improve quality and save money. Whether managed care will achieve its potential as a vehicle for improving coordination of care for older persons remains to be seen. In any event, care for older persons will require such integration, and eventually some reconciliation must be achieved about what constitutes the desired goals of such care. Medicare's move to Accountable Care Organizations (ACOs) represents a step to press for integration at the health program, rather than health plan, level. Its success remains to be determined.

Geriatric care thus implies team care, but teams must be efficient. This concept, in turn, implies trust in other disciplines with special skills and training to undertake the tasks for which they have the requisite skills. Teamwork is successful when each player is confident that the other players will performs their roles competently and in coordination with the others on the team. However, these colleagues should not be expected to operate alone. Good communication and coordination will avoid duplication of effort and lead to a better overall outcome. To play a useful role on the health-care team, physicians need to appreciate what other health professions can do and know how and when to call on their skills. Efficient team care does not involve extensive meetings. It does not mean that everyone needs to be on the same electronic record system. Rather, information can be communicated by various means. However, good team care will not arise spontaneously. Just as sports teams spend long hours practicing to work collectively, so too must health-care teams develop a knowledge and trust of each other's inputs. They need a common language and common playbook. Effective teamwork requires an investment of effort, thus careful thought must be given to when such an investment is justified.

PUBLIC PROGRAMS

Health care, especially that part of it supported by public funds, is now committed to the triple aims enunciated by Donald Berwick (Berwick, 2008):

1. Improving the experience of care
2. Improving the health of populations
3. Reducing per capita costs of health care

To achieve these goals, the system must facilitate enrolling identified populations, who have equal access to universal benefits, from organizations that pursue these goals. He identifies five components for organization involved:

1. Partnership with individuals and families
2. Redesign of primary care
3. Population health management
4. Financial management
5. Macro system integration

The Centers for Medicare & Medicaid Services (CMS) has committed to a major shift to value-based payment across all lines of business by 2018. The new commitment to value, along with a variety of experiments in different approaches to service bundling and capitated payments seen in Medicare, reflect this thinking. Likewise, physician payment is being changed to reflect quality. Questions have been raised about how this will affect geriatrics. The new payment model created under MACRA (Medicare Access and CHIP Reauthorization Act) is described below.

Clinicians caring for older patients must have at least a working acquaintance with the major programs that support older people. We are accustomed to thinking about care of older people in association with Medicare. In fact, at least three parts (called *Titles*) of the Social Security Act provide important benefits for older adults: Title XVIII (Medicare), Title XIX (Medicaid), and Social Services Block Grants (formerly Title XX). Medicare was designed to address health care, particularly acute care hospital services.

The Medicare program is in flux. Changes in the payment system have been introduced to counter what some saw as abuses (certainly expansions) or inefficiencies (and inappropriate incentives) of the previous system. For older people also covered by Medicaid, the latter program essentially filled in the coverage gaps left by Medicare. Medicare was intended to deal with LTC only to the extent that LTC can supplant more expensive hospital care, leaving the major funding for LTC to Medicaid. However, the funding demarcation between acute care and LTC services became blurred.

The distinction in programmatic responsibility between Medicare and Medicaid is a very important one. Whereas Medicare is an insurance-type program to which persons are entitled after contributing a certain amount, Medicaid is a welfare program, eligibility for which depends on a combination of need and poverty. Thus, to become eligible for Medicaid, a person must not only prove illness but also exhaust his or her personal resources—hardly a situation conducive to restoring autonomy.

The pattern of coverage is quite different for the various services covered. Figure 15-2 traces fee-for-service Medicare spending. Managed care, which is not displayed in this figure, has become much more dominant; by 2014 it accounted for more than 20% of all Medicare spending. Part D now accounts for about 15% of all Medicare spending (more if you count what is buried in managed care). As a result, since its inception in 2010, the proportion of fee-for-service payments to hospitals and physicians decreased. Home health care has grown but skilled nursing

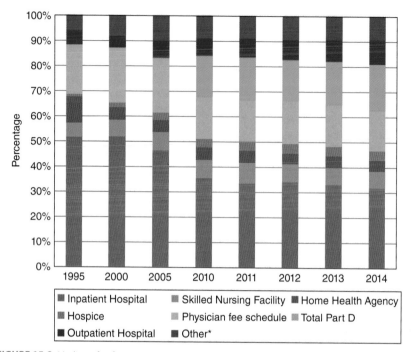

FIGURE 15-2 Medicare fee-for-service expenditures and percentage distribution, by Medicare program and type of service: calendar years 1995–2014. (*Reproduced with permission from Centers for Medicare & Medicaid Services, Medicare Current Beneficiary Survey, Cost and Use.*)

facility care has not. Medicare is a major payer of hospital and physician care but pays for only a small portion of nursing home care, whereas just the reverse applies to Medicaid. (Medicare has played a larger role in nursing home and home health care as the role of PAC has grown.)

MEDICARE

Medicare has four components: Eligibility for Medicare differs for each of its two major parts. Part A (Hospital Services Insurance) is available to all who are eligible for Social Security, usually by virtue of paying the Social Security tax for a sufficient number of quarters. This program is supported by a special payroll tax, which goes into the Medicare Trust Fund. Part B (Medical Services Insurance) is offered for a monthly premium, paid by the individual but heavily subsidized by the government (which pays approximately 70% of the cost from general tax revenues). Almost everyone older than age 65 is automatically covered by Part A. One important exception is older immigrants, who may not have worked long enough to generate Social Security coverage. Part C allows people to enroll in managed care plans, euphemistically called Medicare Advantage; enrollment is optional. Part D covers prescription drugs. Medicare Part D covers medications; all dually eligible (Medicare and Medicare) beneficiaries receive their medications through Part D. For Medicare-only beneficiaries, Part D is elective (but is included in coverage for those who opt for managed care).

The introduction of prospective payment for hospitals under Medicare created a new set of complications. Hospitals are paid a fixed amount per admission according to the diagnosis-related group (DRG), to which the patient is assigned on the basis of the admitting diagnosis. The rates for DRGs are, in turn, based on expected lengths of stay and intensity of care for each condition. The incentives under such an approach (less is better) have a mixed relationship to the goals of geriatrics. Whereas geriatrics addresses the functional result of multiple interacting problems, DRGs encourage concentration on a single problem. Extra time required to make an appropriate discharge plan is discouraged. Use of ancillary personnel, such as social workers, is similarly discouraged. At the same time (as noted in Chapter 5) hospitals are dangerous places for frail older people. The imposition of a prospective payment for hospitals created a new market for what became postacute care (PAC), care that was formerly provided in hospitals but can now be delivered and billed separately by nursing homes, inpatient rehabilitation facilities (IRFs), or home health care. As hospital lengths of stay have decreased, patients are discharged "quicker and sicker," leading to a dramatic growth in PAC.

Many of these former hospital patients are now cared for through home health and nursing homes and IRFs. In effect, Medicare is paying for care twice: It pays for the hospital stay virtually regardless of length and then pays for the posthospital care under PAC.

Currently, payment arrangements for PAC differ by types. IRFs are paid a fixed amount for a rehabilitation stay based on the functional needs of the patient derived from data based on the Functional Improvement Measure (FIM). Home health care is also paid on a different prospective fixed rate basis for up to 60 days of care based on patient characteristics derived from Outcome and Assessment Information Set (OASIS). Skilled nursing facilities, by contrast, are paid a per diem (called resource utilization groups [RUGs]) based on information derived from the Minimum Data Set (MDS). After 20 days patients must pay a copay; 100 days of coverage per episode are allowed.

PAC costs are the fastest-growing aspect of Medicare. Medicare-covered home health care has waxed and waned. Originally intended as a PAC service, it expanded to provide more chronic care, retrenched, and then reemerged as longer-term care after a court case. The prospective payment approach has been applied to PAC as well, but payment for each type of PAC is based on a separate calculation. Thus, three silos were created, with different approaches to providing similar services, each with its own measures of success.

Steps are under way to address this situation. A common assessment tool is being developed for all forms of PAC. New programs that bundle the payments for PAC and even combine hospital and PAC payments are being tested.

The rapid rise in this latter sector has led Medicare to search for solutions. Different types of Medicare prospective payment for the different types of posthospital care have been established. Nursing homes are paid on a per-diem basis, whereas

PART III

home health agencies and rehabilitation units are paid on a per-episode basis. New payment approaches are combining the payment for hospital and posthospital care into a single bundled payment. This approach uses bundled payments, which include costs for hospital and posthospital care, and medical care under several models. It is now being used for joint replacement surgery and will be expanded to coronary by-pass surgery; but a long list of conditions is targeted.

These bundled approaches use what might be thought of as point-of-service capitation, where payments for service packages are grouped rather than as separate payments for each service. Such an approach may make the role of geriatric care more obvious, but this remains to be seen. Focusing on technically complex care may invite some transfer of responsibility to primary care once the major procedure is accomplished and the patient is recuperating. Given the limited supply of geriatricians, it is not clear how big a role they will play in these new arrangements. More likely, investments will focus on using ancillary personnel to coordinate care. For example, medical (or health-care) homes may use case coordinators.

In the past, the payment system was even more paradoxical. The DRG payment was higher for patients with complications, even if those complications arose from treatment during the hospitalization. That approach has been modified to exclude iatrogenic complications, creating a better business case for involving geriatricians in the care of frail patients. Hospitals must now report complications present on admission to avoid having them declared unreimbursable because they arose as part of the hospital care. Likewise, Medicare will not pay for some readmissions within 30 days for the same DRG and imposes a penalty for excessive readmission rates.

The payment systems now in effect create much confusion for Medicare beneficiaries. Although hospitals are paid a fixed amount per case, the patients continue to pay under a system of deductibles and copayments. The majority of Medicare beneficiaries have purchased some form of Medigap insurance to cover these costs, but many variations exist. The picture is even more confused when the Medigap insurance can also cover Part D deductibles and copays.

Managed care is aggressively being pursued as an option to traditional fee-for-service care. Under that arrangement, the managed care organizations receive a fixed monthly payment from Medicare in exchange for providing at least the range of services covered by Medicare. In some areas the managed care plans also charge recipients for an additional premium depending on the regional rates. Despite a slow start, Medicare managed care has increased substantially (from about 7% of beneficiaries in 1995 to about 27% in 2014). The growth in managed care was partly fueled by the introduction of Part D, which covers drugs (see below).

The pricing system used by Medicare to calculate managed care rates reflects the prices paid for fee-for-service care in each county. Managed care organizations are paid a fixed amount calculated on the basis of the average amount Medicare paid for its beneficiaries in that county. This adjusted average per capita cost (AAPCC) varies widely from one location to another.

Because Part C is optional, older persons who are beneficiaries of both Medicaid and Medicare (often called "duals" because of their dual eligibility) may find themselves in different programs for each service. Medicaid programs can compel recipients to enroll in a managed care plan, but Medicare beneficiaries must opt in. Many states are developing managed care programs for these dual eligibles that will entice them to join in hopes of better care coordination.

One apparently successful approach to applying managed care to frail older dual eligibles is PACE (Program for All-Inclusive Care of the Elderly) described earlier. PACE explicitly uses flexible care approaches to reduce the use of institutions (both hospitals and nursing homes). It places great reliance on team care, empowering all members from van drivers on up. Despite its attractiveness, it has proven hard to recruit large numbers of physicians who want to work in such an egalitarian environment. Overall, however, the likelihood of managed care achieving its potential symbiosis with geriatrics appears dim. Ideally, by moving away from fee-for-service (FFS) payment, managed care could provide an environment where many of the principles of geriatrics could be implemented to the benefit of all; but within managed care FFS is still applied, either overtly or under the guise of productivity measures for salaried staff. The performance to date suggests that managed care for Medicare beneficiaries has so far responded more to the incentives from favorable selection (recruiting healthy patients and getting paid average rates), discounted purchasing of services, and barriers to access than to the potential benefits from increased efficiency derived from a geriatric philosophy.

Although Medicare does pay for authorized posthospital services in nursing homes and through home health care, the payment for physicians does not encourage their active participation in postacute care (PAC). For example, while a physician would be paid a fee for daily rounds on a Medicare patient in a hospital, if the patient is discharged to a nursing home the following day, both the rate of physician reimbursement for a visit and the number of visits per week considered customary decrease dramatically. Although physician home visits are still a rarity, payment for these services has increased substantially in recent years. Some physician groups have made a business out of nursing home care and home health care. Increasingly the care of nursing home residents falls to nurse practitioners working as part of geriatric care teams. These teams can play two roles in avoiding hospitalizations: (1) They can provide more effective primary care that prevents an episode that would require a hospital transfer. (2) They can manage events that do arise in the nursing home, thus alleviating the need for a transfer.

Medicare coverage is important to beneficiaries but not sufficient for three basic reasons:

1. To control use, it mandates deductible and copayment charges for both Parts A and B.
2. It sets physicians' fees using a complicated formula called the Resource-Based Relative Value Scale (RBRVS). The RBRVS is designed to pay physicians more closely according to the value of their services as determined both within a specialty and across specialties. Theoretically, both the value of the services provided and the investment in training are considered in setting the rates. This payment

approach was intended to increase the payment for primary care relative to surgical specialties, but, ironically, many geriatric assessment services have been reimbursed at a level lower than before its introduction. Under Medicare Part B, physicians are generally paid less than they would usually bill for the service. (Some physicians opt to bill the patient directly for the difference, but a number of states have mandated that physicians accept "assignment" of Medicare fees, that is, they accept the fee [plus the 20% copayment] as payment in full.)

3. The program does not cover several services essential to patient functioning, such as eyeglasses, hearing aids, and many preventive services (although the benefits for the latter are expanding). Medicare specifically excludes services designed to provide "custodial care"—the very services often most critical to LTC. (However, as noted earlier, the boundary between acute care and LTC exclusions seems to be eroding.) Work is currently under way to change the way physician fee increases are determined. Basically some combination of cost and quality will be used. In lieu of across-the-board increases, payments will be based on physician performance.

Physician payment will change again under the Medicare Access and CHIP Reauthorization Act (MACRA), which goes into effect in 2019 (Clough and McClellan, 2016) using data collected in 2017. It replaces the unsustainable Sustainable Growth Rate formula and represents a welcome step toward paying for value. As part of the press for value-based payment, it enrolls physicians into one of two systems. The predominant one, the Merit-Based Incentive Payment System (MIPS), is a pay-for-performance system that adjusts payments based on four classes of measures derived from prior care.

Payment incentives will be based on four components of MIPS: quality measures, cost reductions, EHR implementation, and practice improvement. The first two components emphasize meeting guidelines and saving money. Presumably those two approaches are complementary. Savings can be achieved by doing less, being more efficient, or reaping benefits from more proactive primary care.

MIPS is basically a payment adjustment system grafted onto fee-for-service payments. MACRA applies only to Medicare fee-for-service population (ie, not PACE, Special Need Populations, Medicare Advantage, VA, etc).

Although details of the program are still evolving, a few elements are clear:

- Clinicians can report either as individuals (based on their National Provider Identifier [NPI]) or as part of a group identified by having a common Tax Identifying Number (TIN).
- In the latter case, clinicians will be rewarded or penalized based on how the organizations they are affiliated with perform.
- Analysis for all MIPS categories would be completely separate. A patient can be seen at multiple facilities, and be qualified for reporting purposes at each. If a patient were to be seen by three different eligible clinicians, then depending on the denominator-eligible criteria that is met, it is possible for the patient encounter under one eligible clinician to meet a certain measure, but another

encounter for the same patient under another eligible clinician could apply to another measure. CMS will evaluate each eligible clinician separately (or group, if they choose to report as a group), based on their denominator-eligible services, as well as their actual reporting/submission that is done (numerator).

- Total per capita or total annual spending for all patients assigned to the MIPS eligible clinicians uses Medicare Spending per Beneficiary which measures all costs around a hospitalization for assigned patients. In other words, the Cost category—previously called "Resource Use"—utilizes claims data to develop measures of cost, mainly for particular episodes of patient care. CMS will do all the work of calculating cost category measures, so clinicians do not need to submit any additional information to get their score.
- All patients treated by a TIN may be involved. All clinicians in the TIN share in the overall TIN performance regardless of whether they were involved with a given beneficiary. Thus, clinicians will be affected by care they may not have given to patients they never met.
- Patients do not enroll in MACRA; they are assigned and may be unaware of what TIN(s) they are in. They have no responsibility (or incentive) to change their behavior. This is a clinician-focused system.
- The first 2 years of MACRA (2017 and 2018) will be spent collecting data. In year 1 of MIPS, clinicians' scores on the cost category will not count toward their overall MIPS score. However, cost will count for 10% in year 2 and 30% in year 3 and beyond. Therefore, clinicians and groups should review their Quality and Resource Use Reports (QRURs). CMS's annual feedback will provide clinicians under MACRA to better understand their performance on these measures. Tasks in the first 2 years must be accomplished to avoid penalties.
- Some quality measures apply to older people (for example, advance directives, medication documentation, alcohol use screening); other quality measures may not be consistent with geriatric precepts (for example, target levels of HbA1c); blood pressure control levels are currently set at 140/90. Specific geriatric quality measures are being promulgated, but are not yet known.

A major expansion of the Medicare program occurred in 2005 with the passage of the Medicare Modernization Act, which included Part D coverage of drugs. This legislation also provides substantial incentives to Medicare Advantage providers and creates a new class of managed care coverage, Special Needs Plans. These are groups of beneficiaries presumed to be at high risk and hence eligible for higher premiums.

The 2010 Patient Protection and Affordable Care Act (PPACA, or more commonly, ACA) was primarily aimed at improving access to care for those currently uninsured. Its direct impact on Medicare is modest but its second order effects have been substantial. The press for value-based purchasing and the support for experimentation with new models of comprehensive care offer at least some hope that reimbursement will more closely align with the philosophy of geriatrics.

Under Part D, the coverage of prescription drugs involves a complicated formula, often referred to as the "donut hole" because of the odd design of benefits. Basically, the patient pays a deductible ($360 in 2016). Then the patient pays a copayment (usually around 25%) on yearly drug costs from $360 to $3,310, and the plan pays the majority of these costs. When the patient has paid $3,310 he or she enters what has been termed "the donut hole," where they must pay 58% of generic drug costs and they get a 55% discount on the cost of brand-name drugs. The donut hole ends when they spend a total of $4,850. At this point drugs are almost completely covered. They pay either a copay of $2.95 for generic drugs and $7.40 for brand-name drugs or a coinsurance of 5%, whichever is greater. Each year, the amount beneficiaries pay while in the donut hole will reduce by a small percentage until 2020, when the coverage gap is planned to be eliminated. In 2020, they will be responsible for only 25% of brand and generic drug costs. This is part of a new law enacted to eliminate the donut hole by 2020.

Part D is administered by a number of drug management firms that offer a confusing array of plans, from a basic plan that covers the Part D pattern to more inclusive coverage that eliminates the donut hole. Of course, the premium cost rises as the coverage expands. Plans are required to cover at least two drugs in each identified category, but the choice of drugs is left to them. Medicare beneficiaries must scramble to find the most affordable plan that covers the drugs they need, but even then there is no guarantee that those drugs will continue to be covered.

As a result of these three factors, a substantial amount of the medical bill is left to the individual. Today, older persons' out-of-pocket costs for health care represent about 12.5% of their income. In general, out-of-pocket costs are less for those in managed care.

MEDICAID

Medicaid, in contrast to Medicare, is a welfare program designed to serve the poor. It is a state-run program to which the federal government contributes (50%–78% of the costs, depending on the state's capita income). In some states, persons can be covered as medically indigent even if their income is above the poverty level if their medical expenses would impoverish them. As a welfare program, Medicaid has no deductibles or coinsurance (although current proposals call for modest charges to discourage excess use). It is, however, a welfare program cast in the medical model.

Ironically, Medicaid was never intended as a major program for older persons. It was designed to cover poor mothers and their children. However, because of a provision that extended coverage to those whose medical costs exceeded most of their income, older persons, especially those in nursing homes, became eligible. They are now a dominant user group.

Medicaid is essentially two separate programs, serving two distinct populations. Since the ACA, this number has risen to three: mothers and children (including a small but expensive subset of children who are severely ill or disabled), elderly persons, and now the rest of the poor population who may be eligible under the ACA depending on states' willingness to participate. Mothers and young children are covered under Aid to Families with Dependent Children (AFDC), whereas persons are eligible if they receive Old Age Assistance or if they qualify for the medically needy program, whereby eligibility is conferred when medical costs—usually nursing homes—exceed a fixed fraction of a person's income.

It is important to appreciate that the shape of the Medicaid expenditures for older people is determined largely by the gaps in Medicare coverage. Medicaid has been described as a universal health program that has a deductible of all your assets and a copay of all your income. Medicaid is the major source of nursing home payments. It requires physicians to certify a patient's physical limitations in order to gain the patient admittance to a nursing home. In some cases, physicians are put in a position of inventing medical justifications for primarily social reasons (ie, lack of social supports necessary to remain in the community).

Because it pays about half of the nursing home costs but covers almost 70% of the residents, Medicaid shapes nursing home policies. The payment discrepancy is explained by the policies that require residents to expend their own resources first. Thus, Social Security payments, private pensions, savings, and the like are used as primary sources of payment, and Medicaid picks up the remainder. However, it does not directly pay for most physician care in the nursing home; that is covered by Medicare. Medicaid would pay the deductibles and copayments and for those services not covered under Medicare. The separation in payment raises policy issues. More aggressive care in nursing homes (paid by Medicaid) can prevent emergency department visits and hospital admissions (paid by Medicare). The nursing homes (and Medicaid) thus underwrite (or cross-subsidize) Medicare savings.

Medicaid also supports home- and community-based LTC services (HCBS). In some states personal care is included as a mandatory Medicaid service under the state's basic Medicaid coverage plan, but in many states HCBS is offered as a waivered service. Under this arrangement, the federal government allows states to use money that would otherwise have gone to nursing homes to fund HCBS. The waiver allows states to offer the service only in specific areas and to limit the numbers of persons enrolled in the program. In theory, these funds are supposed to be offset by concomitant savings in nursing home care. The use of HCBS has greatly expanded over the last decades. Once viewed as simply a cheaper alternative to nursing home care, HCBS is now viewed as the preferred LTC option in many situations (Kane and Kane, 2012). Efforts to use HCBS in preference to nursing homes are being actively pursued by most states motivated by new federal programs.

Whereas going on Medicaid was once seen as a great social embarrassment, associated with accepting public charity, there appears to be a growing sense among many older persons that they are entitled to receive Medicaid help when their health-care expenses, especially their LTC costs, are high. The stigma appears to be displaced by the idea that they paid taxes for many years and are now entitled to reap the rewards. As a result of this shift in sentiment, at least in the states with generous levels of Medicaid eligibility, a burgeoning industry of financial advisers has arisen to assist older persons in preparing to become Medicaid eligible. Because eligibility is usually based on both income and assets, such a step necessitates advance planning. Usually state laws require that assets transferred within 2 or more years (the look-back period varies by state) of applying for Medicaid funds are considered to still be owed. (The situation is more complicated in the case of a married couple, where provisions have been made to allow the spouse to retain part of the family's assets.) This requirement means that older persons contemplating becoming eligible for Medicaid must be willing to divest themselves of their assets at least several years in advance of the time they expect to need such help. This step places them in a very dependent position, financially and psychologically. Much has been made of the "divestiture phenomenon" whereby older people scheme to divest themselves of their assets in order to qualify for Medicaid, but there is no good evidence about the scale of the phenomenon.

The anticipated LTC Medicaid payment crisis resulting from the demographic shifts has prompted enthusiasm for promoting various forms of private LTC insurance, but with very limited success. This coverage, in effect, protects the assets of those who might otherwise be marginally eligible for Medicaid or who simply want to preserve an inheritance for their heirs. Like any insurance linked to age-related events but to a greater degree, LTC insurance is quite affordable when purchased at a young age (when the likelihood of needing it is very low) but becomes quite expensive as the buyer reaches age 75 or older. Thus, those most likely to consider buying it late in life would have to pay a premium close to the average cost of LTC itself and may have prior conditions that render them ineligible. Only a small number of young persons have shown any interest in purchasing such coverage, especially when companies are not eager to add it to their employee benefit packages as a free benefit. Although economic projections suggest that private LTC insurance is not likely to save substantial money for the Medicaid program, several states, sensing a demographic crisis that will affect their Medicaid budgets, have been working hard to find ways to encourage people to save for old age and/or buy insurance by offering linked Medicaid benefits. The enthusiasm for private LTC insurance has declined sharply and many plans have left the market.

But people are retiring with limited funds. The changes in the pension accounting rules several decades earlier prompted most employers to move from a pension plan for retirees (a fixed benefit) to a payment into a retirement account (fixed contribution—the so-called 401[k]). However, the employer contribution is made only when it matches an employee contribution. Many employees fail to contribute because of current demands on their earnings. Hence, they retire with very limited resources; they have a hard time financing their retirement, to say nothing about paying for LTC.

The decision to purchase LTC insurance needs to be made thoughtfully and carefully. People need to understand the actuarial risks and the financial implications. Purchasing this coverage early means investing money in something you will not likely use for some time with the understanding that this money is not recoverable (because it is term insurance). At the least, potential buyers should be encouraged to purchase plans with cash benefits that are not tied to specific services, because the nature of LTC is likely to change considerably. Most LTC insurance is term insurance, meaning that the premiums paid are effectively lost if a person stops paying the premium before any benefits are provided. Failure to pay the premiums results in loss of coverage and forfeiture of all that has been paid to date. Some insurance companies are experimenting with various packages that may entice people to buy some variant of LTC insurance, but the market does not look encouraging.

A specific group of older people of great policy interest are the so-called dual-eligibles, or duals, who are jointly covered by both Medicare and Medicaid. Not surprisingly, they use more care than those in one program alone. They tend to have more problems. They fall into subgroups. Those receiving LTC use more Medicaid funds, whereas those with multiple comorbidities use more Medicare resources. Given the need for better program coordination and concerns about cross-subsidization, states have shown growing interest in using managed care to take on the care of these groups. Federal programs have been initiated specifically to address care for the dual population. Many of these programs involve use of managed care.

OTHER PROGRAMS

The third part of the Social Security legislation pertinent to older persons is Title XX, now administered as Social Services Block Grants. This is also a welfare program targeted especially to those on categorical welfare programs such as Aid to Families with Dependent Children and, more germane, Supplemental Security Income. The latter is a federal program that, as the name implies, supplements Social Security benefits to provide a minimum income. Title XX funds are administered through state and local agencies, which have a substantial amount of flexibility in how they allocate the available money across a variety of stipulated services. The state also has the option of broadening the eligibility criteria to include those just above the poverty line.

Another relevant federal program is Title III of the Older Americans Act. This program is available to all persons over the age of 60 regardless of income. The single largest component goes to support nutrition through congregate meal programs where elderly persons can get a subsidized hot meal, but it also provides meals-on-wheels (home-delivered meals) and a wide variety of other services. Some services duplicate or supplement those covered under Social Security programs; others are unique. Recently, the former Administration on Aging (AoA) supported a number of preventive care initiatives, and the Aging and Disability Resource Centers (ADRC) provided a point of entry into LTC in most states. In 2012, the AoA was reorganized to merge responsibility for all persons with disability. The new organization, the Administration for Community Living, brings together the AoA, the Office on Disability, and the Administration on Developmental Disabilities into a single agency that supports both cross-cutting initiatives and efforts focused on the unique needs of individual groups, such as children with developmental disabilities or seniors with dementia. This new agency will work on increasing access to community supports and achieving full community participation for people with disabilities and older adults.

Table 15-1 summarizes these four programs and their current scope. It is important to appreciate that this summary attempts to condense and simplify a complex and ever-changing set of rules and regulations. Physicians should be familiar with the broad scope and limitations of these programs but will have to rely on others, especially social workers, who are familiar with the operating details.

TABLE 15–1. Summary of Major Federal Programs for Older Patients

Program	Eligible population	Services covered	Deductibles and copayments
Medicare (Title XVIII of the Social Security Act) Part A: Hospital Services Insurance	All persons eligible for social security and others with chronic disabilities, such as end-stage renal disease, plus voluntary enrollees aged 65+ years.	Per benefit period, "reasonable cost" (DRG-based) for 90 days of hospital care plus 60 lifetime reserve days; 100 days of skilled nursing facility (SNF); home health visits (see text); hospice care.*	Full coverage for hospital care after a deductible of about 1 day for days 2–60; then copay for days 61–90. Can use 60 "lifetime reserve" days thereafter. 20 SNF days (after 3-day hospital stay) fully covered; copay for days 21–100; up to 100 days of home health care for homebound persons (after 3-day hospital stay).
Part B: Supplemental Medical Insurance	All those covered under Part A who elect coverage; participants pay a monthly premium.	80% of "reasonable cost" for physicians' services; supplies and services related to physician services; outpatient occupational, physical, and speech therapy; diagnostic tests and radiographs; mammograms; surgical dressings; prosthetics; ambulance; durable medical equipment; home health care not covered under Part A.	Deductible and 20% copayment (no copay after a limit reached).
Part C: Medicare Advantage (MA)	Beneficiaries can opt to enroll in a certified managed care program; enrollment is voluntary.	MA plans must cover at least all Part A and Part B services. They can reduce copayments and may offer additional services. They also provide Part D coverage.	Plans can charge a monthly premium in addition to the Part B premium.

| Part D | Beneficiaries can opt to participate in a standard prescription drug plan. A variety of plans are available through drug benefit companies. Medicaid beneficiaries must be enrolled. Monthly premium varies with coverage arrangement. | Drugs covered in each of a series of mandatory classes but specific drugs vary with each plan. | Annual deductible. Then cost-sharing until the "doughnut hole." Then plan pays 95% of costs above that. |
| Medicaid (Title XIX of the Social Security Act) | Persons receiving Supplemental Security Income (SSI) (such as welfare) or receiving SSI and state supplement or meeting lower eligibility standards used for medical assistance criteria in 1972 or eligible for SSI or were in institutions and eligible for Medicaid in 1973; medically needy, who do not qualify for SSI but have high medical expenses are eligible for Medicaid in some states; eligibility criteria vary from state to state. | Mandatory services for categorically needy: inpatient hospital services; outpatient services; SNF; limited home health care; laboratory tests and radiographs; family planning; early and periodic screening, diagnosis, and treatment for children through age 20. Optional services vary from state to state. Dental care; therapies; drugs; intermediate care facilities; extended home health care; private duty nurse; eyeglasses; prostheses; personal care services; medical transportation and home health care services (states can limit the amount and duration of services). | None, once patient spends down to eligibility level. Spend-down based on income and assets. |

(continued)

PART III

TABLE 15-1. Summary of Major Federal Programs for Older Patients (*continued*)

Program	Eligible population	Services covered	Deductibles and copayments
		Some states use extended home care as part of their state plans. Many home- and community-based services are provided under special waivers that allow limited enrollment.	
Social Services Block Grant (Title XX of the Social Security Act)	All recipients of TANF and SSI; optionally, those earning up to 115% of state median income and residents of specific geographic areas.	Day care; substitute care; protective services; counseling; home-based services; employment, education, and training; health-related services; information and referral; transportation; day services; family planning; legal services; home-delivered and congregate meals.	Fees are charged to those with family incomes >80% of state's median income.
Title III of the Older Americans Act	All persons aged 60 and older; low-income, minority, and isolated older persons are special targets.	Homemaker; home-delivered meals; home health aides; transportation; legal services; counseling; information and referral plus 19 others (50% of funds must go to those listed).	Some payment may be requested.

DRG, diagnosis-related group; TANF, Temporary Assistance for Needy Families.
*Certified hospice providers are paid a preset amount when a patient who is certified as terminal opts for this benefit in lieu of regular Medicare.

LONG-TERM CARE

A proportion of older patients require substantial LTC. There is no uniform definition for LTC, but LTC can be thought of as a range of services that addresses the health, personal care, and social needs of individuals who lack some capacity for self-care. Services may be continuous or intermittent but are delivered for sustained periods to individuals who have a demonstrated need, usually measured by some index of functional incapacity.

Figure 15-3 shows the living arrangements by age for persons over 50. The proportion in group quarters (ie, nursing homes and assisted living facilities) increases with age. More very old people live alone because of spousal death or severe disease. The pattern of LTC has changed substantially over the last decades. HCBS is now a major venue for older persons as well as younger persons with disabilities. Decisions about what kind of LTC is most appropriate can be very complex. A systematic approach to this decision making is described in Chapter 4.

The medical profession plays a supportive role in LTC of older people; most older LTC recipients have underlying chronic diseases that need careful attention. Clinicians are also the gatekeepers. For many services, like admission to a nursing home or home health care, a clinician's order is required. However, most of the LTC in this country is not provided by professionals at all but by a host of individuals loosely referred to as *informal support* (Gaugler and Kane, 2015). These persons may be family, friends, or neighbors. Informal caregivers provide about 85% of

PART III

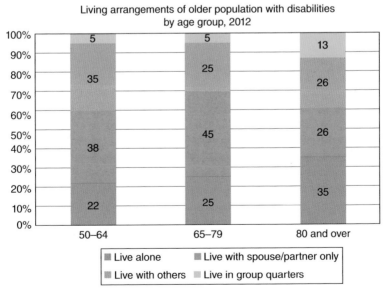

FIGURE 15-3 Living arrangements of older people with disabilities by age group, 2012. (*Data from the Centers for Medicare & Medicaid Services.*)

all care to older adults in the United States (Gitlin and Schulz, 2012). In doing this service they often face great emotional, social, physical, and financial costs (Van Houtven, 2015).

There is no universal definition of a caregiver. Typically caregiving is provided by family members, but it can also be provided by friends and people in the community. It includes many kinds of physical, psychological, emotional, and other types of support. Many caregivers are thrust into caregiving in response to a crisis; there is little time for planning. Caregiving is basically a task performed by women. About two-thirds of those caring for people living with dementia are women, of which about one-third are daughters.

Caregivers play a number of roles in the course of giving care. They serve as advocates. They are care coordinators. They provide direct services. They serve as sentinels to ensure that quality of care is maintained. They recognize and validate feelings experienced by the person living with dementia and they help him or her deal with those emotions and feel supported and cared about in the process.

When working with caregivers and older persons, the principles of person-centered care should apply as much as with any other care relationship. In the context of person-centered care, individual values and preferences are elicited from the older person and, once expressed, guide all aspects of their care, supporting their realistic health and life goals. The essential elements of patient-centered care are summarized in Table 15-2 (a copy of this table also appears in Chapter 3).

In a national survey, only about 5% of adult hospital patients said their preferences and those of their family and caregiver were taken into account when deciding about the patient's discharge health care (2015 National Healthcare Quality and Disparities Report and 5th Anniversary Update on the National Quality Strategy).

Because they are at high risk of physical and mental illness and are essential to caring, caregivers must be protected. Their status should be regularly assessed. The

---

TABLE 15-2. Essential Elements of Person-Centered Care

- Individualized, goal-oriented care plan based on the older person's and caregiver's preferences
- Ongoing review of the older person's and care partner's goals and care plan
- Care supported by an interprofessional team in which the older person and the caregiver are integral
- Assignment of one primary or lead point of contact on the health-care team
- Active coordination among all health-care and supportive service providers
- Continual information sharing and integrated communication
- Education and training for providers and, when appropriate, the older person and caregivers
- Performance measurement and quality improvement using feedback from the older person and caregivers

Data from American Geriatrics Society Expert Panel on Person-Centered Care: Person-Centered Care: A Definition and Essential Elements, *J Am Geriatr Soc.* 2016 Jan;64(1):15-18.

assessment should include the needs and preferences of both the person living with dementia and the caregiver. They should be multidimensional and periodically updated. They should identify both strengths and problems in the caregiving practice. And they should reflect the culturally competent practices appropriate to the caregiver–care recipient dyad. It is also important to encourage caregivers to assess themselves regularly as a basis for more effective self-management of their problems.

Informal care has been and remains the backbone of LTC (Gaugler and Kane, 2015). In many instances, the family (and often nonrelatives) is the first line of support. The ideal program would keep older people at home, relying on family care and bolstering their efforts with more formal assistance to provide professional services and occasional respite care. More than 80% of all the care given in the community comes from informal sources. Surprisingly, this figure seems to remain fairly constant even in countries with more generous provision of formal LTC. Many observers have questioned whether the informal care role, which is largely performed by women, can be sustained as more women enter the labor force and are already managing several roles. Despite dire predictions about its inevitable collapse, there is yet no evidence of serious decline in informal care. It is important to bear in mind that as the age of frailty rises, the "children" of these frail older people may themselves be in their seventh and eighth decades.

The best estimates suggest that about 15% of older adults need the help of another person to manage their daily lives. The good news is that the prevalence of disability among older persons has declined about 1% per year over the last several decades. The improvement is seen in each age group and generally in the lower levels of impairment. At the same time, the proportion of persons who need various levels of assistance increases with age (Fig. 15-4). The summative effect of the relative decline in disability and the substantial growth in the elderly population will produce major increases in the numbers of persons with disabilities (Cutler, 2001). The changes over time are pictured in Figure 15-5. Figure 15-6 shows the various payment sources for covering LTC costs. Medicaid covers about half the costs, Medicare just over a fifth, and out-of-pocket payments represent about a fifth of the costs. Family caregivers are often ill-prepared for the stresses of caregiving. They need support and assistance right from the outset. They have to make difficult decisions about what sort of care is best based on limited information and often great time pressures and anxiety. Caregiver stress can lead to burnout; it can also lead to elder abuse and neglect. Table 15-3 lists some symptoms of potential caregiver stress clinicians should look out for.

Clinicians have a responsibility to be active family advocates and to help them make the best decisions possible. While most clinicians cannot personally direct families to useful resources, they should be able to make informed referrals. They should recognize the spectrum of care options and encourage family members to consider all of them. They should encourage careful consideration of overarching care goals and recognize risk aversion when it arises.

For each person in a nursing home today, there are between one and three persons with equivalent disabilities living in the community. Thus, the first instincts are not

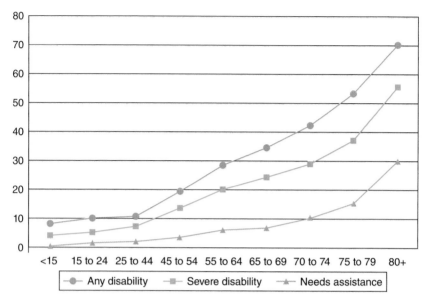

NOTE: The need for assistance with activities of daily living was not asked of children under 6 years.

FIGURE 15-4 Disability prevalence and the need for assistance by age: 2010. (*Reproduced with permission from JCHS tabulations of US Census Bureau, 2012 American Community Survey.*)

always the best. Clinicians have been conditioned to respond to dependent elderly persons by thinking of admission to a nursing home. Because clinicians have great influence, they need to be proactive advocates. Nursing home placement should be the *last* resort, not the first. Physicians should consider the importance of maximizing both quality of care and quality of life. For many frail older persons, the personal price of living in a nursing home is too high. Many would prefer to remain in the community, even if it means taking the risk of getting less care, which is not necessarily the case.

Current practice has succeeded in shifting the balance between institutional care and home- and community-based services to emphasize use of the latter (Kane and Kane, 2012). The waiver programs noted earlier are designed to do just that. Another major factor that has reduced the use of nursing homes has been assisted living. As discussed later, this concept has taken on a variety of meanings as it has been actively marketed.

Why then does our system rely so heavily on the nursing home? Several reasons can be posited. First, nursing homes are available; there are more nursing home beds than acute care hospital beds in this country. Nonetheless, there is usually a waiting list to get in, especially into a relatively good home. (That situation is beginning to change, however. With the growth in alternatives, especially assisted living, for the first time we are seeing substantial numbers of empty nursing home beds.) The

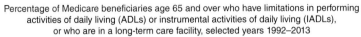

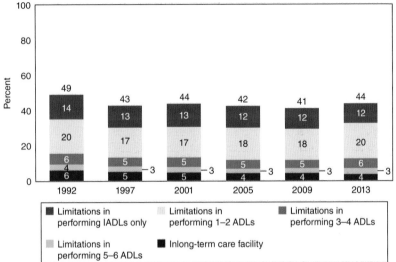

Percentage of Medicare beneficiaries age 65 and over who have limitations in performing activities of daily living (ADLs) or instrumental activities of daily living (IADLs), or who are in a long-term care facility, selected years 1992–2013

■ Limitations in performing IADLs only

▨ Limitations in performing 1–2 ADLs

■ Limitations in performing 3–4 ADLs

▨ Limitations in performing 5–6 ADLs

■ Inlong-term care facility

NOTE: A residence is considered a long-term care facility if it is certified by Medicare or Medicaid; has three or more beds, is licensed as a nursing home or other long-term care facility, and provides at least one personal care service; or provides 24-hour, 7-day-a-week supervision by a caregiver. Limitations in performing activities of daily living (ADL) refer to difficulty performing (or inability to perform for a health reason) one or more of the following tasks: bathing, dressing. eating, getting in/out of chairs, walking, or using the toilet. Limitations in performing instrumental activities of daily living (IADL) refer to difficulty performing (or inability to perform for a health reason) one or more of the following tasks: Using the telephone, light housework, heavy housework, meal preparation, shopping, or managing money. Percentages are age adjusted using the 2000 standard population. Estimates may not sum to the totals because of rounding.
Reference population: These data refer to Medicare beneficiaries.

FIGURE 15-5 Change in ADLs and IADLs from 1992 to 2013. (*Reproduced with permission from U.S. Census Bureau. Survey of Income and Program Participation, May-August 2010.*)

programs to cover LTC services have become a complex maze of eligibility and regulations, which has not encouraged anyone to develop innovative alternatives. The pressure for faster discharge from hospitals has created a new industry of postacute nursing home care. Although changes in Medicare payment have dampened some of the enthusiasm, this sector is still vital.

The emphasis on seeking community-based alternatives to nursing home care has shifted to some extent to developing other mechanisms for providing the combined housing and service functions. Among these are assisted living and adult foster care. Assisted living, in effect, renders the recipient first and foremost a tenant, who has control over her singly occupied living space (eg, a lock on the door and determination about waking and retiring times). In addition to single occupancy, the client's autonomy is reinforced by providing modest cooking and refrigeration facilities,

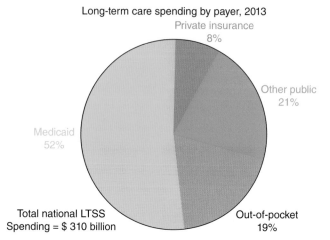

FIGURE 15-6 Long-term care spending by payer, 2013. (*Reproduced with permission from Centers for Medicare & Medicaid Services, Medicare Current Beneficiary Survey, Access to Care.*)

which allow the person to function independently without relying exclusively on the services of the institution (Kane, 2001). However, as assisted living became a more desirable product, it began to lose its identity. A variety of providers have surfaced, many of whom offer very different services under that name. The extent of personal care and nursing assistance varies widely. Some assisted living facilities discharge residents when they become too burdensome (Kane and West, 2005). Many accept only private-pay clients and discharge them when their money runs out. Today, it is hard to know just what one is getting under the rubric of assisted living.

At the same time, there is concern that a preoccupation with a search for alternatives to nursing homes may distract efforts from the sorely needed work to improve

TABLE 15-3. Potential Symptoms of Caregiver Stress

- Depression
- Withdrawal
- Anxiety
- Anger
- Loss of concentration
- Changes in eating patterns
- Insomnia
- Exhaustion
- Drinking or smoking more
- Health problem
- Exacerbations of old ones
- Increased numbers of new ones like colds and flu

the quality of nursing home care. Even in the best situation, a substantial number of older persons will continue to need such care. One scenario for the future holds that the form of nursing homes will change. Many of the residents currently cared for in nursing homes will be treated in more flexible situations, like assisted living, which emphasize living arrangements with nursing and other services brought to the residents on a more individualized basis. Those patients needing more intensive care will be treated in more medically oriented facilities. Alternatively, the playing field can be leveled by changing the current payment arrangements. If services were universally covered and room and board were paid by each recipient, the distinction between nursing homes and community care would effectively disappear.

THE NURSING HOME

Despite its frequent vilification, the nursing home is an important part of the healthcare delivery system for frail older persons. Virtually without planning, it has emerged as the touchstone of LTC. Given its origins as the stepchild of the almshouse and the hospital, it is not surprising that it has enjoyed a poor reputation. Since the passage of the Medicaid legislation in 1965, the nursing home industry has gone through growth and transformation. As a reaction to scandals during the early years, nursing homes are heavily regulated.

Chapter 16 reviews the clinical aspects of nursing home care in more detail. Today's nursing homes serve two different client groups, which complicates any attempt to describe them. Thus, many nursing homes actually provide two types of care: LTC and postacute care (PAC). A substantial portion of nursing home admissions represent short-stay residents who are admitted under Medicare for rehabilitation and recuperation. Many of these residents leave by 21 days, when Medicare imposes a copayment. Almost all are gone by 90 days. For clients admitted from hospitals for rehabilitation, nursing homes function as Medicare posthospital care providers, responsible for administering rehabilitative and restorative services to get these persons back into community living as soon as possible. This line of business is much more lucrative than traditional LTC (often supported by Medicaid), which may last a lifetime.

Persons entering nursing homes for relatively brief periods will have different goals and expectations. They are also different medically, representing a set of PAC diagnoses rather than chronic conditions like dementia. It is thus important to appreciate that descriptions of nursing home samples will differ, depending on whether one is describing an admission cohort, a discharge cohort, or a cross-section.

Many observers consider the term *nursing home* a misnomer. Although these institutions are better staffed and run than in the past, they remain generally somber places that offer their residents neither a great deal of real nursing care nor a very homelike environment.

Although single rooms are increasing, most nursing home residents are still required to share their rooms. There is little privacy and few opportunities to retain control over even small parts of one's life. Fire regulations or nursing home policies often prevent residents from bringing personal furniture into the homes. Nursing homes are smaller and less well-staffed than hospitals, but they are not miniature hospitals. Whereas a hospital has a ratio of greater than three staff for each bed, the nursing home has only about a sixth of that number, and most of those staff are aides. Nursing homes are licensed to provide care that is presumably not available in purely residential facilities that can provide little or no nursing care. But even here the boundaries are blurred. Some forms of assisted living seek to serve a population that heavily overlaps the LTC groups served by nursing homes.

Admission to a nursing home is a function of age. Figure 15-7 illustrates two separate trends in the nursing home utilization picture: (1) There is a sharp rise in the rate of nursing home use with each decade after age 65, such that only about 1% of people aged 65 to 74 are in nursing homes, but 4% of those aged 74 to 85 and 14% of those aged 85 or more are in nursing homes. (2) At the same time, the proportion of older persons who reside in nursing homes has decreased substantially from 1973 to 2004. The greatest change has been seen in the oldest group. Much of this shift can be traced to the use of alternative residential settings. Figure 15-8 contrasts the patterns of institutional care use in 1985 and 2004. Especially among those aged 85+, there was substantial use of alternative residential settings (Fig. 15-9). Figure 15-10 examines this phenomenon from a different perspective by looking at the rate of institutional use for persons at different levels of disability. There is a reduction within each disability group.

Table 15-4 shows the dynamic nature of LTC today. A cohort of persons turning 65 can expect, on an average, to require 3 years of care. Of those who actually use care, the span will be about 4.3 years. Overall, the care will be divided between community care (1.9 years) and facility-based care (1.1 years). For the actual users, the split between community and institutional care is about even, as is the split between time in assisted living and in a nursing home.

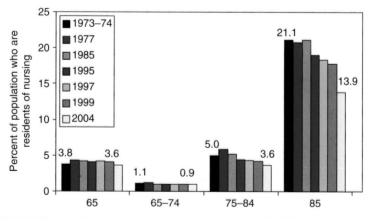

FIGURE 15-7 Change in the rate of nursing home use by age group, 1973–2004. (*Reproduced with permission from KCMU estimates based on CMS National Health Expenditure Accounts data for 2013.*)

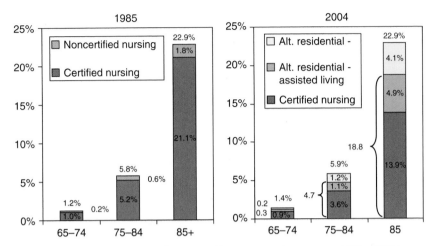

FIGURE 15-8 Use of different types of institutional long-term care by age group, 1985 and 2004. (*Reproduced with permission from 1973-1974, 1997, 1985, 1995, 1997, 1999, and 2004 National Nursing Home Survey.*)

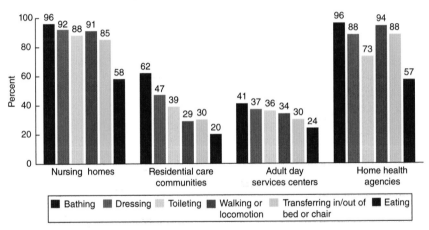

Percentage of users of long-term care services needing any assistance with activities of daily living (ADLs), by sector and activity, 2013 and 2014

NOTE: Long-term care services are provided by paid, regulated providers. They comprise both health care-related and non-health care-related services, including post-acute care and rehabilitation. People can receive more than one type of service. Users of formal long term care include persons of all ages. In nursing homes, 85% of residents were age 65 and over. In residential care communities, 93% of residents were age 65 and over. In adult day services centers, 64% of participants were age 65 and over. Among home health care patients, 83% were age 65 and over. Data were not available for hospice patients participants, patients, or residents were considered needing any assistance with a given activity if they needed help or supervision from another person or used special equipment to perform the activity. See http://www.cdc.gov/nchs/data/series/sr_03/sr03_038.pdf for definitions.
Reference population: These data refer to the resident population.

FIGURE 15-9 ADLs limitations by living situation. Estimates based on CMS National Health Expenditure Accounts data for 2013. (*Reproduced with permission from 1985 and 2004 National Nursing Home Survey and 2002 Medicare Current Beneficiary Survey.*)

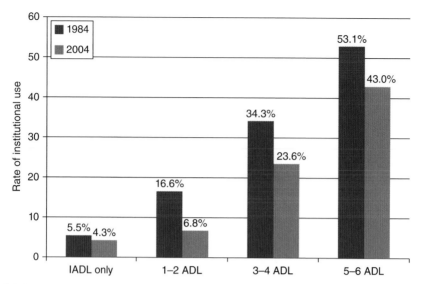

FIGURE 15-10 Institutional use by disability. (*Reproduced with permission from Centers for Disease Control and Prevention, National Center for Health Statistics, National Study of Long-Term Care Providers.*)

Forecasts of nursing home demand must consider the growing number of people who are suffering from diseases that reflect lifestyle choices.

Nursing home residents are distinguishable from older persons living in the community on several basic parameters. In addition to being older, they are more likely to be female, unmarried, and have multiple chronic problems. However, the earlier discrepancy in use by race has disappeared.

TABLE 15-4. Remaining Lifetime Use of Long-Term Supportive Services (LTSS) by People Turning 65 in 2005

Type of care	Avg years of care	% of people using care	Avg years of care among users
All LTSS need	3.0	69	4.3
At home			
Informal care only	1.4	59	2.4
Formal care	0.5	42	1.2
Any care at home	1.9	65	2.9
In facilities			
Nursing facilities	0.8	35	2.3
Assisted living	0.3	13	2.3
Any care in facilities	1.1	37	3.0

Reproduced with permission from Kemper P, Komisar HL, Alecxih L. *Long-term care over an uncertain future: what can current retirees expect? Inquiry.* 2005-2006 Winter;42(4):335-350.

Nursing home users appear to have become more disabled in the last several years. The contemporary nursing home user is older and more disabled than in the past.

Any effort to describe the nursing home resident population must recognize that the nursing home plays multiple roles. It caters to a wide variety of clientele. At least five distinct groups of residents can be identified:

1. Those actively recuperating or being rehabilitated. These are largely persons discharged from hospitals and are expected to have a short course in the nursing home before returning home. This care has been called "subacute" or "transitional." The evidence of the nursing home's capacity to provide effective care of this type is mixed (Kane et al, 1996; Kramer et al, 1997).

2. Those with substantial physical dependencies. These residents need regular and usually frequent assistance during the day. Their care could be managed in the community with sufficient formal and informal support.

3. Those with primarily severe cognitive losses. These people present special management problems because of their behavior and their propensity to wander. Some favor separate facilities for them, primarily to remove them from the environment of those who are cognitively intact. There is no evidence of improvement in the outcomes of demented residents from these "special care units" (Phillips et al, 1997).

4. Those receiving terminal care. This hospice care is directed toward making the person as comfortable as possible. Palliative care is provided, but no heroic efforts are undertaken.

5. Those in a permanent vegetative state. This group is distinguished by its inability to relate to the environment. Care is primarily directed toward avoiding complications (eg, decubitus ulcers).

For those who are sensitive to their environments and likely to be in the nursing home for some time (ie, groups 2 and 4), quality-of-life issues will be at least as salient as traditional quality-of-care issues (Kane, 2001).

Especially in the wake of changing hospital practice and the rise of "subacute care," great care must be exercised in using nursing home data because of the differences in the characteristics of those entering or leaving and those residing at any point in time. The latter are more likely to have chronic problems such as dementia, whereas the former will have problems that either benefit from rehabilitation or are fatal (eg, hip fracture and cancer). This distinction complicates discussions about nursing home patients and may explain the often contradictory findings of research on the total nursing home population.

Payment for nursing home care has been increasingly based on measures that reflect the costs of providing that care. Although this type of payment for postacute care is often called "prospective reimbursement," it is important to recognize that it is quite different from that used with hospitals. Nursing home prospective payment is calculated on a daily rate basis in contrast to the episode basis used for hospitals (and inpatient rehabilitation and home health). Hence as a person's status changes, so does the payment. Medicare payments use a daily prospective payment rate based on case mix (resource utilization groups, or RUGS), and many states are adapting a corresponding approach for Medicaid payments, although the specific systems may use fewer categories.

The most commonly used case-mix system is the resource utilization groups (RUGs). It has been revised several times and is now linked to the Minimum Data Set (MDS), which is the mandated assessment approach for nursing home care. The current RUG-IV creates 66 groups of nursing home residents, each linked to a case-mix index that presumably reflects different levels of staffing needs. This approach has been used by some Medicaid programs and is the basis for Medicare skilled nursing facility payments. Table 15-5 shows the basic components of the RUGs classification approach. A major determining factor is activity of daily living (ADL) needs, but other elements are also considered. The case-mix index generated is then weighted differently for urban and rural areas.

The physician's role in nursing home care is discussed in greater detail in Chapter 16. Suffice it to say here that the nursing home has not been an attractive place for physicians to practice. However, conditions are changing. Clinicians can play a critical role in setting the tone for the care of patients in the nursing home. Clinicians' expectations of professional performance and their advocacy of their patients' needs can be very influential in shaping staff behavior. Some physicians now find nursing home practice attractive because of the lack of office overhead, and the role of the medical director has been professionalized through a certification program of the American Medical Directors Association.

New types of personnel can be used effectively to deliver primary care to nursing home patients. Nurse practitioners and physician assistants deliver high-quality care in this setting (Kane et al, 2003). Medicare regulations covering Part B were altered to allow greater use of physician assistants and nurse practitioners. Similarly, clinical pharmacists are very helpful for simplifying drug regimens and avoiding potential drug interactions.

A Building on the prior successes of using nurse practitioners as key figures to provide primary care to nursing home residents, the Evercare program (now administered by Optum) has developed Medicare managed care risk contracts specifically for long-stay nursing home patients. Under this arrangement, Evercare is responsible for all the residents' Medicare costs (both Part A and Part B) but not their nursing home costs. The underlying concept is that by providing more aggressive primary care, they can prevent hospital admissions (Kane et al, 2003). This approach has been adopted by a variety of programs and is being implemented in settings other than nursing homes, although the savings from avoided hospitalizations are much smaller now.

The nurse practitioners provide closer follow-up and work closely with the nursing home staff to identify problems early. In some cases, Evercare will pay the nursing home extra to increase nursing attention for patients in order to treat that person in the nursing home rather than admitting the patient to a hospital. The theory is that the savings from avoided or shortened hospital stays will offset the added costs of more attentive primary care provided by the nurse practitioners. The apparent success of the Evercare model has spawned similar approaches.

A study by the Institute of Medicine pointed to the need for reforms, many of which were incorporated into the Omnibus Budget Reconciliation Act of 1987

TABLE 15-5. RUG-IV Classification System

Major RUG group	Hierarchical classification*
Rehab Plus Extensive	Ultra high intensity
	Very high intensity
	High intensity
	Medium intensity
	Low intensity
Rehabilitation	Ultra high intensity
	Very high intensity
	High intensity
	Medium intensity
	Low intensity
Extensive Services	Tracheotomy and ventilator/respirator
	Tracheotomy or ventilator/respirator
	Isolation for active infectious disease
Special Care High	Depressed
	Not depressed
Clinically Complex	Depressed
	Not depressed
Behavioral Symptoms and Cognitive Performance	Nursing rehab 2+
	Nursing rehab 0 to 1
Reduced Physical Functioning	Nursing rehab 2+
	Nursing rehab 0 to 1

RUG, resource utilization group.
*Multiple subgroups for each based on activity of daily living scores.
Data from Dey AN. Characteristics of Elderly Nursing Home Residents: Data from the 1995 National Nursing Home Survey. Advance Data from Vital and Health Statistics. Hyattsville, MD: National Center for Health Statistics; 1997.
†From US Census Bureau, 1996.

PART III

(OBRA 1987). The implementation of the OBRA 1987 regulations has produced a number of changes in the way nursing homes are operated. In addition to the standardized assessment mandated in the Minimum Data Set (MDS), the emphasis in regulation has shifted more toward addressing the outcomes of patient care, but some increases in process measures have also been introduced. For example, guidelines for the use of psychoactive drugs have been mandated. All residents admitted and already living in the nursing home must be screened to determine if they are there primarily because of chronic mental illness. If so, a specific plan of care must be developed with appropriate participation from mental health professionals. Those residents who do not require skilled care are supposed to be transferred to more appropriate care settings. More training is mandated for nurses' aides, and the staffing requirements overall have been upgraded.

The new version, MDS 3.0, incorporates more valid assessment in some areas and more focus on the voice and preferences of the residents. Although the MDS was created as an assessment tool, data elements from the MDS have been used to create a series of quality indicators, which are intended to reflect potential areas of poor care in need of further exploration by state surveyors. In a move to foster informed consumer choice, some of these quality indicators are now being posted on websites to provide consumers and their families with better information about the quality of nursing home care. While some states have their own nursing home report cards, the nationally available data set is Nursing Home Compare (www.medicare.gov/NursingHomeCompare/).

New models of nursing home care are being developed despite regulatory constraints on creativity. In some settings, large institutions are being converted into smaller living communities, where residents exert more control over their lives. The Eden Alternative has provided a model for how to humanize nursing home care. The Wellspring Movement is trying to pursue a quality improvement agenda by empowering nursing home staff to take greater responsibility for identifying ways to improve care. Although both are attractive concepts, neither has yet been shown to produce dramatic improvements in residents' quality of care or quality of life. The Green House movement has created a new model of small homelike pods of 10–12 residents, each with a private room and communal space. Universal workers help with all aspects of care, including cooking.

ASSISTED LIVING

Assisted living describes a form of care for many persons who formerly required nursing home care. It is designed to provide services to persons as they require them, in a setting that more closely resembles a person's home. In concept, service recipients need not lose their personhood and their autonomy to get care. Residents still live in institutional settings that house many people within the same facility, thus maximizing efficiency of service delivery. They use common facilities, such as a dining room, but they also retain their privacy. Basically, each resident is treated as a tenant and has control over a living unit. At a minimum, each individually occupied dwelling unit contains space for living and sleeping, a bathroom, and at least minimal cooking facilities. (The stove can be disconnected for those for whom it might pose a serious danger.) Each unit can be locked by the occupant.

Under this approach, control is ideally shifted toward empowering the recipient of care. In contrast to the situation in a nursing home, where residents are expected to conform to the norms of the institution, in an assisted living facility, individualized care is stressed. As the tenant, the resident has control over the use of her space: care providers must be invited in, and care plans must be accepted by the resident. These shifts, while subtle at one level, are fundamental at another. They imply a dramatically altered approach to care, some of which is tangible and some of which is not. The lore of nursing homes is laden with evidence of learned helplessness and enforced dependency. This approach to care is aimed at maximizing a resident's sense of self and independence as much as possible.

Unfortunately, assisted living has been implemented in so many different ways that the name has lost its meaning. Many assisted living facilities offer basic room and board with packages of services. In some instances, the individualized care promised can be obtained only by hiring a personal attendant. There is also a move to provide specialized units for dementia care, often euphemistically called *reminiscence therapy*. These are often locked units.

Especially for persons with chronic disabilities who have retained an appreciation of their environment, such a philosophy of care makes great sense. Examples of such care are becoming more prevalent. Assisted living has been able to serve individuals with extensive disabilities, although most recipients are less impaired. The majority of assisted living exists as a privately paid service. Medicaid in most states has been slow to cover this service, and where it has, it covers only the services component, leaving Social Security and welfare payments to address the room and board costs. This coverage situation can mean that older persons are admitted to assisted living until they use up their resources. Then they are discharged, most likely to a nursing home that accepts Medicaid.

The costs of assisted living are usually less than comparable nursing home care. But one has to be careful comparing costs, especially when an assisted living facility requires that the family purchase their own personal care attendant. One reason that assisted living is less expensive and more flexible is that it has thus far been spared the heavy regulatory mantle laid on nursing homes. Staffing patterns are not as intense or as professionally dictated. Staff performs multiple functions. If it is regulated in the same way, it will inevitably come to resemble nursing home care.

Once again, the form of care is determined by society's willingness to accept some risks. At a minimum, those who receive the care should have an opportunity to choose what kind of care they want to get.

At the same time, assisted living has come under criticisms reminiscent of those addressed at nursing homes in years past. The growth and diversity of models now encompassed by this name make it hard to know just what is being offered by whom. Some standardized taxonomy is needed to allow consumers to make more informed choices. Concerns about quality are frequently expressed, especially with regard to the management of the frailer and more medically complex residents.

HOME- AND COMMUNITY-BASED CARE

We tend to speak of the nursing home and alternatives to it, when we should begin with the premise that older people belong at home and want to be cared for at home. Institutional care will be needed in some cases, when the strain on caregivers is too great, but it should not be the resource of first resort. Our system has not evolved that way, and the resources available for home care are meager, but not so underdeveloped as to be ignored. Even today, most communities have at least some home care services, and more are likely to develop.

Home care involves at least two basic types of care: home health services, and homemaking and chore services. As shown in Table 15-6, different programs provide one or both types. Most older people treated at home require homemaking more than home health services.

Sometimes the differences between the two are purely arbitrary. If we consider that the homemaker replaces or supplements a family member, many of the tasks involved are extensions of home nursing (eg, supervising medication or giving baths). The definitions have emerged to fit the regulations governing a particular program. The physician will usually find that the home health agency is familiar with these regulations and how to deal with them.

Today, there is concern that the criteria for eligibility for these services severely restrict their use. To get home health services for a patient, a physician must certify that the patient is homebound and that intermittent skilled care is likely to produce

TABLE 15-6. Home Care Provided Under Various Federal Programs

	Medicare	Medicaid	Title XX
Eligibility criteria	Must be homebound; need skilled care; need and expect benefit in a reasonable period; need certification by physician	State can use homebound criterion; not limited to skilled care; need certification by physician	Vary from state to state
Payment to provider	Final costs per episode based on functional status, case needs, and diagnoses	Varies with state	Three modes of payment possible: (1) direct provision by government agency, (2) contract with private agency, (3) independent provider
Services covered	Home health services, skilled nursing, physical, or speech therapy as primary services; secondary services (social worker and home health aide) available *only* if primary service is provided; position of occupational therapy in service hierarchy ambiguous*	Limited home health care mandatory; expanded home care optional; personal care in home optional	Wide variety of home services allowed, including home health aide, homemaker, chore worker, meal services

*Occupational therapy is considered an "extended" secondary service, which may continue if needed after primary services are discontinued.

a benefit in a reasonable time. Thus, a large number of dependent older persons who need continuing home nursing but are "custodial" are ineligible unless the physician misrepresents their situation. *Skilled service* is defined as a skilled service offered by a nurse, a physical therapist, or a speech therapist. A recent court case has successfully challenged this restriction and new rules for Medicare home health are likely.

If one of these establishing services is present, the patient may also receive the skilled services of an occupational therapist or medical social worker and/or the services of a home health aide if required by the plan. Medicare has begun to allow home health agencies to continue to serve clients who need case management, thus permitting some cases to remain open longer than the "intermittent" rule might otherwise imply. All reimbursed services must be given by a certified home health agency. (To be certified, the agency needs to offer nursing plus at least one of the five other services.) The requirement for using a certified agency greatly increases the costs of the services, although the assumption is that this certification assures at least a minimal level of professional oversight. A recurring question is how much administrative overhead is affordable as the pressure on the LTC dollar grows.

Medicare-certified home health agencies are required to complete an Outcome and Assessment Information Set (OASIS) form at several stages of care to track outcomes and need for care. This recording burden has proven onerous for many agencies.

Medicaid funds can be used to provide home health care to persons eligible for nursing home care. Home health care under Medicaid must have a physician's authorization, but the patient need not be homebound, and the care need not be "skilled." All agencies delivering home health care under Medicaid must meet Medicare certification standards, but if no organized home health agencies exist in a region, a registered nurse may be reimbursed for the services. Home care is a mandated service under Medicaid, and it can also be part of a waivered service package (ie, services authorized in lieu of nursing home care). In practice, states have often modeled their Medicaid home care benefits after the medically oriented Medicare benefit and thus restricted its use. Under Medicaid, the nursing care is a required component of home health services, and the state has the option to provide physical, occupational, and speech therapy; medical social services; and personal care services. Medicaid allows homemaking assistance on a more generous basis than does Medicare. Personal care services must be prescribed by a physician and supervised by a registered nurse. These services may not be delivered by persons related to the patient. (However, under waiver programs, this restriction is softened to allow some family members to be paid.)

Legislative changes have broadened the permissible use of Medicaid moneys to support a wide variety of LTC services in an effort to reduce nursing home costs. Medicaid home care is a much less medical model that does not require nursing oversight. Much of the care is provided by personal care assistants or homemakers, helping with a variety of basic care chores. A number of states have received waivers to develop this broader package of services in lieu of nursing home care, but most of these waivered services are limited in the numbers of "slots" they are allowed. The waivers have typically require some evidence of budget neutrality, but this requirement has been eased of late. The assumption is that as more care is provided in the community, fewer people will use nursing homes.

Another development has been consumer-directed care, whereby older persons receive cash (or more typically voucher equivalents) to be spent on their care. They can hire whom they wish. The idea is to make the money go further. Consumers get less money but fewer restrictions. Some states provide administrative assistance that handles taxes and workers' compensation.

Despite the growth of home care under Medicaid and the growing number of alternative waiver programs, the bulk of Medicaid LTC funds continue to flow to nursing homes. However, the relative dominance of spending on nursing home care varies widely from state to state.

Additional homemaking services are provided under Title III and Title XX. Title XX provides at least four methods of payment: local public agencies can provide the service directly; they can contract with agency providers (perhaps using competitive bidding); they can purchase services from agencies at negotiated prices; or they can permit the recipient to enter into agreement with independent providers, who do not work for an agency. It is possible to have all these arrangements operating in the same community.

This provision for independent vendors has prompted controversy because maintaining standards is difficult in the absence of any supervisory system or institutional responsibility. Under Title XX, an employment category known as *chore worker* has emerged; although performing functions similar to the home health aide and the homemaker, chore workers do not need to be tightly supervised and cannot be reimbursed under Medicare or Medicaid.

Persons eligible for cash assistance from the state and other persons with low incomes and unmet service needs are eligible for Title XX as long as 50% of a state's annual federal allotment is expended on those receiving cash assistance. Fees are charged to those whose family income exceeds 80% of the state's median income for a family of four.

Home services are one of four priority items under Title III of the Older Americans Act. Although the dollar volume is low, this source is important because means testing (whereby eligibility is set by income) is prohibited for programs under the Older Americans Act, making it possible to target a group that cannot afford private care but is ineligible for Title XX or Medicaid. Generally speaking, the Area Agency on Aging subcontracts for home care services rather than providing them directly. Services vary from area to area but can include personal care, homemaker service, chore service, and service for heavier jobs (eg, minor home repairs or renovations, insect eradication, gardening, and painting). The provisions for assistance under the Area Agency on Aging are sharply limited by their constrained budgets and the competing demands for programs.

The extent of services under these several programs is still limited at present, although enthusiasm for in-home care is growing. Whereas younger persons with disabilities are eager to get out of the house and engage in a full round of social activity, including school and work, older people with disabilities have much lower expectations. Although younger persons with disabilities have long pressed harder for community-care benefits, the total sum of public dollars spent on home care for older clients is beginning to equal that devoted to nursing homes.

Although still a small minority of practice, the number of physicians making home visits has risen. A small industry of physician (and nurse practitioner) home care is developing. A demonstration project is under way to test whether such care is cost-effective for high-risk older persons. But such teams will never achieve the needed cost saving without operating more spartanly.

GETTING THE LTC PEOPLE REALLY WANT

Most discussions about LTC focus on its costs, but we are paying for care we do not want. The first step is to create care that responds to users' goals. The demographic forecast of a rapidly growing older population and stagnant growth of a worker generation strongly argues that we need to find new ways to deliver LTC. This challenge is an opportunity to create a care system that meets the demands of frail older people and their families. They seek a system that reflects care, competence, compassion, respect, dignity, choice, reliability, and responsiveness.

This care needs to include the three basic elements: personal care, medical care for chronic diseases, and housing (see Figure 15-11); but they can be shaped and organized in a variety of ways.

The spectrum of LTC needs is wide. Different groups may need different services. The pyramid shown in Figure 15-12A shows the different levels of personal care interventions that could be required. The higher in the triangle, the more individualized support will be needed for patient care.

Another pyramid (Figure 15-12B) captures the variation in medical care needs. In both instances, a small proportion of people uses a disproportionately large amount

PART III

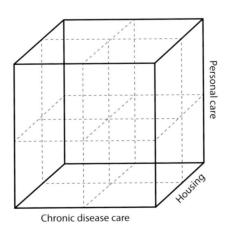

FIGURE 15-11 Core components of long-term care.

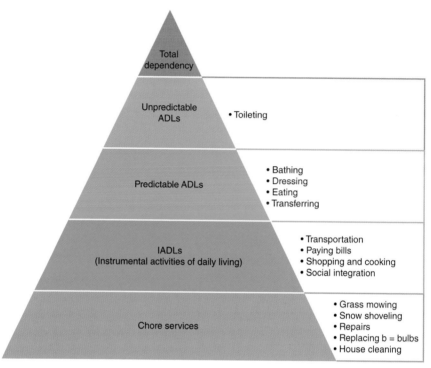

FIGURE 15-12A Personal care pyramid.

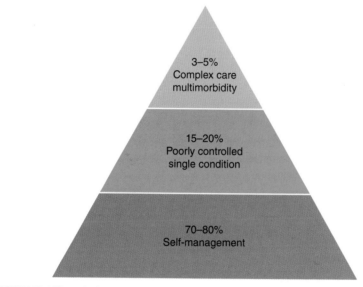

FIGURE 15-12B Medical needs pyramid.

of the care. The two are related but still separate. The spectrum of care needs to serve combinations of both.

OTHER SERVICES

A number of other modes of care can be tapped on behalf of elderly patients. Table 15-7 lists some of these services. However, despite their growing availability, they are still not widely used. The most frequently used service in that set is the senior center, a service designed for the well elderly person.

Day care can fulfill a number of needs. Most day care programs provide some combination of recreational and restorative activity. In contrast to senior centers, which are usually sponsored by recreational departments and targeted at well older adults, day care programs serve persons with limited functional ability. Some are for persons with cognitive impairments. The programs provide supervised activities, which may improve basic ADL skills and social skills. At the very least, they provide an important respite for the primary caregiver and thus may make the critical difference for allowing an older person with impairments to remain at home. To increase efficiency, most programs serve any given client fewer than 5 days a week, usually 2 or 3 days.

Other forms of day care can include a larger medical component. Some areas have developed day hospitals for older adults, where virtually all the services of the hospital are available on an ambulatory basis. Emphasis is usually placed on rehabilitation, especially occupational and physical therapy. The adult day health center is an intermediate model that combines day care with nursing, physical therapy, and perhaps social work. Such sites can also be used for periodic ambulatory care clinics.

A problem common to all day care programs is transportation. It is hard to arrange, expensive, and time-consuming. Special vans are usually needed, and to avoid excessive travel times, services are usually confined to very limited areas.

In many communities, a variety of services exist to help older adults: ombudspersons, peer counselors, mental health clinics, transportation, congregate meal sites, and meals-on-wheels—just to name a few. Availability varies greatly from place to place. Good sources of information are the social work department in a hospital and the Area Agency on Aging.

PART III

TABLE 15-7. Examples of Community Long-Term Care Programs

Home care (home nursing and homemaking)	Caregiver support
Adult day care	Congregate housing
Adult foster care	Home repairs
Assisted living	Meals (congregate and in-home)
Geriatric assessment	
Hospice/terminal care	Respite care
Telephone reassurance	Emergency alarms

The physician cannot be expected to know all the resources available for geriatric patients and will have to rely on other professionals to make appropriate arrangements to take advantage of them. But a physician should have a good sense of what can be done in general and what needs to be done for any particular patient. Often knowing what is needed but not locally available can lead to its development, particularly if responsible professionals take an active role on behalf of their patients.

There is growing interest in providing older people and their families with better information with which to make more informed decisions about LTC choices. Most states have developed some form of web-based information system that provides information about LTC options. Medicare provides online information about the quality of nursing homes (Nursing Home Compare) and home health agencies (Home Health Compare), as well as comparative reports on hospital quality indicators (Hospital Compare). The Administration on Aging and Centers for Medicare & Medicaid Services have jointly funded a network of Aging and Disability Resource Centers (ADRCs) designed to help older persons and their families locate resources and decide what types of LTC are most suitable. ADRCs are located in almost every state. Much of this information is online.

CASE MANAGEMENT

The growing interest in the plethora of community LTC services has sparked some concerns about the need to control use. A frequent answer is *case management*. This term has been widely and variably used. Some people refer to case management as "political pixie dust," because whenever the legislature finds itself proposing a LTC program that will be hard to implement, they call for case management to make it work as desired. The basic components of case management are assessment, prescription, authorization, coordination, and monitoring. Although it is an intrinsically appealing concept, the effectiveness of case management has not been well established. Much of the confusion about the effectiveness of case management can be traced to the confusion about just what is being described. Table 15-8 distinguishes five different types of case management.

Of these five types of case management, eligibility management may be the most common. It is hardly likely to affect care directly. Disease management and chronic care coordination are closely related to the activities of primary care and hence may lead to some concern about role overlap between the case manager and the primary care physician. Disease management is often conducted independently of primary care by an organization contracted by insurance companies. By contrast, chronic care coordination is the basis for proactive primary care. It is possible for physicians to serve as case managers, but most do not have the interest or the resources to perform this task. It is usually more efficient to look to other disciplines to perform this function but to recognize the important role of the physician in the overall care of the

TABLE 15-8. Variations in Case Management

Type of case management	Case manager	Components
Eligibility management	Social worker or nurse	Assessment to see if client reaches threshold for eligibility Care plan Implementations Cursory monitoring for change in status that would affect eligibility
Care coordination	Social worker or nurse	Structured assessment to identify needs Care plan addressing each need Arrange services to meet each need Follow up to ensure services are delivered Reassess periodically and adjust care plan
Utilization management	Usually a nurse	Identify high-volume/high-cost cases Work with high users to change clinical course Monitor intensively Counsel to encourage compliance Seek ways to prevent problems Flag charts to alert clinicians
Disease management	Usually a nurse, possibly an MD	Focus on a single disease Provide reminders Counseling Monitoring Usually not coordinated with primary care
Chronic care coordination	Nurse or nurse practitioner	Establish expected clinical course Monitor salient parameter for each condition followed Patients can do most of the monitoring Communicate with clinicians by phone, web Intervene when actual course differs from expected course Indication for active intervention See clients primarily when their condition changes significantly Can monitor many conditions simultaneously Can address function as well as diseases

PART III

LTC patient. Where a full range of geriatric services is available, case management is usually included.

Regardless of discipline, the case manager faces some difficult tasks. There is often a discrepancy between responsibility and authority. It is very different to prescribe, authorize, or mandate.

Case managers may or may not have the purchasing authority to pay for services they feel are necessary. Case managers may easily find themselves in the same bind as physicians. Specifically, they are expected to serve simultaneously as patient advocates and gatekeepers. The two roles are incompatible. For everyone's peace of mind, it is important to clarify at the outset who is the principal client. Because many decisions involve advocating on behalf of one group over another, this distinction is critical.

Case management has also become a mainstay of managed care. In this context, cases are usually identified based on some risk indicators—either a record of heavy use of services or the presence of risk factors that imply such a pattern in the future. While some case management within managed care is patient centered, operating on the premise that closer care can stave off costly problems, much of it revolves primarily around utilization controls.

Several states have used a program called "cash and counseling." Modeled after successful programs in California and Europe, older persons with disabilities can receive direct cash payments for care, which they can in turn use to purchase services, including from relatives. The preliminary reports have been enthusiastic. Clients have been able to purchase more care for less money with no evidence of untoward effects. In general, these clients are on the low end of the disability spectrum, but the program shows promise. It is, after all, simply creating a situation analogous to what people would do with their own funds. There is still some uneasiness about just how much discretion such programs should allow; many still require limited choices of vendors and evidence that the funds were used for the intended purposes. Nonetheless, these efforts represent a new direction of giving frail older clients more leeway in how to obtain services.

In this chapter we have attempted to summarize a complex array of health services utilized by older adults. There are several important take-home messages related to critical issues raised in the chapter:

- Caring for frail older people is complicated.
- It requires coordination of many services.
- Coordination must be based on shared goals.
- Payment is fragmented.
- Fee-for-service payment is a major barrier to chronic care.
- Long-term care needs to be rethought.

REFERENCES

Agency for Healthcare Research and Quality. 2015 national healthcare quality and disparities report and 5th anniversary update on the national quality strategy. 2015. www.ahrq.gov/research/findings/nhqrdr/nhqdr15/index.html.

American Geriatric Society Expert Panel on Person-Centered Care. *J Amer Geriatr Soc.* 2016;64.

Berwick DM. The science of improvement. *JAMA.* 2008;299(10):1182-1184.

Clough JD, McClellan M. *JAMA.* 2016;35(22):2397-2398.

Cutler DM. Declining disability among the elderly. *Health Aff.* 2001;20(6):11-27.

Gaugler JE, Kane RL, eds. *Family Caregiving in the New Normal.* London: Academic Press; 2015.

Gitlin LN, Schultz R. *Family Caregiving of Older Adults.* Baltimore, MD: Johns Hopkins University Press; 2012:181-204.

Kane RA. Long-term care and a good quality of life: bringing them closer together. *Gerontologist.* 2001;41:293-304.

Kane RL. Finding the right level of posthospital care: "we didn't realize there was any other option for him." *JAMA.* 2011;305:284-293.

Kane RL. Managed care as a vehicle for delivering more effective chronic care for older persons. *J Am Geriatr Soc.* 1998;46:1034-1039.

Kane RL. Meeting the challenge of chronic care. *Drugs of Today.* 2001;37(8):581-586.

Kane RL, Bershadsky B, Bershadsky J. Who recommends long-term care matters. *Gerontologist.* 2006;46(4);474-482.

Kane RL, Chen Q, Blewett LA, Sangl J. Do rehabilitative nursing homes improve the outcomes of care? *J Am Geriatr Soc.* 1996;44:545-554.

Kane RL, Homyak P, Bershadsky B, Flood S. Variations on a theme called PACE. *J Gerontol A Biol Sci Med Sci.* 2006;61:689-693.

Kane RL, Kane RA. HCBS: the next thirty years. *Generations.* 2012;36:131-134.

Kane RL, Keckhafer G, Flood S, Bershadsky B, Siadaty MS. The effect of Evercare on hospital use. *J Am Geriatr Soc.* 2003;51:1427-1434.

Kane RL, Ouellette J. *The Good Caregiver.* New York: Avery; 2011.

Kane RL, West JC. *It Shouldn't Be This Way: The Failure of Long-Term Care.* Nashville, TN: Vanderbilt University Press; 2005.

Kramer AM, Steiner JF, Schlenker RE, et al. Outcomes and costs after hip fracture and stroke: a comparison of rehabilitation settings. *JAMA.* 1997;277:396-404.

Phillips CD, Sloane PD, Hawes C, et al. Effects of residence in Alzheimer disease special care units on functional outcomes. *JAMA.* 1997;278:1340-1344.

Van Houtven K. Informal care and economic stressors. In: Gaugler JE, Kane RL, eds. *Family Caregiving in the New Normal.* London: Academic Press; 2015.

Wieland D. The Program of All-Inclusive Care for the Elderly [PACE]. In: Schulz R, Noelker LS, Rockwood K, Sprott R, eds. *The Encyclopedia of Aging.* 4th ed. New York: Springer Publishing; 2006:973-975.

SUGGESTED READINGS

Boult C, Boult L, Pacala JT. Systems of care for older populations of the future. *J Am Geriatr Soc.* 1998;46:499-505.

Kane RA, Kane RL, Ladd R. *The Heart of Long-Term Care.* New York: Oxford University Press; 1998.

Lachs MS, Ruchlin HS. Is managed care good or bad for geriatric medicine? *J Am Geriatr Soc.* 1997;45:1123-1127.

Morgan RO, Virnig BA, DeVito CA, et al. The Medicare–HMO revolving door—the healthy go in and the sick go out. *N Engl J Med.* 1997;337:169-175.

Sloan J. *A Bitter Pill: How the Medical System Is Failing the Elderly.* Vancouver, BC, Canada: Greystone Books; 2009.

Wunderlich GS, Kohler P, eds. *Improving the Quality of Long-Term Care. Report of the Institute of Medicine.* Washington, DC: National Academy Press; 2001.

CHAPTER 16

Nursing Home Care

The focus of this chapter is the clinical care of nursing home (NH) residents. "Nursing home" refers to facilities that are also often called "skilled nursing facilities", "nursing facilities", and "long-term care facilities". Many older people who would have otherwise been in NHs are now residing in assisted living facilities or in their own homes. Issues discussed in this chapter may also apply to these other settings of care, but the role of the physician and the availability of trained health professionals vary between these setting. Most NHs have two distinct populations. One is there for postacute care (PAC) after a hospitalization. The focus of care for these "patients" is rehabilitation and management of unstable medical conditions, generally with the goal of achieving a higher level of function and discharge back to the community, if feasible. The average length of stay for PAC patients is close to 25 days, but changes in reimbursement are driving even shorter lengths of stay. The second population are long-stayers, who have a stay over 100 days, with an average duration of between 1 and 2 years. The focus of care for these "residents" is managing chronic medical and neuropsychiatric conditions, and maintaining function and a good quality of life.

Management of older people with multiple medical problems and geriatric conditions in the NH setting is challenging for a number of reasons. Although many NHs provide excellent care, the poor quality of care provided in many other NHs has been recognized for decades. Since the Institute of Medicine issued its critical report in 1986 (Institute of Medicine, 1986), and the mandating of the Resident Assessment Instrument in 1987, the overall quality of care has improved. The Centers for Medicare & Medicaid Services (CMS) has instituted several strategies that are designed to improve the quality of NH care. These include the NH Compare website (www.medicare.gov/nhcompare/home.asp), which shows consumers (and NHs) how individual homes perform on surveys and specific quality indicators; the new federal survey process employing the Quality Indicator Survey (QIS; www.cms.gov); the Five-Star Quality Rating System (www.Medicare.gov); and the new requirement in the Affordable Care Act that all NHs must have a Quality Assurance and Performance Improvement (QAPI) program. All of these strategies have limitations, but they are intended to make improvements in care quality. Despite all of these efforts, the U.S. Office of Inspector General issued a report documenting the high frequency of adverse events among NH residents during the first 1 to 2 months of admission. The report documented that about one in three residents suffer an adverse event (including medication-related side effects; adverse events related to the quality of care such as falls, electrolyte disturbances; and infections). Thus, much remains to be done to improve NH care in the United States.

Because typical older NH residents suffer from multiple underlying diseases, good medical care is especially important. Despite the logistical and economic barriers that can foster inadequate medical care in the NH, many straightforward principles and strategies can improve the quality of medical care for NH residents. Fundamental to achieving these improvements is a clear perspective on the goals of NH care, which differ in many respects from the goals of medical care in other settings and patient populations.

Some of the basic demographic and economic aspects of NH care are discussed in Chapters 2 and 15. Ethical issues relevant to NH care and palliative care are discussed in Chapters 17 and 18, respectively.

GOALS OF NURSING HOME CARE

The modern NH serves multiple roles and strives to achieve several basic goals. Table 16-1 lists the key goals of NH care. While the prevention, identification, and treatment of chronic, subacute, and acute medical conditions are important, most of these goals focus on the functional independence, autonomy, quality of life, comfort, and dignity of the patients/residents. Physicians and other clinicians who care for NH residents must consider these goals while the more traditional goals of medical care are being addressed.

The heterogeneity of the NH population results in a diversity of goals for NH care. The population can be subgrouped into six basic types (Fig. 16-1). "Short-stayers" are generally PAC "patients" with goals of care as outlined previously, as opposed to long-stay "residents" who have different goals for their care. In this chapter, in general, "patients" is used to refer to individuals in the NH for PAC, and "residents" is used to refer to individuals who are in the NH long-term due to the differing nature of their conditions and goals for care. While it is not always possible or desirable to isolate these different types of patients and residents geographically, and there is often overlap or change between the types described, subgrouping the NH population in this manner will help the clinician and interdisciplinary team focus the care-planning process on the most critical and realistic goals for individuals.

The underlying social contract implied by NH admission is quite different for each of these groups. In some cases, access to treatment takes precedence over the living environment; in other circumstances, the environment may be the most critical

---

TABLE 16-1. Goals of Nursing Home Care

1. Provide a safe and supportive environment for people who are chronically ill and dependent.
2. Restore and maintain the highest possible level of functional independence.
3. Preserve individual autonomy.
4. Maximize quality of life, perceived well-being, and life satisfaction.
5. Provide effective rehabilitative, medical, nursing, and psychosocial care to individuals discharged from an acute hospital to facilitate their transition to their previous living environment.
6. Provide comfort and dignity for patients who are terminally ill and their loved ones.
7. Whenever possible, stabilize and delay progression of chronic medical conditions.
8. Prevent acute medical and iatrogenic illnesses, and identify and treat them rapidly when they occur.

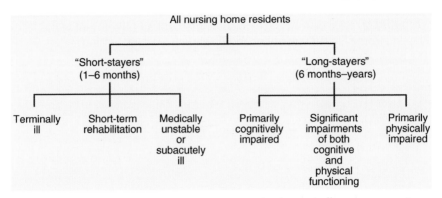

FIGURE 16-1 Categories of individuals in nursing homes. In this chapter, short-stayers are generally referred to as "patients" and long-stayers as "residents" due to the different nature of their conditions and goals for care..

element of care. Those admitted to an NH with the intent of rehabilitation and discharge may be willing to accept a living situation akin to that of a hospital in the expectation that the benefit they receive from treatment will offset any discomfort or inconvenience. For terminally ill persons under the hospice model, the living environment is made as flexible and supportive as possible. Efforts are directed toward making these patients comfortable and permitting them to enjoy, to the extent possible, their last days. For the other groups in the middle of this distribution, attention to both making their living situation comfortable and active primary care are important. Clinicians need to consider the resident's primary goals for their remaining time and avoid overmedicalization. For example, is it necessary to put an 85-year-old type 2 diabetic on an ADA diet when food may be one of her few remaining pleasures? Ideally, a NH should be able to provide what the name implies: active nursing (and medical care) and a homelike environment.

CLINICAL ASPECTS OF CARE FOR NURSING HOME RESIDENTS

In addition to the different goals for care in the NH, several factors make the assessment and treatment different from those in other settings (Table 16-2). Many of these factors relate to the process of care. A fundamental difference in NH care compared to care in other settings is that medical evaluation and treatment must be complemented by an assessment and care-planning process involving staff from multiple disciplines. The integral involvement of nurses' aides in the development and implementation of care plans is crucial to high-quality NH care. Data on medical conditions and their treatment are integrated with assessments of the functional, mental, and behavioral status of the resident in order to develop a comprehensive database and individualized plan of care that reflects the individual's goals.

Several factors complicate medical evaluation and clinical decision making in the NH. Unless the physician has cared for the individual before NH admission, it may

---

TABLE 16-2. Factors That Distinguish Assessment and Treatment in the Nursing Home From Assessment and Treatment in Other Settings

1. The goals of care are often different (see Table 16-1).
2. Specific clinical disorders are prevalent (see Table 16-3).
3. The approach to health maintenance and prevention differs (see Table 16-6).
4. Mental and functional status are just as important, if not more so, than medical diagnoses.
5. Assessment must be interdisciplinary, including:
   a. Nursing
   b. Psychosocial
   c. Rehabilitation
   d. Nutritional
   e. Other (eg, dental, pharmacy, podiatry, audiology, ophthalmology)
6. Sources of information are variable:
   a. Residents often cannot give a precise history due to cognitive impairment.
   b. Family members and nurses' aides with limited assessment skills may provide the most important information.
   c. Information is often obtained over the telephone.
7. Administrative procedures for record keeping in both nursing homes and acute care hospitals can result in inadequate and disjointed information.
8. Clinical decision making is complicated for several reasons:
   a. Many diagnostic and therapeutic procedures are expensive, unavailable, or difficult to obtain and involve higher risks of iatrogenic illness and discomfort than are warranted by the potential outcome.
   b. The potential long-term benefits of "tight" control of certain chronic illnesses (eg, diabetes mellitus, congestive heart failure, hypertension) may be outweighed by the risks of iatrogenic illness in many residents who are very old and functionally disabled.
   c. Many residents are not capable (or are questionably capable) of participating in medical decision making, and their personal preferences based on previous decisions are often unknown (see Table 16-7).
9. The appropriate site for and intensity of treatment are often difficult decisions involving medical, emotional, ethical, economic, and legal considerations that may be in conflict with each other in the nursing home setting.
10. Logistic considerations, resource constraints, and restrictive reimbursement policies may limit the ability of and incentives for physicians to carry out optimal medical care of nursing home residents.

---

be difficult to obtain a comprehensive medical database. Patients/residents may be unable to relate their medical histories accurately or to describe their symptoms, and medical records are frequently unavailable or incomplete, especially those who have been transferred between NHs and acute care hospitals. When acute changes in status occur, initial assessments are often performed by NH staff with limited skills and are transmitted to physicians by telephone or fax. Even when the diagnoses are known or strongly suspected, many diagnostic and therapeutic procedures are associated with an unacceptably high risk–benefit ratio. For example, an imaging study may require sedation with its attendant risks; nitrates and other cardiovascular drugs may precipitate syncope or disabling falls in individuals with baseline postural hypotension; and adequate control of blood sugar may be extremely difficult to achieve without a high risk for hypoglycemia among cognitively impaired diabetics with marginal or fluctuating nutritional intake, who may not recognize or complain of hypoglycemic symptoms.

Further compounding these difficulties is the inability of many individuals to participate effectively in important decisions regarding their medical care because of cognitive impairment. Their previously expressed wishes are often not known, and an appropriate or legal surrogate decision maker has often not been appointed. These issues are discussed further later in this chapter and in Chapter 17.

Table 16-3 lists the most commonly encountered clinical disorders in the NH population. They represent a broad spectrum of chronic medical illnesses; neurological, psychiatric, and behavioral disorders; and problems that are especially prevalent in frail older adults (eg, incontinence, falls, nutritional disorders, chronic pain syndromes). Although the incidence of iatrogenic illnesses has not been systematically studied in NHs, it is likely to be as high as or higher than that in acute care hospitals. The management of many of the conditions listed in Table 16-3 is discussed in some detail in other chapters of this text.

PROCESS OF CARE IN THE NURSING HOME

The process of care in NHs is strongly influenced by numerous state and federal regulations, the highly interdisciplinary nature of NH residents' problems, and the training and skills of the staff members who deliver most of the hands-on care. Federal rules and regulations contained in the Omnibus Budget Reconciliation Act of 1987 (OBRA 1987) and implemented in 1991 placed heavy emphasis on assessment and care planning as a means of achieving the highest practicable level of functioning for each resident. The Minimum Data Set (MDS), now updated to version 3.0, is the foundation of clinical assessment and care planning for individual residents. In addition to the MDS, the goal for the NH stay should be clearly articulated (ie, short-term rehabilitation of medical and nursing management with the goal of returning home; long-term care of chronic conditions; or palliative or hospice care). Detailed guidance for state and federal surveyors has been developed for several clinical care areas, such as unnecessary drugs and urinary incontinence. Failure to adhere to the clinical recommendations contained in the regulations and related surveyor guidance can result in citations and, in some instances, financial penalties for the NH. Failure to appropriately manage medical conditions in the NH puts the facility clinicians, and the medical director at risk for lawsuits.

Physician involvement in NH care and the nature of medical assessment and treatment offered to residents are often limited by logistic and economic factors.

PART III

TABLE 16-3. Common Clinical Disorders in the Nursing Home Population

Medical conditions
  Congestive heart failure
  Degenerative joint disease
  Diabetes mellitus
  Gastrointestinal disorders
    Reflux esophagitis
    Constipation
    Diarrhea
    Conjunctivitis
    Gastroenteritis
Kidney disease (chronic kidney disease, renal failure)
Lung disease (chronic obstructive, emphysema, asthma)
Malignancies
Neuropsychiatric conditions
  Dementia
  Behavioral disorders associated with dementia
    Wandering
    Agitation
    Aggression
    Depression
Neurological disorders other than dementia
  Stroke
  Parkinsonism
  Multiple sclerosis
  Brain or spinal cord injury
Pain: musculoskeletal conditions, neuropathies, malignancy
Geriatric conditions and syndromes
  Delirium
  Incontinence
  Gait disturbances, instability, falls
  Malnutrition, feeding difficulties, dehydration
  Pressure sores
  Insomnia
Functional disabilities necessitating rehabilitation
  Stroke
  Hip fracture
  Joint replacement
  Amputation
Iatrogenic disorders
  Adverse drug reactions
  Falls
  Nosocomial infections
  Induced disabilities
  Restraints and immobility, catheters, unnecessary help with basic activities
    of daily living
Palliative care and end-of-life care

Many physicians who do visit NHs care for relatively small numbers of patients or residents, often in several different facilities. Many NHs, therefore, have numerous physicians who make rounds once or twice per month and focus on visits required by regulations; but they are not generally present to evaluate acute changes in status, and may attempt to assess these changes over the telephone. Increasingly, practice patterns are shifting to a model of physician–nurse practitioner practice teams caring for large numbers of residents in several NHs. Such physician–nurse practitioner teams have been shown to improve care and reduce hospitalization rates (Bakerjian, 2008; Kane et al, 2003; Konetzka et al, 2008; Reuben et al, 1999). Many NHs, especially in rural areas, do not have ready availability of laboratory, radiological, and pharmacy services with the capability of rapid response, further compounding the logistics of evaluating and treating acute changes in medical status. Thus, patients and residents are often sent to hospital emergency rooms, where they are evaluated by personnel who are generally not familiar with their baseline status and who frequently lack training and interest in the care of frail and dependent elderly patients.

Medicare and Medicaid reimbursement policies also dictate certain patterns of NH care. While physicians are required to visit NH residents only every 30 to 60 days, many residents require more frequent evaluation and monitoring of treatment—especially with the shorter acute care hospital stays brought about by the prospective payment system. Many of these visits can be made by a nurse practitioner or physician assistant. While Medicare reimbursement for physician visits in NHs has improved, reimbursement for a routine visit is sometimes inadequate for the time that is required to provide good medical care in the NH, including travel to and from the facility; assessment and treatment planning for residents with multiple problems; communication with members of the interdisciplinary team and the resident's family; and proper documentation in the medical record. Activities often essential to good care in the NH—such as attending interdisciplinary conferences, family meetings, complex assessments of decision-making capacity, and counseling residents and surrogate decision makers on treatment plans in the event of terminal illness—are generally not reimbursable at all in the NH setting. Medicare intermediaries and managed care plans may restrict reimbursement for rehabilitative services for residents not covered under Part A skilled care, thus limiting the treatment options for many residents. Although Medicaid programs vary considerably, many provide minimal coverage for ancillary services that are critical for optimum care. Amid these logistic and economic constraints, expectations for the care of NH residents are high. Table 16-4 outlines the various types of assessment generally recommended for the optimal care of NH residents. Physicians are responsible for completing an initial assessment within 72 hours of admission and for monthly visits thereafter for the next 90 days. Nurse practitioners or physician assistants can perform every other required visit (every 30–60 days) after the first 90 days. More frequent visits are generally necessary for residents admitted on a Medicare Part A skilled nursing benefit. Registered nurses assess new residents as soon as they are admitted and on a daily basis, and they generally summarize the status of each resident weekly. The nationally mandated MDS must be completed within 14 days of admission and updated

TABLE 16-4. Important Aspects of Various Types of Assessment in the Nursing Home

Type of assessment	Timing	Major objectives	Important aspects
Medical initial	Within 72 h after admission	Verify medical diagnoses Medication reconciliation Document baseline physical findings, mental and functional status, vital signs, and skin condition Attempt to identify potentially remediable, previously unrecognized medical conditions Get to know the resident and family (if this is a new resident) Establish goals for the admission and a medical treatment plan	A thorough review of medical records and physical examinations is necessary. Relevant medical diagnoses and baseline findings should be clearly and concisely documented in the patient's record. Medication lists should be carefully reviewed and only essential medications continued. Request for specific types of assessment and input from other disciplines should be made. A database should be established (see example in Fig. 16-2).
Periodic	Monthly or every other month	Monitor progress of active medical conditions Update medical orders Communicate with patient and nursing home staff	Progress notes should include clinical data relevant to active medical conditions and focus on changes in status. Unnecessary medications, orders for care, and laboratory tests should be discontinued. Mental, functional, and psychosocial status should be reviewed with nursing home staff and changes from baseline noted. The medical problem list should be updated.

As needed	When acute changes in status occur	Identify and treat causes of acute changes	Onsite clinical assessment by the physician (or nurse practitioner or physician assistant), as opposed to telephonic consultations, will result in more accurate diagnoses, more appropriate treatment, and fewer unnecessary emergency room visits and hospitalization. Vital signs, food and fluid intake, and mental status often provide essential information. Infection, dehydration, and adverse drug effects should be at the top of the differential diagnosis for acute changes in status.
Major reassessment	Annual	Identify and document any significant changes in status and new potentially remediable conditions	Targeted physical examination and assessment of mental, functional, and psychosocial status and selected laboratory tests should be done (see Table 16-6).
Nursing	On admission, and then routinely with monitoring of daily and weekly progress Complete Minimum Data Set (MDS) within 14 days, update when major change in status occurs and annually; update selected sections quarterly	Identify biopsychosocial and functional status, strengths and weaknesses Develop an individualized care plan Document baseline data for ongoing assessments	Particular attention should be given to emotional state, personal preferences, and sensory function. Careful observation during the first few days of admission is important to detect effects of relocation. Potential problems related to other disciplines should be recorded and communicated to appropriate members of the interdisciplinary care team.

(continued)

PART III

TABLE 16-4. Important Aspects of Various Types of Assessment in the Nursing Home (*continued*)

Type of assessment	Timing	Major objectives	Important aspects
Psychosocial	Within 1–2 weeks of admission and as needed thereafter	Identify any potentially serious psychosocial signs and symptoms and refer to mental health professional if appropriate Determine past social history, family relationships, and social resources Become familiar with personal preferences regarding living arrangements	Getting to know the family and their preferences and concerns is critical to good nursing home care. Relevant psychosocial data should be communicated to the interdisciplinary team. Discharge potential should be assessed.
Rehabilitation (physical and occupational therapy)	Within days of admission and daily or weekly thereafter (depending on the rehabilitation program)	Determine functional status as it relates to basic activities of daily living Identify specific goals and time frame for improving specific areas of function Monitor progress toward goals Assess progress in relation to potential discharge	Small gains in functional status can improve chances for discharge as well as quality of life. Not all residents have areas in which they can reasonably be expected to improve; strategies to maintain function should be developed for these residents. Assessment of and recommendation for modifying the environment can be critically important for improving function and discharge planning.
Nutritional	Within days of admission and then periodically thereafter	Determine nutritional status and needs Identify dietary preferences Plan an appropriate diet	Restrictive diets may not be medically necessary and can be unappetizing. Weight loss should be identified and reported to nursing and medical staff.

Interdisciplinary care plan	Within 1–2 weeks of admission and every 3 months thereafter	Identify interdisciplinary problems Establish goals and treatment plans Determine when maximum progress toward goals has been reached	Each discipline should prepare specific plans for communication to other team members based on their own assessment.
Capacity for medical decision making*	Within days of admission and then whenever changes in status occur	Determine which types of medical decisions the individual is capable of participating in A resident who is still capable of making decisions independently should be encouraged to identify a surrogate decision maker in the event the resident later loses this decision-making capacity If the resident lacks capacity for many or all decisions, appropriate surrogate decision makers should be identified (if not already done)	Residents with varying degrees of dementia may still be capable of participating in many decisions regarding their medical care. Attention should be given to potentially reversible factors that can interfere with decision-making capacity (eg, depression, fear, delirium, metabolic and drug effects). Concerns of the family and health professional should be considered, but the resident's desires should be paramount. The resident's capacity may fluctuate over time because of physical and emotional conditions.
Preferences regarding treatment intensity* and nursing home routines	Within days of admission and periodically thereafter	Determine individuals' wishes as to the intensity of treatment he or she would want in the event of acute or chronic progressive illness	Attempt to identify specific procedures the resident would or would not want. This assessment is often made by ascertaining the resident's prior expressed wishes (if known), or through surrogate decision makers (legal guardian, durable power of attorney for health care, family).

*See Table 16-7 and Chapter 17.

PART III

when a major change in status occurs; several sections must be routinely updated on a quarterly basis. The MDS is intended to assist NH staff in identifying important clinical problems that need further evaluation, management, and monitoring. It is also used as the basis for calculating daily reimbursement rates for residents receiving active rehabilitation under the Medicare Part A skilled benefit by generating a resource utilization group (RUG) that reflects case mix and needed staffing levels (a number of states also use a version of the RUGS for Medicaid payments) and as the basis for calculating various quality measures, including those on the Nursing Home Compare website and those used for the Five-Star Quality Rating System.

The extent of involvement of other disciplines in the assessment and care-planning process varies depending on patients' and residents' problems, the availability of various professionals, and state regulations. Representatives from nursing, social services, dietary, activities, and rehabilitation therapy (physical and/or occupational) participate in an interdisciplinary care-planning meeting. Family members are generally invited, and discussed at this meeting within 2 weeks of admission and quarterly thereafter. The product of these meetings is an interdisciplinary care plan that separately lists interdisciplinary problems (eg, restricted mobility, incontinence, wandering, diminished food intake, poor social interaction), goals for the resident related to the problem, approaches to achieving these goals, target dates for achieving the goals, and assignment of responsibilities for working toward the goals among the various disciplines. These care plans are an important force in driving nursing staff behavior and expectations and should be reviewed by the primary physician.

Staffing limitations in relation to the amount of time and effort required makes intensive interdisciplinary care planning and teamwork challenging in many NHs. Although physicians are too infrequently directly involved in the care-planning meetings in most facilities, they should review the care plan, and may find the team's perspective valuable in setting meaningful and appropriate goals, and planning subsequent medical care.

The general pressure for better documentation of care and assessments should improve the quality of care in NHs, but only if this information is actually used. Federal and state regulations, as well as evolving guidance to surveyors, will inevitably mean that physicians will be asked to make more detailed clinical notes, especially with respect to indicating the underlying reasons for their actions. Electronic health records specific for NHs (typically closely linked to the MDS assessments) are now widely available, and some contain thorough documentation templates that both provide decision support and efficiently improve the clarity and detail of documentation.

STRATEGIES TO IMPROVE MEDICAL CARE IN NURSING HOMES

Better medical care in the NH should lead to fewer serious problems and hence to lower use of emergency rooms and hospitals (Ouslander and Berenson, 2011). Several strategies might improve the process of medical care delivered. Four strategies are briefly described: (1) the use of improved documentation practices; (2) a systematic approach to screening, health maintenance, and preventive practices for the frail, dependent NH population; (3) the use of nurse practitioners or physician assistants; and (4) the use of practice guidelines and related quality improvement activities.

In addition to these strategies, strong leadership of a medical director who is appropriately trained and dedicated to improving the facility's quality of medical care is essential to develop, implement, and monitor policies and procedures for medical services. Certification through the American Medical Directors Association should be encouraged (www.amda.com). The medical director should set standards for medical care and serve as an example to the medical staff by caring for some of the residents in the facility. He or she should also be involved in various committees (eg, quality, infection control) and should try to involve interested medical staff in these committees, as well as in educational efforts through formal in-service presentations, teaching rounds, and appropriate documentation procedures.

Quality indicators, developed through literature review and expert consensus, can be used to track improvements in medical and overall care in the NH setting (Saliba and Schnelle, 2002; Saliba et al, 2004; Saliba et al, 2005). Medical directors should use these indicators and other approaches (eg, Kane, 1998; Mor, 2006) in their quality improvement programs. Publicly reported, MDS-derived quality indicators are available at the CMS Nursing Home Compare website (www.medicare .gov/nursinghomecompare/). Many of these MDS-derived quality indicators are used to calculate the NH Five-Star ratings (www.cms.gov/medicare/provider-enrollment-and-certification/certificationandcomplianc/fsqrs.html). Quality efforts are shifting from external enforcement to greater institutional proactive involvement in quality improvement. CMS now requires all NHs to have a Quality Assurance and Performance Improvement program (QAPI) and provides guidance and tools for these programs on its website (www.cms.gov/Medicare/Provider-Enrollment-and-Certification/QAPI/nhqapi.html).

DOCUMENTATION PRACTICES

As mentioned earlier, electronic health records specific for NHs are now widely available, and when used properly, they can greatly improve clinical documentation. However, many of these records do not have a physician documentation component, and if they do it may be used by only a small proportion of physicians who provide care in the facility. Critical aspects of the medical database should be recorded on a "medical face sheet" in the medical record.

Figure 16-2 shows an example of a format for a medical face sheet. Additional standardized documentation should contain social information, such as individuals to contact at critical times and information about the resident's treatment status in the event of acute illness. These data are essential and should be readily available in one place in the record, so that when emergencies arise, when specialists are involved, or when members of the interdisciplinary team need an overall perspective, they are easy to locate. The face sheet should be copied and sent to the hospital or other

PART III

MEDICAL FACE SHEET

ACTIVE MEDICAL PROBLEMS

1. _____
2. _____
3. _____
4. _____
5. _____
6. _____
7. _____
8. _____

PAST HISTORY

A. Acute hospitalizations since admission to JHA

Diagnoses	Month/Year
1. _____	___/___
2. _____	___/___
3. _____	___/___
4. _____	___/___

NEUROPSYCHIATRIC STATUS

A. Dementia ____ Absent ____ Present
   If present:
   ____ Alzheimer   ____ Mixed
   ____ Multi-infarct ____ Uncertain/Other

B. Psychiatric/behavioral disorders
   1. _____
   2. _____

C. Usual mental status
   ____ Alert, oriented, follows simple instructions
   ____ Alert, *disoriented*, but *can* follow simple directions
   ____ Alert, *disoriented*, *cannot* follow simple directions
   ____ Not alert (lethargic, comatose)

D. Most recent Mini Mental State Score
   ____/30 (Date ____/____/____)

A

FIGURE 16-2 Example of a face sheet for a nursing home record.

FUNCTIONAL STATUS

B. Major surgical procedures *before* admission to JHA

Procedure   Year

1. _____   _____

2. _____   _____

3. _____   _____

4. _____   _____

A. Ambulation
  __ Unassisted
  __ With cane
  __ With walker
  __ Unable
       Transfer: ___ Ind ___ Dep

B. Continence
                        Cont   Inc
  Urine   __   __
  Stool   __   __

C. Basic ADL
                  Ind   Dep
  Bathing   __   __
  Dressing   __   __
  Grooming   __   __
  Feeding   __   __

D. Vision
  __ Adequate for regular print
  __ Impaired—can see large print
  __ Highly impaired—but can get around
  __ Severely impaired—has difficulty getting around

E. Hearing
  __ Adequate
  __ Minimal difficulty
  __ Hears only w/amplifier
  __ Highly impaired—no useful hearing

C. Allergies

1. _____

2. _____

TREATMENT STATUS   (See treatment Status Sheet Note Date ___/___/___)

__ Full code   __ DNR   __ DNR, do no hospitalize   __ No tube feeding

This form completed by _____   Date ___/___/___

B

FIGURE 16-2 (*Continued*)

PART III

health-care facilities when transfers occur. Time and effort are required to keep the face sheet updated. Electronic health records can facilitate incorporating the face sheet into a database and periodic updating.

Medical documentation in progress notes for routine visits and assessments of acute changes is frequently scanty, uninformative, and/or illegible. Statements such as "stable" or "no change" are too frequently the only documentation for routine visits. While time constraints may preclude extensive notes, certain standard information should be documented. The SOAP (*s*ubjective, *o*bjective, *a*ssessment, *p*lan) format for charting routine notes is especially appropriate for NH residents (Table 16-5). Simple forms, flow sheets, or databases with word-processing capabilities can be used to enable physicians to efficiently produce legible, concise, yet comprehensive progress notes. Another tool for documenting change in residents over time is the glidepath approach using flow sheets (see Chapter 4).

Another area where medical documentation is often inadequate relates to decision-making capacity, treatment preferences, and preferences in everyday care for such things as times of meals and bathing. These issues are discussed briefly at the end of this chapter as well as in Chapter 17. In addition to placing critical information in a standardized format in readily accessible locations, it is essential that clinicians

TABLE 16-5. SOAP Format for Medical Progress Notes on Nursing Home Residents

Subjective	New complaints
	Symptoms related to active medical conditions
Objective	General appearance and mood
	Weight
	Vital signs
	Physical findings relevant to new complaints and active medical conditions
	Laboratory data
	Reports from nursing staff
	Progress in rehabilitative therapy (if applicable)
	Reports of other interdisciplinary team members
	Consultant reports
Assessment	Presumptive diagnosis(es) for new complaints or changes in status
	Stability of active medical conditions
	Responses to psychotropic medications (if applicable)
Plans	Changes in medications or diet
	Nursing interventions (eg, monitoring of vital signs, skin care)
	Assessments by other disciplines
	Consultants
	Laboratory studies
	Discharge planning (if relevant)

thoroughly and legibly document all discussions they have had with the patient or resident, family, or legal guardians; they must also document any durable power of attorney for health care about these issues. Failure to do so may result not only in poor communication and inappropriate treatment, but also in substantial legal liability. Notes about these issues should not be removed from the medical record and are probably best kept on a separate page behind the face sheet.

All of these recommendations can and should be incorporated into electronic medical records as NHs increasingly begin to use health information technology.

SCREENING, HEALTH MAINTENANCE, AND PREVENTIVE PRACTICES

A second approach to improving medical care in NHs is developing and implementing selected screening, health maintenance, and preventive practices. Table 16-6 lists examples of such practices. With few exceptions, the efficacy of these practices has not been well studied in the NH setting. In addition, not all the practices listed in this table are relevant for every resident. For example, some of the annual screening examinations are inappropriate for short-term patients or for many long-term residents with end-stage dementia (see Fig. 16-1). Thus, the practices outlined in Table 16-6 must be tailored to the specific NH population, as well as for the individual resident, and must be creatively incorporated into routine care procedures as much as possible to be time-efficient, cost-effective, and reimbursable by Medicare.

NURSE PRACTITIONERS AND PHYSICIAN ASSISTANTS

A third strategy that may help improve medical care in NHs is making greater use of nurse practitioners and physician assistants. This approach appears to be cost-effective in both managed care and fee-for-service settings (Bakerjian, 2008; Kane et al, 2003; Konetzka et al, 2008; Reuben et al, 1999). These health professionals may be especially helpful in carrying out specific functions in the NH setting. Physician assistants and nurse practitioners can bill for services under fee-for-service Medicare; moreover, several states will reimburse their services, and individual facilities and/or physician groups can hire them on a salaried basis. Nurse practitioners may have an especially helpful perspective in interacting with nursing staff about the nonmedical aspects of care. They frequently spend more time with staff educating and explaining aspects of care. They are likely to emphasize function and physical activity, and pay attention to important issues like constipation. Nurse practitioners and physician assistants can be very helpful in implementing some of the screening, monitoring, and preventive practices outlined in Table 16-6 and in communicating with interdisciplinary staff, families, and patients and residents at times when the physician is not in the facility. One of the most appropriate roles for nurse practitioners and physician assistants is in the initial assessment of acute or subacute changes in status. They can perform a focused history and physical examination and can order appropriate diagnostic studies. Several care paths have been developed for this purpose, one of which is shown in Figure 16-3. The use of a similar algorithm for

PART III

TABLE 16-6. Screening, Health Maintenance, and Preventive Practices in the Nursing Home

Practice	Recommended frequency*	Comment
Screening		
History and physical examination	Yearly	Focused examination including rectal, breast, and, in some women, pelvic examination
Weight	Monthly	Generally required
		Persistent weight loss should prompt a search for treatable medical, psychiatric, and functional conditions
Functional status assessment, including gait and mental status testing and screening for depression†	Yearly	Functional status assessed periodically by nursing staff using the Minimum Data Set (MDS)
		Systematic global functional assessment done at least yearly using MDS to detect potentially treatable conditions (or prevent complications) such as early dementia, depression, gait disturbances, urinary incontinence
Visual screening	Yearly	Assess acuity, intraocular pressure, identify correctable problems
Auditory	Yearly	Identify correctable problems
Dental	Yearly	Assess status of any remaining teeth, fit of dentures, and identify any pathology
Podiatry	Yearly	More frequently in diabetics and residents with peripheral vascular disease
		Identify correctable problems and ensure appropriateness of shoes

(continued)

Tuberculosis	On admission and yearly (may vary by state)	All residents and staff should be tested Booster testing recommended for nursing home residents
Laboratory tests Stool for occult blood Complete blood count Fasting glucose Electrolytes Renal function tests Albumin, calcium, phosphorus Thyroid function tests (including thyroid-stimulating hormone level)	Yearly	These tests have reasonable yield in the nursing home population, but the evidence base for their use is limited and testing should be individualized based on how the results will affect the residents function and quality of life, their prognosis, and their preferences

Monitoring in selected residents

All residents Vital signs, including weight	Monthly	More often if unstable or subacutely ill
Diabetes Fasting and postprandial glucose, glycosylated hemoglobin A1c (HbA1c)	Every 1–2 months when stable (fasting) Every 4–6 months (HbA1c)	Fingerstick tests may be useful in initial care after hospitalization, but should not be used for stable residents
Residents on diuretics or with renal insufficiency (creatinine >2 or blood urea nitrogen [BUN] >35): electrolytes, BUN, creatinine	Every 2–3 months	Nursing home residents are more prone to dehydration, azotemia, hyponatremia, and hypokalemia

PART III

TABLE 16-6. Screening, Health Maintenance, and Preventive Practices in the Nursing Home (*continued*)

Practice	Recommended frequency*	Comment
Anemic residents who are on iron replacement or who have hemoglobin <10: hemoglobin/ hematocrit	Monthly until stable, then every 2–3 months	Iron replacement and/or erythropoietin should be discontinued once hemoglobin value stabilizes
Blood level of drug for residents on specific drugs, for example: Anticonvulsants Digoxin Lithium	Every 3–6 months	More frequently if drug treatment has just been initiated
Prevention		
Influenza vaccine	Yearly	All residents and staff with close resident contact should be vaccinated
Oseltamivir, zanamivir	Within 24–48 hours of outbreak of suspected influenza	Residents and staff should be treated throughout outbreak
Zoster vaccination	Once	Selected residents
Pneumococcal/pneumonia bacteremia	Once	
Pneumococcal vaccine		
Tetanus booster	Every 10 years, or every 5 years with tetanus-prone wounds	Many older people have not received primary vaccinations; they require tetanus toxoid, 250–500 units of tetanus immune globulin, and completion of the immunization series with toxoid injection 4–6 weeks later and then 6–12 months after the second injection

Tuberculosis Isoniazid 300 mg/day for 9–12 months	Skin-test conversion in selected residents	Residents with abnormal chest film (more than granuloma), diabetes, end-stage renal disease, hematological malignancies, steroid or immunosuppressive therapy, or malnutrition should be treated
Antimicrobial prophylaxis for residents at risk	Generally recommended for dental procedures, genitourinary procedures, and most operative procedures	Chronically catheterized residents should not be treated with continuous prophylaxis
Body positioning and range of motion for immobile residents	Ongoing	Frequent turning of very immobile residents is necessary to prevent pressure sores Semi-upright position is necessary for residents with swallowing disorders or enteral feeding to help prevent aspiration Range of motion to immobile limbs and joints is necessary to prevent contractures
Infection-control procedures and surveillance	Ongoing	Policies and protocols should be in effect in all nursing homes Surveillance of all infections should be continuous to identify outbreaks and resistance patterns
Environmental safety	Ongoing	Appropriate lighting, colors, and the removal of hazards for falling are essential in order to prevent accidents Routine monitoring of potential safety hazards and accidents may lead to alterations that may prevent further accidents

*Most of the recommendations in this table are relevant to long-stay residents. Frequency may vary depending on resident's condition. Not all recommendations are relevant to every resident.

†The MDS can be supplemented by various standardized tools (see Chapter 3).

PART III

CARE PATH *Symptoms of*
Lower Respiratory Infection

INTERACT
Version 4.0 Tool

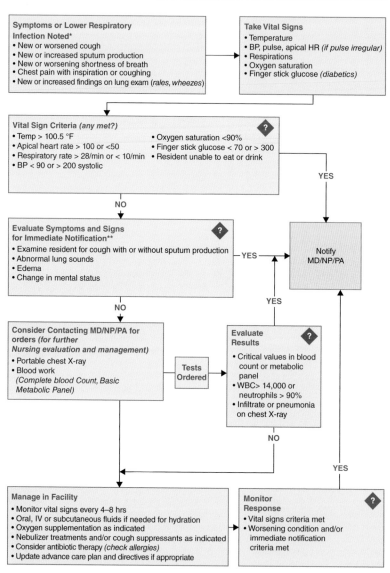

* Refer also to the INTERACT Shortness of Breath Care Path
** Refer also to other INTERACT Care Paths as indicated by symptoms and signs

FIGURE 16-3 Example of an INTERACT VERSION 4.0 care path for managing acute change in condition in a nursing home. (*ADL, activity of daily living; BP, blood pressure; C&S, culture and sensitivity; HR, heart rate; IV, intravenous; NP, nurse practitioner; PA, physician assistant; WBC, white blood cell. ©2011 Florida Atlantic University, all rights reserved. This document is available for clinical use, but may not be resold or incorporated in software without permission of Florida Atlantic University.*)

pneumonia resulted in reduced hospitalizations and related costs in 22 Canadian NHs (Loeb et al, 2006). This strategy enables the onsite assessment of acute change, the detection and treatment of new problems early in their course, more appropriate utilization of acute care hospital emergency rooms, and the rapid identification of residents who need to be hospitalized.

CLINICAL PRACTICE GUIDELINES AND QUALITY IMPROVEMENT ACTIVITIES

Several clinical practice guidelines relevant to NH care have been developed by the American Medical Directors Association (www.amda.com). In addition, quality indicators for a number of conditions have been developed (Saliba et al, 2004). While these guidelines and quality indicators are largely based on expert opinion rather than on controlled clinical trials, they are helpful as a basis for standards of practice that will improve care. Implementation and maintenance of practice guidelines can be difficult in NHs, as it is in other practice settings (Saliba et al, 2005; Schnelle et al, 1997).

Clinical practice guidelines can be useful tools in an overall quality improvement program. NHs are required to have an ongoing quality assurance committee, and as mentioned earlier, a QAPI program is also required. Administrators, directors of nursing, and medical directors must create an environment that provides incentives for ongoing QI activities to maintain these programs over time. This includes active involvement of residents and staff in identifying problems. The Medicare Quality Improvement Organization and Quality Innovation Network programs (www .cms.gov/Medicare/Quality-Initiatives-Patient-Assessment-Instruments/Quality ImprovementOrgs/index.html?redirect=/qualityimprovementorgs/) and the American Medical Directors Association and its journal (*Journal of the American Medical Directors Association*) have substantial resources for assisting NH providers with quality improvement initiatives. In addition, CMS will provide educational resources and tools for NHs to help them meet the QAPI requirement.

POSTACUTE CARE AND THE NURSING HOME—ACUTE CARE HOSPITAL INTERFACE

The increasing acuity and multimorbidity in the NH population, a high incidence of acute conditions, and the need for high levels of skilled postacute care will continue to place increased demands on NHs. Although Medicare fee-for-service rules require that patients admitted to NHs under Part A have a prior 3-day hospital stay (observation stays do not count here), managed care programs (Medicare Advantage) can admit patients with acute but relatively stable conditions (eg, deep vein thrombosis, cellulitis) directly to NHs without a 3-day acute hospital stay. As a result, NHs are providing more and more high-level skilled care. The term *postacute care* has many connotations; for the purposes of this chapter, it refers to skilled care reimbursed by Medicare Part A fee-for-service (or by a capitated or bundled payment system) in a freestanding NH. Caring for patients in a freestanding NH who are recovering from an acute illness and hospitalization intensifies many of the challenges already alluded to in this chapter (see Table 16-2). This level of care requires greater involvement of physicians, nurse practitioners, and physician assistants; nursing staff trained for more acute patients; ready availability of ancillary services such as laboratory, X-ray, and physical and respiratory therapy; and more intensive discharge planning. More-over, Medicare reimbursement for Part A services is paid on the basis of a fixed daily amount based on a RUG category, which covers services ordered by medical staff, including drugs, laboratory tests, X-rays, and therapies. This reimbursement struc-ture requires close cooperation between physicians and NH administrators to make this form of post-acute care economically viable.

As a result of the increasing acuity and frailty of the NH population, transfer back and forth between the NH and acute care hospitals is common. About one in five individuals admitted to a NH from a hospital are readmitted to the hospital within 30 days (Mor et al, 2010). Major reasons for transfer include infection and the need for parenteral antimicrobials and hydration, as well as acute exacerbations of cardio-vascular and pulmonary conditions. Other conditions, such as falls, altered mental status, and behavioral changes that are difficult to manage in the NH are also com-mon. Transfer to an acute care hospital is often a disruptive process for a chronically or subacutely ill individuals and is especially hazardous among those with dementia (Gozalo et al, 2011). In addition to the effects of the acute illness, NH residents are subject to acute mental status changes and a myriad of potential iatrogenic problems. The most prevalent of these iatrogenic problems are related to immobility, includ-ing deconditioning, difficulty regaining ambulation and/or transfer capabilities, hospital-acquired infections, incontinence and catheter use, polypharmacy, delirium, and the development of pressure sores.

NH readmission to a hospital has become a major quality issue with penalties levied against hospitals whose patients have high rates of readmissions. Hospitals are thus increasingly conscious of NH performance in this sphere. Multiple health-care reform initiatives are under way in the United States to reduce unnecessary transfers of NH residents to hospitals, with a particular focus on potentially preventable hos-pital readmissions (Ouslander and Berenson, 2011). Changes in Medicare payment, such as bundled payments and the development of accountable care organizations that include postacute care, will provide potent financial incentives for better coordi-nated care at the NH–hospital interface. Savings from such programs can be shared with providers to make further improvements in care. Expansion of the Programs of All-Inclusive Care for the Elderly (PACE) or statewide programs for dually eligible Medicare and Medicaid beneficiaries will also incentivize better transitional care and will address the problematic cost-shifting that currently occurs between the Medicare and Medicaid programs.

Because of the risks of acute care hospitalization, the decision to transfer a patient or resident to the emergency room or hospitalize a resident must carefully balance a number of factors. A variety of medical, administrative, logistic, economic, and ethi-cal issues can influence decisions to hospitalize NH residents. Decisions regarding hospitalization often boil down to the capabilities of the physician and the NH staff to provide services in the NH, the preferences of the patient or resident and the family, and the logistic and administrative arrangements for acute hospital care. Financial incentives and liability concerns also play an important role. If, for example, the NH staff has been trained and has the personnel to institute intravenous therapy without detracting from the care of the other patients and residents, or if it has arranged for an outside agency to oversee intravenous therapy and there is a nurse practitioner or physician assistant to perform follow-up assessments, individuals with an acute infection who is otherwise medically stable may best be managed in the NH. Hypodermoclysis may be helpful in preventing some acute care transfers (Remington and Hultman, 2007). Better advance care planning and advance directive use can also help avoid unnecessary hospitalization of NH residents with severe impairments (Molloy et al, 2000).

The American Medical Directors Association has developed a clinical practice guideline and related tools on care transitions (www.amda.com/tools/clinical/TOCCPG/index.html), and a quality improvement program (Interventions to Reduce Acute Care Transfers [INTERACT]) with related educational resources and tools has been developed and shown promise in reducing unnecessary hospital transfers (http://interact.fau.edu) (Ouslander et al, 2011). The INTERACT program uses three basic strategies to improve the management of acute changes in condition and prevent unnecessary hospital transfers: (1) proactive identification of conditions before they become severe enough to require hospital care (eg, dehydration, delirium); (2) management of some conditions (eg, pneumonia, congestive heart failure) without transfer when safe and feasible; and (3) improving advance care planning to consider palliative or comfort care as an alternative when the risks of hospitalization may outweigh the benefits.

ETHICAL ISSUES IN NURSING HOME CARE

Ethical issues arise as much or more in the day-to-day care of NH residents as in the care of patients in any other setting. These issues are discussed in Chapter 17. Table 16-7 outlines several common ethical dilemmas that occur in the NH. Although most attention has been directed toward those marginally able to express their preferences, important daily ethical dilemmas also face those who are capable of decision making. These subtler problems are easily overlooked. Physicians, nurse practitioners, and physician assistants providing primary care must serve as strong advocates for the autonomy and quality of life of NH residents.

NHs care for a high concentration of individuals who are unable or questionably capable of participating in decisions concerning their current and future health care. Among these individuals, severe functional disabilities and terminal illnesses are prevalent. Thus, questions regarding individual autonomy, decision-making capacity, surrogate decision makers, and the intensity of treatment that should be given at the end of life arise on a daily basis. These questions are both troublesome and complex, but they must be dealt with in a straightforward and systematic manner to provide optimal medical care in the NH within the context of ethical principles and state

PART III

TABLE 16-7. Common Ethical Issues in the Nursing Home*

Ethical issue	Examples
Preservation of autonomy	Choices in many areas are limited in most nursing homes (eg, mealtimes, sleeping hours).
	Families, physicians, and nursing home staff tend to be paternalistic.
Decision-making capacity	Many nursing home patients and residents are incapable or questionably capable of participating in decisions about their care because of cognitive impairment.
	There are no standard methods of assessing decision-making capacity in this population.
Surrogate decision making	Many nursing home patients and residents have not clearly stated their preferences or appointed a surrogate before becoming unable to decide for themselves.
	Family members may be in conflict, have hidden agendas, or be incapable of or unwilling to make decisions.
Quality of life	This concept is often entered into decision making, but it is difficult to measure, especially among those with dementia.
	Ageist biases can influence perceptions of nursing home residents' quality of life.
Intensity of treatment	A range of options must be considered, including cardiopulmonary resuscitation and mechanical ventilation, hospitalization, treatment of specific conditions (eg, infection) in the nursing home without hospitalization, enteral feeding, comfort, or supportive care only.

*See also Chapters 17 and 18.

and federal laws. NHs should be encouraged to develop their own ethics committees or to participate in a local existing committee in another facility. Ethics committees can be helpful in educating staff; developing, implementing, and monitoring policies and procedures; and providing consultation in difficult cases. Some practical methods of approaching ethical issues are discussed in Chapter 17, and palliative care is discussed in Chapter 18.

REFERENCES

Bakerjian D. Care of nursing home residents by advance practice nurses: a review of the literature. *Res Gerontol Nurs.* 2008;1:177-185.

Gozalo P, Teno JM, Mitchell SM, et al. End-of-life transitions among nursing-home residents with cognitive issues. *N Engl J Med.* 2011;365:1212-1221.

Institute of Medicine. *Improving the Quality of Care in Nursing Homes.* Washington, DC: National Academy Press; 1986.

Kane RL. Assuring quality in nursing home care. *J Am Geriatr Soc.* 1998;46:232-237.

Kane RL, Keckhafer G, Flood S, et al. The effect of Evercare on hospital use. *J Am Geriatr Soc.* 2003;51:1427-1434.

Konetzka RT, Spector W, Limcangco RM. Reducing hospitalizations from long-term care settings. *Med Care Res Rev.* 2008;65:40-66.

Loeb M, Carusone SC, Goeree R, et al. Effect of a clinical pathway to reduce hospitalizations in nursing home residents with pneumonia: a randomized controlled trial. *JAMA.* 2006;295:2503-2510.

Molloy DW, Guyatt GH, Russo R, et al. Systematic implementation of an advance directive program in nursing homes: a randomized controlled trial. *JAMA.* 2000;283:1437-1444.

Mor V. Defining and measuring quality outcomes in long-term care. *J Am Med Dir Assoc.* 2006;7:532-540.

Mor V, Intrator I, Feng V, et al. The revolving door of hospitalization from skilled nursing facilities. *Health Aff.* 2010;29:57-64.

Ouslander JG, Berenson RA. Reducing unnecessary hospitalizations of nursing home residents. *N Engl J Med.* 2011;365:1165-1167.

Ouslander JG, Lamb G, Tappen R, et al. Interventions to reduce hospitalizations from nursing homes: evaluation of the INTERACT II Collaborative Quality Improvement Project. *J Am Geriatr Soc.* 2011;59:745-753.

Remington R, Hultman T. Hypodermoclysis to treat dehydration: a review of the evidence. *J Am Geriatr Soc.* 2007;55:2051-2055.

Reuben D, Buchanan J, Farley D, et al. Primary care of long-stay nursing home residents: a comparison of 3 HMO programs with fee-for-service care. *J Am Geriatr Soc.* 1999;47:131-138.

Saliba D, Schnelle JF. Indicators of the quality of nursing home residential care. *J Am Geriatr Soc.* 2002;50:1421-1430.

Saliba D, Solomon D, Rubenstein L, et al. Feasibility of quality indicators for the management of geriatric syndromes in nursing home residents. *J Am Med Dir Assoc.* 2005;6:S50-S59.

Saliba D, Solomon D, Rubenstein L, et al. Quality indicators for the management of medical conditions in nursing home residents. *J Am Med Dir Assoc.* 2004;5:297-309.

SUGGESTED READINGS

American Medical Directors Association. *Health Maintenance in the Long Term Care Setting Clinical Practice Guideline.* Columbia, MD: American Medical Directors Association; 2012.

Kane RL, West JC. *It Shouldn't Be This Way: The Failure of Long-Term Care.* Nashville, TN: Vanderbilt University Press; 2005.

Morley J, Tolson D, Ouslander J, Vellas B. *Nursing Home Care: A Core Curriculum for the International Association for Gerontology and Geriatrics.* New York, NY: McGraw-Hill; 2013.

Osterweil D, ed. Medical directors role in nursing home quality improvement: an educational symposium of the New York Medical Directors Association. *J Am Med Dir Assoc.* 2007;3(suppl):1-41.

SELECTED WEBSITES (ACCESSED 2017)

American Health Care Association, www.ahcancal.org

American Medical Directors Association (The Society for Post-Acute and Long-Term Care Medicine), www.amda.com

Interventions to Reduce Acute Care Transfers (INTERACT), http://interact.fau.edu

LeadingAge, www.leadingage.org

LTCFocus.org (long-term care), http://ltcfocus.org

National Association of Directors of Nursing Administration in Long-Term Care, www.nadona.org

Nursing Home Regulations Plus, www.hpm.umn.edu/nhregsplus

CHAPTER 17

Ethical Issues in the Care of Older Persons

Ethics is a fundamental part of geriatrics. Ethics, or the provision of ethical care, refers to a framework or guideline for determining what is morally good (ie, right) or bad (ie, wrong). Ethical problems arise when there is conflict about what is the "right" thing to do. This dilemma generally occurs when decisions need to be made whether or not a medical intervention should be implemented and whether or not the intervention is futile. The answers to ethical questions are not straightforward; they involve a complex integration of thoughts, feelings, beliefs, and evidence-based data. Ageism can play a strong role in these decisions. Acknowledging and acting on the wishes of the older individual are a critical component of ethical care.

While ethical dilemmas are central to the practice of medicine itself, the dependent nature of the older adult and the imminence of death raise special concerns. Discussions of ethics and aging seem to focus on the roles of autonomy and cost containment, since a significant portion of the cost of delivering health care is incurred at the end of life.

MAJOR ETHICAL PRINCIPLES

Table 17-1 provides a description of major ethical principles. The ethics of medicine is based on four principles: autonomy, beneficence, nonmaleficence, and justice, which are geared toward maximizing benefits over harm and doing the greatest good for the greatest number. *Autonomy* refers to one's right to control one's destiny, that is, to exert one's will. Obviously, there are limits to how freely such control can be expressed, but for geriatric purposes the principal issue revolves around whether the patient is able to assess the situation and make a rational decision independently. This raises the second concept, *beneficence*, which refers to the duty to do good for others, to help them directly, and to avoid harm. *Nonmaleficence* involves doing no harm and avoiding negligence that leads to harm. Last, *justice* focuses on fairness in the treatment of others.

The principles of autonomy and beneficence can conflict when the patient's wishes and goals are different than that of his or her clinician or other member of the healthcare team. Clinicians can sometimes become paternalistic and undermine the personal autonomy of the individual. For example, an older adult with some cognitive impairment living in a nursing home setting may express the desire to stay in his or her room alone during the day. During this time period, however, he or she makes bad choices (eg, tries to walk independently and falls frequently due to impaired balance). This results in nursing resources being used to evaluate and reevaluate this individual postfalls and thus limiting the amount of time the nurses might spend caring for others. In this situation overriding autonomy might be appropriate as

TABLE 17-1. Major Ethical Principles*

Autonomy
Refers to one's right to control one's destiny, that is, to exert one's will. The principal issue revolves around whether the older adult is able to assess the situation and make a rational decision independently.

Beneficence
Refers to the duty to do good for others, and specifically to avoid harm in the process.

Nonmaleficence
Involves doing no harm and avoiding negligence that leads to harm. Last, justice focuses on fairness in the treatment of others.

Justice
Justice focuses on nondiscrimination and the duty to treat individuals fairly; not to discriminate on the basis of irrelevant characteristics. This involves a duty to distribute resources fairly, nonarbitrarily, and noncapriciously.

*Goal of ethical care: Voiding or minimizing harms and maximizing benefits. The concern and focus should be on preserving and respecting personhood. This is done through recognition of wants, collaboration, play, validating, facilitation, and giving. At the same time, ethics must recognize and deal with competition between organizational/community interests vs individual interests.

acting in the older individual's "best interests" is inconsistent with the greater good of the community.

The ethical decisions and challenges come down to several fundamental issues:

1. Is the patient capable of understanding the dilemma?
2. Is the patient able to express a preference?
3. Are there clear options? Have they been made clear to the patient/family?
4. Has the patient/family received accurate information about the benefits and risks of the options?
5. Are the patient's expectations realistic with regard to treatment decisions?
6. What happens when the patient's preferences are contrary to the preferences of the family or the physician?

COMPETENCE AND INFORMED CONSENT

In the case of older adults, much of the concern is directed toward the issue of whether or not the individual can understand, and remember, the information being provided and whether or not he or she can express an opinion. Individuals who are comatose or who have expressive or receptive aphasia or moderate to severe dementia may not be able to communicate effectively. It is important to preserve autonomy and assess these individuals carefully for what they can understand and communicate.

There is an important difference between the concepts of competence and decision-making capability. A clinician may evaluate a patient's capacity to make decisions, but *competence* is a legal term that implies that the individual has been deemed competent or incompetent by a court of law. Competence refers to a person's ability to act reasonably after understanding the nature of the situation being faced. Someone not competent to act on his or her own behalf requires an agent to act *for* him or her.

In the case of dementia, a person may or may not be capable of understanding and interpreting complex situations and making rational decisions. Intellectual deficits are spotty. A person may get lost easily or forget things but still be able to make decisions with appropriate prompting. The presence of a formal diagnosis of dementia, even by type, may not be a sufficient indicator of the individual's ability to comprehend and express a meaningful preference. Just as it is wrong to infantilize such patients by directing questions to others who are quicker to respond, so, too, might it be inappropriate to prejudge their ability to participate in decisions about their own care.

Determining cognitive ability and decision-making capacity is not easy. One must distinguish memory from understanding. Decisional capacity is predicated on four elements: (1) understanding, or the ability to comprehend the disclosed information about the nature of the situation/medical problem, the procedures involved in testing for example, and the risks and benefits of undergoing or not undergoing testing or treatment; (2) appreciation of the significance of the disclosed information and the potential risks and benefits for one's own situation and condition; (3) reasoning, which involves the ability to engage in a reasoning process about the risks and benefits of a procedure or treatment; and (4) choice, or being able to choose whether or not to undergo further testing or treatment.

There are no cognitive screening tests that are 100% accurate in terms of determining the older adult's decision-making capacity. Screening tools that focus on executive function such as the Clock Drawing Test or the Executive Interview are more likely to be associated with decisional capacity than other measures such as the Mini-Mental State Examination (see Chapter 3). Specific tests have been developed to determine decisional capacity, but these are generally difficult for older adults to complete because they require consideration of hypothetical situations and complex abstract thinking.

One useful and practical criterion for decision making, often used when completing an informed consent process with a resident, is to explain a test or treatment intervention and recheck with the patient after a period of time to be certain that he or she understands the situation and consistently states preferences related to the specific care option. Depending on the setting of care, this may or may not be practical. Ideally, the decision-making process should be structured to allow the individual (and perhaps the family) to review all possible options, understand the risks and benefits associated with each, and identify which outcomes (from a large menu) they would like to achieve. In geriatrics, however, evidence-based information is limited making it difficult to fully and accurately inform older individuals. For example, the impact of a chemotherapeutic agent in a 50-year-old patient in terms of efficacy, side effect profile, and risk will not be the same as it is in a 90-year-old patient. Treatment options for older adults are often not clear-cut in terms of cost–benefit for the older individual, and clinicians may make decisions about which studies or findings to report to the individual in any given situation.

PART III

Although different in nature from treatment-related decisions (eg, surgery), decisions about transitions to alternative levels of care require the same level of serious attention accorded to those about treatments. Other members of the health-care team, such as social workers or nurse case managers, may be the best at delineating the choices and implications of such moves, and older individuals should be referred to these individuals as appropriate. Specific information that needs to be presented includes cost and cost-based alternatives, privacy issues, safety, social issues, and access to appropriate health care.

ADVANCE CARE PLANNING

Advance care planning involves helping patients begin to think about their priorities, beliefs, and values and how they want to be cared for in the face of persistent chronic illnesses and at the end of life. Patients should be encouraged to identify a health-care power of attorney (or health-care proxy or medical power of attorney). The health-care power of attorney is the individual the patient selects to be his or her authorized "agent." The patient can give this agent as much or as little authority as he or she wishes to make independent health-care decisions for the patient. These decisions are not limited to end-of-life decisions. Topics to address include such things as whether to receive cardiopulmonary resuscitation, whether to be put on a respirator, and whether to receive intravenous hydration or artificial nutrition, blood transfusions, organ or tissue donation, or medical devices. Other topics to include might be whether to get transferred to an acute care setting for aggressive interventions, whether to have antibiotics, what type of funeral or memorial service to have, and whether to be buried or cremated. Additional information is also provided in Chapter 18.

ADVANCE DIRECTIVES

The goal of advanced care planning is to develop advance directives (ADs), which are written instructions that are intended to reflect a patient's wishes for health care to guide medical decision making in the event that a patient is unable to speak for herself or himself. ADs vary based on state regulations, and the required forms for formal ADs vary from state to state.

An AD is a legal document that allows patients to convey their decisions about what type of care they want to receive in the event that they are unable to express their wishes. It is important for ADs to be completed as part of a routine care interaction so that these discussions are not occurring during a crisis situation. ADs are helpful ways for patients to give direction to their children, spouse, friend, or identified proxy and simplify the decision-making process for those individuals. ADs can help an adult child feel confident, regardless of the child's own beliefs and desires, that he or she has done what the parent wanted at the end of the parent's life. In a same-sex relationship in which the couple is not legally married, an AD may be the only way in which a couple may be able to ensure who is the decision maker because the other may not have the rights of a spouse.

In contrast to ADs, a living will is simply a written instruction spelling out the treatments you want or don't want if you are unable to speak for yourself and terminally ill or permanently unconscious. The living will is limited because it generally addresses specific clinical situations (vegetative states or terminal illness) and a few treatment options such as cardiopulmonary resuscitation, intubation, implementation of artificial food and hydration, dialysis, or intravenous use. Living wills provide a means to indicate that the patient prefers that heroic measures not be initiated.

The AD is much more inclusive and allows an identified health-care agent or proxy to make medical decisions on the patient's behalf when he or she is not able to do so. A proxy designation can be done by using a durable power of attorney, previously used to transfer control of property. States must specifically extend their durable power of attorney statutes to cover medical decisions. Under this approach, one can specify both the person one wishes to act as agent and the conditions under which such a proxy should be exercised. In geriatrics it is helpful to carefully consider the many decisions that go into and are centered around care in end-of-life situations. Deciding, for example, whether to give an antibiotic treatment or whether to transfer an older individual to the acute care setting for an acute medical event are examples of some of the difficult decisions that must be made at end of life. Guidance from the older individual via ADs indicating his or her preferences is extremely helpful. Table 17-2 shows the components of a durable power of attorney for health care. When the proxy is not certain exactly how the patient might respond in a given situation, the principle of beneficence can be used to guide decisions. The proxy can make medical decisions by weighing the benefits for the patient versus the burdens/risks that might be imposed on him or her to do nothing or to initiate, for example, a specific treatment (eg, excision of a lesion).

The establishment of ADs has been viewed as an effective way in which to spare older adults from unnecessary suffering and is believed to improve the quality of end-of-life care. However, making end-of-life judgments at a time of relatively good health may be challenging because it is hard to conceptualize how one will feel in an acute situation. There is a tendency to believe that older adults, particularly those in their 90s and 100s, have lived a good long life and are ready to die. This should not be assumed. Many of these "old-old" are not necessarily ready to die; they want to receive careful evaluations of their medical problems and discuss treatment options. Thus ongoing discussions between patients and clinicians should be encouraged throughout the aging process. What a patient wants for end-of-life care at 85 years of age may be different at 97 years of age.

Federal law requires that all persons entering a hospital or a nursing home be offered the opportunity to indicate ADs. However, this is not the ideal time to expect the individual to make clear, thoughtful decisions. Too often, this exercise involves asking older persons about possible procedures they would want to have if the occasion arose. Done poorly, the experience can provoke unnecessary anxiety and lead to poor decisions that may be regretted later. Ideally, the health-care provider has discussed establishing an AD with the patient and/or proxy, and all have given time

---

TABLE 17-2. Components of a Durable Power of Attorney for Health Care[*]

Creation of durable power of attorney for health care
　Statement that gives intention and refers to statute(s) authorizing such

Designation of health-care agent
　Statement naming and facilitating access to (address, telephone number) agent; state laws will vary as to who may serve as agent—some states preclude providers of health care or employees of institutions where care is given; person designated as agent should have agreed to assume this role

General statement of authority granted
　Statement about circumstances under which the agent is granted power and indications of the power the agent will have in that event (usually a general statement about right to consent or refuse or withdraw consent for care, treatment, service or procedure, or release of information subject to any specific provisions and limitations indicated)

Statement of desires, special provisions, and limitations
　Opportunity to indicate general preferences (eg, wish not to have life prolonged if burdens outweigh benefits; wish for life-sustaining treatment unless in coma that physicians believe to be irreversible, then no such efforts; wish for all possible efforts regardless of prognosis); opportunity for specific types of things wanted to be done or not done and indications for such actions

Signatures
　Individual dated signature
　Witnesses (better notarized): witnesses cannot be those named as agents, providers of health care, or employees of facilities giving such care

Conditions
　Form should have place where person signing indicates awareness of rights, including the right to revoke the document and the conditions under which the document comes into force; some states require a mandatory maximum period where such a document can be valid without renewal

---

[*]Many state medical associations can provide a copy of a basic form of a durable power of attorney for health care.

and thought to the development of appropriate documents. The acute event requires only that these previously stated decisions be revisited to make sure the choices are consistent with the individual's current philosophy. The advantage of asking new residents in long-term care settings or newly admitted hospitalized patients about their AD is that it prompts the health-care provider to obtain this information and the older individual and/or family to make sure the appropriate forms have been completed. If it is more appropriate to postpone the discussion until the individual has adjusted to the new environment, systems should be in place to be sure the information is obtained at a later date.

Most states have established a process for developing ADs, and standard forms are available on the web for patients and/or families to download and complete (www.everplans.com/articles/state-by-state-advance-directive-forms). Individuals who spend part of the year in one state and part in another should be aware that state laws may vary in terms of criteria around when a living will becomes effective.

With both the living will and the durable power of attorney, there is some potential for misuse. Decisions once made can be difficult to revoke. In addition, it can be difficult to determine when an individual no longer has decisional capacity and the ability to state his or her own health-care preferences. By the same token, physicians need to educate patients and proxies that a course of treatment, once started, need not always be continued. Sometimes a trial of a particular treatment may be attempted and later removed. There is currently no test of mental competence that allows one to change one's mind about a decision to not use life-support systems.

In the absence of any specification of actions or agents, someone must be identified to act for a person who is unable to act on his or her own behalf. There are legal procedures to accomplish this, which vary from state to state. In general, the two major classes of legally empowered agents are conservators and guardians. The latter usually have greater powers. A formal legal decision is needed to establish such a condition.

A critical question is: Who is best qualified to assume that responsibility? Common wisdom suggests that it is the next of kin, but some argue that it should be the person most familiar with the patient's preferences, the person who can most closely estimate what the patient would have wanted. A rarely seen relative might know much less about the patient's wishes or lifestyle than a close friend, clergy, or even the individual's clinician. The choice for who should be the proxy should rest on the level of knowledge possessed. Where there are multiple contenders for the role, the courts may have to decide who is best positioned to know the patient's preferences. This can become contentious. In cases where there is no one appropriate, the court may appoint a public guardian.

Agents, whether designated by durable power of attorney or chosen as the best available person, are vulnerable to pursuing their own interests rather than the patient's. At best, they must make inferences about the patient's wishes from their knowledge of the patient or the choice indicated in the durable power document. Surrogates' decisions may not be congruent with the wishes of the individuals they represent. They can be sincerely torn between acting in what they perceive to be the individual's wishes versus what may actually be their best interests in the given situation. The law typically imposes a standard of conduct on proxies appointed under ADs, proxies qualifying under applicable law, and guardians appointed by a court.

A number of obstacles influence the development of ADs for older adults. These include difficulty older individuals (and/or the proxies) may have in understanding the complexity of the situations that can arise; difficulty in understanding research findings that support medical practice; difficulty for patients, clinicians, and families to discuss death and make end-of-life decisions; and/or difficulty in conceptualizing future treatment preferences. Health-care clinicians, therefore, play a vital role in helping older adults engage in developing ADs and in evaluating geriatric patients' current capacity to give direction about care. Specifically, such direction includes withholding or withdrawing life-sustaining procedures and establishing willingness to receive pain medications, antibiotics, intravenous infusions, and other therapies. A key step in starting the discussion about ADs includes specifically eliciting the older individuals' preferences for medical treatments under a variety of conditions, and encouraging older individuals to specify a proxy and discuss their end-of-life care preferences.

POLST/MOLST

To further facilitate the process of ensuring that patients explicitly express their end-of-life care preferences, State Departments of Health in 38 states have approved the implementation of a clinician order form referred to as Physician Orders for Life-Sustaining Treatment (POLST) or Medical Orders for Life-Sustaining Treatment (MOLST). These forms are easily accessible at www.polst.org/programs-in-your-state/. The forms vary state to state but conceptually are the same. POLST forms can be completed only by physicians, but MOLST forms can be completed by nurse practitioners as well as physicians, allowing for increased access and opportunity to facilitate the completion process. The POLST or MOLST complements the individual's AD and is intended to facilitate end-of-life medical decision making and assure patients' wishes are carried out. It provides standing orders for end-of-life actions based on a person's AD. The order can be used statewide by health-care practitioners and facilities. POLST or MOLST is particularly critical for patients with serious health conditions who (1) want to avoid receiving any or all life-sustaining treatment, (2) reside in a long-term care facility or require long-term care services, and/or (3) might die within the next year. The MOLST or POLST form thus provides guidance to emergency medical personnel during transfers.

Completing the POLST or MOLST begins with a conversation or a series of conversations between the patient, the patient's health-care agent or surrogate, and his or her primary care clinician or specialist with whom he or she has had interactions. The clinician should help delineate the patient's goals for care, review possible treatment options, and facilitate informed medical decision making. There are state-by-state guidelines for how the form is to be completed and what steps to take when changes are made and a new form is completed.

ETHICAL ISSUES TO CONSIDER

Life-and-death decisions attract the greatest attention and have a major impact on cost of care. These decisions include whether to initiate or withdraw treatment or whether to start dialysis, insert an intravenous line for hydration, or insert a feeding tube for artificial nutrition. Certainly, these are important questions posed in the context of real-world situations. Surprisingly, however, they arise much less often than do the less heralded ethical dilemmas that confront clinicians and older patients each day as they decide about discharge from hospitals; make decisions about appropriate levels of care such as nursing home or assisted living; make decisions about screening for diseases such as breast, prostate, or bowel cancer; or recommend therapies. Consideration of the ethics of geriatric care must address the full spectrum of these issues.

Some key points are worthy of special consideration:

- Ethics and law are separate, but overlapping. Ethical guidance may come from a variety of sources, such as national and state professional societies, local and national standards of practice, and other sources. However, health-care professional licensing boards commonly include among licensing standards and grounds for disciplinary action references to "unethical" conduct. Sometimes these are based on external standards that are incorporated into local law, or there may be a specific code of ethics incorporated into the licensing regulations. Health-care clinicians are advised to consider this in the states in which they practice.

- In the area of end-of-life care, state law typically governs. A health-care decisions act or similar law may set out the obligations of health-care clinicians, health-care facilities, patients, and persons who may be authorized to act as proxies for an incapacitated individual. Those statutes and the regulations or interpretations of agencies and attorneys general can affect the expectations imposed on health-care clinicians. Case law may reflect "common law" principles that guide expectations and conduct of health-care clinicians. Any general reading, including a chapter such as this, should be measured against applicable state law.

- Many health-care facilities have "ethics committees," which are interdisciplinary committees empowered to bring together involved staff, independent advisers from various disciplines, and involved family members to provide ethical guidance. Generally the focus of these committees is in three areas: education, consultation, and policy development. Depending on state law, there may be legal protection for health-care clinicians following the recommendations of such committees.

- Informed consent is a routine and fundamental part of provider–patient interactions. A patient who makes an informed decision about health care makes a decision and gives direction that has a continuing effect. Patients have a right to change their minds. For example, a competent individual who refuses otherwise-needed dialysis despite knowing the consequences does not surrender his or her right to reconsider that decision.

- Patients can express their wishes about future health care in several ways. For example, geriatric patients not presently faced with a decision about artificial feeding via a tube may give direction about their future wishes, should that need arise. This may be done in a written form. In some states, state law permits an AD to be made verbally and may subsequently require such directives to be documented in a particular way. For example, these documents may require one or more physician determinations of a particular kind. Specifically, it may be necessary to include a determination of whether the patient was competent at the time an AD was signed, whether the patient is presently competent at the time someone wishes to invoke the document because the patient is incapacitated, and whether the patient is in a particular condition, such as terminal illness, a vegetative state, or some other condition the effect of which is to permit, or not permit, health care to be given, withheld, or withdrawn, even when it is life sustaining.

- State law may set out a process by which, in the absence of an AD from the patient, an individual may act as a surrogate, proxy, or similar title, making health-care decisions for others. This may require a physician determination of competency and evidence that the patient is in a particular clinical condition (eg, terminal).
- State guardianship laws authorize a court to appoint someone as guardian of the person. This is typically based on physician certification of incapacity.
- State law may recognize that health-care clinicians are not only ethically obligated to furnish care, but also empowered to refuse to furnish care that is medically futile and therefore not provided for ethical reasons. Futile care is defined as care that serves no useful purpose. This type of care will not help the patient achieve his or her goals, will not address symptoms, and will not prolong or improve life. Determining when care is futile is often challenging and some have put forward compelling arguments made against the use of the futility principle (Johnston, 2014). The four bioethical principles described in Table 17-1 are generally used to guide the analysis of futile care: respect for autonomy, beneficence, nonmaleficence, and justice. With regard to futile care, it is the principle of justice that is often the most relevant given the limited resources available for health-care services and the role of clinicians in monitoring appropriate use. In the United States, there is not currently a consensus in medicine about the use of unilateral physician decision making concerning medical futility. Alternatively, some clinicians recommend obtaining "informed assent" from a patient or family. In these situations, the patient/family is explicitly offered the choice to defer to clinicians' judgment about withholding or withdrawing life-sustaining therapy. This is particularly useful and helpful to families who do not want to carry the burden of stopping a treatment or dealing with feelings of withholding care from a loved one. In these situations clinicians need to be careful not to make quality-of-life decisions about others.
- There are certain ethical issues that have to be dealt with in health care on a daily basis. These may include (1) prioritizing activities in order of importance, which includes giving preference to one patient over another depending on individual need; (2) maintaining a clear distinction between what is right and wrong; (3) supporting, or not supporting, a patient's decision and choice (even if not in the patient's best interests); (4) not making patients' decisions, or guiding their decisions, on the basis of race, gender, or class; and (5) maintaining the privacy of the patient—but disclosing information where necessary (in case of a crime, for instance, or safety of the patient or community).

END-OF-LIFE CARE

End-of-life care decisions differ from ADs in that the latter address hypothetical situations, whereas the patient is experiencing the implications of end-of-life care when such decisions are made. Completion of the MOLST or POLST may provide some additional and specific guidance to a proxy about specific decisions (eg, the use of antibiotics). Whether being made by the patient or the proxy, the many end-of-life decisions that need to be made are extremely difficult. In the United States, patients/proxies have the right to refuse the initiation (withholding treatment) and the continuation of treatments (withdrawing treatment). These decisions are often based on decisions around comfort and quality of life, and the patient/proxy may decide to transition from aggressive treatment options to symptom management or what is referred to as palliative care. Palliative care (see Chapter 18) is interdisciplinary care that focuses on symptom management to eliminate discomfort and improve quality of life. In palliative care, the treatments provided are not intended to cure the underlying condition and generally focus on management of such things as pain, constipation, nausea, anxiety, and cough.

Substantial controversy surrounds end-of-life care with concerns around cost of care and cost versus benefit for the patient and society as a whole, particularly when the treatment being implemented is futile. As noted earlier, while care is never futile, medical interventions can be futile. In some situations, however, proxies may opt to engage in futile and expensive care.

It is helpful to take a step approach when discussing end-of-life issues with patients and families (deMaine and Dennett, 2014). The steps are provided in Table 17-3. While these discussions take time, they are invaluable to patients and families as well as making sure that the entire health-care team is aware of and comfortable with the care decisions established. Conversely there can be breakdowns in communication when a patient, family, or other member of the health-care team is left out of the decision-making process; when there are attempts to rush these discussions or push patients or families toward a decision; when conflicting opinions are given; when the patient and/or family feel their wishes are being ignored; or when there are issues with regard to the functioning of the family and family communication, differences, or drug and alcohol abuse issues.

THE CLINICIAN'S ROLE IN END-OF-LIFE CARE

Once a decision is made to avoid aggressive life-sustaining interventions, patients and families may benefit from detailed guidance about how to proceed. Clinicians play a vital role in providing this as delineated in Table 17-4. Chapter 18 provides more detailed information about palliative care and ways in which health-care providers can manage unpleasant symptoms, such as pain, nausea, and shortness of breath. In addition to avoiding inappropriate prolongation of dying, other end-of-life tasks include helping the patient achieve a sense of control, relieving burdens, and strengthening relationships with loved ones.

WHEN PATIENTS AND FAMILIES DEFER TO OR DISAGREE WITH CLINICIAN RECOMMENDATIONS

Most older individuals, along with their families, want to have input into end-of-life decisions. In some cases, however, the older individual may ask his or her clinician to make health-care-related decisions. Families or proxies may not want to make

TABLE 17-3. Step Approach to Discussions With Patients Around EOL Care

Steps	Description of activities
Step 1: The meeting	Bring the team together —including the patient and/or family/proxy.
Step 2: The tone	Set the tone of the meeting with values and objectives clearly stated. Focus the discussion around the patient and his or her goals. Reiterate that there are no right or wrong answers.
Step 3: Medical information	Provide medical information about the clinical findings and status objectively. Allow sufficient time for the patient/family to ask questions.
Step 4: Patient preferences	Determine who can speak on the patient's behalf and then have him or her state the patient's goals and preferences and what would be consistent with quality of life for this individual.
Step 5: Medical prognosis	Provide information about prognosis based on what is currently known and available data.
Step 6: Feelings	Ask the patient/family to express their feelings given the imparting of information. This helps the group get a sense of the patient/family concerns and thoughts.
Step 7: Treatment options	Provide the different options for care and treatment including pros and cons for all options.
Step 8: Leadership	Provide a recommendation based on the data, experience, and patient preferences/goals as previously described.
Step 9: Consensus	Make an attempt to reach consensus. The patient or family may need some time to process the information and to consider how the decision will be carried out.
Step 10: Follow-up	Depending on the relationship with the family (an episodic event or longer-term relationship), follow-up should be done after the death of the individual. This can be done via a telephone call or note.

Data from deMaine J and Dennett JM: Communicating with Patients and Families About Difficult End of Life Decisions: A Guide for Medical Providers." *Hamline Law Review* (article 13) 2014;36(2):298-310.

end-of-life decisions for personal or emotional reasons. Moreover, for some families or proxies, these decisions can result in persistent anxiety and depression and long-term feelings of guilt. In these situations, the humane option is to obtain "informed assent" from the family/proxy. The informed assent process allows the clinician to explicitly offer families/proxies the choice to defer to the provider's judgment about withholding or withdrawing life-sustaining therapy or whatever the end-of-life treatment decision might be. When assent is obtained, it should be clearly documented in the patient's medical record.

Alternatively, the clinician may be asked his or her professional and personal opinion about end-of-life decisions for a patient, either by the patient, family, or proxy.

TABLE 17-4. Details and Goals of Care and Symptom Management at the End of Life

Be kept clean

Have a designated decision maker

Have caregivers with whom one feels comfortable and can trust

Know what to expect about one's physical condition at the end of life

Have caregivers who will listen and help manage physical and psychological symptoms

Maintain one's dignity

Have financial affairs in order

Have pain optimally managed

Maintain humor and integrate humor into care and end-of-life challenges

Have an opportunity to say goodbye to loved ones

Experience optimal control of shortness of breath

Experience optimal control of feelings of anxiety

Have appropriate individuals to discuss/express fears

Have opportunities to resolve unfinished business with family or friends

Have opportunities for appropriate levels of physical touch

Have a relationship with providers

Feel reassured that one's family is prepared for the impending death

Ensure the presence of family

Feel reassured that one's end-of-life preferences are known to all providers

Have a plan in place for optimal death (eg, who will be at the bedside, etc)

Provide opportunities for life review

PART III

In these situations, the clinician must decide how actively personal preferences should be voiced. Frequently, this is done in the context of what the clinician might do for his or her mother or family member. Clinicians also continually have to make decisions about what information and how much information to provide to patients/ families or proxies. According to the doctrine of informed consent, clinicians must disclose enough information for the patient to make an "informed" decision. Informed consent laws and principles do not specify, however, exactly how much or what information is the right amount and what exactly must be disclosed. It is difficult to be fully objective in many instances, and the decisions are often not going to be clearly evidence based because the evidence may be variable, not relevant to older adults, or contradictory. Basically, clinicians are obligated to provide the following information: (1) condition being treated; (2) nature and character of the proposed treatment or surgical procedure; (3) anticipated results; (4) recognized possible alternative forms of treatment; and (5) recognized serious possible risks, complications, and anticipated benefits involved in the treatment or surgical procedure, as well as the recognized possible alternative forms of treatment, including nontreatment.

Situations may arise in which the clinician disagrees with the decision of the patient or proxy for ethical reasons. This might occur, for example, if the treatment requested by a patient is believed to be futile based on current research findings, or if the patient refuses care that the clinician feels would be of benefit. These patients can be referred to another clinician, and/or resources such as the health-care facility's ethics committee, social services staff, or agencies that advocate for older adults at the end of life can be contacted.

PHYSICIAN-ASSISTED SUICIDE

Physician-assisted suicide is currently legal in five states in the United States. It is an option for individuals living in Oregon, Vermont, Washington, California, and in Montana based on a court decision. Individuals must be terminally ill with an anticipated length of life of 6 months or less. The method for assisted suicide varies by state but generally involves a prescription from the physician. Physician-assisted suicide is different from euthanasia, which does not include a terminal diagnosis and is not legally supported. Oregon was the first state to legally authorize physician-assisted suicide in 1997 and since that time there has been an increase in the number of prescriptions written and deaths facilitated. In a 2015 report it was noted that 1,327 prescriptions were written and 859 individuals died associated with these prescriptions. It is anticipated that the numbers of assisted-suicide requests will increase as well as the number of states offering this option.

SPECIAL PROBLEMS WITH NURSING HOME RESIDENTS

Nursing home residents present some unique ethical challenges with regard to end-of-life decisions related to care. Older adults are usually admitted to nursing homes because of a reduced capacity to function either physically or mentally. Many suffer from some degree of cognitive impairment. Consequently, there may be some caregivers who assume that their quality of life is miserable and their lives have limited value. Clinicians must be diligent in working to preserve the nursing home resident's personhood. Essentially, nursing home residents should not lose any of their rights as people just because they enter a nursing home. They should be eligible to participate in a full range of activities and to make choices about their lives and their health care at their optimal ability both mentally and physically. Unless the individual has been noted to be without decisional capacity, he or she should be the first one consulted about changes in his or her condition or therapy. Because nursing home residents are vulnerable, special care is needed to protect their rights. The general goal is to maximize the resident's autonomy in making decisions about treatment. A resident's bill of rights (The National Consumer Voice, 2016), which outlines the choices that should be available and the protections that can be sought for residents, has been developed for all individuals in long-term care facilities. Federal law mandates that all nursing homes have written policies that describe the resident's bill of rights.

Clinical decisions in treating long-term care patients pose some of the greatest ethical dilemmas. Beyond the usually considered question of resuscitation, the clinician faces difficult decisions in determining when it is appropriate to transfer a patient from a nursing home to a hospital or when to intervene aggressively to treat changes in physiological status from fluid imbalance or infection. Perhaps one of the most perplexing areas is when to pursue heroic measures to maintain nutritional supports.

Artificial feeding decisions seem to arouse more controversy than other life-sustaining treatment issues, especially when the individual has not clearly stated his or her preferences. There is no evidence to support improved quality of life for individuals through use of a feeding tube. Moreover, the use of a percutaneous endoscopic gastrostomy (PEG) may result in discomfort for the individual and risk of aspiration and the possibility that restraint use may be necessary to avoid self-induced trauma by pulling at the tube. Thus, increasingly, clinicians are suggesting a more humane option, which is to provide "comfort feeding only" (Hanson, 2013). This allows for an individualized approach to helping the individual eat what he or she is able and willing to eat. Moreover, it avoids the negative feelings evoked in clinicians and families/proxies that withholding food and fluid creates. This approach is generally recommended for individuals who have difficulty swallowing due to cardiovascular events or end-stage Parkinson disease.

SPECIAL CASE OF DEMENTIA

As with all nursing home residents, it should not be assumed that residents with dementia no longer have decisional capacity and/or that they have a reduced quality of life. In addition to end-of-life ethical concerns with older adults with dementia, daily ethical issues can arise in the care of these individuals. Ethical decisions arise simply related to providing information around the diagnosis of dementia. For some individuals, it may be devastating to be given this diagnosis, while others want the information to optimize treatment and make plans for the future. The decision of how to proceed in these situations may be best made by taking the lead from the older adult. For example, if the individual is asking about cognitive changes and expressing concern about these changes, then information around a diagnosis will more likely be heard and appreciated. Conversely, if an individual is denying changes and does not want to hear about his or her impairment, then it may be futile to provide the information.

Other care-related issues that commonly create ethical challenges in older adults include such things as refusal of care or resistance to needed care such as bathing, wandering, disinhibited speech or behavior that is upsetting to staff and other residents, or aggressive behavior. Wandering, either deliberate or aimless, can be intrusive for other residents and a significant clinical problem. Ethical issues arise when a resident with dementia invades the privacy and space of another resident, who does not consent to the visit. The balance between the autonomy of the individual who is wandering versus the greater good of the community must be resolved. Ethically based options to manage these situations include such things as moving the resident who wanders or putting up a stop sign on the door to prevent entry. Alternatively, a resident with dementia may refuse to engage in any type of care activity, just wanting to lie in bed. If allowed to make this decision, the individual will be at risk for pressure ulcers, deconditioning, falling, and contractures and will ultimately require higher-level nursing interventions and resources. Preventing these problems would benefit not only the individual in terms of preventing pain and suffering but the community at large. Ethical choices need to be made to resolve the discrepancies between individual choices to engage in certain behaviors and knowingly allowing the resident to engage in behaviors that may cause him or her individual harm.

POLICY ISSUES

Older adults are prime targets for rationing efforts because they consume dispropor-tionately large amounts of medical care and because they are seen as having already lived their lives. At a subtler level, measures of program effectiveness tend to use something equivalent to the quality-adjusted life-year (QALY). This term implies that valuable life must be lived free of dependency. Such proxies for program effec-tiveness incorporate ethical components subtly. Society has not established the base on which to put a value on life lived at some level of dependency. To assume that it has no value, as is implied by active life years, appears to contradict the very purpose for geriatrics, which treats primarily dependent older people. Many older people would actively challenge the tenet that disability implies an absence of quality of life. Persons who are severely disabled at various ages can continue to enjoy pleasant and productive lives. As advocates for their patients, clinicians must be extremely vigilant to how such terms are used both in everyday speech and in analyses. It is important to bear in mind that any measure that uses life expectancy will inevitably be biased against older adults. One that relies on dependency as the primary outcome implies that those who are dependent no longer count; by such logic, disability is equivalent to death. At a time when there is an increased focus on allocation of health-care resources, care must be taken to avoid ageism and assumptions of negative quality of life among those who are cognitively or physically impaired and/or institutionalized.

The role of policy and policy initiatives is critical to encourage the development and use of ADs. In 1991 the Patient Self-Determination Act (PSDA) was established. The PSDA requires that most U.S. hospitals, nursing homes, hospice programs, home health agencies, and health maintenance organizations provide adults, at the time of inpatient admission or enrollment, information about their rights under state laws governing ADs, including (1) the right to participate in and direct their own health-care decisions, (2) the right to accept or refuse medical or surgical treatment, (3) the right to prepare an AD, and (4) information on the provider's policies that govern the utilization of these rights. The patient will be asked to provide his or her advance directive if one has been established. The act prohibits institutions from discriminat-ing against a patient who does not have an AD. The PSDA further requires institu-tions to document patient information and provide ongoing staff and community education on ADs. The law does not state, however, that an AD must be established.

The passage of the PSDA, unfortunately, has had minimal impact on increasing the numbers of individuals with ADs (Van Leuven, 2012). There are many reasons for the lack of uptake and impact in the passage of this policy. There are differences in interpretation and enforcement of the policy across states and settings of care, there is a lack of awareness and understanding among patients and families and a lack of readiness to address the difficult issues presented in ADs and an ongoing unrealistic expectation of the benefit associated with life-sustaining or prolonging care. Further, for patients admitted to the acute care setting for an acute medical or traumatic event, there may not be time or opportunity for the important and time-consuming discussions around ADs to occur. In some of these situations the patient may not be able to communicate and he or she may not have a health-care power of attorney. At the clinician level, there are no established consequences for not working with patients to establish ADs or for not adhering to ADs and clinicians continue to fear litigation by a proxy if all possible tests and treatment are not attempted.

It is possible that the more recent development of policies in now 38 states that require the completion of a MOLST or POLST form in institutionalized individuals will facilitate an increase in addressing ADs and ensuring adherence to the patient's wishes. As of January 2016 the Centers for Medicare & Medicaid Services allows clinicians to bill for advanced care planning during patient interactions. Being able to bill Medicare to establish ADs and the increased number of states recognizing the MOLST or POLST may significantly improve the rate of adherence to completing these important documents.

POLICY AND ETHICAL ISSUES CONCERNING CAREGIVERS

With regard to caregiver-related policy, as shown in Table 17-5, the reauthorization of the Older Americans Act (OAA) is currently under final consideration in the Senate. This bill would provide support and training for caregivers, with resources allocated specifically to help Native American caregivers and those caring for individuals with Alzheimer disease.

Ethically, concerns have been raised around the appropriate role and expectations of caregivers. Informal caregivers provide a significant amount of caregiving at the end of life. In Chapter 15, we noted the central role played by informal caregivers, who constitute the backbone of long-term care. For example, the Family Medical Leave Act asserts that an employee cannot be denied leave if the employee has a medically certified condition or is caring for a covered individual who has a medically certified condition. The question then is, how much of such care should they be expected to provide? What is the nature of the obligation of one generation to another, or even to spouses and siblings from the same generation? A substantial portion of informal care is undoubtedly provided out of love and compassion. This approach works well when it is left up to the family to decide how much care they can give, but what happens when such care becomes mandated? Pressure to control public costs of long-term care could easily lead to demands to require care from families or to require that families pay directly for a certain amount of that care. Clinicians need to be sensitive to the capability of caregivers in any given situation and to caregiver burden and stress.

There are also ethical concerns about the possibility that older persons are manipulating their assets to become unfairly eligible for Medicaid coverage or that younger generations gain control over elders' assets to ensure that funds are left to the next generation through the use of public funding to care for indigents.

PART III

TABLE 17-5. The Older Americans Reauthorization Act of 2016 (S. 192)

This act supports three crucial family caregiver programs:

1. Family Caregiver Support Services program provides a range of support services to approximately 1.4 million family and informal caregivers annually in states, including counseling, respite care, training, and assistance with locating services.
2. Native American Caregiver Support program provides a range of services to Native American caregivers, including information and outreach, access assistance, individual counseling, support groups and training, respite care, and other supplemental services.
3. Alzheimer's Disease Support Services program supports family caregivers who provide countless hours of unpaid care, thereby enabling their family members with dementia to continue living in the community. The program conducts evidence-based interventions and expands the dementia-capable home and community-based services.

Note: The legislation, initially introduced by Senators Lamar Alexander (R-TN), Patty Murray (D-WA), Richard Burr (R-NC), and Bernie Sanders (I-VT), passed the Senate on July 16, 2015. The amended version passed by the House in March 2016 went back to the Senate for consideration. The Older Americans Act makes important investments in creating a well-trained workforce and in providing person- and family-centered care for older Americans.

ELDER ABUSE AND NEGLECT

Although there are numerous support groups and resources available for caregivers of older adults, the stress of caregiving and daily life may result in some type of elder abuse. The National Center on Elder Abuse defines elder abuse as "intentional or neglectful acts by a caregiver or trusted individual that lead to or may lead to harm of a vulnerable older adult." There are several types of elder abuse including physical abuse; financial or material abuse; neglect or abandonment; psychological or emotional abuse; and sexual abuse. It is estimated that 10% of all older adults experience some type of abuse annually.

Although routine screening for elder abuse is not recommended by the U.S. Preventive Services Task Force, it is recommended that ongoing awareness of this growing problem be considered during all patient care interactions. If there are concerns raised than screening can be done with validated tools such as the Elder Abuse Suspicion Index (EASI) (Yaffe et al, 2008). This is a six-item measure that asks older adults directly about specific abusive concerns such as being forced to sign papers, having care withheld, or being touched in ways that were not wanted or hurt physically. If the cognitive status of the patient is not known, then this should be checked prior to completion of the tool.

Given that it is those who are cognitively impaired are at the greatest risk for abuse as they will be unable to accurately recall and report the abuse, assessment of these high-risk individuals for evidence of abuse is critical. Table 17-6 provides examples of common presentations of physical problems that may be indicative of abuse along with confirmatory laboratory findings and risk factors. Physical indicators that

TABLE 17-6. Evidence of Abuse or Neglect

Medical condition indicative of abuse	Physical findings	Laboratory findings	Possible contributing factors
Dehydration	Confusion Nausea and vomiting Dry appearance Orthostatic hypotension Dark, concentrated urine Tachycardia	Elevated serum sodium Elevated BUN/ creatinine ratio to greater than 20 Elevated uric acid Elevated Hgb/Hct	Older individual with urinary incontinence that is dependent in toileting
Malnutrition/ starvation	BMI <21/m² Decline in function Muscle wasting Weight loss	Low serum albumin and prealbumin Low transferrin Anemia Low cholesterol Low total lymphocyte count	Older adult who is dependent in feeding Individual with special dietary needs Financial limitations
Hyper- or hypothermia	Elevated body temperature Septic Dehydration from hyperthermia	Elevated creatinine kinase Elevated thyroid function tests	Inappropriately dressed (over- or underdressed for the weather) Financial limitations impacting heat and air conditioning
Trauma	Fracture Excessive and repeated bruising Subdural hematoma Skin tears Burns/scalds Rhabdomyolysis	Anemia Elevated creatinine kinase Myoglobin in the urine Renal insufficiency— acute Hypokalemia	Fully dependent older adults with cognitive impairment
Drug overdose	Abnormal blood levels of recreational or prescription drugs Sedation Confusion Hypotension Euphoria Depression Decreased respiration	Elevated blood or hair levels of drugs	Fully dependent older adults with cognitive impairment

PART III

(continued)

TABLE 17-6. Evidence of Abuse or Neglect (*continued*)

Medical condition indicative of abuse	Physical findings	Laboratory findings	Possible contributing factors
Sexual assault	Cystocele Decreased anal sphincter function Perineal excoriation Vaginal bleeding and/or excoriation Vaginitis	>100,000 bacteria on a urine culture Abnormal vaginal culture	Fully dependent older adults with cognitive impairment
Overall neglect	Dehydration Malnutrition Fecal impaction Poor hygiene Fungal infections Pressure ulcers Confusion	Elevated serum sodium Elevated BUN/creatinine ratio to greater than 20 Elevated uric acid Elevated Hgb/Hct Low serum albumin and prealbumin Low transferrin Anemia Low cholesterol Low total lymphocyte count	Fully dependent older adults with cognitive impairment Financial limitations

should flag abuse include such things as patterns of injury such as multiple and repeated burns and bruises on the abdomen, neck, and posterior legs—areas that the individual is not likely going to bruise during routine daily activity. Likewise, an unusual or unexplained fracture (ie, no trauma noted), pressure sores, or repeated infections should raise concerns about possible abuse.

If the clinician's concerns about abuse are confirmed, protection of the individual should be considered. This may require hospitalization or institutionalization pending legal investigation. In addition, the clinician will want to alert local social services and the Adult Protect Services program to determine further options for the individual. The National Center for Elder Abuse has a listing of state laws for Adult Protective Services including information about institutional abuse and Long-Term Care Ombudsman Program law.

INTERNATIONAL ASPECTS OF ETHICAL HEALTH CARE

Currently 12% of women and men are aged 60 or over. By 2050 this will increase to over 21%. Thus globally, geriatrics and the assurance of ethical and equitable care for all older adults is a priority. Numerous organizations are working internationally to ensure that this happens. The Global Network of the World Health Organization Collaborating Centres for Bioethics developed a document that reviews international ethical questions related to health, health care, and public health. The document delineates that globally there are concerns about justice and equality with regard to access to health-care resources and the vast differences noted in low-resource countries versus wealthier countries with regard to access to health care. Wealthier countries are challenged to respond and help promote global health equity.

Regardless of resources, older adults, especially frail older individuals, are particularly vulnerable and at risk for being exposed to unethical care, abuse, abandonment, and neglect. There is an appreciation that the current system of health rights in countries around the world does not sufficiently protect the rights and interests of older adults. HelpAge International and the Global Alliance for the Rights of Older People (GAROP) are working toward a convention on the rights of older adults. Specifically HelpAge International is focused on providing a universal position that age discrimination and ageism are morally and legally unacceptable; clarifying governments' human rights obligations toward older people; creating an enforceable monitoring mechanism to hold those in authority accountable for their actions toward older adults; and working to change attitudes so that older adults are recognized as having rights and responsibilities with regard to health care.

GAROP is a collaborative effort of nine organizations: International Network for the Prevention of Elder Abuse (INPEA); International Longevity Centre (ILC) Global Alliance; International Federation on Ageing (IFA); International Association of Homes and Services for the Ageing (IAHSA); International Association of Gerontology and Geriatrics (IAGG); HelpAge International; AGE Platform Europe; Age UK; and AARP International. GAROP has specifically identified the following rights for older adults: the right to freedom from discrimination; freedom from violence; social security; health; work; and property and inheritance. Health-care providers have been encouraged to support these initiatives.

SUMMARY

Ethical issues around care of older people are played out at all levels. Policy issues largely address questions of access and coverage, but these can be influenced by an individual clinician's beliefs about what elements of care are "appropriate" for older people. These beliefs, in turn, can reflect stereotypes. Microethical issues occur at the bedside when decisions about initiating or continuing treatment are made.

These decisions, too, are based on beliefs about appropriateness, including who should have the ultimate word about how much and what kind of care is rendered. Some of these decisions are couched as ethical issues because the requisite facts are not known. When there is evidence of efficacy or futility, the discussion changes, and decisions can be made on more substantial facts. Often, other factors than age are much better predictors of who will likely benefit from a given type of treatment. Great care must be taken to avoid couching rationing decisions as ethical dilemmas. Measures that discount older or frail people will inevitably lead to decisions against treating older persons.

Older adults should not lose their rights to full consideration of options and participation in the decisions that affect their care. The principles of autonomy and beneficence, which form a central part of the ethics of medicine in general, are strained with dependent older persons because the temptation toward paternalism is greater in the presence of the tendency to infantilize frail elderly patients, especially when they cannot readily communicate. Concerns about how to make decisions for persons unable to express their own preferences are often couched in terms of fear of litigation, but the growing body of experience suggests that carefully pursued efforts to establish agency and act accordingly will not put health-care clinicians or institutions at great risk of lawsuits. Rather, there is a risk of litigation if the wishes of the patient are not followed. Finally, it is important to recognize that the life of dependent older persons, especially those in nursing homes, is composed of many little incidents. The daily loss of dignity, privacy, and self-respect may be too readily ignored or may need to be balanced through negotiation based on the needs of the entire community. To be truly the patient's advocate, the health-care provider must be vigilant to these small but critical ethical insults and work toward optimal solutions for the good of all.

Clinicians should bear in mind that ethics is not a "slang" term without a particular meaning or that it simply reflects a set of general principles. Rather, state law may set out ethical standards with particularity. Moreover, clinicians can be effective advocates for patients, both while they are competent and after they are no longer authorized to act for themselves, based on both helping facilitate ADs and making the various clinical findings that are relevant concerning capacity, levels of care needed, and whether the particular care will be clinically effective or, instead, simply futile. Knowledge of the distinctions between types of ADs, how others may act as proxy, and the availability of ethics committees are all important tools. While health-care clinicians do not dictate care, they have not been reduced to passive participants in the process. By understanding both the clinical situation and choices and the ethical and legal context that exists at a particular time, clinicians are empowered to act in an ethical way, in the best interest of patients.

REFERENCES

deMaine J, Dennett JM. Communicating with patients and families about difficult end of life decisions: a guide for medical providers. *Hamline Law Rev.* 2014;36. http://digital commons.hamline.edu/cgi/viewcontent.cgi?article=1020&context=hlr. Accessed April 2016.

Hanson LC. Tube feeding versus assisted oral feeding for persons with dementia: using evidence to support decision-making. *Ann Long Term Care.* 21. www.annalsoflongtermcare.com/article/tube-feeding-versus-assisted-oral-feeding-persons-dementia-using-evidence-support-decision-m. 2013. Accessed April 2016.

Johnston M. Futile care: why Illinois law should mirror the Texas Advanced Directives Act. *Ann Health Law.* 2014;23:27-38.

National Consumer Voice. Resident rights. http://ltcombudsmanorg/issues/residents-rights#what 2016. Accessed April 2016.

Van Leuven KA. Advanced care planning in health service users. *J Clin Nurs.* 2012;21:3126-3133.

Yaffe MJ, Wolfson C, Lithwick M, Weiss D. Development and validation of a tool to improve physician identification of elder abuse: the Elder Abuse Suspicion Index (EASI). *J Elder Abuse Negl.* 2008;20. www.medicine.uiowa.edu/uploadedFiles/Departments/FamilyMedicine/Content/Research/Research_Projects/easi.pdf. Accessed April 2016.

SELECTED WEBSITES (ACCESSED 2017)

Global Alliance for the Rights of Older Persons, www.rightsofolderpeople.org/

National Alliance for Caregiving, Care for the Family Caregiver: A Place to Start, www.caregiving.org/data/Emblem_CfC10_Final2.pdf

National Center on Elder Abuse, What We Do, Research, Statistics/Data "http://ncea.acl.gov/whatwedo/research/statistics.html" ncea.acl.gov/whatwedo/research/statistics.html

State-by-state advance directive forms, www.everplans.com/articles/state-by-state-advance-directive-forms

State-by-state MOLST or POLST forms, www.polst.org/programs-in-your-state/

University of Miami, Geriatrics and Ethics, www.miami.edu/index.php/ethics/projects/geriatrics_and_ethics/

PART III

CHAPTER 18

Palliative Care

Much attention has been focused on the importance of making end-of-life (EOL) care decisions before one is in a crisis situation. Some older adults, however, are ambivalent about what they want at the end of life and may change their minds about treatment options when actually threatened by an illness that can cause death. An option that allows for realistic EOL supportive care without rescinding all efforts at treatment is palliative care. Palliative care is focused on symptom management and relieving suffering and improving quality of life of individuals rather than focusing on cure and lengthening of life. Avoidance of unnecessary, and potentially harmful, tests is initiated, and care is focused on comfort. Palliative care is a philosophy of care that is provided simultaneously with all other appropriate medical management of the patient.

Hospice differs from palliative care. Hospice is a comprehensive care system for patients with limited life expectancy who are living at home or in institutional settings. Hospice is a Medicare benefit that was established in 1982. To be eligible for hospice the patient must have Part A of Medicare and two clinicians must determine that the patient has 6 months or less to live if the disease runs its normal course. For the first 90-day period of care, the primary care clinician and the hospice medical director/hospice physician are required to certify terminal illness. For subsequent certification periods, only the hospice medical director/hospice clinician is required to certify terminal prognosis, unless otherwise specified by state hospice regulations. The clinician must include a brief narrative explanation of the clinical findings that supports a life expectancy of 6 months or less as part of the certification and recertification forms, or as an addendum to the certification and recertification forms. A face-to-face encounter is required for patients entering the third benefit period recertification (at 180 days) and every subsequent benefit period. Services provided through hospice are shown in Table 18-1. Hospice services also include coverage of necessary supplies such as a bedside commode or medications.

Discussing EOL care and decisions about how to approach care at the later stages of an older individual's life are difficult. Usually these discussions occur during a significant change in the patient's condition, following an acute event such as pneumonia or a fall, when a patient is suffering and aggressive treatment is not likely to help that suffering, around an aging milestone such as turning 100, or simply when the patient/family wants to discuss them.

Despite being difficult, having discussions with older patients and their families/caregivers about how they want care managed as they age and at the end of life is a critical aspect of geriatrics. There are numerous resources to help providers with this process (see the Selected Websites at the end of the chapter). Clinicians should use a step approach and discuss prognosis clearly, offer hope as needed, provide evidence-based options, coordinate transitions of care as appropriate through the progression of disease and natural aging, and relieve suffering, both physical and emotional. It is

TABLE 18-1. Hospice Services

Service provided	Description
Nursing	Registered nurses coordinate the care for every patient, provide direct patient care, and check symptoms and medication. Patient and family education is an important part of every visit. The nurse is the link between the patient and his or her family and the physician. The nurse can also help evaluate the patient's condition.
Social services	The social worker provides advice and counseling to the patient and all family members during the crisis period. The social worker assists other care team members in understanding the family dynamics and acts as an advocate for the patient and the family in making use of community resources.
Clinician services	The patient's primary care clinician approves the plan of care and works with the hospice team. In a full hospice program, a hospice medical director is available to the attending physician, the patient, and the hospice care team as a consultant and a resource.
Spiritual/counseling	Clergy and other counselors are available to visit and provide spiritual support to the terminally ill at home. Programs also use churches and congregations to aid the patient and family as requested.
Home health care/ homemaker	Home care aides provide personal care for the patient, such as bathing, shampooing, shaving, and nail care, and homemakers may be available for light housekeeping or meal preparation.
Continuous home health care	If the patient's needs require it or if the family can no longer manage the level of care required around the clock, hospice staff will provide care for 8- to 24-hour periods on a short-term basis.
Therapy/ rehabilitation services	Daily living tasks such as walking, dressing, or feeding oneself can become frustrating and impossible during an illness. Therapists help the patient develop new ways to accomplish these tasks.
On-call team support	A hospice team member is on call 24 hours a day, 7 days a week. If a problem should arise, the team member may offer advice over the phone and, if necessary, make a visit.
Respite care	To provide relief for family members, the hospice may arrange a brief period of in-patient care for the patient.
Bereavement counseling	Bereavement is the time of mourning that we all experience following a loss. The hospice care team works with surviving family members to help them through the grieving process. Support may include a trained volunteer or counselor visiting the survivors at specific periods during the first year, or phone calls and/or letter contact and the opportunity for family members to participate in support groups. The hospice will refer survivors to medical or other professional care if necessary.

TABLE 18-2. A Five-Step Framework for Discussing Care Choices at the End of Life

Step	Description
Step I: Initiating the discussion	Schedule a private location and adequate time for this discussion. Establish a supportive relationship with the patient if appropriate and the family. Establish who is the decision maker. Elicit general thoughts about end-of-life preferences from the patient/decision maker. Plan what you will say to the patient/family. Gather current evidence-based facts/numbers to present (eg, percentage of older adults likely to survive CPR after the age of 80).
Step II: Evaluating the patient/family perspective	Ask the patient/family to state what their thoughts are about the older adult's current status. Ask the patient/family to state their goals in terms of care (eg, focus on life prolongation vs quality of life). Ask if the patient/family is willing to discuss care options.
Step III: Clarifying the prognosis	Provide the facts on current status, life expectancy, and anticipated disease(s) trajectory. If new diagnosis, provide specific detail (eg, this is a malignant melanoma with some evidence of spreading). Deliver information in a straightforward way; don't use euphemisms; use words the patient/family can understand.
Step IV: Identifying end-of-life goals	Provide treatment choices and options with known evidence for outcomes. Focus on care and what will be provided. Establish goals based on all given information.
Step V: Developing a treatment plan	Provide guidance in the development of the plan in terms of recommendations for appropriate treatments. Provide ongoing support to the patient and family for the choices they have made. Ensure that palliative care is initiated in a timely fashion (eg, pain addressed). Clarify and confirm decisions.

CPR, cardiopulmonary resuscitation.

critical to determine what the patient/family wants to know and how much information they want to receive, be prepared to provide care and treatment-related options, be unbiased and open to what the patient/family wants, and be prepared to offer emotional support. Generally there are five steps in the process recommended; these are described below and in more detail in Table 18-2. The steps include:

1. Initiating the discussion
2. Evaluating the patient/family perspectives

3. Clarifying the prognosis
4. Identifying end-of-life goals
5. Developing a treatment plan

A major emphasis during all discussions of EOL care should be on the types of care that will be provided. Statements such as "there is nothing more we can do for you" should be avoided. Rather, the discussion should focus on what types of care interventions will be provided (eg, pain medications, positioning therapies as appropriate, nonpharmacological pain-relieving modalities). Following these steps can help assure that communication is clearly provided, fears are allayed, and the patients are helped to achieve the goals they want at the end of life such as dying with minimal pain.

While it may be difficult to have EOL discussions with patients during the first patient visit, it is helpful to have the discussion early in the clinician–patient relationship. One option is to ask the patient/family if they have had discussions about EOL care and care preferences and, if so, to ask them to bring any documents addressing preferences to the next appointment. If this has not been previously addressed, then a plan to discuss this in more detail at the next visit can be initiated. As noted in Chapter 5, this can also be done during the Welcome to Medicare Visit or Annual Medicare Visit.

For older adults in long-term care settings, one important fact to obtain and clarify during the first visit with a patient involves identifying who will be the primary/first authorized representative to call with changes in the patient's condition (see Chapter 17). When multiple individuals are listed as authorized representatives (eg, all three children) and there are differences of opinion between siblings or caregivers about how treatment should proceed (eg, to go to the hospital or not), the clinician may be asked to facilitate a discussion around the pros and cons of different treatment options. While time-consuming, these conversations can help ease the anxiety experienced among the caregivers and help the entire family feel comfortable with the decisions that are made. The primary care clinician may need to help families explain difficult situations to a patient. Examples include such things as helping a patient with mild cognitive impairment understand that refusing dialysis may result in death. The clinician may also have to anticipate for families or interpret behavioral responses to interventions for families of individuals who are not able to verbally express their thoughts (eg, pulling out tubes or turning down feedings may be indicative of refusal).

THE SLOW MEDICINE APPROACH

Slow medicine is a philosophy of care that was developed to help older adults and their families and caregivers manage some of the changes that occur with aging and the declines that commonly occur (McCullough, 2008). Slow medicine is a commonsense approach to care of older adults in which careful consideration is given to the pros and cons of each treatment option. The underpinning of slow medicine is a sustained relationship with a primary care clinician whom the patient and family come to trust. This sustained relationship allows time for EOL issues to be broached and revisited, a situation in stark contrast to the requirement that such topics be broached on admission to a medical facility. Decisions are strongly based on quality-of-life factors, comfort, and the risk of doing more harm than good with any given intervention. In many situations in geriatrics, a "tincture of time" may in fact be the best approach as it allows for the symptoms associated with a clinical problem to resolve prior to initiating an intervention that may cause harm (eg, an antibiotic with side effects). The slow medicine philosophy can be used to help with decisions around prevention practices (eg, use of statins) as well when managing acute situations.

GUIDANCE PROVIDED BY CHOOSING WISELY INFORMATION

Older adults and/or families often request that tests and treatments be provided for themselves or their loved ones that may not necessarily be of benefit to them. In addition, clinicians may recommend tests and procedures based on guidelines and data provided for younger individuals or as a way to cover all possible outcomes. Increasingly, there are beliefs and concerns over testing and subsequent harm to older adults. In response to these concerns, the American Board of Internal Medicine Foundation joined with nine leading medical specialty societies to develop a list of tests and procedures that should not be recommended for patients across the aging continuum. Currently there are 70 lists available from numerous specialty and aging groups as well as pediatrics, nursing, and physical therapy. The goal of choosing wisely is to help health-care providers and patients and families think about and talk about undergoing expensive interventions that are not likely to be beneficial for optimizing quality of life. Most recently the *Choosing Wisely* campaign encouraged participating societies to identify clinicians, or teams of clinicians, whose work in their respective specialties represents significant contributions to advancing the goals of the *Choosing Wisely* campaign by encouraging conversations about avoiding unnecessary care. These contributions will help demonstrate the best ways to disseminate this information and use it in real-world clinical care.

FRAILTY AND A PALLIATIVE CARE FOCUS

Unlike in other areas of medicine, in geriatrics there is not likely to be a single diagnosis that contributes to cause of death. Rather, we are managing multiple comorbidities and frailty. Frailty, which is caused by age-related physiological decline and/or a combination of disease states, has been defined as a diminishing capacity to manage stress with subsequent risk of negative outcomes in terms of physical health and function. Frailty is associated with a progressive decline in function that impacts quality of life and thus raises patient/family interests and provider inclination to discuss palliative care. Frailty is commonly associated with the following symptoms: loss of strength, weight loss, decreased physical activity and poor endurance, and slowing of performance. There may be associated changes in cognition, balance, and emotional health with subsequent falls, trauma, and depression. Identification, understanding, and acknowledgment of frailty are important for patients and families. Moreover, given the many factors and lack of a cure for frailty, it is a useful stepping stone for discussing palliative care. Table 18-3 provides an overview of common signs and symptoms of frailty that can be used to establish evidence for this condition.

PART III

TABLE 18-3. Signs and Symptoms of Frailty

Patient symptom	Objective finding/sign
Decreased appetite/loss of weight	A greater than 5% loss of body weight in the past year A loss of 10 lb or more not intended Clothes no longer fitting
Weakness and less able to do what he or she used to do	A decline in grip strength if prior testing had been done Time to walk 15 ft at usual pace (slow ≥7 seconds for men or tall women; ≥6 seconds for others)
Fatigue	A decrease in usual activities
Pain	Rate pain on a scale of 0 to 10 and explore if pain interferes with normal activity
Depression	Evaluate patient for affect (appearing sad or blue) Ask patient directly if he or she is depressed
Falls	Observe gait changes and risk for falls based on function

The Clinical Frailty Scale (available at www.bcguidelines.ca/pdf/frailty_csha.pdf) can be used to determine evidence of frailty from severely frail (completely dependent on others for the activities of daily living, or terminally ill) to Very fit (robust, active, energetic, well motivated, and fit; these individual commonly exercise regularly and are in the most fit group for their age).

Unfortunately, when considering EOL and speaking with patients and families the issue of frailty and the combined impact of frailty and new diagnosis or change in a prior comorbid conditions is not discussed. This information is critical, however, as the treatment options and outcomes for single disease states (eg, heart failure, aortic stenosis, metastatic melanoma) have not been tested and established for frail older adults. Treatments that may work well for younger individuals may have less benefit for frail older adults who often will not return to baseline function and cognitive status following many medical and surgical interventions. Moreover, these individuals are likely to have many fewer years of life expectancy to experience treatment benefit even if it does occur. It is important to be avoid providing treatment options without full disclosure of the risks noted when provided to a frail older adult. To ensure the most accurate and useful discussions and best decisions about EOL care in the face of frailty, four principles should be followed as described in Table 18-4.

ESTABLISHING A PALLIATIVE CARE APPROACH

Depending on the setting of care, a palliative care approach can be initiated and established in different ways. Some acute and long-term care settings have established palliative care teams that include members from a variety of disciplines (eg, nursing, medicine, social work, pastoral services) to facilitate the discussions (as addressed earlier) and initiate the palliative care orders. This might include discontinuing certain procedures or treatments (eg, stopping intravenous fluids) and focusing on managing

TABLE 18-4 Principles for End-of-Life Decision Making in Frail Older Adults

Principle	Description	Support/rational for the principle
Principle 1	Provide a comprehensive geriatric assessment	To optimally evaluate function, both physical and cognitive, as these are both critical to ongoing quality of life.
Principle 2	Provide complete and accurate information about prognosis	Patients and families cannot make good decisions unless they understand how being frail may impact their response to any type of treatment.
Principle 3	Provide the long-term impact (risks and benefits) of care decisions	To understand specifically what the treatment option may mean in terms of benefits and risks.
Principle 4	Encourage patients and families to seek answers to useful decision-making questions	Examples: • Which health conditions are easily treatment and which are not? • How will frailty make treatment risky? • How can symptoms be safely and effectively managed? • How will the proposed treatment improve or worsen function and cognition?

PART III

unpleasant symptoms experienced by the older patient. Some settings may use a preset order form to facilitate the implementation of a palliative care approach. Order forms generally address in detail what patients and/or families want done, or not done, with regard to palliative management. Decisions are made around routine care activities such as vital signs, weights, assessment of intake and output, glucose monitoring, and lab work. In addition, decisions may be made to continue or stop all rehabilitation services and some or all medications. Last, forms provide treatment options for common symptoms that may occur as part of EOL care including management of pain, shortness of breath, anxiety, nausea, agitation, constipation, and excessive secretions.

CULTURAL CHALLENGES AND PALLIATIVE CARE

Culture influences individuals' decisions about EOL care decisions. There are, however, more similarities than differences between ethnocultural groups and what they believe palliative care involves. Increasingly there is recognition that EOL care cuts across assumed cultural beliefs with individuals requiring and wanting the same focus on alleviation of symptoms such as pain and shortness of breath. Given the heterogeneity among individuals and the increasing focus on patient-centered care combined with cultural competence and sensitivity, it is important to not generalize and assume what an individual is likely to want at EOL based on his or her cultural group.

Conflicts may occur due to differing beliefs, communication styles, and goals, and this may impact the patient–provider relationship. Understanding and addressing the

TABLE 18-5 Assess ABCDE to Determine Level of Cultural Influence in EOL Decisions

Activity	Relevant information to obtain	Interview question to guide interaction
Attitudes	What attitudes does this ethnic group have regarding providing diagnostic information and prognosis? What attitudes do they have toward death?	Educate yourself about the commonly noted cultural beliefs of the group and ask specifically if the patient holds those beliefs.
Beliefs	What are the patient's religious and spiritual beliefs?	Obtain information about beliefs of the group/common religions and ask specifically about EOL beliefs.
Context	Review with the patient/family the context of their lives (eg, if they are newly immigrated; their language skills; their degree of integration with cultural group and community).	Ask specific questions about birth place, living location, education, and life history.
Decision-making style	What decision-making styles are generally followed by the patient/family?	Be familiar with cultural group preferences and specifically ask if they maintain those beliefs.
Environment	What environment do they currently live in? Is it culturally diverse? What resources are available?	Be familiar with culturally based environments in the area and available resources.

patient's cultural beliefs without making assumptions is critical to ensuring optimal palliative care. It is critical to ask patients and/or families about their cultural beliefs and expectations and to discuss these in an open format. Basic cultural information can be obtained through a number of resources (American Geriatrics Society Ethnogeriatrics Committee, 2016; Brangman and Periyakoil, 2014). In addition, the ABCDE (attitudes, beliefs, context, decision making, and environment) approach (McPhee et al, 2011) can be used to guide health-care providers in managing cultural issues associated with palliative care (Table 18-5). Obtaining information, for example, about EOL customs or religious rituals and providing assurance to patients and families that these customs and rituals will be respected can help optimize the palliative care experience.

MANAGEMENT OF SYMPTOMS IN PALLIATIVE CARE

Symptoms such as pain, shortness of breath, anxiety, and fatigue, among others, can cause distress as people age with chronic or life-threatening illnesses. These symptoms can all be addressed using a palliative care approach with a variety of pharmacological and nonpharmacological interventions. An overview of treatment options is provided in Table 18-6 for many of these symptoms, and the most prevalent symptoms are described in more detail in the following sections.

PAIN

Pain management will vary based on the cause and whether or not this is acute versus chronic pain. The goal is to treat pain proactively and to find the minimum dose of medication or medication combined with nonpharmacological treatment that can prevent the pain. Older adults may fear pain at the end of life, and assurance is needed that their pain will be managed using a variety of approaches. Recommendations for pain management are discussed in detail in Chapter 10. With regard to palliative care, however, pain management decisions need to consider the entire patient/family situation. For example, because a caregiver is not available to provide frequent dosing of a medication, a decision may be made to use a long activity medication or a subcutaneous method of administration versus an injection or frequent oral treatment. Despite an interest in taking a palliative care approach, some older adults and/or family members may continue to fear use of opioids due to concerns about addiction or a fear that use of morphine will lead to death. In these situations, education to help patients and families work through these feelings should be initiated. In addition, patients and families should be helped to understand that there may be side effects to opioid use that can likewise be managed. These include such things as nausea and vomiting, sedation, delirium, respiratory depression, constipation, multifocal myoclonus, and seizures. Alternatively, there are some patients who may choose to avoid the use of medications due to these side effects and these requests should be honored and supported. In these situations, nonpharmacological approaches to manage pain should be considered. As appropriate to the pain management needs of the patient opioid dosage can be decreased, and adjuvant coanalgesic medications and treatments can be added (Table 18-7). Innovative approaches such as the use of a Toolbox for pain management (eg, patient access to a variety of treatment options within the home setting) can help ensure optimal pain management (Rosenberg et al, 2015). As described in Chapter 10, nonpharmaceutical interventions can also be initiated and these include such things as positioning, heat or ice, music or other types of distractions, acupuncture, and massage.

CONSTIPATION

Constipation is a common symptom that often needs to be managed during palliative care treatment. Constipation is addressed in detail in Chapter 8. As with use of opioids, patients and families need to be assured that the patient need not worry about dependence on a laxative. Moreover, preventive measures for constipation such as increasing fluid and fiber may be useful for prevention of constipation but are not likely to be effective to treat acute symptoms of constipation. Rather, drug therapy of the patient's choice should be considered. For example, a patient who wants immediate relief may want to get a suppository versus an oral agent. Once constipation is identified as a problem, preventive treatment should be initiated with increases

TABLE 18-6. Management of Symptoms Noted at End of Life

Symptom	Management
Myoclonus	Treat underlying cause of myoclonus if possible (may be due to opioid use).
	Maintain adequate hydration.
	Rotate to alternate opioid.
	Give low-dose lorazepam or a benzodiazepine.
Dyspnea	Use opioids (small, frequent doses as needed for opioid-naïve patients).
	Use benzodiazepines if anxiety is present.
	Use glucocorticoids or bronchodilators for bronchospasm.
	Use antibiotics if it is believed that a bacterial infection is exacerbating dyspnea and treatment will likely improve symptoms.
	Use oxygen only when hypoxia is present and patient finds it helpful.
	An open window or fan may be comforting.
	Consider patient position, including measures such as elevating the head of the bed and sitting up in a chair.
	Encourage physical activity as tolerated.
	Consider complementary treatment, including acupuncture or massage.
Fatigue/ apathy	Consider pharmacological treatment options including methylphenidate (Ritalin) 2.5 mg twice daily (in morning and at noon) and increase up to 30 mg/day.
	Use modafinil (Provigil) 50–100 mg/day to start; this can be increased to 100–200 mg/day.
	Ensure that fatigue is normal and suggest energy-conservation methods.
	Employ sleep hygiene measures to facilitate optimal nighttime sleep.
Cough	Consider etiology (infection, bronchospasm, effusions, lymphangitis, cardiac failure) and treat accordingly.
	Use opioids for cough suppression, particularly if cough prevents the patient from sleeping.
	Use other antitussives such as guaifenesin or dextromethorphan.
	Use glucocorticoids if it is believed that the cough is due to irritation or is inflammatory in nature.
	Use bronchodilators as appropriate (eg, for bronchospasm) and beneficial such as albuterol 2–3 inhalations every 4–5 hours.
	Use diuretics if it is believed that the cough may be due to congestive heart failure and fluid overload.
Excessive secretions	Do not suction.
	Use scopolamine transdermal patch, 1.5 mg (start with one or two patches; if ineffective, switch to 50 μg/h continuous IV or SQ infusion and double the dose every hour, up to 200 μg/h).

(continued)

TABLE 18-6. Management of Symptoms Noted at End of Life (*continued*)

Symptom	Management
	Use glycopyrrolate, 1–2 mg PO or 0.1–0.2 mg IV or SQ every 4 hours; or 0.4–1.2 mg/day continuous infusion.
	Use atropine, 0.4 mg SQ every 15 minutes PRN; atropine eyedrops can be given orally as well.
	Use hyoscyamine, 0.125–0.25 mg PO or SL every 4 hours.
	Monitor for excessive fluid intake and reduce intake as acceptable to the patient.
Delirium	Review for underlying cause of the delirium (Chap. 6) and eliminate if possible.
	If symptoms are upsetting to the patient or put him or her or others at danger, pharmacological interventions such as antipsychotic medications in low dosages and/or sedative hypnotics for hyperactive delirium may be helpful; hypoactive delirium may respond to treatments consistent with fatigue as delineated above.
Fever	Use antimicrobials if infection is the cause of the delirium and if treatment is consistent with goals of care and does not cause additional symptoms (eg, diarrhea, nausea).
	Use antipyretics such as acetaminophen either orally or rectally.
	Bathe with tepid or cool water as tolerated by the patient.
Depression	Use antidepressants, depending on the situation (they are less likely to be immediately effective).
	Consider counseling, pastoral or otherwise, if acceptable to the patient.
Pain	Initiate pharmacological interventions as described in Chapter 10 and Table 18-7.
	Consider nonpharmacological interventions including positioning, distraction, music, acupuncture, massage, laughter, or lifelong patient preferences for management and coping with pain.
Hemorrhage	Decrease visualization of excessive external bleeding from patient and family by using dark (vs white) towels.
	Treat associated anxiety that may occur due to the bleeding (see above management of anxiety with lorazepam or other anxiolytic).

IV, intravenous; PO, oral; PRN, as needed; SL, sublingual; SQ, subcutaneous.

in fiber, fluid, and physical activity as tolerable and possible and/or regular laxative use. Dosing of laxatives and use of combination drugs will likely need ongoing management.

Lubiprostone, Naloxegol, and Methylnaltrexone are all treatment options for opioid-induced constipation. Naloxegol and Methylnaltrexone should be reserved for when other laxatives are not effective. Methylnaltrexone is given subcutaneously while the others are orally administered. It should be noted, however, that

TABLE 18-7. Adjuvant Pharmacologic Treatments for Pain Management

Drug group	Route	Pain indication	Additional information
Nonsteroidal anti-inflammatory drugs	Oral Topical	Neuropathic Visceral Bone Inflammatory	May cause gastrointestinal or renal side effects
Corticosteroids	Oral Intravenous	Spinal/nerve compression Neuropathic Bone	May cause gastrointestinal symptoms, hyperglycemia, or psychosis
Benzodiazepines	Oral (liquid or tablet) Intramuscular	Anxiety associated with the pain	May cause sedation or confusion/delirium and alter function
Anesthetics	Intravenous Topical	Intractable pain Neuropathic pain	May cause gastrointestinal side effects, confusion, urinary retention, headache, or anxiety For topical agents monitor for skin reaction
Anticonvulsants	Oral	Neuropathic pain	May cause confusion, change in function, sleepiness, or edema
Antidepressants	Oral	Neuropathic pain Chronic pain	Tricyclic antidepressants have anticholinergic properties and can cause confusion, orthostatic hypotension, constipation, urinary retention; dual reuptake inhibitors of both serotonin and norepinephrine serotonin can cause hyponatremia and confusion and can take up to 6 weeks to be effective
Muscle relaxants	Oral	Skeletal muscle spasm Akathisia	Use short term only due to side effects of sedation and increasing risk of muscle weakness and falls

Methylnaltrexone can exacerbate the emetic property of morphine (Stettler and Zulian, 2013). In acute bowel obstruction, attempts should be made to disimpact the patient manually and/or with enemas and prevent reoccurrence. Alternatively, Octreotide, which is a synthetic analog of somatostatin, can be used to manage the symptoms of bowel obstruction. The inhibitory effect of Octreotide on peristalsis and gastrointestinal sections reduces bowel distention and the secretion of water and sodium by the intestinal epithelium and this reduces the patient's symptoms of vomiting and pain.

DIARRHEA

Diarrhea, defined as the passage of more than three unformed bowel movements within 24 hours, is also a common symptom that requires management when engaging in palliative care. Diarrhea may be due to malignancy, prior cancer-related treatment (eg, radiation), side effects from drugs used to manage other symptoms at the end of life, or long-term chronic problems (eg, irritable bowel syndrome). For new-onset diarrhea, it is useful to rule out or treat any underlying cause such as impaction, drug side effects, or infection. Treatment should include bulking agents and over-the-counter agents such as loperamide. Bulking agents and Questran can be particularly effective if the patient is able and willing to ingest these in adequate amounts.

NAUSEA AND VOMITING

Nausea and vomiting should be evaluated to determine whether an underlying cause can be identified and attempts made to eliminate the cause. Nausea may be due to central causes in the chemoreceptor trigger zone of the brain. Conversely, peripherally caused nausea is mediated in the gastrointestinal system and the vestibular system. Receptors, including serotonin, dopamine, histamine, and acetylcholine, are involved in mediating nausea. There are basically five classes of antiemetic drugs: antidopaminergic drugs, antiserotonergic drugs, antihistamines, anticholinergics, and neurokinins. In addition, there are a group of adjunctive drugs that, although not directly antiemetics, treat specific causes of nausea (such as hyperacidity or gut dysmotility). Matching treatment to what is assumed to be the underlying cause should be the first line of treatment. For example, dopamine-mediated nausea is probably the most common form of nausea and the most frequently targeted for initial symptom management. Treatment options include dopamine agonists such as haloperidol. Conversely, when the nausea is assumed to be due to a sluggish gut then the use of metoclopramide may be effective. Ondansetron and other serotonin 5-hydroxytryptamine-3 receptor antagonists are dopaminergic antagonists and act in the chemoreceptor trigger zone along with the peripheral areas to decrease nausea. They are most effective for chemotherapy-induced nausea and less effective for opioid-induced nausea. Antihistamines are helpful in situations in which it is believed the vestibular system is involved. Last, corticosteroids can further augment the treatment of nausea, particularly when there are concerns about increased intracranial pressure.

DECREASED APPETITE AND WEIGHT LOSS

Decreased appetite and weight loss may impact quality of life for older adults. If, however, the patient is not bothered by these symptoms, there is no need to treat the problem. If appetite and weight loss are concerns of the family or caregivers, then education can be provided about the advantages to decreased intake (eg, energy conservation, decreased bowel and bladder function). It is critical, however, when addressing appetite and oral intake to explore the cultural beliefs in this area. There are some cultures, for example, that believe the individual cannot pass into heaven on an empty stomach.

Addressing symptoms that can impact appetite may be beneficial in terms of optimizing intake. Symptoms that can impact appetite include such as things as mouth dryness, which can be managed with moist compresses and ointment such as Vaseline. Appetite may be pharmaceutically induced with corticosteroids, some antidepressants (eg, mirtazapine), megestrol, the use of the marijuana congener dronabinol, or a glass of wine or a cocktail prior to eating. Nonpharmaceutical appetite stimulates include focusing on food preferences and ensuring that eating experiences are in pleasant situations and settings.

SHORTNESS OF BREATH

Dyspnea, or shortness of breath, is particularly common in patients with chronic obstructive pulmonary disease or end-stage cardiac disease. The cause of the underlying dyspnea may be multifactorial and difficult to determine. There is a physiological interaction between chemoreceptors in the respiratory tract and central nervous system, upper airway receptors, stretch receptors in the chest wall, irritant receptors in the airway epithelium, and C fibers in the alveolar walls and blood vessels, and psychiatric symptoms (eg, anxiety) that can exacerbate dyspnea. Patients may experience benefits from direct use of oxygen via nasal cannula or face mask, increased oxygen in the patient's immediate environment, or having a fan blow cool air on the patient. Pharmacotherapy can include use of benzodiazepines to control the associated anxiety. Opioids are used to decrease respiratory drive and also to decrease the associated anxiety. These two treatment options (benzodiazepines and opioids) can be used together to provide a synergistic effect and allow for lower dosages of each drug group and thus less side effects experienced from either agent.

EXCESSIVE SECRETIONS AND COUGH

Excessive secretions that the patient can't expectorate can be particularly bothersome to both the patient and the family/caregivers. Rather than have the patient endure the discomfort of suctioning, pharmacological treatment can be initiated. Treatment includes use of anticholinergic agents such as hyoscyamine or atropine given orally.

The excessive secretions experienced by a patient may result in a cough. Alternatively, patients may cough at the end of life due to mucus, blood, foreign material, or stimulation of the receptors in the airway due to some type of irritation. Symptomatic treatment will vary based on the cause. For example, if the patient is in heart failure, the use of additional diuretics may help resolve the cough. Antibiotics appear to be useful if it is believed that an upper respiratory infection and excessive mucus are stimulating the cough. Cough suppressants such as dextromethorphan can be helpful in decreasing cough centrally without causing significant side effects. Elixirs with codeine may be used if the patient can tolerate these without side effects.

PSYCHIATRIC SYMPTOMS: ANXIETY, DEPRESSION, HALLUCINATIONS, AND DELIRIUM

Anxiety, delirium, depression, hallucinations, and associated agitation are not unusual, particularly as patients near the end of life. These symptoms are bothersome to patients and even more so to families and caregivers who witness them and are providing the ongoing management of the patient. If the patient is not bothered by the symptom (eg, the hallucinations are not unpleasant), then no treatment is required, and assurance and support for families and caregivers can be provided. Management of these problems is discussed in detail in Chapters 6, 7, and 14. Treatment should generally be initiated in the most expedient way possible with consideration of quality-of-life factors associated with symptoms experienced and treatment side effects (eg, sedation from anxiolytics).

Challenging situations often arise in which treatment for one symptom at the end of life results in another unpleasant symptom such as delirium. For example, opioids used to decrease pain may cause significant changes in cognition and delirium. It may be helpful to change pain treatment regimens by switching to another opioid or a different route of administration (eg, use of a patch versus oral treatment).

INTERNATIONAL ASPECTS OF PALLIATIVE CARE

There is an increasing interest in the implementation of palliative care approaches internationally given global aging. The International Association for Hospice and Palliative Care was developed with an international perspective designed to avoid promoting a single unique palliative care model. Rather the goal was to encourage and enable each country, according to its resources and conditions, to develop its own model of palliative care provision. This allows developing countries to take advantage of what has been learned in more affluent countries.

Internationally, countries are aware that, despite cultural challenges and differences, there will likely be a need for palliative care. China is particularly interested in teaching providers about palliative care given the large number of older adults, the limited use of opioids and a cultural aversion to having anyone but family provide care. Moreover, there is evidence in China of a change in cultural beliefs regarding death. Although traditionally it was believed to be sacrilegious to talk about death, current surveys among Chinese elderly indicate that they prefer to be informed of the diagnosis if they have a terminal illness and prefer to receive medical treatment that focuses on comfort. Japan, recognizing their great need for palliative care as well revised their position statement on End-of-Life Care for the Elderly (The Japanese Geriatric Society Ethics Committee et al, 2014).

There is also some interest internationally among speciality organizations to address palliative care as it relates to a certain disease state. For example, palliative care in dementia was recently addressed by the European Association for Palliative Care using input from an International panel of experts. Other areas of international palliative care interest are in nephrology and chronic obstructive pulmonary disease.

PART III

While there is interest in palliative care internationally, it is also recognized that there are big differences in the quality of and access to palliative care between countries. This is particularly noted between affluent and less developed countries. The United Kingdom has been recognized as having the top rankings in the Quality of Death Index (Burki, 2015). The Quality of Death Index was developed by the Economist Intelligence Unit to rank countries according to their provision of EOL care. The United Kingdom has the longest history of providing palliative care and served as an example for many other countries in terms of how to provide this type of care across a variety of settings. Australia and New Zealand came second and third while Chile and Mongolia were the best at providing palliative care among low- and middle-income countries. These countries all showed evidence of a national policy to support palliative care, strong public awareness of this philosophy of care, financial resources allocated to palliative care, and wide availability of opioids. Internationally, it has been recognized that all countries are preparing for the expected future demand and need for palliative care and are allocating resources to facilitate this approach.

CONCLUSION

Providing patients with the opportunity to receive palliative care is a critical aspect of geriatrics and is as important as the diagnosis and management of acute medical problems. Decisions of when to consider palliative care may occur at different points in time for each patient. Offering this approach as an option for patients and their caregivers/loved ones should always be considered. Ongoing discussions may be needed, and decisions may be revisited throughout the course of aging. Understanding cultural differences and exploring patient and family knowledge, goals, and expectations are important aspects of palliative care. Most importantly, providers should remind patients and their families/caregivers that palliative care does not mean *no* care. Rather, focusing on treatment and the many ways in which we can treat symptoms that occur during the aging process should be emphasized. Although discussions around palliative care approaches and management often require significant time and energy on the part of the provider, the benefits are great. Patients and families are often spared unnecessary and unpleasant symptoms, and health-care providers have the opportunity to focus exclusively on comfort and symptom management.

REFERENCES

American Geriatrics Society Ethnogeriatrics Committee. Achieving high-quality multicultural geriatric care. *J Am Geriatr Soc.* 2016;64:255-260.

Brangman S, Periyakoil VS, eds. *Doorway Thoughts: Cross-Cultural Health Care for Older Adults.* New York, NY: American Geriatrics Society; 2014.

Burki TK. Variation in palliative care standards worldwide. *Lancet Oncol.* 2015;16:e533.

Japanese Geriatric Society Ethics Committee, Iijima S, Aida N, et al. Position statement from the Japan Geriatrics Society 2012: end-of-life care for the elderly. *Geriatr Gerontol Int.* 2014;14:735-739.

McCullough D. *My Mother, Your Mother: Embracing "Slow Medicine": The Compassionate Approach to Caring for Your Aging Loved Ones.* 2008.

McPhee SJ, Winker MA, Rabow MW, Pantilat SZ, Markowitz AJ. *Care at the Close of Life.* New York, NY: McGraw-Hill; 2011.

Rosenberg JP, Bullen T, Maher K. Supporting family caregivers with palliative symptom management: a qualitative analysis of the provision of an emergency medication kit in the home setting. *Am J Hospice Palliative Med.* 2015;32:484-489.

Stettler A, Zulian GB. Unexpected side effect of methylnaltrexone. *J Palliative Med.* 2013;16:1168.

SUGGESTED READINGS

Balaban RB. A physician's guide to talking about end-of-life care. *J Gen Intern Med.* 2000;15(3):195-200. www.ncbi.nlm.nih.gov/pmc/articles/PMC1495357/. Accessed April 2016.

Coyle N, Manna R, Johnson Shen M, et al. A communication skills training module for oncology nurses. *Clin J Oncol Nurs.* 2015;19(6):697-702.

SELECTED WEBSITES (ACCESSED 2017)

American Academy of Hospice and Palliative Medicine, www.aahpm.org

Choosing Wisely, www.choosingwisely.org/

Department of Health and Human Services, Administration for Community Living, www.aoa.acl.gov/AoA_Programs/Tools_Resources/diversity.aspx and www.aoa.acl.gov/AoA_Programs/Tools_Resources/diversity.aspx#cultural

National Hospice and Palliative Care Organization, www.nhpco.org

National Institute on Aging, Working with Diverse Older Patients, www.nia.nih.gov/health/publication/talking-your-older-patient/working-diverse-older-patients

PART III

Selected Internet Resources on Geriatrics

ORGANIZATIONS

AARP (formerly American Association of Retired Persons)	www.aarp.org
Administration for Community Living	https://aoa.aci.gov
Alzheimer's Association	www.alz.org
Alzheimer's Disease Education and Referral Center	www.nia.nih.gov/alzheimers
AMDA—The Society for Post-Acute and Long-Term Care Medicine	www.paltc.org
American Academy of Home Care Medicine	www.aahcm.org
American Academy of Pain Medicine	www.painmed.org
American Geriatrics Society	www.americangeriatrics.org
American Geriatrics Society Foundation for Health in Aging	www.healthinaging.org
American Health Care Association	www.ahca.org
American Pain Society	www.americanpainsociety.org
American Parkinson Disease Association	www.apdaparkinson.org
American Society of Consultant Pharmacists	www.ascp.com
American Society on Aging	www.asaging.org
A Place for Mom	www.aplaceformom.com
Arthritis Foundation	www.arthritis.org
British Geriatrics Society	www.bgs.org.uk
Canadian Geriatrics Society	www.canadiangeriatrics.ca
Centers for Disease Control and Prevention	www.cdc.gov
Center to Advance Palliative Care	www.capc.org
Geriatric Fast Facts	www.geriatricfastfacts.com
Gerontological Advanced Practice Nurses Association	www.gapna.org
Gerontological Society of America	www.geron.org
LeadingAge	www.leadingage.org
Medicare	www.medicare.gov
National Adult Vaccination Program	www.navp.org
National Association for Continence	www.nafc.org
National Association of Area Agencies on Aging	www.n4a.org
National Association of Directors of Nursing Administration in Long-Term Care	www.nadona.org

National Association of Nutrition and Aging Services Programs — www.nanasp.org

National Council on Aging — www.ncoa.org

National Institute on Aging — www.nia.nih.gov

National Parkinson Foundation — www.parkinson.org

Nurses Improving Care for Healthsystem Elders — www.nicheprogram.org

CLINICAL TOPICS—FOR PROFESSIONALS

ADVANCE CARE PLANNING

Coalition for Compassionate Care of California — http://coalitionccc.org

The Conversation Project — http://theconversationproject.org

Decision Guide: Go to the Hospital or Stay Here? — www.decisionguide.org

National Hospice and Palliative Care Organization, Caring Connections educational materials — www.nhpco.org

National POLST Paradigm, POLST (Physician Orders for Life-Sustaining Treatment) form — http://polst.org

ALZHEIMER DISEASE

2014–2015 Alzheimer's Disease Progress Report: Advancing Research Toward a Cure — www.nia.nih.gov/alzheimers/publication/2014-2015-alzheimers-disease-progress-report/introduction

CARE TRANSITIONS

Bridge Model — www.transitionalcare.org/the-bridge-model

Care Transitions Program — www.caretransitions.org

Interventions to Reduce Acute Care Transfers (INTERACT) — https://interact.fau.edu

National POLST Paradigm, POLST (Physician Orders for Life-Sustaining Treatment) form — http://polst.org

Project Re-Engineered Discharge (Project RED) — www.bu.edu/fammed/projectred

Society of Hospital Medicine, Better Outcomes by Optimizing Safe Transitions (BOOST) program — www.hospitalmedicine.org/Web/Quality_Innovation/Mentored_Implementation/Project_BOOST/About_BOOST.aspx

Transitional Care Model — www.transitionalcare.info

DELIRIUM

American Delirium Society

www.americandeliriumsociety.org

Hospital Elder Life Program (HELP) for Prevention of Delirium

www.hospitalelderlifeprogram.org

DIABETES CARE

American Diabetes Association home page for health care professionals

http://professional.diabetes.org/?loc=bb-dorg

FALL PREVENTION

Centers for Disease Control and Prevention, STEADI (Stopping Elderly Accidents, Deaths and Injuries)

www.cdc.gov/steadi

GENERAL

ABIM Foundation, Choosing Wisely campaign

www.abimfoundation.org

Alternative Medications for Medications in the Use of High-Risk Medications in the Elderly and Potentially Harmful Drug–Disease Interactions in the Elderly Quality Measures

http://onlinelibrary.wiley.com/doi/10.1111/jgs.13807/full

American Geriatrics Society 2015 Updated Beers Criteria for Potentially Inappropriate Medication Use in Older Adults

http://onlinelibrary.wiley.com/doi/10.1111/jgs.13702/full

Guiding Principles for the Care of Older Adults with Multimorbidity: An Approach for Clinicians

www.ncbi.nlm.nih.gov/pmc/articles/PMC4450364

GERIATRIC EMERGENCY DEPARTMENT

Geriatrics Emergency Medicine training for health professionals

www.geri-em.com

GERIATRICS EDUCATION

The Portal of Geriatrics Online Education

www.pogoe.org

HEALTHY AGING

Centers for Disease Control and Prevention, The State of Aging and Health in America

www.cdc.gov/aging/data/stateofaging.htm

HEARING IMPAIRMENT

American Academy of Audiology, Hearing Loss

www.audiology.org

LOW VISION

American Academy of Ophthalmology

www.aao.org

American Glaucoma Society

www.glaucomaweb.org

Foundation Fighting Blindness

www.blindness.org

Macular Degeneration Foundation www.eyesight.org
Macular Degeneration Partnership www.amd.org

MEDICATIONS
American Society of Consultant Pharmacists www.ascp.com

PACE PROGRAM
Medicaid.gov, Program of All-Inclusive Care for www.medicaid.gov/medicaid/
the Elderly (PACE) ltss/pace/index.html

PAIN MANAGEMENT
American Society for Pain Management Nursing www.aspmn.org
Pharmacological Management of Persistent Pain in www.americangeriatrics
Older Persons, American Geriatrics Society Panel on .org/files/documents/2009_
the Pharmacological Management of Persistent Pain Guideline.pdf
in Older Persons (PDF)

PALLIATIVE CARE
GeriPal: A Geriatrics and Palliative Care Blog www.geripal.org

PARKINSON DISEASE
American Parkinson Disease Association www.apdaparkinson.org

URINARY INCONTINENCE
National Association for Continence www.nafc.org

CLINICAL TOPICS—FOR PATIENTS

ALZHEIMER DISEASE
National Institute on Aging, Alzheimer's Disease www.nia.nih.gov/Alzheimers/
Fact Sheet Publications/adfact.htm

DEPRESSION
Depression and Bipolar Support Alliance www.ndmda.org
National Institute of Mental Health, Older Adults www.nimh.nih.gov/health/
and Depression publications/older-adults-and-
depression/index.shtml

GENERAL
Aging with Dignity, Five Wishes www.agingwithdignity
.org/5wishes.html
American Geriatrics Society Foundation, Health www.healthinaging.org
in Aging

A Place for Mom, Nursing Home Checklist	http://nursing-homes .aplaceformom.com/articles/ nursing-home-checklist
Medicare.gov, Nursing Home Compare	www.medicare.gov/ nhcompare/home.asp

HEARING IMPAIRMENT

Healthy Hearing	www.healthyhearing.com

LOW VISION

American Macular Degeneration Foundation	www.macular.org
Glaucoma Research Foundation, What is Glaucoma?	www.glaucoma.org/glaucoma
Macular Degeneration Foundation	www.eyesight.org
Macular Degeneration Partnership	www.amd.org
National Eye Institute, Facts About Age-Related Macular Degeneration	https://nei.nih.gov/health/ maculardegen/armd_facts

MEDICATIONS

AMDA—The Society for Post-Acute and Long-Term Care Medicine, Top 10 Particularly Dangerous Drug Interactions in Post-Acute /Long-Term Care	www.paltc.org/top-10- particularly-dangerous-drug- interactions-paltc

PAIN MANAGEMENT

Pain (PDQ): Supportive Care-Patients Geriatric Pain, developed by Keela Herr at the University of Iowa	https://geriatricpain.org/

PARKINSON DISEASE

National Institutes of Health, Parkinson's Disease information page	https://nihseniorhealth .gov/parkinsonsdisease/ whatisparkinsonsdisease/01 .html

APPENDIX

INDEX

Page numbers followed by *f* indicate figures; *t* indicate tables.

AAA. *See* abdominal aortic aneurysm
AAPCC. *See* adjusted average per capita cost
AARP International, 519
abdominal aortic aneurysm (AAA), 111*t*
acarbose, 4
ACC. *See* American College of Cardiology
Accountable Care Organizations (ACOs), 430
   in chronic disease management, 103
ACD. *See* anemia of chronic disease
ACE inhibitors. *See* angiotensin-converting
      enzyme inhibitors
acetaminophen, 161
ACOs. *See* Accountable Care Organizations
ACOVE. *See* Assessment Care of Vulnerable Elders
acquired immunodeficiency syndrome (AIDS), 361
activities of daily living (ADLs), 30–31
   assessment for, 62
   day care for, 465
   Medicare and, 31*f*, 449*f*
   NH and, 39*t*
   RUGs and, 456
   stroke and, 317
acute incontinence, 207, 219
acute myocardial infarction (AMI).
      See myocardial infarction
acute pain, 282
acyclovir, 370
AD. *See* Alzheimer disease
ADA. *See* American Diabetes Association
adherence, with medications, 407–410, 410*t*
adjusted average per capita cost (AAPCC), 434
ADLs. *See* activities of daily living
Administration for Community Living, 441
Administration on Aging (AoA), 441
ADRC. *See* Aging and Disability Resource Centers
β-adrenergic antagonists, for IHSS, 322
α-adrenergic blockers
   for BPH, 232
   for overflow incontinence, 233
β-adrenergic blockers, for atrial fibrillation, 323
ADs. *See* advance directives
adult foster care, 449–450
advance directives (ADs), 25, 164, 502–508
   in chronic disease management, 83
   geriatric consultation and, 70
   PSDA for, 514
advanced care planning, 164, 502
adverse drug reactions, 410–416, 412*t*–415*t*
   confusion from, 141
   dementia and, 152*t*
   in NH, 40
   from ophthalmic solutions, 387*t*

AFDC. *See* Aid to Families with Dependent Children
Affordable Care Act. *See* Patient Protection
      and Affordable Care Act
African Americans. *See* blacks
ageism, 107
age-related macular degeneration (AMD), 385–388
aggression
   with cognitive impairment, 141
   with vascular depression, 172–173
aging
   anabolic hormones and, 356–357
   biological, 16–17
   BMI and, 65–66
   cardiovascular disease and, 301
   chronic disease management and, 33
   chronological, 4
   defined, 3
   depression and, 170–173, 172*t*
   diabetes and, 335–336
   disability and, 24–25
   disease and, 15–16
   environmental factors and, 5, 18
   frailty and, 12–13
   hallmarks of, 6–12, 7*t*–10*t*
   hearing impairment and, 390, 392, 393*t*
   hyperparathyroidism and, 355
   instability and, 243–246
   kidneys and, 418*t*
   loss in, 18
   medications and, 416–419, 416*t*
   multimorbidity and, 14
   normal, 4, 5–6
   orthopedic problems and, 30
   process of, 3–5
   resilience and, 13–14
   retirement and, 18
   sensory impairment and, 30
   sleep and, 177
   taste and, 401
   UI and, 205
   variability in, 18
   workers and, 23, 24*f*
Aging and Disability Resource Centers
      (ADRCs), 441, 466
agitation
   with cognitive impairment, 141
   with delirium, 143
   with depression, 180
   with serotonin syndrome, 194
AHA. *See* American Heart Association
Aid to Families with Dependent
      Children (AFDC), 438, 441

AIDS. *See* acquired immunodeficiency syndrome
akathisia, from psychotropic drugs, 422
alcohol
    abuse, screening for, 114*t*, 121
    atrial fibrillation and, 323
    confusion from, 141
    dementia and, 151, 152*t*
    depression and, 180
    diet and, 360
    falls and, 249
    geriatric consultation and, 70
    hypertension and, 304
    normal aging and, 5
    polyneuropathy and, 401–402
    Pra and, 70
    UI from, 209*t*
aldosterone blockers
    for CHF, 325
    for MI, 319
alexithymia, 173
allopurinol, 271
alpha blockers, 249
alpha tocopherol, 129
Alzheimer disease (AD), 153–154
    death from, 24, 27, 28*f*
    depression and, 178
    diagnosis of, 150*t*–151*t*
    medications for, 161–162
    prevention of, 128–129
Alzheimer's Association, 121, 128, 162, 163
amantadine, 275
ambulatory care, for geriatric patients, 36, 37*t*
AMD. *See* age-related macular degeneration
American Academy of Neurology, 313
American Academy of Orthopaedic Surgeons, 251
American Cancer Society, 120
American College of Cardiology (ACC), 126–127
    on hypertension, 306
American College of Physicians, 99, 100*t*
American College of Surgeons, 72
American Diabetes Association (ADA), 335, 336
American Geriatrics Society, 17
    Choosing Wisely of, 99, 100*t*, 527
    on falls, 251
    on pain management, 281
    on preoperative evaluations, 72, 73*t*
American Heart Association (AHA), 126–127
    on hypertension, 306
    on stroke, 312, 313
American Thoracic Society, 369
aminoglycosides, 395
anabolic hormones, 356–357
anemia
    depression and, 178, 185
    fatigue from, 51
    malnutrition and, 66
    stem cell exhaustion and, 11
    vitality decrease and, 357–361, 358*t*
anemia of chronic disease (ACD), 359
    Epo and, 361
anesthesia, 74

angina pectoris, 317
angiotensin-converting enzyme
      inhibitors (ACE inhibitors)
    atrial fibrillation and, 323
    for CHF, 325
    diabetes and, 343
    for hypertension, 308–310, 315
    for MI, 319
    UI from, 209*t*
angiotensin-receptor blockers (ARBs), 308, 310
    aging and, 4
    atrial fibrillation and, 323
    for CHF, 325
    diabetes and, 343
    for heart failure, 325
angle-closure glaucoma, 385
anhedonia, 185
anhidrosis, 372
ankle-brachial index, 326, 326*t*
Annual Wellness Visit, Medicare and,
      67, 69*t*–70*t*, 109, 119*t*
    for psychosocial problems, 121
ANP. *See* atrial natriuretic peptide
antibiotics, 367
    hearing impairment from, 395
anticholinergics
    for nausea and vomiting, 535
    UI from, 209*t*
anticoagulants
    for atrial fibrillation, 323
    for cardiovascular disease prevention, 126–127
    for stroke, 313
anticonvulsants, 285
antidepressants, 190–198, 191*t*–193*t*, 196*t*.
    See also tricyclic antidepressants
    for bipolar affective disorder, 198
    falls and, 249
    treatment approaches for, 193*t*
antiemetics, 535
antihistamines, 535
antimuscarinic drugs, 228–232
antinuclear antibody, 401
antioxidants
    AMD and, 387
    vitamins as, 362
antiplatelet therapy, 327
antipsychotics, 420–423, 420*t*
    for bipolar affective disorder, 198
    for dementia, 161
    for depression, 192*t*–193*t*
    falls and, 249
    immobility from, 265
    UI from, 209*t*
antithrombotic therapy, 323
antitumor agents, 67*t*
anxiety
    in EOL, 537
    falls and, 249
    hearing loss and, 393*t*
    PD and, 275
    weight loss from, 51

AoA. *See* Administration on Aging
aortic stenosis
  calcium and, 319–321
  falls and, 254
  preoperative evaluation for, 74
apathy
  with cognitive impairment, 141
  with delirium, 143
  with depression, 178
  immobility and, 265
  screening for, 121, 123*t*
apixaban, 323
appendicitis, 367
appetite, in EOL, 535–536
ARBs. *See* angiotensin-receptor blockers
Area Agency on Aging, 163
  day care and, 465
  HCBS and, 462
arginine vasopressin (AVP), 205–207
arthritis. *See also* osteoarthritis
  ambulatory care for, 37*t*
  depression and, 172
  rheumatoid, 361
aspiration pneumonia
  PD and, 275
  PVD and, 327
  stroke and, 316
aspirin
  cardiovascular disease and, 114*t*
  for cardiovascular disease prevention, 126–127
  hearing impairment from, 395
  for hip fractures, 273
  for MI, 318
  for stable angina, 317
  for stroke, 313, 315
assessment
  for ADLs, 62
  of cognitive impairment, 64, 139–141, 140*t*
  of delirium, 139–141
  of dementia, 139–141, 155–159, 157*t*, 159*t*
  for falls, 251–254
  for function, 17
  functional
    geriatric consultation and, 70
    for geriatric patients, 59–64, 61*t*, 62*t*
  of geriatric patients, 43–76, 45*f*, 46*t*
    caregiver assessment for, 75–76, 75*t*
    with chronic disease management, 89
    for environmental factors, 64
    functional assessment for, 59–64, 61*t*, 62*t*
    geriatric consultation for, 67–72, 71*t*–72*t*
    laboratory tests for, 57–59, 58*t*
    for malnutrition, 65–67, 67*t*
    Medicare and, 67
    Medicare Annual Wellness
      Visit and, 67, 69*t*–70*t*
    in NH, 475–482, 478*t*–481*t*
    for pain, 64–65, 65*t*, 66*f*
    patient history for, 47–54, 48*t*–50*t*
    physical examination for, 54–57, 55*t*–57*t*
    for physical functioning, 62–64, 62*t*

preoperative evaluation for, 72–74, 73*t*
  for prevention, 108*t*
  screening questions for, 52*t*–53*t*
  for weight, 65–66, 67*t*
of hearing, 391–392, 391*t*, 392*t*
of hypertension, 303–304, 303*t*
of immobility, 267–269, 268*t*
of outpatient geriatric patients, 45
of UI, 212–219, 213*t*, 222*f*
Assessment Care of Vulnerable Elders
    (ACOVE), 102, 102*t*
  for falls, 251
assisted living, 449, 458–459
  NH and, 454
atherosclerosis
  diabetes and, 343
  hypertension and, 303–304
  infective endocarditis and, 368
atrial fibrillation, 16, 322–323
  heart failure and, 325
  hypothyroidism and, 352
  IHSS and, 322
  stroke and, 314, 315
atrial natriuretic peptide (ANP), 205–207, 324
auditory system, 390, 391*t*
autonomy, 499
AVP. *See* arginine vasopressin

back pain, 114*t*
bacteriuria, 369–370
  screening for, 114*t*
  UI and, 215–217
balance. *See also* gait and balance assessment
  diet and, 267
  falls and, 125, 246
  immobility and, 265
  muscle weakness and, 246
  NH and, 38
  physical activity for, 295
barbiturates, 356
bariatric surgery, 365
basic activities of daily living, frailty and, 12
Beck Depression Inventory (BDI), 122*t*
bed rest
  immobility and, 263
  risk factors with, 133, 134*t*
Beers Criteria, 134, 415
behavior change, for prevention, 124
behavioral disturbances, NH and, 40
beneficence, 499
benign prostatic hyperplasia (BPH)
  UI and, 205, 212, 232
  urinary tract infections and, 366
bereavement, depression and, 170, 173
Berwick, Donald, 430
best practices
  for function, 17
  health span and, 4
beta-blockers
  for atrial fibrillation, 323
  cardiovascular disease and, 23–24

beta-blockers (*Cont.*):
  for cardiovascular disease prevention, 127
  for CHF, 325
  for heart failure, 325
  for hypertension, 307–308, 315
  for hypothyroidism, 351–352
  for MI, 319
  for stable angina, 317
bethanechol, 233
bevacizumab, 388
biofeedback, 224
biological aging
  function and, 17
  person-centered care and, 16–17
biopsychosocial needs, 17
bipolar affective disorder, 170–171
  management of, 195–198
bisphosphonates
  cardiovascular disease and, 24
  normal aging and, 5
  for osteoporosis prevention, 128, 129*t*
blacks (African Americans)
  AD in, 153
  cultural competence for, 94
  life expectancy of, 28
  prostate cancer in, 357
  women, frailty of, 13
bladder
  cancer of
    obesity and, 365
    screening for, 115*t*
  normal urination and, 202–203
  UI and, 205, 210–211, 211*t*
bladder record, for UI, 213–214, 215*f*
bladder retraining, 225*t*, 226–227, 227*t*
bladder training, 221–222, 225*t*
blindness, 382–389
blood urea nitrogen (BUN), 356
body mass index (BMI), 125, 336
  aging and, 65–66
BPH. *See* benign prostatic hyperplasia
bradycardia, 127
bradykinesia, 422
breast cancer
  obesity and, 365
  screening for, 111*t*, 115*t*
BUN. *See* blood urea nitrogen
bupropion, 190, 195
burden-of-illness measures, for chronic
    disease management, 89

CAD. *See* coronary artery disease
caffeine, 209, 209*t*
calcium
  aortic stenosis and, 319–321
  hyperparathyroidism and, 355
  mitral annulus and, 321
  normal aging and, 5
  for osteoporosis prevention, 128
  vitality decrease and, 361–362

calcium channel blockers
  for hypertension, 308, 315
  for stable angina, 317
  UI from, 209*t*
caloric intake, 364
CAM. *See* complementary and alternative
    medicine; confusion assessment method
Canadian Study of Health and
    Aging (CSHA), 12–13
cancer. *See also specific types*
  death from, 27, 28*f*
  NH and, 39*t*
  obesity and, 365
  prevention of, 120–121
  telomerase inhibitors for, 11
  weight loss from, 51
carbamazepine, 198
cardiac arrhythmias, 322–324
  falls and, 250, 252
  hypothermia and, 372
  OSA and, 177
cardiac output
  cardiovascular disease and, 301
  depression and, 178
  stress and, 6
cardiovascular disease, 301–327, 326*t*–327*t*
  aging and, 301
  aspirin and, 114*t*
  cardiac output and, 301
  CVD and, 326
  death from, 27, 28*f*
  decreases in, 23–24
  falls and, 248
  prevention of, 126–127
  screening for, 114*t*
  statins for, 5
Cardiovascular Health Study, 13
cardiovascular system
  aging and, 7*t*
  stress and, 6
CARE. *See* Continuity Assessment
    Record and Evaluation
caregivers, 32
  for chronic disease management, 89
  clinical glidepath and, 87
  day care and, 465
  defined, 447
  for dementia, 159, 162–163, 446–447
  depression of, 173
  elder abuse by, 516–518, 517*t*–518*t*
    cognitive impairment and, 70
    emergency room visits and, 72
    Pra and, 70
    screening for, 116*t*
  ethics for, 515–516
  geriatric patient assessment and, 51
  motivation of, 60
  stress on, 75–76, 75*t*, 449, 451*t*
  UI and, 225*t*, 227–228
carisoprodol, 285

carotid artery stenosis (CAS), 111t
carotid endarterectomy, 316
carotid sinus sensitivity, 250
CAS. *See* carotid artery stenosis
case management
    in chronic disease management, 87–89
    in LTC, 466–468, 467t
case managers, 88
cataracts, 383–384, 384t
catechol-O-methyltransferase inhibitors, 275
catheters
    for UI, 219, 234–235, 235t
    urinary tract infections from, 366
CBC. *See* complete blood count
CBT. *See* cognitive behavior therapy
CDC. *See* Center for Disease
        Control and Prevention
cell-mediated immunity, 366–367
cells, 11
cellular senescence, 10t, 11
centenarians, 11
Center for Disease Control and
        Prevention (CDC), 285
    on cataracts, 383
    on diabetic retinopathy, 388
    on glaucoma, 384
    on infections, 368
Center for Epidemiologic Studies Depression
        Scale (CES-D), 122t, 184
Centers for Medicare & Medicaid
        Services (CMS), 161, 437, 466
    on NH, 467, 483
central adiposity, 66
central nervous system (CNS)
    falls and, 250
    hyperthermia and, 372
    SIADH and, 356
cerumen, 395
cervical cancer, 112t, 120
CES-D. *See* Center for Epidemiologic
        Studies Depression Scale
CHD. *See* coronary heart disease
chemotherapy, 121
CHF. *See* congestive heart failure
chloramphenicol, 359
chlorpropamide, 356
chlorzoxazone, 285
cholesterol, screening for, 114t
cholinesterase inhibitors, 123
    for AD, 161–162
    falls and, 249
    UI from, 209t
chondroitin
    for degenerative bone disease prevention, 128
    for OA, 270
Choosing Wisely, 99, 100t, 527
chore worker, 466
chromatin, 11
chronic disease management, 3, 79–103, 80t
    ACOVE for, 102, 102t

aging and, 33
caregivers for, 89
case management in, 87–89
clinical glidepath for, 84–87, 86f
computer technology for, 99–102
cultural competence in, 94–95
decision making in, 92–94, 93t
for diabetes, 343, 347
EOL in, 83–84
expected and actual care for, 81–82, 82f
hospitalization in, 93
increases for, 27
infections and, 367
long-term care (LTC) for, 88, 463f
LTC for, 447, 463f
Medicare for, 33f, 88–89
multimorbidity with, 79, 80–81, 80f
in NH, 80, 94
outcomes of, 95–98, 96t–98t
teams for, 89–91, 91t, 92t
technology for, 98–102
transitional care for, 82–83
variation in, 99
chronic kidney disease (CKD)
    EPO for, 360–361
    multimorbidity and, 14
chronic obstructive pulmonary disease (COPD)
    ambulatory care for, 37t
    death from, 27, 28f
    hospitalization for, 33, 34f
    screening for, 115t
chronic pain, 282
    herpes zoster and, 120
chronological aging, 4
cilostazol, 327
CIND. *See* cognitive impairment, not dementia
citalopram, 190
CKD. *See* chronic kidney disease
Clinical Frailty Scale, 12–13, 528
clinical pathways, 87
Clock Drawing Test, 501
clonidine, 310
clopidogrel
    for MI, 318
    for PVD, 327
    for stroke, 315
Clostridium difficile, 133, 369
CMS. *See* Centers for Medicare
        & Medicaid Services
CNS. *See* central nervous system
cocaine, 304
cochlear implants, 399, 400t
cognitive behavior therapy (CBT), 189, 423
cognitive impairment, 15–16. *See also*
        Alzheimer disease; delirium; dementia
    with antidepressants, 190
    assessment of, 64, 139–141, 140t
    competence and, 500–502
    delirium and, 149t
    depression and, 170

cognitive impairment (*Cont.*):
  differential diagnosis for, 141–143
  elder abuse and, 70
  falls and, 246
  in geriatric syndromes, 15
  hearing loss and, 393*t*
  immobility and, 265
  NH and, 38, 39*t*, 457
  prevention of, 128–129
  from psychotropic drugs, 422
  reversible conditions for, 152*t*
  screening for, 121–123
cognitive impairment, not dementia (CIND), 142
colchicine, for gout, 271–273
colorectal cancer
  fiber and, 364
  NSAIDs and, 114*t*
  obesity and, 365
  screening for, 112*t*, 120
community-acquired pneumonia, 367
comorbid illness. *See* multimorbidity
compensatory care, 429
competence, 500–502
complementary and alternative medicine (CAM)
  for delirium, 145, 145*t*
  for depression, 187*t*
complete blood count (CBC)
  for infections, 369
  for polyneuropathy, 401
compression of morbidity, 4, 28
computer technology, for chronic
    disease management, 99–102
confusion, 141
  stress and, 6
  sundowning with, 147
confusion assessment method (CAM), 139–140
congestive heart failure (CHF)
  ambulatory care for, 37*t*
  confusion from, 141
  fatigue from, 51
  hospitalization and, 133
  hyperthyroidism and, 354
  immobility and, 265
  malnutrition and, 67*t*
  medications for, 325
  preoperative evaluation for, 73–74
  UI and, 209
  weight loss from, 51
Consensus Development Conference, 60
constipation
  depression and, 178
  diet for, 236–237
  fecal impaction and, 236
  fecal incontinence and, 236
  immobility and, 267
  medications for, 238*t*
  from opioids, in EOL, 531–535
consumer-directed care, 462

Continuity Assessment Record and
  Evaluation (CARE), 63–64
COPD. *See* chronic obstructive pulmonary disease
Cornell Depression Scale, 182, 184
Cornell Scale for Depression in Dementia, 122*t*
coronary artery bypass graft, 317–318
  hospitalization for, 33
  preoperative evaluation for, 74
coronary artery disease (CAD)
  heart failure and, 325
  multimorbidity and, 14
  subclinical hyperthyroidism and, 347
coronary heart disease (CHD)
  screening for, 112*t*
  subclinical hypothyroidism and, 352
corticosteroids
  for gout, 271
  for HZ, 370
  for pain, 285
corticotrophin, 271
cough, in EOL, 536
Coumadin. *See* warfarin
COX-2. *See* cyclooxygenase-2 selective inhibitors
CPK. *See* creatinine phosphokinase
creatinine, 6, 356
creatinine phosphokinase (CPK), 351
CSHA. *See* Canadian Study of Health and Aging
cultural competence
  in chronic disease management, 94–95
  in palliative care, 529–530, 530*t*
cyclobenzaprine, 285
cyclooxygenase-2 selective inhibitors (COX-2), 285
cyclosporine, 304
CYP. *See* cytochrome P450
cystoceles, 214–215, 218*f*
cytochrome P450 (CYP), 194, 417

dabigatran, 323
day care, 469
death. *See also* end-of-life care
  from Alzheimer disease, 24
  from bacteriuria, 369
  from cardiovascular disease, 24
  from falls, 243
  frailty and, 12, 13
  from infections, 367
  leading causes of, 24, 25*f*, 27, 28*f*
  from obesity, 365
degenerative joint disease. *See also* arthritis
  falls and, 246
  prevention of, 127–128
dehydration
  delirium and, 149*t*
  depression and, 178
  falls and, 252
  NH and, 40
delirium, 139–164
  assessment of, 139–141
  common causes of, 147–148, 147*t*

complementary and alternative
  medicine for, 145, 145*t*
depression and, 145, 146*t*
diagnostic criteria for, 143–144, 143*t*
in EOL, 537
hearing loss and, 393*t*
hypo- and hyperactive, 143
from medications, 148, 148*t*
precipitating factors for, 144*t*
predisposing factors for, 144*t*
psychosis and, 145, 146*t*
risk factors for, 149*t*
dementia, 139–164. *See also* Alzheimer disease
alcohol and, 151, 152*t*
assessment of, 139–141, 155–159, 157*t*, 159*t*
bipolar affective disorder and, 171
caregivers for, 159, 162–163, 447–448
causes of, 152*t*
clinical features of, 154*t*
competence and, 501
confusion from, 141
decreases in, 23
defined, 149
depression and, 172, 178
diagnosis of, 150*t*–151*t*
EOL for, 513–514
functional incontinence and, 212
management of, 159–165, 160*t*, 164*t*–165*t*
medications for, 161–162
patient history for, 157–158
PD and, 275
physical examination for, 158
prevention of, 128–129, 162
psychotropic drugs for, 422
reminiscence therapy for, 462
reversible conditions for, 152*t*
screening for, 112*t*, 123
symptoms of, 156–157, 156*t*
types of, 152–155
UI and, 203
urgency incontinence and, 229–231
dementia with Lewy bodies (DLB), 152–153
demethylchlortetracycline, 356
dental disease, 67*t*
depression, 169–198. *See also* antidepressants
aging and, 170–173, 172*t*
ambulatory care for, 37*t*
causes of, 172, 172*t*
with chronic disease management, 89
with cognitive impairment, 141
delirium and, 145, 146*t*
dementia and, 152*t*
diabetes and, 336
in EOL, 537
falls and, 249
fatigue from, 51
geriatric consultation for, 71*t*
in geriatric syndromes, 15
hearing loss and, 393*t*

immobility and, 265
insomnia and, 174–177, 176*t*, 423
malnutrition and, 67*t*
management of, 186–198, 198*t*
from medications, 178, 180*t*
medications for, 188
multimorbidity with, 177–178, 179*t*
PD and, 275
screening for, 115*t*, 121, 122*t*,
  169–170, 180–185, 184*t*–185*t*
signs and symptoms of, 173–178, 175*t*
suicide and, 170, 171*t*
weight loss from, 51
depressive pseudodementia, 151–152
desipramine, 195–196
deterioration, in normal aging, 5–6
detrusor hyperactivity with impaired
  contractility (DHIC), 211
diabetes
aging and, 335–336
ambulatory care for, 37*t*
anabolic hormones and, 356
chronic disease management for, 343, 347
CVD and, 326
death from, 28*f*
depression and, 178
diet for, 110
heart failure and, 325
hospitalization for, 348*f*–349*f*
hypertension and, 305, 306
immobility and, 265
infections and, 366
medications for, 337–338, 339*t*–342*t*
multimorbidity with, 14, 343, 344*t*–346*t*
NH and, 39*t*
obesity and, 335, 337
polyneuropathy and, 401–402
preoperative evaluation for, 74
screening for, 116*t*
stroke and, 312, 314
vitality decrease and, 335–347, 344*t*–347*t*
diabetic ketoacidosis (DKA), 347
diabetic neuropathy, 212
diabetic retinopathy, 388–389
diagnosis-related groups (DRGs), 433, 435
NH and, 457
diarrhea, in EOL, 535
diet (nutrition). *See also* malnutrition
aging and, 18
alcohol and, 360
AMD and, 387
for cognitive impairment prevention, 128–129
for constipation, 236–237
depression and, 178
for diabetes, 110
food additives and, 364
functional deficit and, 362–363
for hypertension, 306–307
immobility and, 267

diet (nutrition) (*Cont.*):
   normal aging and, 5
   obesity and, 126
   for prevention, 109, 125–126
   screening for, 116*t*
   vitality decrease and, 361–365
Dietary Guidelines for Americans, 125
dietary supplements, 363
   herbal, 304
digoxin
   for atrial fibrillation, 323–324
   beta-blockers and, 127
   for CHF, 325
   for heart failure, 325
   malnutrition and, 67*t*
diltiazem, 127
   for atrial fibrillation, 323
disability
   aging and, 24–25
   assisted living for, 462–463
   from falls, 243
   geriatric consultation for, 71*t*
   of geriatric patients, 28–31
   handicap and, 29
   life expectancy and, 28
   NH and, 454, 456*f*
   prevalence of, 448–449, 449*f*
   prevention of, 129–131
   rates of, 24
disease. *See also* chronic disease management
   aging and, 15–16
   frailty and, 12
   management of, 88
   in NH, 476*t*
diuretics
   for heart failure, 325
   thiazide, for hypertension, 307–308, 307*t*, 315
   UI from, 209*t*
divalproex sodium, 198
diverticulosis, 358
dizziness
   falls and, 248, 249
   prevention of, 107
DKA. *See* diabetic ketoacidosis
DLB. *See* dementia with Lewy bodies
DNA, 6, 10*t*
donepezil, 162
dopamine, 274, 275
dopamine agonists, 275
dopaminergic agents, 275
DRGs. *See* diagnosis-related groups
drop attacks, 249
drugs. *See* medications
duloxetine, 190, 195, 232, 402
durable power of attorney, 503, 504*t*, 505
dyslipidemia, 343
dyspnea (shortness of breath), 51, 59, 323
   in EOL, 536

EASY. *See* Exercise and Screening for You
ECG. *See* electrocardiogram

echocardiography
   for IHSS, 322
   for mitral annulus calcification, 321
ECT. *See* electroconvulsive therapy
Eden Alternative, 462
effective care, 99
Eighth Joint National Committee
      (JNC8), 305
elder abuse, 516–518, 517*t*–518*t*
   cognitive impairment and, 70
   emergency room visits and, 72
   Pra and, 70
   screening for, 116*t*
electrocardiogram (ECG)
   for hypertension, 304
   for hypothermia, 371
   for mitral valve prolapse, 322
   for stroke, 313
electroconvulsive therapy (ECT)
   for bipolar affective disorder, 198
   for depression, 187*t*, 189–190
electrolytes
   depression and, 178
   hypothermia and, 372
electromyography (EMG), 224
emergency room visits, elder abuse and, 72
EMG. *See* electromyography
encephalitis, 152*t*
endocrine system, aging and, 9*t*
end-of-life care (EOL), 3
   ADs and, 505–506
   anxiety in, 537
   appetite in, 535–536
   care choices for, 525*t*
   in chronic disease management, 83–84
   cough in, 536
   delirium in, 537
   for dementia, 513–514
   depression in, 537
   diarrhea in, 535
   ethics of, 411, 508–514
   family and, 509–512
   hallucinations in, 537
   nausea and vomiting in, 535
   in NH, 512–513
   opioid-induced constipation in, 531–535
   pain management in, 531, 534*t*
   palliative care for, 523–538
   physicians in, 509–512
   shortness of breath in, 536
   slow medicine in, 526–527
   symptom management in, 511*t*
   weight loss in, 535–536
End-of-Life Care for the Elderly, 537
environmental factors
   aging and, 5, 18
   dementia from, 152*t*
   disability from, 30
   in disability prevention, 120
   for falls, 246–248, 248*t*, 259
   geriatric consultation and, 70

geriatric patient assessment of, 64
    for immobility, 263
EOL. *See* end-of-life care
epigenetic alteration, aging and, 10*t*
eplerenone, 310
EPO. *See* erythropoietin
ePrognosis, 89
erythropoietin (EPO), 360–361
escitalopram, 190
estrogen
    for dementia prevention, 162
    for stress incontinence, 232–233
    UI and, 205
ethacrynic acid, 395
ethanol, 359
ethics
    ADs and, 502–508
    advance care planning and, 502
    for caregivers, 515–516
    competence and, 500–502
    of EOL, 411, 508–514
    geriatric patients and, 499–520
    informed consent and, 500–502
    international aspects of, 518–519
    for NH, 495–496, 496*t*
    policy issues with, 514–515
    principles of, 499–500, 500*t*
European Association for Palliative Care, 537
Evercare, 461
executive function
    dementia and, 150
    depression and, 185, 188
Executive Interview, 501
exercise. *See* physical activity
Exercise and Screening for You (EASY), 125
exhaustion, frailty and, 12
ezetimibe, for MI, 319

Faces Pain Scale-Revised (FPS-R), 66*f*
falls, 243–259, 259*t*–260*t*
    assessment for, 251–254
    balance and, 125, 246
    causes of, 246–251, 247*t*
    death from, 243
    disability from, 243
    environmental factors for, 246–248, 248*t*, 259
    frailty and, 13
    gait, 254, 255*t*
    gait and balance assessment for,
        246, 254, 255*t*–256*t*, 401
    hearing loss and, 393*t*
    immobility and, 243, 267
    management of, 257–259, 257*t*–259*t*
    medications and, 249–250
    in NH, 39*t*, 40, 243, 248*t*
    patient history for, 251, 252*t*
    physical examination for, 251–252, 253*t*
    prevention of, 107, 243
    screening for, 116*t*
    visual impairment and, 384
famciclovir, 370

family
    in chronic disease management, 93–94
    dementia and, 159, 163–164
    EOL and, 509–512
    hearing loss and, 393*t*
    informal support by, 448
    LTC by, 449–450
fatigue, 51
    with chronic disease management, 89
    depression and, 178, 185
    diabetes and, 336
fecal impaction
    constipation and, 236
    delirium from, 148
    immobility and, 267
    stroke and, 316
    UI and, 207
fecal incontinence, 236–238, 238*t*–239*t*
    causes of, 236*t*–237*t*
fee-for-service (FFS), 436
feet
    falls and, 253
    immobility and, 263
    polyneuropathy and, 402
FFS. *See* fee-for-service
fiber
    colorectal cancer and, 364
    for constipation, 236–237
fibrinolytics, 313–314
FIM. *See* Functional Improvement Measure;
        Functional Independence Measure
Five-Star Quality Rating System, 471, 482
folate deficiency, 359–360
fondaparinux, 273
food additives, 364
FPS-R. *See* Faces Pain Scale-Revised
fractures. *See also* hip fractures
    PAC for, 36
    visual impairment and, 384
frailty
    aging and, 12–13
    with chronic disease management, 89
    geriatric patient assessment and, 51
    immobility and, 13
    mitochondria and, 11
    obesity and, 365
    palliative care and, 527–528, 528*t*, 529*t*
    Pra and, 70
    preoperative evaluation for, 74
    QALYs and, 29
    vitality decrease and, 333–334
free radical theory, 364
Fries, J. F., 28
function
    biological aging and, 17
    geriatric patient assessment for, 62–64, 62*t*
    immobility and, 268–269
    preventative care for, 129–131
functional assessment
    geriatric consultation and, 70
    for geriatric patients, 59–64, 61*t*, 62*t*

functional deficit
  with chronic disease management, 89
  depression and, 170
  diet and, 362–363
  from immobility, 266–267
functional dependence
  frailty and, 13
  geriatric syndromes and, 15
Functional Improvement Measure (FIM), 434
functional incontinence, 211t, 212
Functional Independence Measure (FIM), 63
furosemide, 395

gabapentin
  for HZ, 370
  for polyneuropathy, 402
  UI from, 209t
gait and balance assessment, 63, 246, 251
  for falls, 254, 255t
  for polyneuropathy, 401
  Up and Go Test for, 253–254, 255t–256t, 336
galantamine, 162
GAROP. See Global Alliance for the
    Rights of Older People
gastroesophageal reflux
  antimuscarinic drugs and, 228
  weight loss from, 51
gastrointestinal system, aging and, 8t
Gawande, A., 18–20
gene expression, aging and, 11
genomic instability, aging and, 10t
geriatric consultation, 67–72, 71t–72t
Geriatric Depression Scale, 74, 122t, 180, 184
geriatric patients
  ambulatory care for, 36, 37t
  anesthesia for, 74
  assessment of, 43–76, 45f, 46t
    caregiver assessment for, 75–76, 75t
    with chronic disease management, 89
    for environmental factors, 64
    functional assessment for, 59–64, 61t, 62t
    geriatric consultation for, 67–72, 71t–72t
    laboratory tests for, 57–59, 58t
    for malnutrition, 65–67, 67t
    Medicare Annual Wellness
        Visit and, 67, 69t–70t
    in NH, 475–482, 478t–481t
    for pain, 64–65, 65t, 66f
    patient history for, 47–54, 48t–50t
    physical examination for, 54–57, 55t–57t
    for physical functioning, 62–64, 62t
    preoperative evaluation for, 72–74, 73t
    for prevention, 108t
    screening questions for, 52t–53t
    for weight, 65–66, 67t
  demographics and epidemiology of, 23–40
  disability of, 28–31
  ethics and, 499–520
  growing numbers of, 26–28
  health services for, 427–468
  PAC for, 34–36, 36t

person-centered care for, 51, 54t
  services for, 33–37
geriatric syndromes, 14–15
geriatrics model of care, 4
gerontological aging, 4
gerontology, 3
geroscience hypothesis, 4
ginkgo biloba, 162
glaucoma, 384–385
  antimuscarinic drugs and, 228
  screening for, 116t
glitazones, 209t
Global Alliance for the Rights of Older
    People (GAROP), 519
glomerular filtration rate
  for hypertension, 304
  normal aging and, 6
glucosamine
  for degenerative bone disease prevention, 128
  for OA, 270
glucose
  anabolic hormones and, 356
  polyneuropathy and, 401
  stroke and, 314
gonorrhea, 116t
Good Palliative-Geriatric Practice, 415
gout, 271–272
grandiosity, with bipolar affective disorder, 171
Green House, 458
grip strength, 12, 74
group care, 88
growth hormone, 11, 357
Guillain-Barré syndrome, 401

habit training, for UI, 225t, 228
hallucinations, in EOL, 537
Hamilton Depression Rating Scale, 122t
HAND. See HIV-associated
    neurocognitive disorders
handicap, 29
Hayflick, L., 6
HCBS. See home- and community-
    based LTC services
HCCs. See hierarchical clinical conditions
headache, with serotonin syndrome, 194
health insurance, 25
Health Insurance Portability and
    Accountability Act (HIPAA), 101
health promotion, 110
health services. See also hospitalization; long-term
    care; Medicaid; Medicare; nursing homes
  for geriatric patients, 427–472
  public programs, 430–444, 442t–444t
health span, 4
Healthy People 2020, 108, 110t
hearing
  aging and, 9t
  assessment of, 391–392, 391t, 392t
  auditory system for, 390, 391t
  geriatric consultation for, 71t
  in geriatric syndromes, 15

impairment, 389–400
    aging and, 392, 393*t*
    delirium and, 149*t*
    depression and, 172
    health implications of, 393*t*
    localization and, 394
    loudness and, 394
    rehabilitation for, 395–399
    screening for, 116*t*
    speech and, 394
    strategies to improve communication, 400*t*
    sensitivity of, 393–394
hearing aids, 395–399, 397*t*–399*t*
Hearing Handicap Inventory for the
    Elderly-Screening, 390
heart attack. *See* myocardial infarction
heart disease. *See* cardiovascular disease
heart failure, 324–326. *See also*
    congestive heart failure
    hospitalization for, 33, 34*f*
heart murmurs, 320, 320*t*
    with IHSS, 322
heat stroke, 372–373, 372*t*, 373*t*
HelpAge International, 519
hematuria, 215
heparin
    for atrial fibrillation, 323
    for hip fractures, 272–273
hepatic encephalopathy, 152*t*
hepatitis B, 116*t*
hepatitis C, 117*t*
herbal supplements, hypertension and, 304
herpes simplex, 117*t*
herpes zoster (HZ), 120, 370
HHA. *See* home health care
HHS. *See* hyperosmolar hyperglycemic state
hierarchical clinical conditions (HCCs), 435
hip fractures, 18
    cataracts and, 384
    decreases in, 23
    from falls, 243, 250, 259
    immobility from, 272–273, 273*f*
    NH and, 37
    preoperative evaluation for, 72
HIPAA. *See* Health Insurance Portability
    and Accountability Act
Hispanics
    cultural competence for, 94
    life expectancy of, 28
histone, 11
HIV. *See* human immunodeficiency virus
HIV-associated neurocognitive disorders
    (HAND), 152*t*, 401
home- and community-based LTC
    services (HCBS), 439, 445–446,
    459–465, 460*t*
    Medicare for, 461
home health care (HHA), 37*t*
Home Health Compare, 470
homeostenosis, 5, 13–14
hormone replacement therapy, 113*t*, 187*t*

hospice care, 524*t*
    in chronic disease management, 84
    Medicare for, 523
    in NH, 458
    palliative care and, 523
Hospital Compare, 466
Hospital Elder Life Program, 148
hospitalization
    ADs in, 503–504
    bacteriuria with, 369
    in chronic disease management, 93
    cost of, 33
    daily cost of, 448
    day care in, 465
    for diabetes, 348*f*–349*f*
    discharge planning for, 135–136
    for EOL, 513
    falls and, 243
    frailty and, 13
    in HIPAA, 101
    incontinence in, 207
    Medicare and, 431
    NH and, 39–40
    PAC and, 493–495
    readmission for, 33, 34*f*
    risk factors of, 130, 131*t*
Housing Enabler, 18
Howell, Timothy, 17
human immunodeficiency virus (HIV), 117*t*
hydralazine, 310, 325
hyperactive delirium, 143
hypercalcemia, 178, 207
hypercapnia, 152*t*
hypercholesterolemia, 317
hyperglycemia, 207, 337
hyperlipidemia, 310–311, 314
hyperosmolar hyperglycemic state (HHS), 347
hyperparathyroidism
    depression and, 178
    hypertension and, 304
    vitality decrease and, 355
hypersexuality, 171
hypertension, 301–310, 304*t*
    ambulatory care for, 37*t*
    assessment of, 303–304, 303*t*
    atrial fibrillation and, 323
    CAD and, 317
    diabetes and, 343
    heart failure and, 325
    management of, 304–310
    medications for, 306*t*, 307–310, 309*t*
    multimorbidity and, 14
    NH and, 39*t*
    stroke and, 312, 315
    thiazide diuretics for, 307–308, 307*t*
hyperthermia, 372–373, 372*t*, 373*t*
hyperthyroidism, 354
    atrial fibrillation and, 323
    depression and, 178
    subclinical, 355
hypoactive delirium, 143

hypochondriasis, depression and, 180
hypochromic anemia, 359, 360*t*
hypoglycemia
  dementia and, 152*t*
  diabetes and, 337
  falls and, 249
hyponatremia, 178, 356
hypothermia, 371–372, 371*t*
hypothyroidism, 350–352
  depression and, 185
  fatigue from, 51
  hypothermia and, 371
  subclinical, 352, 353*f*
hypoventilation syndrome, 365
hypoxia
  dementia and, 152*t*
  depression and, 178
  OSA and, 177
HZ. *See* herpes zoster

IADLs. *See* instrumental activities of daily living
IAGG. *See* International Association of
    Gerontology and Geriatrics
IAHSA. *See* International Association of
    Homes and Services for the Ageing
iatrogenesis. *See also* adverse drug reactions
  falls and, 243
  in geriatric syndromes, 15
  LTC and, 134–135
  prevention of, 131–133, 132*t*
idiopathic hypertrophic subaortic
    stenosis (IHSS), 322
IFA. *See* International Federation on Ageing
IGF-1. *See* insulin-like growth factor 1
IHSS. *See* idiopathic hypertrophic
    subaortic stenosis
IL-6. *See* interleukin 6
ILC. *See* International Longevity Centre
immobility, 295*t*–296*t*
  assessment of, 267–269, 268*t*
  causes of, 263–265, 264*t*
  complications of, 265–267, 266*t*
  falls and, 243, 267
  frailty and, 13
  function and, 268–269
  in geriatric syndromes, 14
  from hip fractures, 272–273, 273*f*
  management of, 266–281
  muscle weakness and, 266, 269*t*
  from OA, 269–272, 271*t*
  occupational therapy for, 293, 295*t*
  from pain, 281–292
  from PD, 273–275
  physical activity for, 292
  physical therapy for, 293
  pressure sores from, 267, 278–281, 279*t*, 280*t*
  from psychotropic drugs, 422
  rehabilitation for, 292–295, 293*t*–294*t*
  from stroke, 263, 267, 275–278

immune deficiency, 15
immunizations
  for HZ, 370
  for influenza, 107, 367–368
  for pneumonia, 107
  for prevention, 109, 119–120
IMPACT. *See* Improving Medicare Post-Acute
    Care Transformation Act of 2014
impotence, 15
Improving Medicare Post-Acute
    Care Transformation Act of
    2014 (IMPACT), 63–64
incipient dementia bipolar affective
    disorder and, 171
incontinence, 201–235. *See also* fecal
    incontinence; urinary incontinence
  geriatric consultation for, 71*t*
  in geriatric syndromes, 15
  NH and, 40
infection
  confusion from, 141
  depression and, 178
  in geriatric syndromes, 15
  hyperthyroidism and, 354
  in LTC, 368–369
  NH and, 40
  from pressure sores, 281
  stress and, 6
  from urinary catheters, 219
  vitality decrease and, 365–370, 366*t*, 368*t*
infective endocarditis, 368
  mitral valve prolapse and, 322
inflammaging, 12
inflammatory markers
  intracellular communication and, 12
  sarcopenia and, 14
influenza
  death from, 27, 28*f*
  immunization for, 107, 120, 367–368
informal support, 445, 448
  in NH, 457
Information and Communication Technologies,
    for cognitive impairment, 123
informed consent, 411, 500–502
INH. *See* isonicotinic acid hydrazide
Initial Preventive Physical Examination
    (IPEE), 67, 68*t*
inpatient rehabilitation facilities (IRFs),
    34–35
  immobility, 293
  Medicare and, 434
INPEA. *See* International Network for
    the Prevention of Elder Abuse
insomnia
  depression and, 174–177, 176*t*, 423
  in geriatric syndromes, 15
  sedative–hypnotics for, 421*t*, 423
  with serotonin syndrome, 194
  weight loss from, 51

instability
  aging and, 243–246
  falls and, 250, 252
  in geriatric syndromes, 14
instrumental activities of daily
    living (IADLs), 30–31
  cognitive impairment assessment and, 141
  frailty and, 12
  hearing loss and, 393*t*
  Medicare and, 31*f*
  sarcopenic obesity and, 14
insulin-like growth factor 1 (IGF-1), 11
  anabolic hormones and, 356
  protein and, 125–126
integumentary system, aging and, 7*t*
intellectual impairment. *See* cognitive impairment
INTERACT. *See* Interventions to
    Reduce Acute Care Transfers
interleukin 6 (IL-6), 14, 172
International Association for Hospice
    and Palliative Care, 537
International Association of Gerontology
    and Geriatrics (IAGG), 519
International Association of Homes and
    Services for the Ageing (IAHSA), 519
International Federation on Ageing (IFA), 519
International Longevity Centre (ILC), 519
International Network for the Prevention
    of Elder Abuse (INPEA), 519
International Osteoporosis Foundation, 363
Interventions to Reduce Acute Care Transfers
    (INTERACT), 40, 492*f*, 495
intracellular communication, aging and, 10*t*
intraocular pressure, 381
intrinsic sphincter deficiency (ISD), 210
IPEE. *See* Initial Preventive Physical Examination
IRFs. *See* inpatient rehabilitation facilities
iron deficiency anemia, 358–359
irritable colon, 15
Isaacs, Bernard, 25
ischemic heart disease
  ambulatory care for, 37*t*
  preoperative evaluation for, 73
ISD. *See* intrinsic sphincter deficiency
isolation
  in geriatric syndromes, 15
  hearing loss and, 393*t*
  malnutrition and, 67*t*
isoniazid, 359
isonicotinic acid hydrazide (INH), 369

JNC8. *See* Eighth Joint National Committee
justice, 499

Kaiser Pyramid, 43, 44*f*
Kegels (pelvic floor exercises)
  for fecal incontinence, 237
  for UI, 223–224, 225*t*

kidney. *See also* chronic kidney
    disease; renal insufficiency
  aging and, 418*t*
  cancer, obesity and, 365
  disease, PAC for, 36
  medication excretion by, 418–419
  normal aging and, 6
Kuchel, G., 13

lamotrigine, 198
laxatives, 236, 237
lead, 359
leukocytosis, 367
levothyroxine (Synthroid), 351–352
lidocaine, 370
life expectancy, 4
  disability and, 28
  increases to, 5, 27–28
  with MI, 318
  normal aging and, 5
  obesity and, 24
  retirement and, 26
life span, 4, 11
lifestyle. *See also* diet; physical activity; weight loss
  aging and, 18
  for cognitive impairment prevention, 128–129
  diabetes and, 335
  health promotion for, 110
  for hypertension, 306
  in normal aging, 5
Listeria monocytogenes, 368
lithium, 198
living will, 503, 505
localization, hearing impairment and, 394
loneliness
  hearing impairment and, 393*t*
  screening for, 121, 122*t*
long-term care (LTC), 26, 428, 445–451.
    See also caregivers; nursing homes
  case management in, 466–468, 467*t*
  for chronic disease management, 88, 447, 463*f*
  computer technology for, 101–102
  discharge planning for, 135–136
  by family, 449–450
  getting services people want, 467–469, 464*f*
  in HIPAA, 101
  infections in, 368–369
  Medicaid for, 440, 441–442, 449
  Medicare for, 433, 445, 449, 460–461
  outcomes for, 96
  risk factors of, 134–135
  social support for, 31–32
  spending by payer, 450*f*
  tuberculosis in, 369
long-term care hospital (LTCH), 37*t*
long-term supportive services (LTSS), 454*t*
loss, in aging, 18
loss of function, in normal aging, 5–6
loudness, hearing impairment and, 394

low back pain, 114*t*
low molecular weight heparin, 272–273
LTC. *See* long-term care
LTCH. *See* long-term care hospital
Lubiprostone, 533
lung cancer, 117*t*, 120
Lyme disease, 152*t*

MACRA. *See* Medicare Access and
    CHIP Reauthorization Act
Major Depression Inventory, 122*t*
major depressive episode, 181–182, 182*t*
malnutrition
    geriatric consultation for, 71*t*
    geriatric patient assessment for, 65–67, 67*t*
    in geriatric syndromes, 15
    MNA for, 126
    NH and, 40
    PD and, 275
    risk factors for, 67*t*
    tuberculosis and, 369
managed care, 430
    Medicare and, 431
    in NH, 460–461
Mant, J., 325
MAOIs. *See* monoamine oxidase inhibitors
MCI. *See* mild cognitive impairment
MDRD. *See* Modification of Diet in Renal Disease
MDS. *See* Minimum Data Set
Medicaid, 438–441
    assisted living and, 458–459
    eligibility for, 440–441
    for HCBS, 461–462
    hearing aids and, 397
    for LTC, 436, 437–438, 445
    for NH, 38, 455, 473
    for nursing homes (NH), 436
    PACE and, 429
    waiver programs for, 448
medical fact sheets, in NH, 483–486, 484*f*–485*f*
medical needs pyramid, 464*f*
Medical Orders for Life-Sustaining
    Treatment (MOLST), 506, 515
Medicare, 432–438, 433*f*. *See also* Annual
    Wellness Visit; Welcome to Medicare Visit
    ADLs and, 31*f*, 449*f*
    AMD and, 388
    for chronic disease management, 33*f*, 88–89
    health expenditures with, 26–27, 27*f*
    hearing aids and, 397
    for hospice care, 523
    IADLs and, 31*f*
    IPPE and, 67, 68*t*
    for LTC, 433, 445, 449, 460–461
    medications and, 407, 437–438
    multimorbidity and, 14
    for NH, 38–39, 459, 460–461, 473, 482
    PACE and, 429, 435
    PPACA and, 25, 437

    rehabilitation and, 294
    stroke and, 275
Medicare Access and CHIP Reauthorization
    Act (MACRA), 436, 437
Medicare Advantage, 432, 437
Medicare Current Beneficiary Survey, 88
Medicare Modernization Act, 437
medications, 405–423, 423*t*. *See also*
    adverse drug reactions; iatrogenesis
    absorption of, 416
    for AD, 161–162
    adherence with, 407–410, 410*t*
    aging and, 4, 416–419, 416*t*
    for CHF, 325
    for constipation, 238*t*
    delirium from, 148, 148*t*
    for dementia, 161–162
    for depression, 188, 190–198
    depression from, 178, 180*t*
    for diabetes, 337–338, 339*t*–342*t*
    distribution of, 416–417
    excretion, 417–418
    falls and, 249–250
    hearing impairment from, 395
    for hypertension, 306*t*, 307–310, 309*t*
    immobility and, 265
    insulin/IGF-1 signaling pathway, 11
    malnutrition and, 67*t*
    Medicare and, 438–439
    metabolism of, 417
    My Medicine Record for, 408*f*–409*f*
    for overactive bladder, 230*t*–231*t*
    for pain, 285, 286*t*–291*t*, 292
    for PD, 275, 276*t*–277*t*
    prescribing, 419, 419*t*
    tissue and receptor sensitivity to, 418–419
    for UI, 228–233, 230*t*–231*t*
    UI from, 209*t*
Medigap, 434
memantine, 162
memory loss, 71*t*
meningitis, 152*t*, 368
meperidine, 194, 285
Merit-Based Incentive Payment
    System (MIPS), 436, 437
metabolic syndrome, 170
metformin, 4
methylation, 11
Methylnaltrexone, 533–534
mild cognitive impairment (MCI), 142, 142*t*, 149
Mini Nutritional Assessment (MNA), 126
Mini-Cog, 139–141
    for dementia, 155
    for diabetes, 336
Mini-Mental State Examination, 74, 501
Minimum Data Set (MDS), 63, 433, 457, 477, 482
    computer technology for, 101
    NH and, 459
MIPS. *See* Merit-Based Incentive Payment System

mirabegron, 232
mirtazapine, 190, 195
mitochondria, aging and, 10*t*, 11
mitral annulus calcification, 321
mitral insufficiency, 321
mitral valve prolapse, 321–322
MNA. *See* Mini Nutritional Assessment
Modification of Diet in Renal
     Disease (MDRD), 418
MOLST. *See* Medical Orders for
     Life-Sustaining Treatment
monoamine oxidase inhibitors
     (MAOIs), 190, 191*t*, 195
     for PD, 275
mood stabilizers, 196
motivation
     of caregivers, 60
     for disability prevention, 130–131
     frailty and, 74
     for rehabilitation, 170
multi-infarct dementia, 155, 156*f*, 178
multimorbidity
     aging and, 14
     with chronic disease management,
         79, 80–81, 80*f*
     with depression, 177–178, 179*t*
     with diabetes, 343, 344*t*–346*t*
     frailty and, 12
     hospitalization and, 133
     in NH, 40, 471–472
     self-care and, 16
multiple organ system failure, 13–14
multiple sclerosis, 212
muscle relaxants, 285
muscle strength/weakness
     balance and, 246
     with chronic disease management, 89
     falls and, 246, 254
     immobility and, 266, 269*t*
     for OA, 270
musculoskeletal system, aging and, 8*t*
My Medicine Record, 408*f*–409*f*
myelodysplasia, 11
myocardial infarction (MI, heart
     attack), 317–319, 318*t*
     confusion from, 141
     heart failure and, 324–325
     hospitalization for, 33, 34*f*
     immobility and, 267
     OSA and, 177
     preoperative evaluation for, 74
     stroke and, 314
myopia, 381
MyPlate, 125, 126*f*
myxedema coma, 352–354, 353*t*

Naloxegol, 533
National Health and Nutrition
     Examination Survey, 390

National Institute for Health and Clinical
     Excellence (NICE), 24, 304–306
     on heart failure, 324
National Institutes of Health, 60
National Long-Term Care Survey, 24
National Osteoporosis Foundation
     (NOF), 265, 363
National Provider Identifier (NPI), 436
nausea and vomiting, in EOL, 535
nephritic syndrome, 28*f*
nephritis, 28*f*
nephrosis, 28*f*
Neupro. *See* rotigotine
neurokinins, 535
neurological system, aging and, 7*t*
NF-kB transcription factor, 12
NH. *See* nursing homes
NICE. *See* National Institute for Health
     and Clinical Excellence
nocturia, 203, 209
     falls and, 251
     weight loss from, 51
NOF. *See* National Osteoporosis Foundation
nonalcoholic liver disease, 401
nonmaleficence, 499
non-ST elevation acute coronary
     syndrome, 318–319
nonsteroidal anti-inflammatory drugs (NSAIDs)
     colorectal cancer and, 114*t*
     for dementia prevention, 162
     for gout, 271
     hypertension and, 304
     for OA, 270
     for pain, 285
norepinephrine and dopamine
     reuptake inhibitors, 190
norepinephrine reuptake inhibitors, 190
normal aging, 4, 5–6
nortriptyline, 195–196
NPI. *See* National Provider Identifier
NSAIDs. *See* nonsteroidal anti-inflammatory drugs
nurse practitioners, in NH, 461, 477, 487, 493
Nursing Home Compare, 458, 466, 482
nursing homes (NH), 37–40, 39*t*,
     449–458, 454*t*, 471–496
     ADs in, 503–504
     for chronic disease management, 94
     chronic disease management in, 80, 94
     clinical care in, 473–475, 474*t*
     clinical practice guidelines for, 493
     cognitive development in, 139
     cognitive impairment and, 38, 39*t*, 457
     daily cost of, 452
     disability and, 454, 456*f*
     diseases in, 476*t*
     distinct resident groups in, 457–458
     documentation in, 483–486
     DRGs and, 457
     EOL in, 512–513

nursing homes (NH) (*Cont.*):
 ethics for, 495–496, 496*t*
 falls in, 39*t*, 40, 243, 248*t*
 fecal incontinence in, 236
 frailty and, 13
 geriatric patient assessment in, 475–482, 478*t*–481*t*
 goals of, 472–473, 472*t*
 hospice care in, 458
 improvements to care in, 482–493
 informal support in, 457
 as last resort, 448
 managed care in, 459–460
 Medicaid for, 38, 440, 459, 477
 medical fact sheets in, 483–486, 484*f*–485*f*
 Medicare for, 434, 459, 460–461, 477, 482
 multimorbidity in, 471–472
 nurse practitioners in, 487, 493
 obesity and, 365
 PAC in, 34–36, 36*t*, 451, 471
  hospitalization and, 493–495
  Medicare and, 430, 432
 patient types in, 473*f*
 payment for, 455
 permanent vegetative state in, 455
 physician assistants in, 460, 487, 493
 physicians in, 459–460, 475–477
 prevention in, 487, 488*t*–491*t*
 quality improvement activities for, 493
 rehabilitation in, 457
 risk for admission to, 452, 452*f*
 social support and, 32
 UI in, 228
 use by age group, 453, 453*f*, 454*f*
 vitamin D in, 362
nutraceuticals, for OA, 270
nutrient-sensing deregulation, aging and, 10*t*, 11
nutrition. *See* diet
nystagmus, 249

OA. *See* osteoarthritis
OAA. *See* Older Americans Act
OASIS. *See* Outcome and Assessment Information Set
obesity, 14
 ambulatory care for, 37*t*
 AMD and, 387
 atrial fibrillation and, 323
 diabetes and, 335, 337
 hypertension and, 304
 life expectancy and, 24
 MNA for, 126
 OSA and, 177
 vitality decrease and, 365
OBRA 1987. *See* Omnibus Budget Reconciliation Act of 1987
obstructive sleep apnea (OSA), 176–177
 atrial fibrillation and, 323
 dementia and, 152*t*

hypertension and, 304
 obesity and, 365
occupational therapy, 293, 295*t*
Octreotide, 534–535
Older Americans Act (OAA), 442, 515, 516*t*
 HCBS and, 462
Omnibus Budget Reconciliation Act of 1987 (OBRA 1987), 457
open-angle glaucoma, 385
ophthalmic solutions, adverse drug reactions from, 387*t*
opioids
 constipation from, in EOL, 531–535
 serotonin syndrome and, 194
oral cancer, 117*t*
orthopedic problems, aging and, 30
orthopnea, 51
orthostatic hypotension
 from beta-blockers, 127
 falls and, 249
 immobility from, 265
OSA. *See* obstructive sleep apnea
osteoarthritis (OA)
 immobility from, 269–272, 271*t*
 obesity and, 365
osteopenia, 127
osteoporosis
 bisphosphonates for, 5
 hypothyroidism and, 352
 immobility and, 265
 obesity and, 365
 prevention of, 107, 127–128
 screening for, 113*t*
 vitamin D and, 363
otosclerosis, 395
ototoxic medication, 395
Outcome and Assessment Information Set (OASIS), 63, 433
 for HCBS, 465
outcomes
 of chronic disease management, 95–98, 96*t*–98*t*
 computer technology for, 101
 measurement of, 428*f*
outpatient geriatric patients
 assessment of, 45
 medications for, 407
ovarian cancer, 113*t*, 115*t*
overactive bladder, 212
 falls and, 251
 medications for, 230*t*–231*t*
overflow incontinence, 212, 233

PAC. *See* postacute care
PACE. *See* Program for All-Inclusive Care for the Elderly
PAD. *See* peripheral arterial disease
pain
 geriatric patient assessment for, 64–65, 65*t*, 66*f*
 health span and, 4

immobility from, 281–292
management of, 283*t*–284*t*
   in EOL, 531, 534*t*
medications for, 285, 286*t*–291*t*, 292
stress and, 6
palliative care
   for cancer, 121
   in chronic disease management, 84
   cultural competence in, 529–530, 530*t*
   for EOL, 523–538
   establishing approach to, 528–529
   frailty and, 527–528, 528*t*, 529*t*
   international aspects of, 537–538
   symptom management in, 530–537, 532*t*–533*t*
pancreatic cancer
   depression and, 178
   obesity and, 365
   screening for, 117*t*
parathyroid disease, 178. *See also*
      hyperparathyroidism
Parkinson disease (PD)
   confusion from, 141
   dementia and, 158
   depression and, 172, 178
   falls and, 250, 254
   immobility and, 263–265, 273–275
   medications for, 275, 276*t*–277*t*
   UI and, 203
Parks and Novelli checklist, 76
paroxetine, 190
Patient Health Questionnaire (PHQ), 76, 122*t*
   for depression, 182–185, 184, 336
patient history
   for dementia, 157–158
   for falls, 251, 252*t*
   for geriatric patient assessment, 47–54, 48*t*–50*t*
   for immobility, 267
   for prevention, 123–124
   for UI, 214*t*
Patient Protection and Affordable Care
      Act (PPACA), 25, 427, 437
   in chronic disease management, 103
   Medicaid and, 438
   on NH, 471
Patient Self-Determination Act (PSDA), 514
PCI. *See* percutaneous coronary intervention
PD. *See* Parkinson disease
PEARLS. *See* Program to Encourage Active,
      Rewarding Lives for Seniors
PEG. *See* percutaneous endoscopic gastrostomy
pelvic floor exercises (Kegels)
   for fecal incontinence, 237
   for UI, 223–224, 225*t*
pelvic prolapse, 212, 214–215
pentoxifylline, 327
percutaneous coronary intervention (PCI), 318
percutaneous endoscopic gastrostomy (PEG), 513
percutaneous transluminal coronary
      angioplasty, 33, 74

performance
   in normal aging, 5–6
   obesity and, 14
periodontal disease, 67*t*
peripheral arterial disease (PAD), 113*t*
peripheral neuropathy, 265
peripheral vascular disease (PVD), 326–327
permanent vegetative state, 458
pernicious anemia, 360
persistent incontinence, 210–212, 211*t*
persistent pain, 282
personal care pyramid, 464*f*
person-centered care
   biological aging and, 16–17
   by caregivers, 446
   essential elements of, 446
   for geriatric patients, 51, 54*t*
pertussis, 120
phagocytes, 366–367
pharmacodynamic changes, 418–419
phenotypes, frailty, 12–13
pheochromocytoma, 304
PHN. *See* postherpetic neuralgia
PHQ. *See* Patient Health Questionnaire
physical activity (exercise)
   aging and, 18
   with chronic disease management, 89
   for cognitive impairment, 123
   for cognitive impairment prevention, 129
   for depression, 187*t*, 189
   for falls, 257
   frailty and, 12, 74
   for hypertension, 306
   for immobility, 292
   NH and, 40
   normal aging and, 5
   obesity and, 126
   for OSA, 177
   for PD, 275
   for prevention, 107, 109, 124–125, 124*t*
   for PVD, 327
   screening for, 116*t*, 125
physical examination
   for dementia, 158
   for falls, 251–252, 253*t*
   for geriatric patient assessment, 54–57, 55*t*–57*t*
   for hypertension, 303
   for prevention, 123–124
   for UI, 213, 214–215, 217
physical therapy
   for immobility, 293
   for polyneuropathy, 402
physician assistants, in NH, 456, 487, 493
Physician Orders for Life-Sustaining
      Treatment (POLST), 506, 515
physician-assisted suicide, 512
physicians
   in EOL, 509–512
   for HCBS, 463

physicians (*Cont.*):
LTC and, 470
in NH, 455–456, 475–477
physiological reserve
frailty and, 12
homeostasis and, 14
PMR. *See* polymyalgia rheumatica
pneumonia. *See also* aspiration pneumonia
community-acquired, 367
death from, 27, 28*f*, 367
hospitalization for, 33, 34*f*, 133
immunization for, 107, 120
PAC for, 36
pulse oximetry for, 369
POLST. *See* Physician Orders for Life-
Sustaining Treatment
polydipsia, 336
polymyalgia rheumatica (PMR), 270–271
polyneuropathy, 401–402
gait and balance assessment for, 401
polyuria
diabetes and, 336
UI and, 207–208
postacute care (PAC), 34–36, 36*t*, 453, 471
hospitalization and, 493–495
Medicare and, 434, 436
postherpetic neuralgia (PHN), 120, 370
postural hypotension
diabetes and, 307
falls and, 246, 249, 252
immobility and, 267
postvoiding residual (PVR), for UI, 213, 217–218
potassium, 306
PPACA. *See* Patient Protection and
Affordable Care Act
PPS. *See* prospective payment system
Pra. *See* Probability of Repeated Admissions
preference-sensitive care, 99
pregabalin, 209*t*
preoperative evaluation, 72–74, 73*t*
preoperative evaluation for, 74
presbycusis, 392
presbyopia, 381
pressure sores
from immobility, 267, 278–281, 279*t*, 280*t*
PD and, 275
stroke and, 316
prevention, 107–136, 109*t*
of Alzheimer disease, 128–129
behavior change for, 124
of cancer, 120–121
cancer screening for, 120–121
of cardiovascular disease, 126–127
challenges to, 110
of degenerative joint disease, 127–128
of dementia, 128–129, 162
diet for, 109, 125–126
of disability, 129–131
of falls, 107, 243

geriatric patient assessment for, 108*t*
of hyperlipidemia, 310
of hyperthermia, 373
of iatrogenesis, 131–133, 132*t*
immunizations for, 109, 119–120
in NH, 487, 488*t*–491*t*
of osteoporosis, 107, 127–128
patient history for, 123–124
physical activity for, 124–125, 124*t*
physical examination for, 123–124
prophylactic medications for, 126–127
of stroke, 314–315
Prevnar-13, 120
primary degenerative dementia, 155, 156*f*
primary prevention, 107, 109
Probability of Repeated Admissions
(Pra), 70–72, 72*t*, 88
probenecid, 271
problem-solving therapy (PST), for
depression, 188, 189
Program for All-Inclusive Care for the
Elderly (PACE), 429–430, 435–436
Program to Encourage Active, Rewarding
Lives for Seniors (PEARLS), 189
prompted voiding, for UI, 225*t*, 228, 229*t*
prospective payment system (PPS), 34
prostate cancer
obesity and, 365
screening for, 113*t*, 120
prostatic enlargement. *See* benign
prostatic hyperplasia
protein
aging and, 11
IGF-1 and, 125–126
immobility and, 267
malnutrition and, 66–67
vitality decrease and, 361–362
proteostasis, aging and, 10*t*, 11
PSDA. *See* Patient Self-Determination Act
pseudoephedrine, 232
pseudohypertension, 304
pseudoparkinsonism, 422
PST. *See* problem-solving therapy
psychosis
delirium and, 145, 146*t*
PD and, 275
psychotherapy
for bipolar affective disorder, 198
for depression, 187*t*, 188, 189
psychotropic drugs, 420–423
for dementia, 161
UI from, 209*t*
PTD. *See* verteporfin photodynamic therapy
pulmonary edema, 74
pulmonary embolism
falls and, 248
stroke and, 316
pulse oximetry, 369
PVD. *See* peripheral vascular disease

PVR. *See* postvoiding residual
pyridoxine, 359

QALYs. *See* quality-adjusted life-years
QAPI. *See* Quality Assurance and
    Performance Improvement
QIS. *See* Quality Indicatory Survey
Quality and Resource Use Reports (QRURs), 437
Quality Assurance and Performance
    Improvement (QAPI), 471, 483
Quality Indicator Survey (QIS), 471
Quality of Death Index, 538
quality of life
    dementia and, 164
    geriatric patient assessment and, 51
    geriatric syndromes and, 15
    hearing loss and, 393*t*
    in NH, 458
    obesity and, 365
    prevention and, 110
quality-adjusted life-years (QALYs),
    28–29, 514

ranibizumab, 388
rapamycin, 4, 11
RBRVS. *See* Resource-Based Relative Value Scale
RDW. *See* red cell distribution width
REACH II Risk Appraisal, 76
Reconciliation Act, 25
red cell distribution width (RDW), 357
"red flag" signs, 16
rehabilitation. *See also* inpatient
    rehabilitation facilities
    depression and, 170
    for hearing impairment, 395–399
    for immobility, 292–295, 293*t*–294*t*
    for MI, 319
    motivation for, 170
    in NH, 457
    for stroke, 316–317, 316*t*, 317*t*
rehabilitation therapists, 64
reminiscence therapy, 459
renal blood flow, 6
renal insufficiency
    malnutrition and, 67*t*
    preoperative evaluation for, 74
reproductive system, aging and, 8*t*
reserpine, 67*t*
resilience, 13–14
resource utilization groups (RUGs),
    433, 456, 457*t*, 482
Resource-Based Relative Value Scale
    (RBRVS), 435–436
respiratory system, aging and, 7*t*
restless leg syndrome (RLS), 176–177
retirement
    aging and, 18
    life expectancy and, 26
Reuben's Physical Performance Test, 63

rheumatoid arthritis, 361
rheumatoid factor, 401
rib fractures, 243
rivaroxaban, 323
rivastigmine, 162
RLS. *See* restless leg syndrome
Rosalynn Carter Institute, 162
rotigotine (Neupro), 275
RUGs. *See* resource utilization groups

sarcopenia
    with chronic disease management, 89
    homeostasis and, 14
    prevention of, 125
Savvy Caregiver Program, 162
schizophrenia, 170
Screening Tool of Older Persons'
    Potentially Inappropriate Prescriptions
    (STOPP), 134, 415
Screening Tool to Alert Doctors to Right
    Treatment (START), 134
secondary prevention, 107–108
sedative–hypnotics, 420–423, 421*t*
    depression and, 180
    falls and, 249
    immobility from, 265
    UI from, 209*t*
selective serotonin reuptake inhibitors
    (SSRIs), 191*t*–192*t*
    for depression, 190, 194
    for pain, 285
    serotonin syndrome from, 194
self-care
    frailty and, 13
    multimorbidity and, 16
self-help groups, 131
sensitivity, of hearing, 393–394
sensory impairment, 381–402, 402*t*.
    See also hearing; vision
    aging and, 30
    confusion from, 141
sepsis, 371
septic arthritis, 367
serotonin antagonist/reuptake inhibitors, 190
serotonin norepinephrine reuptake
    inhibitors (SNRIs), 190
    for pain, 285
serotonin reuptake enhancers, 190
serotonin syndrome, 194
sertraline, 190
sexually transmitted infections (STIs), 117*t*
Short Form-36 (SF-36), 63
Short Scale to Measure Loneliness, 122*t*
shortness of breath (dyspnea), in EOL, 536
SIADH. *See* syndrome of inappropriate
    secretion of antidiuretic hormone
sick sinus syndrome, 324, 324*t*
sideroblastic anemia, 359
Sigma Theta Tau Geriatric Pain, 281

skilled nursing facility (SNF), 37*t*
  for immobility, 293–294
skilled service, 461
skin cancer, 117*t*
sleep. *See also* insomnia; obstructive sleep apnea
  aging and, 177
  for cognitive impairment prevention, 129
  depression and, 170
  deprivation of, delirium and, 149*t*
  disorders
    dementia and, 152*t*
    PD and, 275
slow medicine, 526–527
smell
  aging and, 9*t*
  malnutrition and, 67*t*
smoking
  AMD and, 387
  CAD and, 317
  cessation of, 107, 108, 118*t*
    for MI, 319
  cognitive impairment prevention and, 129
  CVD and, 326
  diabetes and, 343
  hypertension and, 306
  multimorbidity and, 14
  normal aging and, 5
SNF. *See* skilled nursing facility
SNPs. *See* special needs populations
SNRIs. *See* serotonin norepinephrine
    reuptake inhibitors
SOAP. *See* subjective, objective, assessment, plan
social life, aging and, 5
Social Security. *See also* Medicare
  Title XX of, 441, 462
  workers paying for, 23
Social Services Block Grants, 441
social support
  depression and, 173
  for geriatric patients, 31–32, 32*f*
  NH and, 38, 39*t*
  with technology, for disability prevention, 131
Society of Thoracic Surgeons (STS), 321
socioeconomic status
  depression and, 173, 188
  malnutrition and, 67*t*
sodium
  as food additive, 364
  hypertension and, 306
somatic cells, 4
somatrophic axis, 11
special needs populations (SNPs), 435
speech, hearing impairment and, 394
spinal cord injury, 212
SPRINT trial, 305–306
SSRIs. *See* selective serotonin reuptake inhibitors
St. John's wort, 194
stable angina, 317
Staphylococcus aureus, 366

START. *See* Screening Tool to Alert
    Doctors to Right Treatment
statins
  for cardiovascular disease prevention, 127
  for hyperlipidemia, 311
  for MI, 319
  normal aging and, 5
stem cell exhaustion, 10*t*, 11
STIs. *See* sexually transmitted infections
STOPP. *See* Screening Tool of Older Persons'
    Potentially Inappropriate Prescriptions
Streptococcus pneumoniae, 367, 368
stress
  on caregivers, 75–76, 75*t*, 447, 450*t*
  frailty and, 13
  homeostenosis and, 13–14
  normal aging and, 6
  resilience and, 13–14
stress incontinence, 210, 211*t*
  estrogen for, 232–233
stroke, 18, 311–317, 312*t*, 313*t*
  AD and, 155
  confusion from, 141
  death from, 27, 28*f*
  decreases in, 23
  depression and, 172, 177
  falls and, 248, 250
  hospitalization for, 34*f*
  hyperthyroidism and, 354
  immobility from, 263, 267, 275–278
  multimorbidity and, 14
  NH and, 39*t*
  PAC for, 36
  prevention of, 314–315
  rehabilitation for, 316–317, 316*t*, 317*t*
  UI and, 203
Stroke Aphasic Depression
    Questionnaire, 182, 184–185
STS. *See* Society of Thoracic Surgeons
subacute care, 458–459
subclinical hyperthyroidism, 355
subclinical hypothyroidism, 352, 353*f*
subdural hematoma, from falls, 243, 250
subjective, objective, assessment,
    plan (SOAP), 486, 486*t*
substance abuse
  dementia and, 152*t*
  depression and, 170, 173
  Pra and, 70
sugar, 364
suicide
  depression and, 170, 171*t*
  physician-assisted, 512
  screening for, 118*t*
sundowning, with confusion, 147
supply-sensitive care, 99
syncope, 248, 250
syndrome of inappropriate secretion of
    antidiuretic hormone (SIADH), 356

Synthroid. *See* levothyroxine
syphilis
    dementia from, 152*t*
    screening for, 118*t*

T$_3$. *See* triiodothyronine
T$_4$. *See* thyroxine
tachyarrhythmia, 354
tachycardia syndrome, 324
tardive dyskinesia, 422
taste, 401
    aging and, 9*t*
    malnutrition and, 67*t*
TAVR. *See* transcatheter aortic valve replacement
Tax Identifying Number (TIN), 436, 437
TCAs. *See* tricyclic antidepressants
technology
    for chronic disease management, 98–102
    social support with, for disability
        prevention, 131
telomerase, 11–12
telomerase inhibitors, 11
telomeres, aging and, 6, 10–11, 10*t*
temperature regulation, 370–373
tertiary prevention, 108
    for cancer, 121
testosterone, 357
tetanus, 120
therapeutic window, 80–81, 81*f*, 132*f*
thiazide diuretics, for hypertension,
    307–308, 307*t*, 315
thyroid disease. *See also* hyperthyroidism;
        hypothyroidism
    dementia and, 152*t*
    depression and, 178
    hypothermia and, 371
    screening for, 113*t*
    vitality decrease and, 347–355, 350*t*
thyroid-releasing hormone (TRH), 347
thyroid-stimulating hormone (TSH)
    hyperthyroidism and, 354
    hypothyroidism and, 351
    polyneuropathy and, 401
    subclinical hyperthyroidism and, 347
    subclinical hypothyroidism and, 352
thyroxine (T$_4$), 347
    hyperthyroidism and, 354
TIA. *See* transient ischemic attack
TIBC. *See* total iron-binding capacity
ticagrelor, 318
TIN. *See* Tax Identifying Number
tinnitus, 394–395
Title XX, of Social Security, 441, 462
tophi, 271
total iron-binding capacity (TIBC), 358
touch, 9*t*
tramadol
    for pain, 285, 292
    serotonin syndrome and, 194

transcatheter aortic valve replacement (TAVR), 321
transient incontinence, 207, 219
transient ischemic attack (TIA),
    246, 311–317, 314*t*
    atrial fibrillation and, 323
    falls and, 250, 254
transitional care, for chronic disease
    management, 82–83
TRH. *See* thyroid-releasing hormone
tricyclic antidepressants (TCAs),
    190, 191*t*, 194–195, 197*t*
    for polyneuropathy, 402
    serotonin syndrome from, 194
    UI from, 209*t*
triiodothyronine (T$_3$)
    hyperthyroidism and, 354
    hypothyroidism and, 347
    subclinical hyperthyroidism and, 347
TSH. *See* thyroid-stimulating hormone
tuberculosis, 369
tympanic membrane, 391–392
tympanosclerosis, 395

UI. *See* urinary incontinence
unfractionated heparin, 272–273
Up and Go test, 253–254, 255*t*–256*t*, 336
uremia, 152*t*
urethritis, 205, 207
urgency incontinence, 210, 211*t*
    dementia and, 229–231
    falls and, 251
    medications for, 228
urinalysis, 213, 369
urinary incontinence (UI)
    adverse effects of, 202
    aging and, 205
    assessment of, 212–219, 213*t*, 222*f*
    bacteriuria with, 370
    behavioral interventions for,
        221–228, 225*t*–226*t*
    catheters for, 219, 234–235, 235*t*
    causes and types of, 204–212
    criteria for specialist referral for, 220*t*–221*t*
    fecal incontinence and, 236
    management of, 219–236, 223*t*, 224*t*
    from medications, 209*t*
    medications for, 228–233, 230*t*–231*t*
    persistent, 210–212, 211*t*
    physical examination for, 213, 214–215, 217
    prevalence of, 202*f*
    reversible factors in, 207–210, 208*t*, 209*t*
    surgery for, 233–234
urinary retention, 207, 212
    delirium from, 148
    immobility and, 267
urinary system, aging and, 8*t*
urinary tract infections, 133
    antibiotics for, 367
    from catheters, 366

urinary tract infections (*Cont.*):
  delirium from, 148
  UI and, 207
urination, normal, 202–204, 203*t*, 204*f*
  peripheral nerves and, 205*f*
U.S. Preventive Services Task Force
      (USPSTF), 109, 111*t*–118*t*
  on dementia, 139
  on diabetes, 335
  on hearing assessment, 391
  on vitamin D, 363

vaginitis, UI and, 205, 207
valacyclovir, 370
value-based purchasing, 25
valvular heart disease, 319–322
variation
  in aging, 18
  in chronic disease management, 99
vascular dementias, 155, 156*f*
vascular depression, 172–173
vascular ectasia, 358–359
vascular endothelial growth factor (VEGF), 388
vasopressin, vitality decrease and, 355–356
VEGF. *See* vascular endothelial growth factor
venlafaxine, 190, 195
verapamil, 127
verteporfin photodynamic therapy (PTD), 388
vertigo, 249
vision
  aging and, 9*t*
  aids for, 389*t*
  geriatric consultation for, 71*t*
  in geriatric syndromes, 15
  impairment, 382–389
    delirium and, 149*t*
    signs and symptoms of, 386*t*
  physical and functional changes
      to, 381–382, 382*t*
  screening for, 113*t*
visual acuity, 252, 381
Visual Analog Scale, for depression, 182, 185
vitality decrease, 333–373, 373*t*–374*t*
  anabolic hormones and, 356–357
  anemia and, 357–361, 358*t*
  diabetes and, 335–347, 344*t*–347*t*
  diet and, 361–365
  frailty and, 333–334
  hyperparathyroidism and, 355
  infection and, 365–370, 366*t*, 368*t*
  obesity and, 365
  temperature regulation and, 370–373
  thyroid disease and, 347–355, 350*t*
  vasopressin and, 355–356
vitamin B₁ deficiency, 152*t*
vitamin B₁₂ deficiency, 359–360, 401

vitamin D, 362–363
  deficiency
    dementia and, 152*t*
    vascular depression from, 172
  falls and, 254, 257
  for immobility, 267
  normal aging and, 5
  for OA, 270
  for osteoporosis prevention, 128
  screening for, 118*t*
vitamin E, 129, 162
vitamins
  for prevention, 118*t*
  vitality decrease and, 361–362
Vulnerable Elders-13, 88

waist-to-hip ratio, 66
walking speed
  with chronic disease management, 89
  frailty and, 12, 74
warfarin (Coumadin)
  for atrial fibrillation, 323
  for mitral annulus calcification, 321
weight, geriatric patient assessment for, 65–66, 67*t*
weight loss, 51
  for diabetes, 337
  diabetes and, 335
  in EOL, 535–536
  frailty and, 12, 74
  geriatric consultation for, 71*t*
  for OA, 270
  for obesity, 365
  for OSA, 177
Welcome to Medicare Visit, 119*t*
  for EOL, 526
  for hearing, 390
  for vision, 383, 383*t*
Wellspring Movement, 458
white blood cell count
  for infections, 369
  stress and, 6
Wisconsin Star method, 17
women
  blacks, frailty of, 13
  as caregivers, 446
  frailty of, 13
  in informal support, 448
  life expectancy increases in, 28
  pelvic floor exercises for, 223–224
workers, aging and, 23, 24*f*
World Health Organization, 29
  on ethics, 519

Yale Single Item Depression Screening Tool, 185*t*

Zarit Burden Interview, 76
Zung Depression Scale, 122*t*, 184

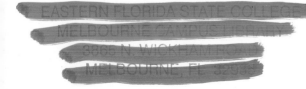